HANDBOOK OF
PEDIATRIC
PRIMARY CARE

HANDBOOK OF
PEDIATRIC PRIMARY CARE

Marilyn P. Chow, R.N., M.S., P.N.P.
Assistant Clinical Professor, Department of Family Health Care
Nursing, University of California, San Francisco

Barbara A. Durand, R.N., M.S., P.N.P.
Associate Clinical Professor, Co-Director
Pediatric Nurse Practitioner Program, Department of Family Health
Care Nursing, University of California, San Francisco

Marie N. Feldman, R.N., B.S., P.N.P., C.N.
Formerly Pediatric Nurse Practitioner, Kaiser Permanente Medical
Clinics, San Francisco, and Clinical Instructor
Department of Family Health Care Nursing, University of California,
San Francisco.

Marion A. Mills, R.N., B.S., P.N.P., C.N.
Pediatric Nurse Practitioner, Pediatric and Adolescent Clinics, University of California, San Francisco.

A WILEY MEDICAL PUBLICATION
JOHN WILEY & SONS
New York • Chichester • Brisbane • Toronto

Library of Congress Cataloging in Publication Data:

Main entry under title:
 Handbook of pediatric primary care.

 Includes index.
 1. Pediatric nursing—Handbooks, manuals, etc.
2. Pediatrics—Handbooks, manuals, etc. 3. Ambulatory
medical care for children—Handbooks, manuals, etc.
4. Nurse practitioners—Handbooks, manuals, etc.
I. Chow, Marilyn P. [DNLM: 1. Pediatric nursing—
Handbooks. 2. Primary nursing care—Handbooks.
3. Nurse practitioners—Handbooks. WY159 H236]

RJ245.H33   610.73'62   78-19731
ISBN 0-471-01771-X

Printed in the United States of America

10 9 8 7 6 5 4 3 2 1

DEDICATION

To my parents, Alice and Bill, and to John.

Marilyn Chow

To my parents, with appreciation and awe.

Barbara Durand

To my friends and mentors, Drs. Henry Shinefield
and S. Robert Burnip.

Marie Feldman

To Marian C. Fraticelli and Kathryn M. Rudnicki.

Marion Mills

Preface

One of the major changes in the delivery of health care during the last ten years has been the increasing emphasis on provision of primary care services as a way to improve, maintain, and promote the total health of individuals. With this shift in emphasis, the nursing profession has advocated and supported the development of more responsible and accountable nursing roles in primary care, largely through the nurse practitioner movement. Pediatric nurse practitioners (PNPs) were the first such group to assume a major role in the provision of primary care services by delivering comprehensive well-child care to children and to their families.

The impetus for this handbook came from our discovery that traditional resources are not appropriately directed to the specific demands of PNP practice. There are no resources which combine content on primary care plus management from a family-oriented perspective in a compact and practical format. This finding was validated by colleagues who consistently complained that an appropriate resource handbook was unavailable for use in the clinical setting. Basic nursing texts do not provide the nurse practitioner with the depth of knowledge necessary to practice, and medical texts go beyond the needs of primary care.

This handbook is designed specifically for use in the clinical setting by practicing nurse practitioners who deliver comprehensive pediatric primary care from a health-oriented, family-centered approach. It is a resource book with a wealth of practical information on primary care for children. Although the content is directed to the PNP, it will be useful as well to physicians and other health professionals who provide pediatric primary care, including other nurses (e.g., school nurses, office nurses, family nurse practitioners, maternity nurse practitioners, and perinatal nurse specialists), physician assistants, and child health associates.

With the increasing emphasis on primary care in the undergraduate and graduate nursing curricula, we believe that this book will be a useful supplement or reference book for nursing students preparing to practice pediatrics in primary health care settings. We also anticipate that students in other health professional schools will find this book to be a comprehensive introduction to pediatric primary care. Finally, since we believe that parents are the true primary managers of their children's care and should be as fully informed as possible, we think that this book can serve as a useful resource for selected parents.

In planning the content for this book, we asked ourselves: What information does the PNP need to provide primary care in the ambulatory setting, including the home? What information is important to have available immediately? What questions and problems are commonly raised by parents? The result is a blend of content taken from actual clinical experience and from information available in texts, journals, and other published resources.

This handbook is unique in that it goes beyond basic nursing knowledge into those areas of primary care where the functions of medicine and nursing are integrated. The authors are PNPs who, individually and collectively, have extensive experience in clinical practice and in the education of PNPs.

The Handbook is divided into two major parts: Part I, Assessment and Management of the Healthy Child, and Part II, Assessment and Management of Common Clinical Problems. Each chapter identifies essential content for assessment and management of a specific area of primary care and discusses the common clinical problems that occur in ambulatory settings. We have included only those problems which we consider common and important in practice. Information on one topic is consolidated into a specific chapter whenever possible. For example, epiglottitis is discussed in Chapter 18, The Respiratory System, even though it is a true emergency

(Chapter 30). All chapters include heavy emphasis on counseling and teaching parents and pertinent resource information.

The reader will note that there is not a specific chapter devoted to growth and development. This was a deliberate decision based on our belief that knowledge of growth and development is the underlying framework from which all child health care is approached. Thus, content on growth and development is integrated throughout the book. Specific developmental assessment tools are found in Chapter 25, The Neuromuscular System.

Part I includes not only traditional ambulatory pediatric content such as history-taking, physical examination, immunizations, well-child schedules, and nutrition but also extensive information on parent-child interaction, feeding approaches, common well-child problems, normal developmental stresses, adolescence, and family planning. Chapters on accident prevention and safety and on health education are included to specifically address the counseling and teaching needs of parents.

Part II defines the illness component of our practice. The content is written with the strong belief that collaboration with physicians and other health professionals is an essential element of our practice and strengthens the quality of health care available to children and to their families. We have presented guidelines for referral and specified the assessment and management role of the PNP. The suggested interventions are meant to be used as *guides*, *not* as complete answers. In addition to a systems approach to the content, we have included chapters on approach to illness and to medications, language and learning disabilities, allergies, emergencies, sudden infant death syndrome, failure to thrive, and child abuse. The Handbook is organized to be most efficiently used through the index. Extensive cross referencing within the text allows for quick, easy access to needed information.

Acknowledgments

Numerous persons deserve acknowledgment in the total effort that went into this book. We wish to recognize Doris E. Dunbar (R.N.) and Donald L. Fink (M.D.) for their foresight and leadership in the development of the PNP Program at the University of California, San Francisco. We express our sincere appreciation to the following people who reviewed and critiqued specific portions of the manuscript.

Thomas Bell, M.D., Lecturer, Mental Health and Community Nursing and Clinical Instructor of Pediatrics, UCSF.

James Brevis, M.D., Chief of Orthopedics, Kaiser Permanente Medical Center, San Francisco.

John C. Dower, M.D., Professor of Pediatrics, UCSF.

Donald German, M.D., Allergist, Kaiser Permanente Medical Center, San Francisco.

Yolanda Gutierrez, M.S., Assistant Clinical Professor, Nutritionist, Family Health Care Nursing, UCSF.

Julien I. Hoffman, M.D., Professor of Pediatrics, UCSF.

Charles E. Irwin Jr., M.D., Director, Adolescent Program, Assistant Professor of Pediatrics, UCSF.

Paula Johnson, R.N., M.S., P.N.P., Assistant Clinical Professor,

Pediatric-Child Study Unit and Family Health Care Nursing, UCSF.

Marion A. Koerper, M.D., Assistant Clinical Professor of Pediatrics, UCSF.

Robert H. Levin, Pharm.D., Associate Clinical Professor of Pharmacy, UCSF.

Delmer J. Pascoe, M.D., Clinical Professor of Pediatrics and of Ambulatory and Community Medicine, UCSF, and Director of Pediatric Ambulatory Services, San Francisco General Hospital.

Jane Phillips, M.D., Assistant Clinical Professor of Pediatrics and Lecturer in Family Health Care Nursing, Co-Program Director of PNP Program, UCSF.

Linda Raybin, B.A., for her special knowledge of learning disabilities.

D. Stewart Rowe, M.D., Associate Clinical Professor of Pediatrics, UCSF.

Peter Sommers, M.D., Assistant Clinical Professor of Pediatrics and of Ambulatory and Community Medicine, San Francisco General Hospital.

Earl L. Stern, M.D., Associate Clinical Professor of Ophthalmology, UCSF.

David Weinberg, M.D., Dermatologist, Palo Alto.

We also wish to express our gratitude to Dorothy Walker, R.N., P.N.P., C.N. for preparing Chapter 9, Accident Prevention and Safety; and to Margaret Oakley for typing the manuscript. Our special thanks go to our editor, Cathy Somer, who provided the enthusiasm, energy, and support that were critical to the completion of this project.

Marilyn Chow
Barbara Durand
Marie Feldman
Marion Mills

Foreword

The timeliness of this book is evident when one considers the growth and maturity of the nurse practitioner concept. After a number of years of moving in divergent directions, medicine and nursing have come together in collaborative work in the interest of providing the best primary health care for children and for families. With the possible exception of critical care, this development represents the most successful collaboration between nursing and medicine to date. As a result, new and different resources will be in demand.

We welcome the publication of *Handbook of Pediatric Primary Care*, which, in our opinion, fills a need not met by standard pediatric and nursing texts. This book will be of use not only to pediatric nurse practitioners and family nurse practitioners caring for children but to any clinician—physician, physician assistant and health associate, dentist, clinical pharmacist, child psychologist, and others—who deals on a day-to-day basis with the full range of primary child health care problems.

The value of the Handbook comes from the wide range of problems discussed. Such common problems as diaper rash and excessive cerumen are frequently a challenge to clinicians but are usually omitted from textbooks. Diagnostic information is presented in a practical and clear format, and the reader is directed to further references and available resources.

Of special merit are the discussions of management, which are concise, practical, and specific. Discussions of alternative modes of diaper service and factors in compliance and family cooperation in medication giving are examples of the practical content covered. Counseling and family education are regularly included in each management plan, as are developmental aspects.

Both diagnostic and management sections reflect an appropriate collaborative interdependence between nurses, physicians, and other clinicians in providing comprehensive care to children. Of equal importance is the reflection of the collaborative role between the clinician and the family which is essential in the successful delivery of primary care.

The authors are unusually well qualified to write this book. All are experienced nurse clinicians who were among the pioneers in the development of expanding nursing roles in child health care. They include some of the first nurse practitioners, and all have been involved in active clinical practice and teaching in the University of California San Francisco Pediatric Nurse Practitioner Program. They have also been clinical teachers of medical students, pediatric residents, and fellows. This extensive experience in clinical practice and teaching is the basis of the day-to-day practicality of the Handbook.

As the former Co-Program Directors of the Pediatric Nurse Practitioner Program, University of California San Francisco, we have had the pleasure and privilege of working with the authors as colleagues since 1971. It is gratifying to see their knowledge and skill made available to many others through this book.

Doris E. Dunbar, R.N.
Associate Clinical Professor
Maternal-Child Nursing
University of California
San Francisco

and

Donald L. Fink, M.D.
Professor of Pediatrics and
Ambulatory and Community Medicine
University of California
San Francisco

Contents

HANDBOOK OF
PEDIATRIC
PRIMARY CARE

ASSESSMENT AND MANAGEMENT OF THE HEALTHY CHILD

The nurse practitioner exercises professional judgments and accepts responsibility for the delivery of primary health care. Mutual trust and collaboration among health care providers and families form the bases for effective delivery of quality care. Incorporated in this framework of care are the concepts of prevention, health promotion, and health maintenance. Teaching and counseling are strongly emphasized.

Delivery of primary care requires a continuous relationship between the health professional and the family. The child and family are the primary focus and they are encouraged to become responsible partners in their care.

Part I provides information necessary to maintain and to promote the *health* of the child from birth through adolescence and to assess and to manage specific common concerns and conditions of the healthy child. It also presents pertinent information for parent-child teaching and counseling.

1

Child Health Assessment

The provision of pediatric primary care requires mastery of the knowledge and skills of data gathering, namely, the history and the physical examination, and the ability to communicate this information through the chart to other health professionals. This chapter provides general guidelines for the interview, history, physical examination, and problem-oriented record.

INTERVIEW GUIDE

Mastery in the art of interviewing requires the ability to weave observation and communication skills into an accurate picture of a situation. The interview sets the stage for future contacts with the family and allows for the reciprocal transfer of pertinent information between the family and primary care provider. In addition, it is an excellent opportunity to learn about the family's attitudes toward health and their strengths and vulnerabilities and to provide appropriate health teaching and counseling.

Interview

The expectations of the client and the nurse practitioner are clarified so each person understands what is expected and what can be provided. The nurse practitioner must listen carefully to the parent and to the child and, in particular, must observe the non-verbal messages. It is essential to use open-ended questions, to avoid the use of technical language, and to be aware of personal biases. If the child is older, the child may be interviewed separately from the parent.

Questions to Ask Yourself as the Interviewer

IMMEDIATE ENVIRONMENT

Does everyone look relaxed? Does the parent look rushed? How is the child responding to me? How does the child react in this situation? How does the child use the play equipment?

PRESENT CONCERNS

Is this the problem? Is the information accurate and reliable? What do the parent and child expect from me? What are the parent and the child trying to tell me? What does this tell me about the family's style of interaction?

OBSERVATIONS

What are the facial expressions, body gestures, tone of voice, and tone of the replies? Are there signs of stress, anxiety, and anger reactions? What are the family's responses to them?

HEALTH HISTORY GUIDE

The history is a longitudinal and cumulative process. The amount and type of history information obtained depends on the purpose of the visit and on the concerns of the parents. This section discusses the components of the history data base. For a discussion of an acute problem history, the reader is referred to Chapter 13, Assessment of the Presenting Symptom.

Obtaining a complete health history (see Table 1) on the first visit is time consuming because an initial base of information is collected in addition to eliciting the present concerns. The initial data base varies according to the age of the child, but it includes information in areas that are stable and unlikely to change such as family health history, past medical history, and developmental milestones. Some health care facilities have successfully developed parent questionnaires as a way of solving this problem. In facilities where questionnaires are unavailable the nurse practitioner may find it necessary to gather the health history over a period of time. The purpose of the visit, the interval since the last visit, and the presenting concerns will determine the type and amount of information collected.

Present Concerns

Elicit the chief concerns of the visit and obtain a detailed history of each one. Indicate how each concern affects the child's ability to function (eat, sleep, play) as appropriate. *Remember:* A parent or child's first stated concerns may not be the primary reason for the visit. In eliciting the concerns of the parent, the parent and the child are allowed to tell their story from their own perspectives. An opening question might be: Tell me what has been concerning you about Jennifer? Other questions to ask are: What brings you here this particular day? What worries you most and why? What do you think would be helpful? What ideas do you have about the cause of the problem?

Table 1
Summary of Health History

1. Identifying information
   Name
   Address
   Phone Number
   Clinic Number
2. Present concerns
3. Family profile
   Age and health status of family members
   Familial and communicable diseases
   Socioeconomic background
   Support system
4. Child profile
   Past medical history
      Gestation
      Birth history
      Neonatal period
      Immunizations and laboratory tests
      Infectious diseases
      Operations/hospitalizations
      Accidents
      Allergies
      Current medications
      Review of systems
         Head
         Skin
         Eyes, ears, nose, throat
         Dentition
         Heart and lung
         Blood
         Gastrointestinal
         Genitourinary
         Skeletal
         Neuromuscular
   Personality
      The child as a person
      Interaction
   Development
      Language
      Fine motor
      Gross motor

Nutrition
Sleep
Elimination
School
Past utilization of health care
Special concerns of the adolescent
24-hour history

Family Profile

Obtain information about the age and health status of the family (natural parents, grandparents, relatives, and siblings), familial and communicable diseases (e.g., diabetes, epilepsy, hypertension, sickle cell anemia, tuberculosis), the chronological order of each pregnancy, and socioeconomic background (education, occupation, religious affiliation). Draw a kinship diagram (see Figure 1) and indicate the age and health status of each individual. Note factors such as the physical environment and cultural and social values that will influence the diagnosis, treatment, and management. Useful questions include: How would you describe your own health? Are there any serious illnesses in the family such as convulsions, diabetes, heart disease, hypertension, mental problems, or tuberculosis? Is this your first pregnancy? Who else shares your household? Do you live in an apartment or house? What kind of work do you do? Your spouse? What year of school did you complete?

SUPPORT SYSTEMS

Elicit information on the parent's style of coping and whether supportive resource people are available. Suggested questions are: How do you manage? Who and what are sources of pressure or support for you? For your child? How do you react to all these pressures? How does your child react? What do you do when things get rough? Do you ever have time for yourself? Are there extended

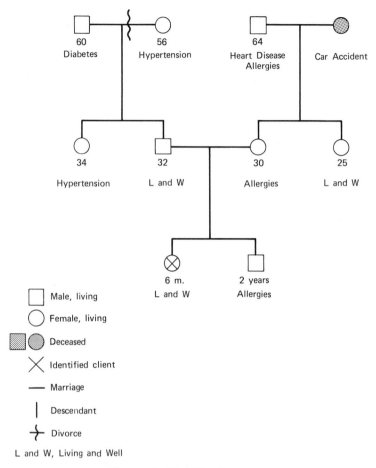

Figure 1. Kinship diagram.

family or close adult relationships in your life? In the child's? Do you get any help caring for your child? With whom do you talk when you have a problem? Who is your chief critic?

Child Profile

Obtain information that provides a picture of the child's strengths and vulnerabilities, roadblocks and frustrations, and style of coping with problems.

PAST MEDICAL HISTORY

Obtain information that establishes the relationship of gestational and perinatal events and past health problems to the child's present state of health.

Gestation. Questions to ask include: In what month did you start prenatal care? How was your health during the pregnancy? Were there any unusual stresses during the pregnancy? Illnesses? Accidents? X-rays? Special diets? Hospitalizations? Medications? How many months did the pregnancy last?

Birth history. See Chapter 4, Assessment of the Newborn. Questions to ask include: How many hours was the labor? Was any anesthesia used? What type of delivery was it (breech, cesarean section, vaginal)? Was the birth of the baby unusual? What was the baby's condition at birth? Did the baby have any trouble breathing? Was the baby's color yellow? What was the birth weight? Was anyone else present at the delivery? How soon after the birth did the parent(s) touch the baby?

Neonatal period. See Chapter 4, Assessment of the Newborn. Questions to ask are: Did the baby have any problems in the nursery? Was the baby's color ever "yellowish" or blue? Did the baby have any problems with feedings? When did the baby go home? Did the mother and baby go home together? What was the baby's weight at discharge? Did the baby have any illnesses or problems in the first month of life?

Immunizations and laboratory tests. See Chapter 2, Immunizations, and Chapter 20, The Hematopoietic System. Questions to ask are: Has the baby received any "baby shots?" At what age? Did the child have any reactions to the immunizations? If yes, can you describe them? Has the child ever had a tuberculin test? What was the reaction? Has the child had any other skin tests? Has the child ever had a blood test? What was the result? Has the child been screened for sickle cell anemia? G-6-PD?

Infectious diseases. See Chapter 29, Infectious Diseases. Questions to ask include: Has the child had chickenpox? Has the child had measles? Has the child had mumps? Has the child had any streptococcal infections?

Operations/hospitalizations. Describe each one by diagnosis, indications for surgery or for hospitalization, results, and known residual problems. Questions to ask include: Has the child ever had any operations? If yes, for what reasons? What happened? How is the child now? Has the child ever spent any time in the hospital? For what reasons? What was the child's response during the hospitalization? Is the problem resolved?

Accidents. See Chapter 30, Emergencies. Questions to ask include: Has the child ever had an accident? What happened? Can you describe what occurred? What was done for the child? How did the child respond?

Allergies. See Chapter 28, Allergies. Questions to ask include: Is the child allergic to any foods? If yes, what types of food? What is the reaction? Has the child had any reactions to insect bites, medications, immunizations? What happened?

Current medications. What medications do you give your child regularly? Is your child receiving any medications for any illnesses?

Review of systems. Record problems not previously identified according to the body part or system. List the symptoms, treatments, and known sequelae.

HEAD. Does your child complain of headaches? Has your child ever fallen and remained unconscious? (See Chapter 30, Head Injury.)

SKIN. See Chapter 15, The Skin. Has your child ever had a severe skin reaction? Has your child ever been treated for a skin infection? What was the diagnosis and treatment?

EYES, EARS, NOSE, AND THROAT. See Chapter 16, The Eye, and Chapter 18, The Respiratory System. Do your child's eyes ever cross? Does your child have trouble seeing? Can your child see the chalkboard at school? Do the eyes tear excessively? Does your child have trouble reading? In what position and distance does your child watch television? Does your child have frequent earaches? Ear infections? Do you think your child has trouble hearing? Has your child been screened for vision or hearing? If yes, what were the results? Does your child have persistent nosebleeds? Does your child have nasal congestion or stuffiness? Does your child have frequent streptococcal sore throats?

DENTITION. See Chapter 17, The Mouth and Teeth. How many teeth does your child have? Has your child ever had any extra teeth removed? When was your child's last dental check-up? Is your child a thumbsucker? Do you have trouble understanding your child's speech? (See Chapter 26, Language and Learning Disabilities.)

HEART AND LUNG. See Chapter 19, The Heart, and Chapter 18, The Respiratory System. Does your baby have trouble finishing a 3- to 4-ounce bottle of milk without tiring? Does your child have any trouble breathing? Describe what occurs. Does your child turn blue? Does your child have trouble with active participation in playground activities? Does your child tend to self-limit play activities?

BLOOD. See Chapter 20, The Hematopoietic System. Has your child ever been anemic? Has your child ever had a blood transfusion? Describe the circumstances.

GASTROINTESTINAL. See Chapter 21, The Gastrointestinal System. Does your child have problems with diarrhea? Constipation? Does your child have black, tarry stools? Has your child ever complained of anal itching? Does your child complain of stomachaches?

GENITOURINARY. See Chapter 22, The Urinary System, and Chapter 23, The Genitalia. Does your child have a strong urinary stream? Does your child have urinary frequency? Has your child complained of pain on urination? When was your child toilet trained? Does your child sleep through the night without wetting the bed? *For females over 10* (see Chapter 10, Health Care of the Adolescent): At what age did menstruation start? Note date, frequency, duration, and intensity. Do you have any vaginal discharge? Itching?

SKELETAL. See Chapter 24, The Skeletal System. Has your child ever broken any bones? Has your child ever sprained any joint? Has your child complained of pain, redness, or swelling around the joints?

NEUROMUSCULAR. See Chapter 25, The Neuromuscular System. Has your child ever had convulsions? Has your child ever had a fainting spell? Does your child have tremors? Twitches? Blackouts? Dizzy spells? Frequent headaches? Does your child have night terrors? Sleepwalk? Has your child complained of weakness in the extremities? Does your child appear awkward and clumsy?

PERSONALITY

The child as a person. Elicit descriptions of the child's personality (activity, attention span, intensity of reactions, adaptability, strengths, sensitivities, fears, crying patterns, impulse control, and frustration levels) and independence (eating, separation, self-care, responsibilities, special and outside interests, and talents). Questions to ask include: How would you describe Jennifer? How does she spend the day? What do you see as her strengths and vulnerabilities? How would you describe her ability to handle new situations? Does your child withdraw or actively participate? Is your child easily frustrated? What happens when this occurs? What upsets her? Can you describe her behavior? What calms her down? How would you compare her to the siblings? What does she do when you leave? What activities does she engage in outside of the home?

Interaction. See Chapter 5, Assessment of Parent-Child Interaction, and Chapter 8, Common Problems of Infancy and Childhood. Elicit descriptions of the quality of the interaction with family members and peers, limit-setting, and discipline. Questions to ask include: Can you leave the children alone in a room together? How would you describe the older child's behavior to the baby? When was the first time you had to discipline your child? Do you remember what happened? How often do you find that you need to discipline your child? (If a situation presents itself in which the parent attempts to discipline the child ask: Does that usually work?). Does your child have playmates?

DEVELOPMENT

See Chapter 25, The Neuromuscular System.

Language. See Chapter 26, Language and Learning Disabilities. Elicit information about communication patterns, comprehension, speech, and reading. Questions to ask include: Can you understand your child? Does your child follow directions? Does your child get confused? Does your child repeat words? Does your child stutter?

Fine motor. Elicit information about manual dexterity, drawing, dressing, tying, and writing. Questions to ask include: Does your child scribble? Can your child use a pencil? Can your child tie shoe laces? Button clothes? Does your child have difficulty writing school assignments?

Gross motor. Inquire about developmental landmarks such as sitting alone, standing, walking, riding a tricycle or bicycle. Questions to ask include: What does your child do for fun? Does your child enjoy playing on the playground in the schoolyard? Does your child have trouble manipulating the parallel bars? Does your child have any difficulty walking? Running? How old was your child when she used a tricycle?

NUTRITION

See Chapter 6, Nutrition in Infancy and Childhood, and Chapter 7, Feeding in Infancy and Childhood. Elicit information according to age, presence of illness, and symptoms. Minimum information includes an evaluation of feeding during the first year and present nutritional status. Determine the gross quantification of protein, iron, and vitamin intake for crucial ages such as infancy and adolescence. If the parent is a poor historian, obtain a detailed 24-hour nutrition history of the day before this visit. Questions to ask include: How would you describe your child's appetite (good, poor)? How would you describe the eating environment at home? What is the feeding schedule? What kind of milk does the child drink? How much is consumed in 24 hours? How is the milk prepared? What solids does the child eat (fruit, vegetables, sweets) and in what quantities? Does the child self-feed? Can the child use utensils? Does the child drink from a cup? How do you handle the messiness? Is the child taking any vitamins?

SLEEP

Obtain information about the length of sleep and naps and about the character of sleep. Questions to ask are: Do you think your child is getting enough sleep? How many hours in a 24-hour period? When does your child awaken and go to bed? Does your child take naps during the day? How long are they? Does the child awaken at night? If yes, how often? What do you do? Does the child have any nightmares or night terrors?

ELIMINATION

See Chapter 8, Common Problems in Infancy and Childhood. Inquire about patterns and toilet training. Questions to ask are: What are the child's bowel patterns? Frequency? Does the child complain of any discomfort? Is the child toilet trained? At what age was this accomplished? Does the child have any "accidents"? If so, is it during the day or night? How often does it happen?

SCHOOL

See Chapter 26, Language and Learning Disabilities. Inquire about the ability to function in school. Questions include: What grade is your child in? Does your child like school? What is the favorite school subject? The least favorite? Has your child missed much school? What are your expectations as a parent for your child's school performance? Is your child enrolled in a special class?

PAST UTILIZATION OF HEALTH CARE

Where has the child usually gone for health care? How often do you take your child to a health care facility? For what reasons?

SPECIAL CONCERNS OF THE ADOLESCENT

See Chapter 10, Health Care of the Adolescent.

24-HOUR HISTORY

Obtain a detailed hourly history if the information is vague and contradictory. Questions might be: What is a typical day like for your child? What time did your child awaken yesterday? What happened then? When did you serve breakfast? And then what happened?

PHYSICAL EXAMINATION

A skillful physical examination is done with a minimum of trauma to the child. It is done with sensitivity to the child's behavior, activity level, and responses, and it takes advantage of opportunities such as crying by quickly looking into the mouth.

Usually a child under 2 years of age is best examined on the lap of the parent. Whenever possible time is allowed for the child to manipulate the intrusive instruments. At some point during the examination the child should be completely undressed to enable a thorough look.

There are four basic techniques: auscultation, palpation, percussion, and observation. Of these four techniques, systematic, thorough observation is the most important one.

This section provides information on the general physical examination. See Table 2 for a summary of the physical examination. For more detailed information on physical examination techniques and physical findings according to body system, the reader is referred to the appropriate chapter.

Table 2
Summary of Physical Examination

Measurements and vital signs
General condition
Skin
Lymph nodes
Head
   Face
   Eyes
   Ears
   Nose
   Mouth
   Throat
Neck
Chest and lungs
Heart
Abdomen
Genitalia
Rectum and anus
Skeletal
Neuromuscular

Measurements and Vital Signs

Obtain the following measurements: height, weight, head circumference, temperature, respiration rate (see Chapter 18), pulse rate (see Chapter 19), and blood pressure (see Chapter 19). Table 3 approximates the height and weight of infants and children, and Table 4 lists the expected increments of head circumference in average full-term infants.

General Condition

Note appearance (alert, happy, sick, distressed, pained), activity level (lethargic, playful, active, tired), development, and behavior in relation to age and state of nutrition.

Table 3
Mnemonics (Weech) for Approximate Height and Weight of Infants and Children

(a) At birth:	Weight (W) in lb	= 7 lb 6 oz (7.35 lb)
(b) From 3 to 12 months:	W (lb)	= age (mo) plus 11
(c) From 1 to 6 years:	W (lb)	= (age [yr] × 5) plus 17
(d) From 6 to 12 years:	W (lb)	= (age [yr] × 7) plus 5

> Note: (c) and (d) give the same value (47 lb) at 6 years. 48 lb is a closer approximation of average. The following mnemonic is suggested: "Up to 5: 5A[a] plus 17. From 7 on: 7A plus 5. At 6: use either one, but add 1."

(e) At birth:	Length = 20 in	
(f) At one year:	Length = 30 in	
(g) From 2 to 14 years:	Height (in) = (age [yr] × 2½) plus 30	

Source: From V. C. Vaughan and R. J. McKay, *Nelson Textbook of Pediatrics,* 10th ed., p. 25, © 1975 by the W. B. Saunders Company, Philadelphia.
[a]A = age [yr]

Table 4
Head Circumference in Term Infants[a]

Period	HC Increments	
First 3 months	2 cm/month =	6 cm
4–6 months	1 cm/month =	3 cm
6–12 months	0.5 cm/month =	3 cm
First year		12 cm

Source: Reprinted with permission from J. A. McMillan, et al, *The Whole Pediatrician Catalog,* (Philadelphia: The W. B. Saunders Company, © 1977), p. 6.
[a] Expected head circumference (HC) during infancy can be estimated by remembering that the average full-term infant will show the following increments in head growth.

Skin (see Chapter 15, The Skin)

Inspect *color* (jaundice, pallor, cyanosis), *hair* (texture, location, distribution), *nails* (clubbing, unusual markings), *lesions* (color, type, location, distribution, shape, size); observe for *purpura, petechiae, hemangiomas, scarring, mongolian spots, pigmentation, evidence of trauma;* palpate for *temperature* (hot, cold), *texture* (edematous, rough, moist, clammy), *turgor*, and *lesions.*

NOTE

1. Fingernails are replaced every 5-1/2 months and grow an average of 0.1 mm/day between the fifth and thirtieth year of life.
2. Toenails are replaced every 18 months.

Lymph Nodes

Inspect and palpate for *tenderness, consistency* (soft, hard), *size, shape, location, mobility, temperature,* and *inflammation.* Palpate the suboccipital, preauricular, anterior cervical, posterior cervical, submaxillary, sublingual, axillary, epitrochlear, and inguinal lymph nodes.

NOTE

Normal ranges of lymph node sizes and characteristics:

1. Nodes up to 3 mm
2. Nodes up to 1 cm in the cervical and inguinal area
3. Nodes that are nontender, cool, and mobile

Head (see Chapter 4, Assessment of the Newborn)

Inspect and palpate for *shape, size, symmetry* (paralysis, weaknesses), *fontanels* (measurements, tension, intracranial pressure, delayed or premature closure), *sutures* (overriding), *molding, prominences* (cephalohematoma, caput succedaneum, frontal "bossing"), *lesions, craniotabes, position, movement,* and *dilation of veins.*

NOTE

1. Measurement of the head circumference is best done with a flexible, narrow steel tape measure placed around the largest occipital-frontal circumference. Check for accuracy by repeating this procedure a second time; take the largest of the two measurements if there is a difference.

2. Transillumination of the head is done in a completely darkened room using a standard flashlight with a soft rubber collar attached to the lighted end placed flush against the skull at various points.

3. The mean anterior fontanel for the newborn is 2.1 cm with 2SD above and below, 0.6 and 3.6 cm respectively. The anterior fontanel closes between 4 to 26 months. See Figure 2 for the mean anterior fontanel size during the first postnatal year.

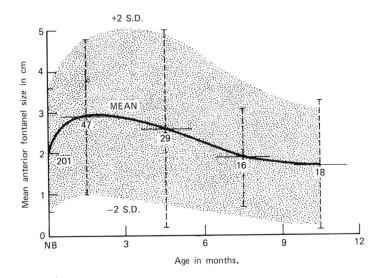

Figure 2. Mean anterior fontanel size during the first postnatal year. Beyond the newborn period (NB) the data are averaged at 3-month intervals with the number of individuals in each group indicated. (From G. A. Popich and D. W. Smith, "Fontanels: Range of Normal Size," *J Pediatr* 80:749–752, 1972.)

Face

Inspect for size, shape, symmetry, positioning of eyes, nose, mouth in relation to each other, paralysis, mandibular size, swelling, hypertelorism, and palpate for sinus tenderness.

Eyes (see Chapter 16, The Eye)

Observe external eye for *shape, symmetry, placement, lid* (ptosis, epicanthic fold, paralysis, crusting, edema, nodules, scaling, discharge, symmetry), *conjunctiva, sclera* (icterus, hemorrhages), *cornea, pupil* (color, symmetry, round, reaction to light, and accommodation); inspect for *conjugate gaze, extraocular movements* (nystagmus), test for *visual acuity;* inspect internal eye for *red reflex* and *fundus.*

NOTE

1. To see the red reflex in a sleepy infant, place the infant over the parent's shoulder.
2. Tearing starts several weeks after birth.

Ears (see Chapter 18, The Respiratory System)

Inspect the *pinna* (shape, size, malformations, placement, skin tags, swelling, tenderness), *canal* (patency, discharge, narrowing, redness, pain, cerumen), *tympanic membrane* (short process, umbo, long process, light reflex, color, bullae, bulging, foreign bodies, perforation, retraction, mobility); test hearing (see Chapter 26).

NOTE

1. To visualize the tympanic membrane be sure the child's head is tilted *away* from the examiner toward the other shoulder, and insert the speculum toward the child's eyes.

2. Tuning fork tests are used to distinguish between conductive and sensorineural hearing loss in a cooperative older child; however, they are difficult to interpret.

- The Weber test is done by striking the tuning fork and placing the handle on the center of the forehead. The child is asked to indicate in which ear the sound can be heard. Normally, the sound should not lateralize to one ear more than to the other.
- The Rinne test is done by striking the tuning fork and placing the handle first on the mastoid process and then on the external ear without interfering with the sound waves. The child is asked to indicate when the sound disappears in each position. Normally, the child should hear the sound louder near the ear canal than on the mastoid bone (+ Rinne) since air conduction is longer than bone conduction. If the sound is heard best on the mastoid bone, the Rinne test is negative.

Nose (see Chapter 18, The Respiratory System)

Inspect external nose for *shape* (straight), *nares* (symmetry, flare, discharge). Inspect internal nose for *color of mucosa* (pale, boggy, edematous, reddened), *turbinates, discharge* (purulent, bloody, crusty, amount), *foreign body, polyps, tumors,* and *perforation.*

Mouth (see Chapter 17, The Mouth and Teeth)

Inspect *lips* (symmetry, paralysis, fullness, thinness, cleft, fissures, pallor, color), *mucosa* (bleeding, Stensen's duct, Koplik's spots, petechiae), *gums* (bleeding, discoloration, swelling), *dentition* (number, malocclusion, caries, discoloration, mottling, notching), *uvula, palates* (high arching, Epstein's pearls, cleft), *tongue* (geographic, color, coated, deviation, fissures, protuberant), *mandibular size, salivary glands* (parotid, submandibular, sublingual); note *breath odor* (see Table 1 in Chapter 17) and *mouth breathing.*

NOTE

1. Salivary production begins at 3 months of age.

Throat (see Chapter 17, The Mouth and Teeth, and Chapter 18, The Respiratory System)

Inspect *color of mucosa, tonsils* (exudate, inflammation, size, color), *voice* (pitch, hoarseness, stridor, grunting), and *cry* (shrill, high-pitched, whiny, weak, hoarse, aphonia).

Neck

Note *positions* (torticollis, opisthotonos), *control, range of motion, stiffness, webbing;* palpate for *cysts, sternocleidomastoid muscle masses* (shape, size, location, mobility), and *thyroid* (size, tenderness, texture, nodules).

Chest and Lungs (see Chapter 18, The Respiratory System)

Inspect for *color* (cyanosis), *respirations* (quality, depth, effort, rate, rhythm, *type of breathing* (abdominal, costal), *chest size, symmetry, shape* (pectus excavatum, "barrel chest," slope), *breast* (areola, nipple placement, spacing, presence or absence in relation to age), *respiratory distress* (expiratory grunting, nasal flaring, retractions), *dyspnea* (restlessness, apprehension, rib retractions), cough; palpate the *general chest configuration, breasts* (see Chapter 10), *scapulas, clavicles;* auscultate the breath sounds (presence or absence, intensity, quality, duration, vesicular, bronchovesicular, bronchial) and note abnormal chest sounds (rales, rhonchi, wheezes, pleural friction rub); percuss for dullness and lung size.

NOTE

1. Respirations:
   - Ratio of respiration to pulse should be 1:4.
   - Short periods of apnea can be normal in newborns.
   - Respiratory movement is abdominal until around 7 years of age when it becomes predominantly costal.
2. Auscultation:
   - Sound is best conducted through solid matter, passes less well through water, and least well through air (Delaney, 1975).
   - To check for transmitted breath sounds, block the nasal passages.
3. Breasts:
   - Breasts usually develop asymmetrically.
   - They are examined after the menstrual period so premenstrual engorgement and tenderness will not be misleading.

Heart (see Chapter 19, The Heart)

Observe activity level (fatigability); inspect *color* (pallor, cyanosis), *clubbing, prominent veins, precordial bulging;* palpate for the point of *maximal impulse* (PMI), *pulses* (femoral, radial), presence of *thrills* or *heaves;* auscultate *heart sounds* (S_1, S_2, rate, rhythm), *murmurs* (location, rhythm, radiation, intensity, timing, quality, pitch, effect of positional change).

NOTE

1. Thrill is best detected with the edge of the palm.
2. In the young child the apex beat is outside the nipple line in the fourth interspace; in the older child it is more nearly in the adult position.
3. The key to auscultation is to listen to one heart sound at a time:
   - Aortic valve is best heard in the second right intercostal space.

- Pulmonic valve is best heard in the second left intercostal space.
- Tricuspid valve is best heard in fifth right intercostal space near the sternum.
- Mitral valve is best heard in fifth left intercostal space near the midclavicular line.
- S_1 is louder at the apex.
- S_2 is louder at the base.
- Bell of stethoscope detects low frequency sounds.
- Diaphragm of stethoscope detects high frequency sounds.

Abdomen

Inspect *size, shape, symmetry, protuberance, distention, distended veins, guarding, facial expression, body movements of child;* palpate for *softness, rigidity, tenderness, masses* (note location, size, consistency, tenderness, mobility, fluctuation), *liver, spleen, bladder, umbilicus, kidneys, hernias, diastasus rectus,* and *rebound tenderness;* auscultate *bowel sounds* (tympanitic, dull, absent).

NOTE

1. In examining a child with a complaint of a tender abdomen, do not begin the examination with the tender area. While doing the examination, observe the child's reactions: Is the child guarding? Is it voluntary or involuntary?
2. A cough may bring out bulge in hernias of the abdominal wall.

Female Genitalia (see Chapter 23, The Genitalia)

Inspect external genitalia for *color, labia* (majora, minor), *clitoris, urethral meatus, pubic hair* (presence or absence); note *odor,* presence of *adhesions, bleeding, discharge, ulcerations, edema, imperforate hymen;* inspect *vagina* and *cervix;* palpate the *uterus;* note *position of uterus, presence of foreign body,* and *discharge.*

NOTE

1. A pelvic examination is usually not done until puberty.
2. A small amount of bloody discharge is normal in newborns up to 1 month of age.

Male Genitalia (see Chapter 23, The Genitalia)

Inspect the external genitalia for *penis* (size, glans, shape), *foreskin* (circumcision, retraction, phimosis, paraphimosis), *urethra* (ulceration, position of meatus), *scrotum* (hydrocele, hernia), *pubic hair;* palpate *testes, epididymis, spermatic cord.*

Rectum and Anus (see Chapter 21, The Gastrointestinal System)

Inspect muscle tone, sensation, patency; note presence of foreign body, bleeding, fissures, skin tags, pilonidal dimple, stool, and masses.

NOTE

1. Examine the anus with the fifth finger, noting sphincter tone.

Skeletal (see Chapter 24, The Skeletal System)

Observe *gait* (opposing arm and leg swing, normal heel-to-toe gait), *posture, symmetry;* examine *spine and back* (body alignment, curvature, rigidity, CVA tenderness, tufts of hair, lesions, pilonidal dimple, kyphosis, scoliosis), *joints* (range of motion, edema, tenderness, redness, nodules, abnormal prominences), *hips* (abduction, internal rotation), *knees* (length, contour), *forefoot* (adduction), *fingers and toes* (number, spacing, length, curvatures, webbing, clubbing).

Neuromuscular (see Chapter 25, The Neuromuscular System, and Chapter 26, Language and Learning Disabilities)

Observe *mental status* (orientation, alertness), *motor development* (Romberg's sign, ability to do knee bend, to hop, to walk on toes and heels, to maintain the arms held forward, to grip the examiner's fingers), *muscle tone* (strength, symmetry, spasticity, hypotonia, hyperreflexia), *cerebellar function* (gait, posture), *sensory* (light touch on the limbs, stereognosis in the hands, pain and vibration in hands and feet), *reflexes* (see Tables 1 and 2 in Chapter 25), and *cranial nerves* (see Chapter 25, Cranial Nerve Function).

LABORATORY AND SCREENING RESULTS

Results of laboratory tests (e.g., CBC, UA) and screenings (e.g., sickle cell, G-6-PD, vision, and hearing) are usually recorded after the physical examination.

PROBLEM-ORIENTED HEALTH RECORD

Problem-oriented recording is the current form of written communication among health professionals. While there are variations in the implementation of the problem-oriented form of recording, this chapter offers a foundation from which to build expertise with it. Figure 3 diagrams the problem-oriented system, and Figure 4 outlines the schema of the problem-oriented record. A summary of the format for recording visits is listed in Table 5.

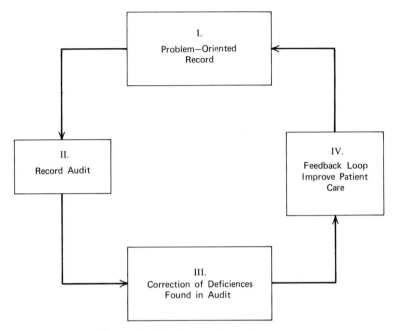

Figure 3. Problem-oriented system.

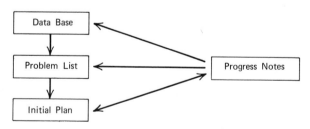

Figure 4. Schema of problem-oriented record.

Table 5
Format for Recording Visits

INITIAL VISIT
1. Identifying information—date of visit
2. History (see Table 1)
3. Physical examination (see Table 2)
4. Laboratory and screening results
5. Problem #1—health supervision (Note: The entire problem list is written on the master problem list located at the front of the record.)
    Initial plan
        Immunization
        Nutrition
        Growth and development
        Safety
6. Problem #2
    Initial plan
        Diagnostic
        Therapeutic
        Patient education
        Follow-up
SUBSEQUENT VISITS
1. Date, problem title and number
2. Subjective
3. Objective
4. Assessment
5. Plan
    Diagnostic
    Therapeutic
    Patient education
    Follow-up

Data Base

It is the first component of the problem-oriented system. It consists of *standardized* and *defined* elements of the history, physical examination, and laboratory tests. The nurse practitioner gathers the information as soon as possible so the problem list can be completed. The comprehensive initial data base is located at the front of the record. Interval data are located within the body of the chart.

COMMON QUESTIONS

How are changes recorded in the areas of health supervision, such as nutrition and growth and development which obviously change as the child grows?
There are two alternatives:

- Write a progress note under Problem #1 including specific changes in areas of health supervision such as nutrition and growth and development; or
- Use a periodic update data base sheet designed specifically for well-child care.

How is the initial data base updated?
It is either updated in the progress notes or updated on the initial data base form.

What is an "incomplete data base"?
This term is used when it is not possible for the defined data base to be completed, as in an emergency. In such a situation the term should be listed as problem #1 to serve as a reminder that the problem(s) may be dealt with out of context.

Problem List

It is the *index* to the record. It is located at the front of the record to provide an overall perspective of the client's problems. Usually the provider who obtains the initial data base formulates the problem list. Other health professionals may also add to the list as other problems develop. Each problem is numbered and titled on the master problem list (see example in sample record).

COMMON QUESTIONS

What is a problem?
A situation identified by either client or health provider that requires management.

How are problems formulated for the problem list?
A problem statement:

- Does not contain "rule-outs," "probably," or question marks ("Rule-out" is an approach to the solution of a problem and so belongs under Initial Plans.)
- Does not state any guesses
- Is a symptom, a finding, or a diagnosis
- Is specific
- Is stated at the highest level of understanding
- Is stated succinctly
- Reflects only what is known from reviewing the data base

How are problems categorized?
They are categorized by type and status.

Type:

1. Medical—physiologic finding, symptom, or abnormal lab value ("Probable," questionable diagnoses, and "rule-outs" are not included here.)
2. Social—finances, housing, employment
3. Psychiatric
4. Environmental

Status:

1. Active problem: currently requiring management
2. Inactive or resolved problem: one that either no longer requires management or is stable but may recur
3. Temporary problem: minor problem that is identified in progress notes; may be listed on the "short-term problem list" using letters rather than numbers for identification.

Are temporary or short-term problems listed on the problem list?

There are two options:

1. Use a separate sheet titled "short-term problem list." See example in sample record; or
2. Note problems in progress notes using letters to identify them as temporary. If a problem has more than two entries in the progress notes, a decision is made about listing the problem on the problem list.

How are changes recorded on the problem list?
The following are examples of common changes:

1. Reformulation of problems
   Corrected statement

Date	No.	Title
8/7/78	3	hgb 9.0 gm/dl

8/8/78 ⟶ Iron deficiency anemia

Combination of problems

Date	No.	Title
9/6/78	4	acute abdominal pain
9/6/78	5	nausea
9/6/78	6	elevated WBC

9/7/78 ⟶ #4 Appendicitis

Once a problem number has been used, it cannot be used again; so in the above example, numbers 5 and 6 cannot be reused.

2. Change of status

Date	No.	Title	Date resolved
8/7/78	3	hgb 9.0 gm/dl	11/8/78 Iron deficiency anemia

8/8/78 ⟶

Initial Plan

It organizes the plan of management for the problem. It is written when the problem is first identified by the health care provider. The components of the initial plan are:

1. *Diagnostic:* A list of probable causes and specific plans to rule out each cause
2. *Therapeutic:* Palliative or curative measures for alleviation of the problem
3. *Patient education:* Explanation of the problem and therapeutics

4. *Follow-up:* Plans for the client to return to health care facility

Each plan is numbered and titled according to corresponding problem number and title on the problem list. Subsequent plans are written in the progress notes for each problem. See progress notes written in the sample record.

Progress Notes

They are the mechanism for monitoring the progress of each problem. Progress notes are divided into three types: narrative notes, flow sheets, and discharge summaries.

NARRATIVE NOTES

They are commonly referred to as "SOAP" notes. The format is:

Date, Title, and Number of Problem
*S*ubjective: interval history from client regarding problem
*O*bjective: information gathered from physical, lab, and screening tests
*A*ssessment: conclusion or comparison stated to level of knowledge. It is the sum of subjective and objective information.
*P*lan: given above, a description of plans

The narrative notes are written with attention to previous progress notes. See sample record for examples.

FLOW SHEETS

They are used to monitor several variables at a glance to understand the client's progress. They are usually for routine care or for monitoring stable diseases, such as diabetes. Examples include vital signs and medication sheets.

DISCHARGE SUMMARY

If the client decides to change care providers, each problem is summarized by problem number, title, and plans.

SAMPLE RECORD

NAME   Juliette D.

BIRTHDATE   12/10/1976

CHART NO.   00-00-00

MASTER PROBLEM LIST

DATE ONSET	NO.	ACTIVE PROBLEMS	INACTIVE/ RESOLVED PROBLEMS	DATE RESOLVED
6/12/78	1	Health supervision		
6/12/78	2	Hgb 9.0 gm/100 ml Iron deficiency anemia		12/78
6/12/78	3		H/O PDA	3/77
6/12/78	4	Inadequate housing		12/78

NAME   Juliette D.

BIRTHDATE   12/10/76

CHART NO.   00-00-00

SHORT-TERM PROBLEM LIST

LETTER	PROBLEM	DATES OF OCCURRENCE
A	Upper respiratory infection	6/77 9/77 1/78
B	Acute otitis media	2/78
C	Tinea corporis	3/78

NAME ___Juliette D.___

BIRTHDATE ___12/10/76___

CHART NO. ___00-00-00___

Date: 6/12/78

PRESENT CONCERNS: well-child visit; no particular problems or questions

FAMILY PROFILE:

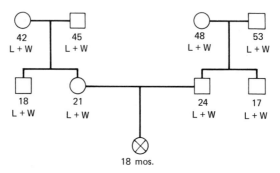

Parents in good health; no significant family medical history; family lives in studio apartment across from maternal grandmother; father employed as baker; no stated financial difficulties; health insurance through employer.

Mother completed tenth grade and father completed high school.

Extended family reported to be positive support system; mother expresses desires to get out more frequently by herself.

CHILD PROFILE:

Past Medical History

Gestation: 1st pregnancy for P_1G_1 woman who initiated care in third month of pregnancy; attended Lamaze classes; no illnesses or unusual strains during pregnancy.

Birth history: 12-hr labor, vaginal delivery with paracervical block given; infant delivered spontaneously. Mother breast-fed in delivery room.

Neonatal period: BW 6 lb 10 oz; spontaneous cry; no respiratory difficulties; jaundice on 2nd day. F/u with blood tests

(Continued)

34

revealed no further problems. Mother and child discharged on third day.

Immunizations: DPT × 3 and OPV × 3; M-M-R at 15 months; tine test and screening tests done.

Infectious disease: None.

Operation/hospitalization: None.

Accidents: None.

Current medications: None.

Review of systems: Negative except for the following:

Skin: History of "ringworm" in March 1978, treated with Tinactin cream.

Ear, Nose, Throat: 3 episodes of "colds," treated with ↑ fluids, and acetaminophen prn. Dates were 6/77, 9/77, 1/78. One episode of acute otitis media bilaterally in February, treated with Ampicillin and a decongestant.

Heart: Mother states a heart murmur noted at the first well-child visit. Family told that murmur was due to transition from fetal circulation to independent circulation. Normal ECG. Mother told murmur "was gone" at 3 months of age.

Personality: Very active, "happy" child; cries little. Seems to adapt well to changes in environment; extremely inquisitive, and parents attempt to set limits but, at times, get very frustrated.

Development: Sat alone at 6 months; stood alone at 10 months; took first steps at 11 months; walks up steps; drinks from cup without spilling much; eats with hands; content to play by herself at times; very verbal, can say 2 words such as "bye-bye"; seems to hear well; plays with small objects.

Nutrition: 8 oz whole milk x 5/ day; three meals a day but eats little fruits, meats, vegetables; no vitamins or minerals taken.

Sleep: Sleeps well, usually from 8:00 PM to 7:00 AM; nap 1/day for 1½ hours. Sleeps in own bedroom.

Elimination: BM x 1/day; usually after breakfast; normal consistency.

Past utilization of health care: Formerly seen by private pediatrician, Dr. L. Brolyn, on Mission St.

PHYSICAL EXAMINATION: Ht 82 cm; Wt 12.5 kg; HC 46.5 cm; HR: 116; RR: 30.

General appearance: Well-developed child in no acute distress who clung to mother during the exam.

(Continued)

35

Skin: Fair; nailbeds pink; good turgor; hair evenly distributed; without lesions.

Head: Normocephalic, symmetrical; AF and PF closed.

Lymph nodes: None palpable.

Eyes: Grossly normal; PERRLA; cover test normal; red reflex noted bilaterally; sclera and conjunctiva clear.

Ears: N1 position; light reflex and bony landmarks seen bilaterally.

Nose: No abnormalities noted; mucosa pink; no bleeding noted; clear, watery discharge seen.

Mouth and throat: 8 teeth present; dentition normal; moist mucous membranes; tongue shows no deviation; uvula rises symmetrically.

Neck: Supple, without adenopathy or masses.

Chest: No evidence of respiratory distress; lungs clear throughout.

Heart: NSR; PMI at 4th ICS, MCL. No thrills; heart sounds S_1 and S_2 nl. No murmurs noted; femoral pulses palpated bilaterally.

Abdomen: Soft without tenderness, without masses; liver, spleen not palpable.

Genitalia: Nl female; external structures intact; no discharge or foul odor.

Rectum and anus: No lesions noted: Good sphincter tone.

Skeletal: No obvious deformities; straight spine; full ROM of extremities.

Neuromuscular: Alert, responsive child; see DDST for development; cranial nerves II-XII normal.

Parent-child interaction: Mother responsive to child's needs; able to set limits but needs much support with this; child responds warmly to mother . . . .

LABORATORY AND SCREENING RESULTS:
Hemoglobin: 9.0 gm/100 ml
Urinalysis: ph 5
        neg. for glucose, ketone, protein, blood
        0–1 WBC/HPF
        0 RBC/HPF

(Continued)

PROBLEMS
Problem: #1—health supervision

a. Yearly screening tests
   Initial Plan
       Diagnostic: UA, CBC, tine test—done.
       Therapeutic: None.
       Pt. education: Discussed with parent the rationale for
           these tests.
       Follow-up: Will call results to parents.

b. Immunizations not up-to-date
   Initial Plan
       Diagnostic: None.
       Therapeutic: Given DPT booster in ® anterior lateral
           thigh and OPV.
       Pt. education: Reviewed with parent the immunization
           schedule, side effects of DPT, and support measures.

Follow-up: 1. Discussed return for DPT and OPV boosters prior
to entering school. 2. Send for records from private physician.

c. Accident prevention
   Initial Plan
       Diagnostic: None.
       Therapeutic: Dispense Ipecac.
       Pt. education: Discuss common accidents of toddlers
           and safety measures to prevent them. Telephone no. of
           clinic and ER given to mother. Advised her to call in
           case of ingestion.
       Follow-up: Discuss at next well-child visit in 6 months.

d. Growth and development
   Initial Plan
       Diagnostic: None.
       Therapeutic: None.
       Pt. education: Anticipatory guidance re: independence
           and autonomy of child, toilet training; discussed lan-
           guage stimulation.
       Follow-up: Discuss at next well-child visit in 6 months.

(Continued)

Problem: #2—hemoglobin of 9.0 gm/100 ml
Initial Plan
    Diagnostic: R/O anemia, probably iron deficiency anemia—obtain CBC, blood smear, and retic. count.
    R/O blood loss—obtain stool guaiac.
    Therapeutic: No medication at this time.
    Pt. education: 1. Discuss lab finding and need for further blood tests to identify cause of low hgb. 2. ↓ milk to 24 oz/day. Suggest offering food before milk to encourage the child to eat more. 3. Review sources of iron-containing foods. List given to mother.

    Follow-up: 1. Obtain further lab studies today. 2. Call mother re results and future plans.
Problem: #4—inadequate housing
Initial Plan
    Diagnostic: None.
    Therapeutic: Support move to a larger apartment.
    Pt. education: None.
    Follow-up: Check on progress next well-child visit.

PROBLEM PROGRESS FORM

Patient name ___Juliette D._____ Date ___8/15/78_____

Chart No.: 00-00-00

Problem: #2—hemoglobin of 9.0 gm/100 ml ⟶ iron deficiency anemia

Subjective: Mrs. D. is regularly giving iron-containing foods such as meats, eggs, beans, raisins. She has noted that Juliette's BMs are black; Juliette does not "like the medicine, but I mix it with her juice."

Objective: Repeat hgb today is 11.0 gm/100 ml; Retic. count was 3%.

Assessment: Problem resolving.

Plan: Therapeutic: Continue to include iron-containing foods in diet.

(Continued)

Continue Fer-In-Sol 1.2 cc tid X 1 month.

Pt. education: Reassure mother that problem is resolving and continue with diet supports; review side effects of Fer-In-Sol.

Follow-up: Encourage Mrs. D. to call if any questions or changes; repeat hgb in May at next well-child visit.

Problem: #4—inadequate housing

Subjective: The apartment situation is the same. Space is totally inadequate for 3 persons. Mrs. D. has not found time to look for a larger place but plans to look this weekend. She's pessimistic that she'll find something that she can afford.

Objective: Made home visit last week. Apt. is well kept despite lack of space. No medicines or household toxins are kept where children can get them.

Assessment: Problem unstable.

Plan: Have arranged for Mrs. D. to speak with Center social worker about possible housing resources.

Follow-up: Will contact Mrs. D. by phone in 2 weeks.

PROBLEM PROGRESS FORM

Patient Name __Juliette D.__ Date __12/16/78__

Chart No.: 00-00-00

Problem: #1—health supervision

Subjective:

a. *Family:* Warm, stimulating environment in home. Mrs. D. has been spending more time with Juliette on weekends and is getting out herself more than before.

b. *Child Rearing:* Mrs. D. no longer having significant concerns. Has been using discipline more judiciously and consistently.

c. *Nutrition:* Well-balanced diet with adequate sources of protein. Mrs. D. has tried cutting down on sweets and has ↑ iron-containing foods for whole family.

d. *Development:* See Denver Developmental Screening Test in chart. Normal language development for age. Toilet training completed.

(Continued)

e. *Child Safety:* Mrs. D. has not been able to get harness auto restraint for Juliette.

f. *Immunizations:* Complete for age. Will need boosters before starting kindergarten.

g. *Dental:* Brushing teeth with help from mother.

Objective: Ht 87 cm; Wt 13.75 kg; HC 49.5 cm. See growth chart. Physical exam normal.

Assessment: Problem is stable. I feel that things are going relatively well in family at present.

Plan:

1. Encourage to get auto harness restraint and to keep Juliette in back seat until then.
2. Suggestions for fostering language development given.
3. RTC in 6 months.

Problem: #4—inadequate housing

Subjective: Parents found 1-bedroom apartment. Rent is a little more than they expected to pay, but they feel they can manage.

Objective: None.

Assessment: Problem resolved.

Plan: None.

Resource Information

There are many audiovisual resources available for learning the skills of the physical examination. Only selected ones are presented here.

Eye

1. Colenbrander Ophthalmoscopy Mannequin: Model with slides for simulating normal and abnormal conditions of the eye.
2. Ophthalmoscopy Unit: Self-instructional units for ophthalmology
   Part I: Tape/slide and handouts
   Both items 1 and 2 are available from:
   Hansen Ophthalmic Development Laboratory, P. O. Box 613, Iowa City, IA 52240.

Heart

1. CARDIAC AUSCULTATION RECORDS, HEART SOUNDS
   Merck, Sharp and Dohme, West Point, PA 19486.
2. INDEX OF HEART SOUNDS AND MURMURS
   National Medical Audiovisual Center, Video Duplication Service, 1600 Clifton Road, N.E., Atlanta, GA 30333.
3. HEART SOUNDS ACCESS TAPE
   American College of Cardiology, 9650 Rockville Pike, Bethesda, MD 20014.
4. RECORDING OF STETHOSCOPIC HEART SOUNDS
   Service of Roerig, Division of Pfizer, Inc., 235 E. 42nd Street, New York, NY 10017.
5. SOUNDS OF PEDIATRIC CARDIOLOGY PEDIATRICS, Vol. 18, No. 5
   Audio Digest Foundation, 1250 So. Glendale Avenue, Glendale, CA 91205.
6. STETHOSCOPIC HEART RECORD, HEART RECORDINGS, Columbia 91B02058, (Collector Series)
   Columbia Special Products, 51 West 52nd Street, New York, NY 10019.

Physical Examination

1. Series on Physical Assessment of the Well Adult (cassette slides)
   Wiley Biomedical, John Wiley & Sons, Inc., 605 Third Avenue, New York, NY 10016.

References

Alexander, M. and M. Brown. *Pediatric Physical Diagnosis for Nurses.* New York: McGraw-Hill, 1973.

Alexander, M. and M. Brown. "Physical Examination, Part 2: History-Taking." *Nursing 73* 3:35–39, August 1973.

Alexander, M. and M. Brown. "Physical Examination, Part 3: Examining the Skin." *Nursing 73* 3:39–43, September 1973.

Bates, B. *A Guide to Physical Examination.* Philadelphia: Lippincott, 1974.

Berni, R. and H. Readay. *Problem-Oriented Medical Record Implementation.* St. Louis: Mosby, 1974.

Bonkowsky, M. "Adapting the Problem Oriented Medical Record to Community Child Health Care." *Nurs Outlook* 20:515–518, August 1972.

Delaney, M. "Examining the Chest, Part 1: The Lungs." *Nursing 75* 5:12–14, August 1975.

Delaney, M. "Examining the Chest, Part 2: The Heart." *Nursing 75* 5:41–46, September 1975.

Froelich, R. E. and F. M. Bishop. *Clinical Interviewing Skills.* St. Louis: Mosby, 1977.

Gane, D. "Sparky: A Success Story." *Am J Nurs* 73:1176–1177, July 1973.

Hurst, J. W. and H. K. Walker, editors. *The Problem Oriented System.* New York: Medcom Press, 1972.

Malasanos, L., et al. *Health Assessment.* St. Louis: Mosby, 1977.

McMillan, J. A., P. I. Nieburg, and F. A. Oski. *The Whole Pediatrician Catalog.* Philadelphia: Saunders, 1977.

Popich, G. A. and D. W. Smith. "Fontanels: Range of Normal size." *J Pediatr* 80:749–752, May, 1972.

Stewart, R. and C. McGill. "Maximizing the Nursing Role in Public Health." Excerpt on teaching aids from Report of Work Conference Series sponsored by The University of Texas School of Nursing at San Antonio, 1974.

Waring, W. W. and L. O. Jeansonne III. *Practical Manual of Pediatrics.* St. Louis: Mosby, 1975.

Weed, L. *Medical Records, Medical Education, and Patient Care.* Cleveland: Press of Case Western Reserve University, 1970.

Woody, M. and M. Mallison. "The Problem Oriented System for Patient Centered Care." *Am J Nurs* 73:1168–1175, July 1973.

2

Immunizations

The use of immunizations to control and to prevent specific infectious diseases is an established component of comprehensive health care. In fact, the antibody formation induced by immunizing agents is the most specific tool the practitioner has to prevent illness. Nurse practitioners involved in primary care of infants and children will be participating in the planning and implementation of immunization programs and in the education of families and communities regarding the rationale for immunizations. It must be kept in mind that, although familiar to health professionals, immunization procedures and their rationale are not necessarily understood by parents and families. To provide the preventive and protective benefits of immunizations to the largest possible number of children and individuals at risk, it is essential that primary care providers conduct the teaching necessary to ensure the fullest informed participation of their clients.

This chapter presents information on immunization procedures and content necessary to understand and to explain the need for such procedures. See Chapter 29, Infectious Diseases, for discussion of common infections in childhood. Concepts of immunology are discussed also in Chapter 28, Allergies.

IMMUNITY

Definitions

IMMUNITY

Immunity refers to the resistance of the body to the effects of harmful agents. See also Chapter 28, Allergies.

Humoral immunity. This refers to the circulating immunoglobulins (IgA, IgG, and others) which are the predominant antibodies in many infections, especially bacterial infections.

Cell-mediated immunity. This is another part of body defense mechanisms that operates against those agents (viruses, certain bacteria, protozoa, and fungi) that are not affected by humoral antibodies once they enter host cells, and that are capable of intracellular survival and growth.

ANTIGEN

An antigen is a substance not normally present in the body which, when introduced, stimulates production of an antibody that reacts specifically with it.

ANTIBODY

An antibody is a protein that is produced in response to invasion by a foreign agent and that reacts specifically with it.

Types of Protective Immunity

ACTIVE IMMUNITY

Active immunity is long-lasting immunity produced by natural or artificial stimulation so the body produces its own antibodies.

Natural active immunity. This is produced by an attack of the specific disease (e.g., measles).

Artificial active immunity. This is produced by the introduction of vaccines and toxoids (e.g., measles vaccine).

PASSIVE IMMUNITY

Passive immunity is a state of temporary nonsusceptibility to certain microorganisms produced by provision of ready-made antibodies.

Natural passive immunity. This is produced by the maternal transfer of specific antibodies through the placenta to the fetus.

Artificial passive immunity. This is produced by injection of specific antibodies of the following types:

1. Human immune serum globulin (gamma globulin). It is prepared from pooled plasma for general use and is given to reduce the severity of disease or to prevent the disease.
2. Specific human immune serum globulin. This is prepared with known antibody content for a specific illness (e.g., tetanus immune globulin).
3. Animal antiserum or antitoxin. This is prepared from animal serum (horses, cows) and carries with it the danger of foreign serum reactions. It is not given without testing to determine hypersensitivity. An example is tetanus antitoxin.

Types of Agents Conferring Active Artificial Immunity

TOXOID

A toxoid is a bacterial toxin that has been treated by heat or by chemicals to decrease its virulence without destroying its ability to stimulate antibody production (e.g., tetanus, diphtheria).

VACCINE

A vaccine is a suspension of attenuated or killed microorganisms. There are several forms:

1. Killed bacteria (e.g., typhoid, pertussis)
2. Killed virus (e.g., Salk polio)
3. Live attenuated virus (e.g., measles, mumps, rubella, Sabin polio, smallpox)

ADJUVANTS

Adjuvants are substances added to the immunizing agent to enhance the antigenic effect (e.g., alum, aluminum phosphate, aluminum hydroxide). These "depot" antigens retain the antigens at the depot site and release them slowly thus enhancing the response by prolonging contact. They are given intramuscularly and are more likely to produce local reactions at the site of injection. DTP is a depot antigen.

FLUID TOXOIDS AND VACCINES

These have no adjuvant and are more rapidly absorbed so they produce a more rapid secondary response. That is why fluid tetanus toxoid is given following injury in persons who have completed the initial series.

Intervals Between Immunizations

INTERVALS BETWEEN DOSES

Primary response. After the first injection (DTP is an example), antibody is produced relatively slowly and in small concentration but the antibody-producing mechanisms are so altered that with subsequent injection of the same antigen they recognize and remember the antigen and react with the secondary response.

Secondary response. Once the body recognizes the antigen, antibodies are produced much faster and in higher concentration than after the first injection. In other words, the system is capable of responding with increased intensity to future challenges by the same antigen.

Interruption in a series. Due to the secondary response phenomenon, if the initial series is interrupted, *regardless of length of time elapsed*, the series does *not* have to be restarted.

BOOSTERS

Once the initial series is completed and sound immunity is achieved, all that is necessary is to keep the concentration of antibody at a reasonable level by subsequent "boosters" at appropriate times of increased risk. The response is usually excellent.

LIVE VIRUS VACCINES

It has been demonstrated that live virus vaccines can be given simultaneously with excellent antibody responses and no increase in reactions (e.g., measles-mumps-rubella, trivalent oral poliovirus vaccine). However, when giving single live virus vaccines at different times, at least 1 month should elapse between administration.

Initiation of Artificial Immunization in Infancy

IMMUNE STATUS OF THE NEWBORN

The neonate and young infant is at risk for infection because the immune system is poorly developed at birth and too immature to respond with sufficient antibody production. The passive transfer of maternal antibodies to the fetus provides the infant with resistance to infectious diseases for the first few weeks or months after birth. This protection is only against diseases for which the mother has developed sufficient antibodies and is only temporary. An adequately immunized mother passively transfers antibodies to the infant for measles, diphtheria, tetanus, and poliomyelitis. Little to no pertussis immunity is transmitted through the placenta.

AGE TO BEGIN IMMUNIZATIONS

In the normal infant the immune system is capable of responding with adequate antibody production by 2 months of age, and this is the recommended age to begin artificial immunizations.

UNIMMUNIZED CHILDREN

Occasionally children will be encountered who have had no immunizations and whose exposure to on-going primary care services is doubtful. In such situations, when the likelihood of follow-up poses serious question, it is valid to administer *simultaneously* the following agents:

- DTP (or Td if the child is over 6 years of age)
- TOPV
- M-M-R
- Tine test

Contraindications to Routine Immunization

GENERAL RULES

1. Any acute febrile illness is reason to defer any immunization. Minor infections not associated with fever are not contraindications according to the American Academy of Pediatrics. However, if such a child receives an immunization and subsequently develops fever in the next 24 to 48 hours, it is difficult to assess etiology, especially by telephone, and will require an additional visit to the health care facility for evaluation. Children with upper respiratory symptoms on an allergic basis are safe candidates for immunization.
2. Persons with the following conditions are not immunized routinely, especially with live virus vaccines, and medical con-

sultation is required before instituting any immunization procedures:

- Pregnant women
- Persons with leukemia, lymphoma, or other generalized malignancy
- Persons on immunosuppressive therapy (e.g., steroids, irradiation, antimetabolites, alkylating agents)
- Persons with immunodeficiency diseases (e.g., children with cellular immunodeficiencies must not receive BCG or live virus vaccines due to the risk of overwhelming infection)
- Persons with marked sensitivity to eggs, chickens, or neomycin. Such persons are theoretically at risk to live virus vaccines prepared in media containing these substances. Although hypersensitivity reactions to egg and chicken vaccine products have not been reported, and it is considered safe to administer these vaccines, consultation should be obtained if marked sensitivity exists.
- Persons who have had recent administration of immune serum globulin, plasma, or blood. It is advised to wait three months before administering immunizations.

SPECIFIC CONTRAINDICATIONS

These are discussed under each specific immunizing agent in "Guide for Use of Common Immunizing Agents." See below.

IMMUNIZATION SCHEDULES

Considerations in Planning Immunizations

Recommendations for immunizations are meant to be general guidelines and may need to be modified to meet individual or community needs. Factors to be considered include:

1. Risk of a particular disease for an individual or special population (e.g., pertussis in infants, rubella in pregnant women)

2. Risk of the disease for the "herd" or community at large (e.g., polio)

3. Time when optimum immune effect can be obtained (e.g., measles at 15 months of age)

4. Time when risk from the vaccine is minimal (e.g., diphtheria toxoid in childhood)

5. Legal requirements (e.g., in California all children are required to have DTP, polio, and measles immunizations before entry into nursery schools, day care centers, and public schools)

Table 1
Recommended Schedule for Active Immunization of Normal Infants and Children

2 mo	DTP[a]	TOPV[b]
4 mo	DTP	TOPV
6 mo	DTP	TOPV[c]
1 yr		Tuberculin Test[d]
15 mo	Measles,[e] rubella[e]	Mumps[e]
1½ yr	DTP	TOPV
4–6 yr	DTP	TOPV
14–16 yr	Td[f]—continue every 10 years	

Source: Reprinted with permission from American Academy of Pediatrics, *Report of the Committee on Infectious Diseases*, 18th ed., (Evanston, Ill., 1977).

[a]DTP: diphtheria and tetanus toxoids combined with pertussis vaccine.

[b]TOPV: trivalent oral poliovirus vaccine. This recommendation is suitable for breast-fed as well as bottle-fed infants.

[c]The third dose of TOPV is optional but may be given in areas of high endemicity of poliomyelitis.

[d]Frequency of repeated tuberculin tests depends on risk of exposure of the child and on the prevalence of tuberculosis in the population group. For the pediatrician's office or outpatient clinic, an annual or biennial tuberculin test, unless local circumstances clearly indicate otherwise, is appropriate. The initial test should be done at the time of, or preceding, the measles immunization.

[e]May be given at 15 months as measles-rubella or measles-mumps-rubella combined vaccines.

[f]Td: combined tetanus and diphtheria toxoids (adult type) for those more than 6 years of age, in contrast to diphtheria and tetanus (DT) toxoids which contain a larger amount of diphtheria antigen. *Tetanus toxoid at time of injury:* For clean, minor wounds, no booster dose is needed by a fully immunized child unless more than 10 years have elapsed since the last dose. For contaminated wounds, a booster dose should be given if more than 5 years have elapsed since the last dose.

Concentration and Storage of Vaccines
Because the concentration of antigen varies in different products, the manufacturer's package insert should be consulted regarding the volume of individual doses of immunizing agents.

Because biologics are of varying stability, the manufacturer's recommendations for optimal storage conditions (e.g., temperature, light) should be carefully followed. Failure to observe these precautions may significantly reduce the potency and effectiveness of the vaccines.

Recommended Schedules

The Committee on Infectious Diseases of the American Academy of Pediatrics recommends immunization schedules for children and periodically revises them as new knowledge emerges. Table 1 gives the current recommendations for normal infants and children, and Table 2 gives data for children not immunized in infancy.

Informed Consent

Currently there is much discussion and concern surrounding the issue of informing clients and parents of the possible side effects of

Table 2
Primary Immunization for Children Not Immunized in Early Infancy[a]

Under 6 Years of Age	
First visit	DTP, TOPV, tuberculin test
Interval after first visit	
1 mo	Measles,[b] mumps, rubella
2 mo	DTP, TOPV
4 mo	DTP
10–16 mo or preschool	DTP, TOPV
Age 14–16 yr	Td—repeat every 10 yr

6 Years of Age and Over	
First visit	Td, TOPV, tuberculin test
Interval after first visit	
1 mo	Measles, rubella, mumps
2 mo	Td, TOPV
8–14 mo later	Td, TOPV
Age 14–16 yr	Td—repeat every 10 yr

Source: Reprinted with permission from American Academy of Pediatrics, *Report of the Committee on Infectious Diseases,* 18th ed., (Evanston, Ill., 1977).

[a]Physicians may choose to alter the sequence of these schedules if specific infections are prevalent at the time. For example, measles vaccine might be given on the first visit if an epidemic is underway in the community.

[b]Measles vaccine is not routinely given before 15 months of age (see Table 1).

immunizations. Parents *should* be informed of risks and benefits. Efforts are under way by the Committee on Infectious Diseases of the American Academy of Pediatrics to help practitioners present clear and understandable information on risk/benefit factors without causing unnecessary alarm or jeopardizing preventive health programs. Similar efforts could be undertaken in communities by practitioners and parents to determine reasonable approaches to informed consent.

COMMON IMMUNIZING AGENTS

Immunizations are such a routine part of health maintenance care that they are, perhaps, given too "routinely." On-going research and study continually result in new data which affect immunization procedures in terms of administration, efficacy, and safety. The Guide for the Use of Common Immunizing Agents, which follows, provides current information on the administration of routine immunizing agents. Current recommendations for immunization against other diseases (e.g., cholera, plague, rabies, typhoid, typhus, yellow fever) can be obtained by consulting local health departments. Active immunization against tuberculosis and influenza and passive immunization against hepatitis, measles, and varicella-zoster infections are discussed in Chapter 29, Infectious Diseases.

GUIDE FOR THE USE OF COMMON IMMUNIZING AGENTS

DTP

AGENTS

Diphtheria toxoid, tetanus toxoid, and pertussis vaccine combined with aluminum phosphate adsorbed.

(Continued)

AGE TO ADMINISTER

Begin at 2 months of age. Do not give over 6 years of age.

TECHNIQUE OF ADMINISTRATION

Primary Course: 3 doses of 0.5 cc each at 8 week intervals followed by a fourth dose of 0.5 cc approximately 1 year after the third dose.

Booster Dose: One dose of 0.5 cc at 4 to 6 years of age (prior to school entrance). Thereafter use Td 0.5 cc every 10 years.

All doses are given intramuscularly in the mid-lateral thigh muscles.

COMMENTS

• The fourth dose is an integral part of the basic immunizing course. Basic immunization cannot be considered complete until the fourth dose has been given.

• Reactions

1. Local reaction. Redness, induration, and/or a nodule may develop at the injection site. Discomfort may be relieved by placing the child in a soothing warm bath. Nodules occasionally persist for several weeks. Rotate injection sites during the primary course.

2. Systemic reaction. Mild to moderate temperature elevations and irritability may occur soon after injection and usually do not persist past 24 to 48 hours. If severe febrile or local reactions occur modification of the schedule and dosage must be considered. Fractional doses of one half to one fourth of the recommended dose may be given. Parents should be fully informed of possible reactions and questioned carefully at subsequent visits about occurrence and nature of reactions. Treatment of reactions is usually not indicated but acetaminophen may be prescribed for fever over 38.5°C.

3. Pertussis. Before giving pertussis vaccine a history of central

(Continued)

nervous system problems should be ruled out. Pertussis vaccine should not be repeated if any CNS disorder (convulsions, prolonged screaming, prolonged drowsiness) develops after a DTP injection. The series is continued using DT.

- Exposure to disease. Upon exposure to diphtheria or pertussis an emergency booster dose of the appropriate single antigen is indicated unless the fourth dose or a booster dose has been given within the past year. Since the too-frequent use of tetanus toxoid has resulted in an increased incidence of hyperimmunity and severe reactions, the current recommendations for tetanus prophylaxis are presented in Table 3.

DT—Pediatric

AGENTS

Diphtheria toxoid and tetanus toxoid combined with aluminum phosphate adsorbed.

Table 3
Guide to Tetanus Prophylaxis
in Wound Management

History of Tetanus Immunization (Doses)	Clean, Minor Wounds		All Other Wounds	
	Td^a	TIG^b	Td	TIG
Uncertain	Yes	No	Yes	Yes
0–1	Yes	No	Yes	Yes
2	Yes	No	Yes	No^c
3 or more	No^d	No	No^e	No

Source: Reprinted with permission from S. Krugman, et al, *Infectious Diseases of Children*, 6th ed., (St. Louis: C. V. Mosby, 1977), p. 488.
^{a}Td: adult type tetanus-diphtheria toxoid.
^{b}TIG: tetanus immune globulin.
^{c}Unless wound is more than 24 hours old.
^{d}Unless more is than 10 years since last dose.
^{e}Unless more is than 5 years since last dose.

(Continued)

AGE TO ADMINISTER

Do not give over 6 years of age.

TECHNIQUE OF ADMINISTRATION

Same as for DTP.

COMMENTS

- DT—pediatric is for use in infants and young children under 6 years of age when contraindications to the use of pertussis vaccine exist.
- It contains a larger amount of diphtheria antigen than Td.

Td—Adult Type

AGENTS

Diphtheria toxoid and tetanus toxoid combined with aluminum phosphate adsorbed.

AGE TO ADMINISTER

For children over 6 years of age and adults.

TECHNIQUE OF ADMINISTRATION

Primary Course: 2 doses of 0.5 cc each at 8-week intervals followed by a third dose of 0.5 cc 6 to 12 months after the second dose

Booster Dose: One dose of 0.5 cc at 14 to 16 years and thereafter every 10 years

(Continued)

COMMENTS

- It contains no pertussis vaccine since the risk of the disease decreases with age.
- It contains less diphtheria antigen since reactions to diphtheria antigen increase with age.

OPV

AGENTS

Poliovirus vaccine, live, oral, trivalent
Poliovirus vaccine, live, oral, type 1
Poliovirus vaccine, live, oral, type 2
Poliovirus vaccine, live, oral, type 3

AGE TO ADMINISTER

Begin at 2 months. Do not give to persons over 18 years.

TECHNIQUE OF ADMINISTRATION

Primary Course: 2 doses at 8-week intervals within the first 6 months of life followed by a third dose at 18 months of age

Booster Dose: One dose at 4 to 6 years of age (prior to school entrance)

Primary Course for Children and Adolescents under 18 years of age: 2 doses at 8-week intervals followed by a third dose 8 to 14 months later (see Table 2)

COMMENTS

- TOPV (Sabin) is suitable for breast-fed infants. It is not necessary to withhold breast-feeding before or after giving TOPV.
- Vaccine must be kept frozen. If unopened vaccine thaws it may be refrozen provided the temperature does not exceed 8°C

(Continued)

(46°F) during the thaw period. See manufacturer's insert for details.

- There are reportedly no reactions to the vaccine.
- Population at risk. The widespread use of polio vaccines and especially the mass vaccinations of the early 1960s have provided mass immunity. OPV simulates natural infection so antibodies develop. OPV also induces local immunity in the intestinal tract which prevents the wild virus from multiplying and spreading (see Chapter 29, Poliomyelitis). Therefore, the quantity of wild virus circulating in the general population has been reduced and has resulted in "herd immunity" (i.e., a barrier is present in the community to protect susceptible individuals). Eighty percent of the community (herd) must be immune to provide an effective barrier to the wild virus. Thus, the use of vaccines, while reducing and even eradicating polio, makes it essential that all infants and children be immunized. The wild virus population has declined and no longer will contribute significantly to maintaining immunity. If a significant number of children are not vaccinated, especially in the 0 to 4 year age group, they will be susceptible to the wild virus; the wild virus could circulate among them and result in epidemics when a virulent strain is introduced.
- Epidemics. These can be controlled by giving the monovalent vaccine of the same serotype as that causing the outbreak.
- Risks of the vaccine. Live virus persists in the GI tract of the vaccinee for 4 to 6 weeks after vaccination, and cases of paralytic disease in vaccinees and their contacts have appeared. In 1975–76 there were reported each year two cases of paralytic illness in household contacts of infants given TOPV. These occurred at a rate of approximately one per 12.5 million doses of vaccine given. Also during 1975–76, seven cases of paralytic illness occurred in children who received the oral vaccine. On investigation it was discovered that all these children had unusual immunodeficiency disorders. Consequently the use of inactivated poliovirus vaccine (Salk) is now recommended for children with immune deficiency diseases and their siblings and for adults over 18 years of age who have had no previous polio

(Continued)

immunization and require it because of risk of exposure in an endemic area (AAP, 1976).

- See Contraindications to Routine Immunization, this chapter.

Measles

AGENTS

Measles virus vaccine, live, attenuated
Also in combination:
   Measles-rubella virus vaccine, live, attenuated
   Measles-mumps-rubella virus vaccine, live, attenuated

AGE TO ADMINISTER

Begin at 15 months of age. See below, Comments.

TECHNIQUE OF ADMINISTRATION

One subcutaneous injection. Vaccine supplied as a single dose vial of lyophilized vaccine with a disposable syringe containing diluent. Inject total volume of reconstituted vaccine.

COMMENTS

- Inactivated measles vaccine, first licensed in 1963, is no longer recommended and is no longer available in the United States, for the following reasons:

   1. The immunogenic and protective effects of the vaccine were transient.
   2. Atypical measles including symptoms of high fever, edema of the extremities, and pneumonitis occurred on exposure to measles virus later on.

- Live vaccines used commonly today are further attenuated forms of the original Enders-Edmonston B strain.

(Continued)

- Vaccine is prepared by growing virus in chick embryo cultures and theoretically should not be given to individuals who are hypersensitive to eggs, but no serious adverse effects have been reported in egg-sensitive children.

- One injection confers long-lasting immunity. Antibody titers are lower than those following natural measles, but the protection is durable according to follow-up evidence which now extends 14 to 15 years.

- Reactions. The vaccine produces a mild or inapparent non-communicable infection. Fifteen percent of vaccinated children have symptoms which include fever, faint rash, and minor toxicity. Symptoms usually occur 5 to 12 days after vaccination. Significant central nervous system reactions, thought to be associated with measles vaccine, occur approximately once for every million doses.

- Recent outbreaks. Cases of measles have been reported in groups of children and adolescents who:

  1. Have never had measles and have never received live attenuated measles vaccine

  2. Received live attenuated vaccine before 12 months of age

  3. Received live measles vaccine that had been inactivated by exposure to light, inadequate refrigeration, or use of wrong diluent (Do not store vaccine in refrigerator door.)

  4. Received too large a dose of gamma globulin with the measles vaccine when immunized before 1969

  5. Received killed measles vaccine

- Indications for measles immunization and re-immunization are as follows:

  1. Routine measles immunization should be deferred until about 15 months of age. This is a recent recommendation based on studies that show that seroconversion rates of 80 to 85 percent occur in children immunized at 12 months, as compared with seroconversion rates of more than 95 percent in children immunized after 13 to 14 months of age (Krugman, 1977, p. 6).

(Continued)

2. Measles vaccine should be given any time after 6 months of age during measles outbreaks. A second vaccination should then be given after 15 months of age.

3. If doubt exists about the details of immunization status, another inoculation of measles vaccine should be given.

4. Children vaccinated with simultaneous administration of gamma globulin at any age should be revaccinated.

5. Children vaccinated with inactivated vaccine should be reimmunized.

6. Children who were vaccinated before 13 months of age should be re-immunized (Shinefield, 1977, p. 13). (There is not universal agreement on this point.)

• Tuberculin testing

1. It is recommended that tuberculin testing be done prior to administration of measles vaccine because of the hazard of the possible exacerbation of undiagnosed, untreated tuberculosis (see Chapter 29, Tuberculosis). Since this possibility is remote, and since the value of protection against natural measles exceeds the theoretical hazard of exacerbation of tuberculosis, the recommended procedure should not interfere with community-wide immunization programs where the risk of natural measles is high.

2. Measles vaccine may alter immune mechanisms and temporarily depress tuberculin sensitivity. This could result in a false-negative tuberculin test. If measles vaccine precedes TB testing, 4 to 6 weeks should elapse before administering a tuberculin test.

3. It has been demonstrated recently that it is valid to administer M-M-R vaccine and tuberculin skin testing simultaneously.

• Live measles vaccine can usually prevent the disease if administered within 2 days after exposure to natural measles.

• Children with underlying illness that contraindicates the use of live vaccine should be protected on exposure by the use of immune serum globulin. See Table 3 in Chapter 29.

(Continued)

Rubella

AGENTS

Rubella virus vaccine, live, attenuated

Also in combination:
Measles-rubella virus vaccine, live, attenuated
Mumps-rubella virus vaccine, live, attenuated
Measles-mumps-rubella virus vaccine, live, attenuated

AGE TO ADMINISTER

Begin at 15 months. Do not give to pregnant women. See below, Comments.

TECHNIQUE OF ADMINISTRATION

Same as for measles.

COMMENTS

- The vaccine was licensed in 1969. Primary rationale for use is to prevent congenital rubella syndrome (see Chapter 29). Two population groups are targets for immunization:

  1. Children between the ages of 15 months to 12 years of age to reduce the spread of natural rubella infection
  2. Susceptible nonpregnant women on a selective basis (See below.)

- Vaccination of women of childbearing age (including adolescents):

  1. Perform serologic testing—hemagglutination inhibition test (HI titer)
  2. If rubella antibodies are present and immunity is confirmed, do not vaccinate. A titer of 1 : 10 or higher indicates adequate protection.

(Continued)

3. If susceptible and nonpregnant, vaccination is advised only if the woman understands that she *must not* become pregnant for at least 2 months after vaccination. An acceptable method of contraception must be followed.
4. An ideal time to vaccinate susceptible women is in the immediate postpartum period.

- Reactions and side effects:
  1. Fever and rash occur rarely
  2. Transient arthritis and arthralgia occur frequently in women who are vaccinated but rarely in children. It occurs 2 to 4 weeks post vaccination.
  3. Three types of rubella vaccine are used in immunization programs: those prepared either in duck embryo, rabbit kidney, or human diploid cell cultures. The strain prepared in dog kidney cell culture was associated with a greater incidence and severity of arthritis, arthralgia, and neuropathy and has now been removed from distribution. This has reduced concerns about these side effects to a minimum.

- Communicability. After vaccination, rubella virus is shed and excreted from the pharynx for 2 or more weeks but a number of studies have confirmed that immunized children are not contagious. There is no contraindication to the use of rubella vaccine in children of pregnant mothers. In fact, susceptible children of pregnant mothers *should* be immunized.
- Risk of vaccine to the fetus. This issue is not completely resolved. Attenuated virus has been recovered from fetal tissue. There is also evidence that women inadvertently vaccinated shortly before or after conception have delivered live infants without evidence of congenital rubella syndrome. In the study by Modlin (1975) none of the live-born infants of susceptible immunized mothers had evidence of congenital rubella (see also Chapter 29, Rubella).
- Re-infection. Re-infection can and does occur more commonly after vaccination than after natural rubella. Viremia has *not* been detected during re-infection. Consequently it is unlikely that fetal infection will occur in association with re-infection.

(Continued)

- Pregnant woman exposed to rubella. When a pregnant woman whose immune status is unknown is exposed to rubella two facts must be established:

    1. Whether or not the woman is immune to rubella
    2. If not immune, whether or not she has contracted the current infection

The procedure recommended is as follows:

    1. Obtain an HI titer as soon as possible (within 1 week of exposure).
    2. If antibodies are present in adequate amounts the woman can be reassured.
    3. If antibody is not detectable, gamma globulin may be given and a second HI titer obtained 4 weeks later. If antibodies are then detectable it indicates current rubella infection. Gamma globulin has not proven effective in preventing rubella, but it is worth the try if abortion is not an acceptable alternative.
    4. If more than 1 week has elapsed before the first blood specimen is obtained, the presence of antibodies may indicate past *or* current infection. Thus a second specimen should be obtained 1 to 2 weeks later to check for a rising antibody titer indicative of current infection.
    5. The way to avoid this stressful situation is by vaccinating all children between 15 months and 12 years of age and by encouraging women of childbearing age to have baseline antibody titer determinations performed.

Mumps

AGENTS

Mumps virus vaccine, live, attenuated
Also in combination:
    Mumps-rubella virus vaccine, live, attenuated
    Measles-mumps-rubella virus vaccine, live, attenuated

(Continued)

AGE TO ADMINISTER

Begin at 15 months of age.

TECHNIQUE OF ADMINISTRATION

Same as for measles.

COMMENTS

- Because mumps vaccine is available in combined form with measles and rubella vaccines, it should be considered for use at 15 months of age. Otherwise it should be used in susceptible children approaching puberty, in adolescents, and in adults, particularly males who have no history of mumps. See Chapter 29.
- There are no known serious side effects of this vaccine. Occasionally a mild, brief fever develops.

Smallpox

AGENT

Active, live vaccinia virus (nonattenuated).

AGE TO ADMINISTER

Not recommended as routine procedure for individuals residing in the United States. See Comments.

TECHNIQUE OF ADMINISTRATION

Vaccine supplied as glycerinated vaccine or lyophilized vaccine.

Primary Vaccination: A small drop of vaccine is placed on the outer aspect of the upper arm. A series of pressures (8–10) is

(Continued)

made with a sterile needle held parallel to the skin, thereby depositing vaccine under the superficial skin. Excess vaccine is wiped away with dry sterile gauze. No dressing is necessary.

COMMENTS

- Successful vaccination depends on the use of a potent vaccine and correct technique. A successful "take" will produce a slowly growing area of erythema after 4 to 5 days which reaches maximal size in 8 to 14 days, acquires a vesicular appearance which then scabs, and usually leaves a recognizable scar. If no vesicle appears do not assume the individual is immune. Repeat the vaccination using another lot (batch) of vaccine.

- Re-vaccination. A similar technique is used but 25 to 30 pressures are recommended. Reaction should consist of vesicular or pustular lesion or definite palpable induration surrounding a central lesion. In endemic areas re-vaccination is recommended every 3 years.

- Routine vaccination is no longer recommended by the U.S. Public Health Service, the American Academy of Pediatrics, and the World Health Organization. Rationale includes the following:

  1. There have been no documented cases of smallpox in the United States since 1949.

  2. Importation is the only way a case could occur and public health surveillance measures are very effective.

  3. The risks of vaccination outweigh the risks of contracting the disease. In 1968, nine persons died as a result of vaccination. Six of these deaths occurred in primary vaccinees, two in re-vaccinees, and one in a contact.

  4. As of 1977 the only country in the world endemic for smallpox is Ethiopia.

- Vaccination is recommended for:

  1. Travelers to endemic countries
  2. Health personnel
  3. International Certificate of Vaccination is required for entry

(Continued)

into most countries of Africa, Asia, and Central and South America.

- Precautions:

    1. Persons with eczema should not be vaccinated nor exposed to vaccinated individuals.
    2. If an individual with eczema requires vaccination it is accompanied with a prophylactic dose of Vaccinia Immune Globulin. Consult with a physician before vaccinating.
    3. Do not vigorously cleanse the vaccination site. Danger of skin abrasions and subsequent larger area for virus innoculation result. Do not use alcohol to cleanse the skin. Use acetone.
    4. Do not vaccinate anyone with acute skin lesions (e.g., poison ivy, burns, impetigo).
    5. See Contraindications to Routine Immunization, this chapter.

- Vaccination of young infants:

    1. In a situation of high risk infants over 2 months of age could be vaccinated after medical consultation. Complication rates appear to be twice as high for children under one year of age.
    2. Young children traveling with parents to countries requiring smallpox vaccination for entry can be spared vaccination by providing a letter from medical authorities advising against vaccination.

DELIVERY OF IMMUNIZATION SERVICES

Current Immunization Status

Immunization levels against polio, measles, rubella, mumps, diphtheria, pertussis, and tetanus have seriously declined among 1- to 4-year-old children. National surveys in 1974 and 1975 indicated

Table 4
Immunization Levels: 1974 and 1975

	Percentage of Preschool Children (1 to 4 years) Adequately Immunized	
Disease	1974	1975
DTP	73.9	75.2
Polio[a]	63.1	64.8
Measles	64.5	65.5
Rubella	59.8	61.9
Mumps	39.4	44.4

Source: U.S. Immunization Surveys, 1964–1975, Center for Disease Control, Immunization Division, Atlanta, Georgia, 30333.
[a] Among nonwhite urban children current levels were only 47.0 percent in 1974.

that approximately 5.3 million of the nearly 13.2 million 1- to 4-year-old children are inadequately immunized. See Table 4.

Efforts to Improve Immunization Levels

1. Legislation. Laws have been enacted in 38 states and are pending in several more requiring specific immunizations prior to school entry.
2. Accurate reporting of cases to local health departments. This is an important yet frequently overlooked responsibility.
3. Accurate record keeping. Permanent records at health facilities as well as provision of records to parents help to identify children at risk.
4. Education of parents and communities.
5. Provision of funds to health department to purchase vaccines.
6. Continued surveillance by health providers of the immunization status of every child they see.

Resource Information

1. Local health departments.
2. Manufacturers' inserts. These contain complete information on the use of each specific vaccine.

3. Committee on Infectious Diseases, American Academy of Pediatrics. Their report, the "Red Book," is frequently updated, is very complete, and can be purchased by writing to AAP, P.O. Box 1034, Evanston, IL 60204.

4. Advisory Committee on Immunization Practices (ACIP), U.S. Public Health Service, Center for Disease Control, Atlanta, GA 30333. Telephone: 404-633-3311. They also publish *Morbidity and Mortality Weekly Reports*, an excellent resource for developing and revised recommendations.

References

American Academy of Pediatrics, Committee on Infectious Diseases. "Poliovirus Immunization Re-examined." *News and Comments* 27(12), December 1976.

American Academy of Pediatrics. *Report of the Committee on Infectious Diseases*, 18th ed. Evanston, Ill., 1977.

Barrett-Connor, E. "Advice to Travelers." *West J Med* 123:22–30, July 1975.

Brandling-Bennett, A. D., et al. "The Risks of Rubella Vaccination in Pregnancy." *Contemp Obstet Gynecol* 4:77–80, July 1974.

Brickman, H. F., et al. "Timing of Tine Tests in Relation to Immunizations." *Pediatrics* 55:392–396, March 1975.

Deforest, A., et al. "The Effect of Breastfeeding on the Antibody Response of Infants to Trivalent Oral Poliovirus Vaccine." *J Pediatr* 83:93–95, July 1973.

Francis, B. J. "Current Concepts in Immunizations." *Am J Nurs* 73:646–649, April 1973.

Hodges, F. B. "Public Health Report: Recent Developments in Immunization." *California Medicine* 117:71–73, August 1972.

Horstmann, D. M. "Rubella: The Challenge of Its Control." *J Infect Dis* 123:640–654, June 1971.

Kempe, C. H. "The End of Routine Smallpox Vaccination in the United States." *Pediatrics* 49:489–491, April 1972.

Krugman, S. "Present Status of Measles and Rubella Immunization in the United States: A Medical Progress Report." *J Pediatr* 78:1–16, January 1971.

Krugman, S. "Present Status of Measles and Rubella Immunization in the United States: A Medical Progress Report." *J Pediatr* 90:1–12, January 1977.

Krugman, S., et al. "Combined Live Measles, Mumps, Rubella Vaccine." *Am J Dis Child* 121:380–381, May 1971.

Krugman, S. and S. Katz. "Rubella Immunization: A Five-Year Progress Report." *N Engl J Med* 290:1375–1376, June 13, 1974.

Krugman, S., R. Ward, and S. Katz. *Infectious Diseases of Children*, 6th ed. St. Louis: Mosby, 1977.

Kulenkampff, M., et al. "Neurological Complications of Pertussis Inoculation." *Arch Dis Child* 49:46–49, January 1974.

Marcuse, E. K. and M. G. Grand. "Epidemiology of Diphtheria in San Antonio, Texas, 1970." *JAMA* 224:305–310, April 16, 1973.

Modlin, J. F., et al. "A Review of Five Years Experience with Rubella Vaccine in the United States." *Pediatrics* 55:20, January 1975.

Ross, L. A. R. and A. S. Yeager. "Measles Encephalitis in an Immunized Child." *J Pediatr* 90:156–157, January 1977.

Shinefield, H. "Meeting of Committee on Infectious Diseases, Chapter 1, A.A.P." *California Pediatrician*, Summer 1977, p. 13.

Witte, J. J. "Recent Advances in Public Health: Immunization." *Am J Public Health* 64:939–944, October 1974.

3

A Comprehensive Schedule for Well-Child Care

Recognizing the parents as the true providers of child health care, health professionals assist them in parenting by offering guidance, counseling, and teaching. For this reason health visits are not equated with immunization schedules. Families need individual attention; some will function with fewer visits; some, especially first-time parents, will need longer visits, and/or extra visits. The goals in planning for comprehensive child health care are:

- To recognize that routine health supervision enhances the optimal physical, intellectual, emotional, and social growth of the child
- To provide direct services to clients and families via a caring relationship and a nonfragmented, communicative approach
- To direct families toward responsible parenting through education in childrearing practices, knowledge of normal child development and emotional needs, awareness of preventive measures such as immunization schedules, safety precautions, and illness care
- To develop self-confident parents through the provision of encouragement, reassurance, and other measures supportive of the parenting role

Toward better preventive pediatric care it is recommended that parents be encouraged to visit the pediatric primary health care provider prenatally to discuss similarities and differences of child-care philosophies, options for health care, and knowledge of services of a public health nurse. This relationship is especially recommended for first-time parents who need help soon after the infant's birth.

The following schedule is considered an outline for content of the health visit at different ages. The reader is referred to appropriate chapters for complete information regarding specific topics.

FIRST VISIT

Health Assessment

See Table 1.

Counseling

PHYSICAL CARE

Discuss:

- Bathing and the use of lotions, powders, and soaps. See Chapter 15, General Care of the Skin, and Care of the Diapers.
- Care of the cord. See Chapter 4, Physical Care of the Newborn.
- Elimination. Discuss patterns and colors of stools. See Chapter 8, Stool Patterns.
- Safety. See Chapter 9, Accident Prevention and Safety.
- Out-of-doors. See Chapter 15, Sunburn, Prevention.
- Equipment. Discuss need to obtain car seat (Chapter 9) vaporizer (Chapter 18), and other equipment appropriate for age.
- Illness prevention. Discuss early rashes and their care (see Chapter 15, Miliaria, Diaper Rashes), colds, and the need for protection from infection in the early months.

Table 1
Health Assessment at First Visit

Health History Physical Exam	Nutrition	Development	Laboratory Procedures Immunizations
Parental concerns	Assess caloric needs for optimum growth: 100–110 cal/kg/day	Two-weeks: sucking and rooting reflexes, Moro Reflex and tonic neck reflex (TNR)	Urine ferric chloride for PKU
Prenatal history			Discuss with parents
Birth history	Discuss need for iron, vitamins, fluoride		Discuss immunization schedule and its importance
Neonatal history		Sensitive to light and noise	
History of familial diseases	Discuss current feeding methods	One month: responds to bell, eyes follow to midline, regards face, lifts head when prone	
Interval history			
Family and social history			
Length, weight, and head circumference			
Complete physical exam			
Discussion of normal variants and abnormal physical findings with parents			

- Protocol of visits. Discuss the components of child health care and immunization schedules.

EMOTIONAL AND MENTAL DEVELOPMENT

Discuss:

- Gratification of basic infant needs; contact such as holding, singing and talking to, fondling, and rocking; and sucking needs such as amount of time and when to use the pacifier, non-nutritive breast or bottle sucking
- Differences in infant temperament and the part these play in parental understanding of the infant's behavior. See Chapter 8, Psychological Needs in Infancy.

STIMULATION

Infants at this age need and enjoy:

- Being moved through space (kinesthesia). A cradle, rocking-chair, carriage, or automobile can be used.
- Sucking to ease discomfort and tension. If the infant needs more non-nutritive sucking, fingers or a pacifier may be used. It may be necessary at times to hold the pacifier in the infant's mouth.
- Having physical contact with the mother, father, or caretaker. The infant should be held, fondled, walked, rocked, and talked or sung to.
- Changing position
- Observing a mobile

PARENT-CHILD RELATIONSHIP

Discuss:

- Parental expectations in reference to crying, feeding, elimination, sleeping, and spoiling
- The importance of mother-child attachment

PARENTING

Discuss:

- The shift in the family from two to three members and its meaning to the family
- The need for adopting a philosophy of child care which is mutually agreed upon by parents
- The importance of help in the home for cooking, cleaning, and to relieve the mother for the care of the child
- The need to consider time for the mother's own needs and for rest
- Her feelings of inadequacy, anxiety, resentments, and isolation
- Realistic expectations of the parents for themselves and each other as parents and the changes in their relationship
- The importance of the father's understanding of the physical and emotional changes occurring in the mother and the need for his support
- Active participation of the father in the care of the child as part of his role
- The father's needs and availability of support

NURSE PRACTITIONER GOALS

These goals include:

- Providing health education about infant care and development
- Recognizing this period as one of greatest apprehension and anxiety for the parents about assuming the responsibility of a dependent infant
- Providing an atmosphere supportive of responsible parenting and a free exchange of ideas
- Listening well and answering all questions fully
- Observing the interactions of the parents with their child and assessing parental understanding of the child's temperament and/or behavior
- Identifying potential and high-risk situations such as extreme parental frustration or anger, and faulty parental bonding

- Examining one's own feelings about the family
- Discussing family planning
- Assessing the parents' understanding of the health care system and encouraging both parents to accompany the child to the health visit
- Encouraging the parents' attendance at parenting groups or classes

VISIT AT 5 TO 9 WEEKS

Health Assessment

See Table 2.

Counseling

PHYSICAL CARE

This includes a review of the first visit and discussion of the following:

- Sleep patterns and sleeping arrangements
- The meaning of illness, colds, and fever. Teach the use of the thermometer, and when to call for medical care.
- Accident prevention appropriate for age

EMOTIONAL AND MENTAL DEVELOPMENT

Review basic psychological needs and discuss:

- The child's continued gratification of these needs
- Attachment and its meaning to the infant and mother
- The parents' observations of the child's temperament

Table 2
Health Assessment at 5 to 9 Weeks

Health History Physical Exam	Nutrition	Development	Laboratory Procedures Immunizations
Parental concerns	Assess caloric needs for optimum growth	5 weeks: rooting, Moro, and TNR	Diphtheria, tetanus, pertussis vaccine (DTP)
Interval history to include past illnesses, eating, sleeping, elimination, behavior	Discuss parental attitudes and expectations re: solids	May "smile"	Trivalent oral polio vaccine (TOPV)
Family and social history	Discuss need for water	Fist to mouth	
Length, weight, and head circumference		Follows light; tracks sound	
Complete physical exam		9 weeks:	
Discussion of findings with parents		Smiles	
		Vocalizes	
		Hands to midline	
		Listens	
		Follows light past midline	
		Holds head up 90° in prone position	

STIMULATION

The 5- to 9-week-old child needs and enjoys:

- A mobile to watch, later a mirror placed in the crib, and pictures of faces
- A change of scenery. The infant seat may be propped and moved about.
- Non-nutritional sucking of fingers or pacifier
- A prone position to allow lifting of the head. This should occur several times a day.
- Crib devices which are semi-rigidly supported and strong enough to withstand abuse. Rattles and hand toys are not good at this age.
- Opportunities to be held, rocked, talked and sung to, and to have parents repeat the noises which are made by the infant.

PARENT-CHILD RELATIONSHIP

Discuss:

- Need for taking time to enjoy and observe the movements, reactions, rhythm, and uniqueness of the child

PARENTING

Repeat from first visit as necessary and discuss:

- The mother's need for rest, relaxation, and exercise. She may need help with organizing the day. Discuss her feelings about how things are going.
- The father's role as supportive. How does he see his role? Discuss his need to become familiar with the infant by gentle handling and playing.
- The parents' need to occasionally be away from the infant for short periods of time. If the mother returns to work there needs to be joint responsibility for planning care of the infant and care of the home.

NURSE PRACTITIONER GOALS

These include:

- Providing support and reassurance to the parents. In this early period the family rhythm is set by the child. The parents may be worn out from too little sleep. They may feel resentment at the constant attention needed by the infant. They need to know that the infant becomes more secure with their care and therefore easier to manage.
- Encouraging participation in parenting groups or classes

VISIT AT 2-1/2 TO 4 MONTHS

Health Assessment

See Table 3.

Counseling

PHYSICAL CARE

Discuss:

- The need for an organized day and consistency of care
- Sleep and napping needs
- Drooling as a sign of salivary gland maturation and the infant's inability to swallow excessive saliva. It is not necessarily teething.
- The use of jumpers, walkers, and high-chairs when the head is held erect

EMOTIONAL AND MENTAL DEVELOPMENT

Review basic psychologic needs and discuss:

- Gratification of basic needs

Table 3
Health Assessment at 2½ to 4 Months

Health History Physical Exam	Nutrition	Development	Laboratory Procedures Immunizations
Parental concerns Interval history Family and social history Length, weight, and head circumference Complete physical exam Discussion of findings with parents	Continued need for iron-enriched formula Digestive system now mature enough to handle solids Introduction of cereal, fruits at 4 mo Teething biscuits may be used; avoid wheat products.	2½ mo: holds head and chest to 90° in prone position Laughs, babbles TNR and Moro reflex diminishing 4 mo: holds head erect and steady in sitting position Bears weight on legs May roll over	DTP and TOPV #2

- Use of the pacifier. The infant may not be as dependent on the pacifier at about 4 months. This is a good time to watch for clues to discontinue its use.

STIMULATION

The 2-1/2- to 4-month-old infant needs and enjoys:

- Being talked to, played with affectionately, and moved about to various parts of the house. Playpens and cribs are not advisable for long periods of time.
- Looking at mirrors. These should be of good stainless steel placed about 4 to 5 inches from the child. This is a particularly good device for the diapering table.
- Handling, pulling, and grabbing at crib devices
- Kicking and thumping at a large stuffed toy tied to the foot of the crib

PARENT-CHILD RELATIONSHIP

It is helpful to figure out the infant's "life-style." Discuss:

- The infant's patterns. Has the infant fairly regular patterns? Is the infant easily satisfied or does he/she react strongly?
- The infant's developing temperament. Awareness of the infant's temperament and how the parents deal with it is a key aspect of how smoothly the child's development will proceed. A good reference for parents is *Infants and Mothers* by T. Berry Brazelton (New York: Delacorte Press, 1969).

PARENTING

Discuss:

- Sharing of child care. The father may diaper and bathe the infant to overcome his fear of handling the infant.

NURSE PRACTITIONER GOALS

These remain the same as the first visit with the addition of:

- Reassuring the parents that they are doing a good job

VISIT AT 6 MONTHS

Health Assessment

See Table 4.

Counseling

PHYSICAL CARE

Discuss:

- Accident prevention appropriate to age
- Teething and use of teething toys and crackers
- Use of jumpers, swings, and walkers with caution. They should not be used for long periods of time and should be safely constructed.
- Care of upper respiratory infections and mild diarrhea

EMOTIONAL AND MENTAL DEVELOPMENT

Discuss:

- The need for answering all cries within a reasonable period of time
- Stranger anxiety and what it means to members of the family
- Attachment to certain objects as normal, such as blankets and toys

Table 4
Health Assessment at 6 Months

Health History Physical Exam	Nutrition	Development	Laboratory Procedures Immunizations
Parental concerns	Limit milk to 24 oz/24 hr	Laughs, babbles	DTP and TOPV #3
Interval history	Discuss iron-containing	Passes object hand to hand	
Family and social history	foods, finger foods	and mouths objects	
Length, weight, and head circumference	Advise waiting to wean until after 1 year	Tooth eruption Turns to voice	
Complete physical exam including eye cover test for strabismus	Discuss fluoride, avoidance of sugared foods	Rolls over, may get to sitting	
Discussion of findings with parents		Beginning stranger anxiety Stronger attachment to mother	

- Consistency, continuity, and sameness. This is very helpful in enabling the infant to start to develop some beginning sense of self-identity.

STIMULATION

This age child needs and enjoys:

- Being physically active
- Hearing sounds, those of others and his/her own. Talk to the infant about what is occurring at the moment.
- Grabbing, pulling, and dropping objects
- Moving about. Allow child space to roam, to roll over, and to crawl, preferably on a blanket on the floor.
- Using walkers and jumpers. These are used with caution. They should be safe and not used for long periods of time.
- Playing with safe small objects, stuffed toys, and jack-in-the-box toys

PARENT-CHILD RELATIONSHIP

The child's personality changes with assumption of the upright position. Discuss:

- Stranger anxiety. This may create problems within the family since the infant prefers the mother at this time.
- Parents' attitudes toward messiness, food play, and spoiling

PARENTING

Discuss:

- Time away from the child for short periods of time. This is not a time for prolonged separation.
- Feelings about getting up at night
- Differences of opinion between parents on child-raising philosophy
- Problems regarding family planning if necessary

NURSE PRACTITIONER GOALS

These include:

- Continuing to provide appropriate health education
- Reassuring parents in reference to their concerns
- Expressing empathy toward their frustrations in handling infant behavior
- Recognizing that some families need more or longer visits

VISIT AT 9 MONTHS

Health Assessment

See Table 5.

Counseling

PHYSICAL CARE

Discuss:

- Accident prevention appropriate to age
- Safe area for child to move about without restricting exploration and satisfaction of normal curiosity
- Caries prevention. Cleaning teeth daily with gauze, and no bottles at bedtime or nap with milk or fruit juices
- Use of Ipecac
- Disadvantages of early toilet training. It is better to wait until the child is ready.
- Reasons for not weaning from breast or bottle too early

Table 5
Health Assessment at 9 Months

Health History Physical Exam	Nutrition	Development	Laboratory Procedures Immunizations
Parental concerns	Advise 3 meals/day	Jabbers, babbles	Hematocrit, hemoglobin, and RBC indices
Interval history	May introduce cup if child ready; advise waiting to wean until after 1 yr	Thumb-finger grasp	Sickle cell and G-6-PD screening
Family and social history		Imitates speech sounds	No immunizations if up to date
Length, weight, and head circumference	Normal drop in appetite	Plays pat-a-cake	
Complete physical exam including hearing assessment (infant should turn head at least 45° to locate sound)	Restriction of sugared foods, milk, and juices in bedtime bottles	May pull to stand and/or crawl	
Discussion of findings with parents			

EMOTIONAL AND MENTAL DEVELOPMENT

Discuss:

- Need for feeling loved and cared for
- Separation anxiety
- Night-crying. Difficulty in putting infant down for nap and at bedtime, and the need for bedtime rituals
- Need for satisfaction of normal curiosity. This is not a time for repeated "no's."

STIMULATION

The 9-month-old child needs and enjoys:

- Imitation of sounds. These should be answered in kind by the parent.
- Space to crawl about, to touch, and to explore
- Large balls, boxes, blocks, stack toys, jack-in-the-box toys
- Hide-and-seek and peek-a-boo games

PARENT-CHILD RELATIONSHIP

Discuss:

- The child's continuing preference for the mother
- Need to respond to the child such as picking up dropped toys, playing peek-a-boo

PARENTING

Discuss:

- Feelings and ideas toward weaning, toilet training, masturbation, discipline, and the need to set limits
- Availability of parenting groups or classes

NURSE PRACTITIONER GOALS

These include:

- Reassuring and educating parents about their concerns
- Treating their concerns with respect and empathy

VISIT AT 12 MONTHS

Health Assessment

See Table 6.

Counseling

PHYSICAL CARE

Discuss:

- Accident prevention. House should be made toddler-safe.
- Caries prevention. Clean child's teeth daily with gauze.
- Illness care. Teach bed care, diet, throat examination, and symptoms of an ear problem.

EMOTIONAL AND MENTAL DEVELOPMENT

Discuss:

- The development of the child's strong will
- The need for dependence-independence
- Learning to distinguish between self and parent
- Increased growth of ego. "I am me"
- The expression of curiosity which aids in the child's intellectual development

Table 6

Health Assessment at 12 Months

Health History Physical Exam	Nutrition	Development	Laboratory Procedures Immunizations
Parental concerns	Review basic food groups, table foods, and amounts appropriate for age	Indicates wants	Urinalysis
Interval history		Drinks from cup	Hemogram if not obtained sooner
Family and social history		Pincer grasp	Tuberculin test
Length, weight, and head circumference	Lessened appetite	May use spoon	
Complete physical exam	Milk limited to 16–20 oz/24 hr	Ma-ma, da-da	
Discussion of findings with parents	Avoidance of sugared foods and drinks	Crawls, walks holding on or alone	

STIMULATION

This child needs and enjoys:

- Being read to
- Naming and pointing to features, such as nose, eye
- Roaming and being allowed to touch, to investigate, and to manipulate objects
- Playing in water and sand with appropriate toys
- Playing and holding dolls and stuffed toys
- Sorting, piling, and dumping small objects from a box

PARENT-CHILD RELATIONSHIP

Discuss:

- The parents' feelings toward "education" versus development, discipline-punishment, setting of limits, and temper tantrums
- Development of autonomy. This begins the age of exploration and sometimes creates a conflict or battle of wills between the parent and the child. The mother may be threatened by the independence shown by her baby or may expect too much in terms of "good" behavior from the child.
- Demands of supervising a mobile infant. How does the mother feel about the constant picking up of toys, and the full-time job of protecting this beginning toddler?

PARENTING

Discuss:

- Any conflicts of opinion between the parents concerning child-rearing practices
- Changes in parental relationships. The child's need for constant supervision drains energy and emotional reserve. There should be an awareness of the need to maintain closeness and emotional contact with each other, not just in the parental role but in giving to each other as adults.

NURSE PRACTITIONER GOALS

These goals include:

- Helping parents to recognize and to deal with their frustrations
- Being alert for signs of anger and resentment toward child
- Re-emphasizing developmental processes as normal

VISIT AT 15 TO 18 MONTHS

Health Assessment

See Table 7.

Counseling

PHYSICAL CARE

This includes:

- Accident prevention appropriate to age
- Cleaning teeth with gauze or soft brush daily. The child may wish to imitate adult brushing teeth. May pay first visit to dentist.
- Beginning toilet training if child indicates readiness
- Management of colds and complications, diarrhea, and constipation

EMOTIONAL AND MENTAL DEVELOPMENT

Discuss:

- Age of negativism as a natural aspect of development
- Age of curiosity. Parents should not use repeated "no's."

Table 7
Health Assessment at 15 to 18 Months

Health History Physical Exam	Nutrition	Development	Laboratory Procedures Immunizations
Parental concerns	Review basic food groups	More than 5–6 words	Measles, mumps, and rubella (M-M-R) vaccine at 15 months
Interval history	Stress need for iron and avoidance of sugared foods and drinks	Uses spoon	
Family and social history		Scribbles on paper	
Height and weight	May feed self	Points to one or more parts of body	DTP and TOPV #4 at 18 months if #3 was given at 6 months
Complete physical exam		Climbing, running	
Discussion of findings with parents			

- Importance of intellectual development at this age
- Beginning interest in peers
- Nursery school

STIMULATION

This child needs and enjoys:

- Push-pull toys, large and small balls, and dolls
- Sand, water, and paper to play with
- Noisy and manipulative toys
- Books and being read to
- Climbing, running, especially out-of-doors
- Encouragement of curiosity

PARENT-CHILD RELATIONSHIP

Discuss:

- Period of egocentrism in the child which makes it difficult for the child to appreciate other's point of view
- Permissiveness versus overpermissiveness, handling of discipline, and setting of limits
- The use of substitution and positive reinforcement in place of frequent "no's"
- Sibling relationships. This age child may show hostility to an older sibling.

PARENTING

Discuss:

- Attitudes toward coping with negativism, temper tantrums, and obedience
- Intellectual interests of the child such as books, toys, equipment. This is a key time to encourage the child to explore and for the parents to react enthusiastically to his discoveries. Take the time

to explain how things work. Intrigue and stretch the child's observations of the world without pushing.

NURSE PRACTITIONER GOALS

These include:

- Continuing to provide education re: care and development
- Continuing to offer reassurance
- Assessing parental needs for support measures
- Assessing parents' knowledge of safety precautions
- Identifying high-risk situations

VISIT AT 2 YEARS

Health Assessment

See Table 8.

Counseling

PHYSICAL CARE

Discuss:

- Accident prevention appropriate for age
- Care of the teeth. They should be brushed and flossed daily. Primary dental visit may be made.
- Toilet training should be in progress for most children
- Sleeping problems

Table 8
Health Assessment at 2 Years

Health History Physical Exam	Nutrition	Development	Laboratory Procedures Immunizations
Parental concerns	Review basic food groups and appropriate amounts for age	May talk well and follow directions	Urinalysis if not done earlier
Interval history	Reduce milk intake to 16 oz/24 hr	Purposeful markings on paper	
Family and social history	Discuss importance of proper snacks (low sugar, high protein)	Balances 4 blocks	
Height, weight, and head circumference		Performs simple household tasks	
Complete physical exam		Later may throw ball overhand	
Discussion of findings with parents			

EMOTIONAL AND MENTAL DEVELOPMENT

Discuss:

- The need for being with peers and the importance of nursery school
- Nightmares versus night terrors related to fears
- Autonomy-dependency conflict. This child is still interested in the mother (or primary parent-figure) but becomes less "clingy" at age 2½.
- Development of pride in personal accomplishment

STIMULATION

This child needs and enjoys:

- Practicing skills on small objects, such as fill and dump toys, stacking toys, blocks, and pencils and crayons
- Exploring the nonsocial world such as playing with the telephone, puppets, and household items
- Carrying on a conversation, being read to, and pretend reading
- Telling stories and singing
- Pretend activity, such as dressing up in adult clothes and playing house
- Playing out-of-doors with sand, water, slides, balls, swings, and climbing equipment
- Watching television

PARENT-CHILD RELATIONSHIP

Discuss:

- The child's moving toward his/her own way of trying to do things. Constant "no's" from the child are not indications of stubbornness but attempts to develop autonomy. Parents need to use alternatives, substitution, and positive reinforcement and should not expose themselves to a battle of wills.

PARENTING

Discuss:

- Coping methods used by parents
- Need for parents to understand that the child must explore and practice constantly

NURSE PRACTITIONER GOALS

These include:

- Encouraging the use of nursery school for relief for the mother and social development of the child

VISIT AT 3 YEARS

Health Assessment

See Table 9.

Counseling

PHYSICAL CARE

Discuss:

- Accident prevention appropriate for age
- Dental care. First visit to the dentist should be scheduled, if not already done, and visits should be every 6 months through time of tooth eruption and period of excessive dental caries (ages 4 to 8).
- Local park or out-of-doors play for release of energy. Nursery school should be encouraged.

Table 9
Health Assessment at 3 Years

Health History Physical Exam	Nutrition	Development	Laboratory Procedures Immunizations
Parental concerns	Review basic food groups and appropriate amounts for age	Talks well, uses plurals	Tuberculin skin test.
Interval history		Jumps, runs	Urinalysis for girls
Family and social history	Discuss proper snack foods	Pedals tricycle	Hemoglobin or hematocrit
Height and weight; blood pressure	Eating patterns are influenced by family members	Washes and dries hands	
Complete physical exam		Separates from mother easily	
Vision screening			
Hearing screening			
Language screening (DASE, Denver Articulation Screening Examination)			
Discussion of findings with parents			

- Care of illness, symptoms of common cold and complications, and when to call for medical care
- Lapses in bladder and bowel control

EMOTIONAL AND MENTAL DEVELOPMENT

Discuss:

- Sexual curiosity. Answers should be appropriate to the questions. Parents should examine their own attitudes.
- Sibling and peer rivalry
- Beginning of early fears, such as bodily injury, and of imagination, such as imaginary friends
- Interest in language. Child shows ability to notice small details and discrepancies
- Ability to anticipate consequences and the ability to deal with abstractions

STIMULATION

This child needs and enjoys those activities enjoyed by the 2-year-old child as well as:

- Getting dressed by self and performing small household tasks
- Growing plants in cans
- Throwing, catching, and playing ball
- Climbing a rope ladder
- Stringing objects, finger-painting, and using play dough
- Creating own art work at drawing board or block building
- Sewing cards and using blunt scissors
- Riding a tricycle
- Going for excursions, such as a bus ride, the zoo, shopping

PARENT-CHILD RELATIONSHIP

Discuss:

- Period of high activity level for child which is wearing to the mother

- Need for youngsters to climb, jump, and run and need for channels to release energy
- Need to permit child to develop at own pace. There is no advantage to pushing nor to overindulgence.

PARENTING

Discuss:

- Role of father in nighttime contact such as playing, reading, bathing, and performing bedtime rituals
- Need of mother for relief from constant care. Nursery school or cooperative child care should be encouraged.

NURSE PRACTITIONER GOALS

These include previous goals and:

- Providing education, support, and anticipatory guidance
- Reinforcing parental strengths and resources
- Encouraging joint decision making regarding child health care

VISIT AT 4 YEARS

Health Assessment

See Table 10.

Counseling

PHYSICAL CARE

Discuss:

- Accident prevention appropriate to age

Table 10
Health Assessment at 4 Years

Health History Physical Exam	Nutrition	Development	Laboratory Procedures Immunizations
Parental concerns	Review basic food groups and appropriate amounts for age	Knows first and last names	Hematocrit and RBC indices
Interval history		Copies circles and crosses	Tuberculin skin test, if not done at 3 years
Family and social history	Continued need for iron-containing foods	Understands prepositions and opposites	
Height and weight; blood pressure	Avoidance of sugared snacks and drinks	May dress self	
Complete physical exam		Separates from mother easily	
Vision screening		Heel to toe walk	
Hearing screening			
Discussion of findings with parents			

- Dental care. Visits to the dentist should be made every 6 months during the period of greatest carious activity, 4 to 8 years of age.
- Recreation, such as going to the local park or out-of-doors activity for release of energy. There is a need for nursery school or excursions.
- Toileting. Forty percent of 4-year-olds continue to bedwet.

EMOTIONAL AND MENTAL DEVELOPMENT

Discuss:

- The process of refinement of abilities rather than the emergence of new abilities at this age
- Need for the child to learn place in the family, as a child with parents, and to accept the boundaries between children and adults
- Need for socialization of the child. The child can no longer function by just listening or voicing own needs and wishes. Parents and society make demands and this presents conflicts. There is a slow process of helping the child to become "socialized" to participate outside of the home.

STIMULATION

This child needs and enjoys those activities enjoyed by the 3-year-old as well as:

- More peer activity
- Challenge from nursery school and increased excursions, such as bus, train, or plane rides; visits to zoo, airfields, and fire stations
- An increased interest in sports

PARENT-CHILD RELATIONSHIP

Discuss:

- Limits set by parents. These are essential to help the child in the

struggle to deal with inner feelings. Disappointments, frustrations, and delay are all part of growing up.
- Methods of handling the child's egotism. It is important to avoid destroying it or creating a battle of wills. Parents should help youngsters to cope by encouraging them to experiment with new tasks. Parents should not "push" development or "cop out" by leaving children alone (overpermissiveness).

PARENTING

Discuss:

- Problems within the family which may be disturbing to the child or may be the source of behavioral problems. Family problems may stem from disagreements on methods of discipline, marital problems, older members in the family, sibling rivalry, divorce, moving, or death.

NURSE PRACTITIONER GOALS

These include:

- Continuing to listen well
- Examining own attitudes about the family
- Helping parents to identify needs for support. The practitioner supports what parents are doing whether permissive or strict as long as extremes are being avoided, the approach is consistent, and the child is adapting well to the approach being used.

VISIT AT 5 TO 10 YEARS

Health Assessment

See Table 11.

Table 11
Health Assessment at 5 to 10 Years

Health History Physical Exam	Nutrition	Development	Laboratory Procedures Immunizations
Parental and client concerns Interval history: illnesses, injuries, major changes in life-style Review of systems Family and social history Weight, height, blood pressure, pulse, and respiration A complete physical is done Discuss the findings with the parent and client Screening: visual acuity and audiogram, language (DASE)	Basic food groups: milk, 3 servings; meat (including poultry, fish, eggs, peanut butter, dried beans), 4 servings; fruits, vegetables, 4 servings; breads, cereals, 4 servings Food likes and dislikes Types of food used for snacking Sugar intake Other considerations: milk fortified with vitamin D; iodized salt; whole grain or enriched breads and cereals; evaluate calcium, fluoride, iron source	5 to 6 years: balance on one foot for 10 seconds; backward heel to toe walk; draws person with greater than 6 parts; performs self-care activities 6 to 9 years: latency period of physical and psychological growth; questions about sex and conception 9 to 11 years: concrete thinking continues: judges thoughts only in reference to own experience, learns by trial and error Beginning growth spurt: females at approximately 9-½ years and males at approximately 10-½ years Females: beginning growth of pubic hair and breast budding; tomboy activities Males: male-dominated social activity	DTP and trivalent OPV boosters are given between 4 and 6 years of age Tuberculin testing every 3 years Routine urinalysis and complete blood count if not done within the last 3 years

Counseling

Health teaching is directed toward the client when appropriate for age.

PHYSICAL CARE

This includes:

- Maintenance of self-hygiene with frequent washing of oily skin and hair
- Oral hygiene: brushing after meals and at bedtime; flossing once a day
- Outdoor activity for exercise

EMOTIONAL AND MENTAL DEVELOPMENT

Discuss:

- Talking out problems with family members
- Needs of child: positive input from family, setting of appropriate limits and after school chores
- Parents interest in and participation in school activities
- Importance of peer relationships and group activities
- Outdoor activities as a method to reduce tension and stress

STIMULATION

Discuss:

- Conversing with child to explore thoughts, feelings, and daily activities
- Going on family trips and doing projects at home: cooking, games, handicrafts
- Instructing in the telling of time, traffic rules, remembering phone number, address

PARENT-CHILD RELATIONSHIP

Discuss:

- Family's ability to grant some autonomy to the child in decision making: choosing own clothes, planning leisure activities
- Importance of chores in helping to establish feelings of responsibility and accomplishment
- Family and child's readiness for separation and school
- Approach to discussion of sexual matters with child

NURSE PRACTITIONER GOALS

These include:

- Being an advocate for the child
- Providing health education about nutrition, development, safety
- Being aware of signs of family dysfunction: noncommunication, school phobia, scapegoating
- Communicating with family and school officials if learning problems are present

VISIT AT 11 TO 14 YEARS

Health Assessment

See Table 12.

Counseling

PHYSICAL CARE

Discuss:

- Routine hygiene and skin care

Table 12
Health Assessment at 11 to 14 Years

Health History / Physical Exam	Nutrition	Development	Laboratory Procedures / Immunizations
Past history: birth, maternal medications during pregnancy, developmental milestones, illnesses, injuries, immunizations, communicable diseases, family history Present history: client and parental concerns, history of presenting concern, nutrition; social: relationships with peers, school marks, social interests, future goals, sexual information and activity Review of systems Complete physical exam is done including weight, height, blood pressure, pulse, and respiration; pelvic exam if indicated Screening: visual acuity and audiogram	See Table 11 for basic food groups Eating habits: number of regular meals a day, snacking pattern and types of food; use of crash diets, fasting, food fads; source of protein and iron; knowledge of balanced food choices; availability of nutritious snacking foods	Hormonal influences: as a defense mechanism against changing body image there are increased somatic complaints Males: beginning growth of pubic hair, enlargement of testicles; wet dreams Females: continued breast development, growth of axillary and pubic hair Thought process: beginning of abstract thinking to manipulate concepts outside of own experience; self-centered (egocentrism); feelings of autonomy, mood swings, antisocial behavior Family: negativism as a manifestation of rejection of parents' values and seeking own identity, testing of parental controls, beginning emancipation from family Peers: importance of peer group for psychologic support and social development See Chapter 10, Health Care of the Adolescent	Td and TOPV boosters TB test Routine urinalysis Complete blood count (CBC) Rubella titer (females) VDRL Pap smear and gonorrhea cervical culture if sexually active (females) Sickle cell screening if indicated

107

- Daily oral hygiene and periodic dental exams
- If sexually active, knowledge of contraception and protection against venereal disease

EMOTIONAL AND MENTAL DEVELOPMENT

Discuss with the client:

- Emancipation from parents and other adults: activities away from the family, decisions made by self
- Feelings about self: smart, dumb, popular, physical appearance
- Normalcy of being moody, needing time alone
- Importance of peer group participation for validation of feelings
- Attitude towards smoking, alcohol, drugs
- Feelings about the opposite sex
- Availability of family members to listen to client's concerns
- Need for balance between client's own handling of responsibilities and consistent, fair limit setting when responsibilities cannot be managed

PARENT-CLIENT RELATIONSHIP

Discuss:

- Family conflicts and how resolved
- Parental frustration at adolescent behavior
- Client's developmental need for some independence

PEER RELATIONSHIPS

Discuss:

- Importance of socializing with peers to aid in increasing self-esteem through validation of own feelings
- Constructive outlets for socializing

NURSE PRACTITIONER GOALS

These include:

- Accepting client: nonjudgmental attitude and the absence of moralizing
- Discussing school progress and problems
- Helping client see responsibility for own actions, successes, and failures

VISIT AT 15 TO 18 YEARS

Health Assessment

See Table 13.

Counseling

The client is the primary focus. Parents are usually seen separately or with the client if special circumstances indicate.

PHYSICAL CARE

Discuss:

- Routine hygiene and skin care
- Daily oral hygiene and periodic dental exams
- If sexually active, knowledge of contraception and protection against venereal disease
- Protection against injuries in contact sports
- Safe driving habits

Table 13

Health Assessment at 15 to 18 years

Health History Physical Exam	Nutrition	Development	Laboratory Procedures Immunizations
Health history (see Table 12) A complete physical exam. is done including weight, height, blood pressure, pulse, and respiration; pelvic exam if indicated Screening: visual acuity and audiogram	Basic food groups (see Table 11) Eating habits (see Table 12)	Hormonal influences: continued development of secondary sexual characteristics Males: increased size of penis, testes, scrotum; growth of body hair, voice and skin changes Females: enlarged breasts, broadened pelvic bones, growth of body hair, menstruation Thought process: use of formal logic in solving problems; feelings and goals directed away from self toward idealistic causes; future goals become more clear Family: movement away from family into own relationships and activities; views family's morals and culture with criticism because of idealism Peers: regular group social activity and/or individual dating See Chapter 10, Health Care of the Adolescent	Td and OPV boosters if not given within the last 10 years Routine urinalysis and CBC if not done within the last 3 years Rubella titer (females) VDRL Pap smear and gonorrhea cervical culture if sexually active (females) Sickle cell screening if indicated

EMOTIONAL AND MENTAL DEVELOPMENT

Discuss client's:

- Perception of self: feelings of belittlement, inferiority, superiority, attitude towards body image
- School adjustment and progress
- Relationship with the opposite sex
- Feelings about smoking, alcohol, drugs
- Preparation and anxiety about future goals
- Feelings about leaving family

PARENT-CLIENT RELATIONSHIP

Discuss:

- Degree of autonomy client is allowed in the home
- Types of limit setting
- How family conflicts are resolved

NURSE PRACTITIONER GOALS

These include:

- Accepting client: nonjudgmental attitude, absence of moralizing
- Encouraging planning for future goals
- Helping client take responsibility for own actions

References

Brazelton, T. B. *Infants and Mothers*. New York: Delacorte, 1967.

Brown, M. S. and M. A. Murphy. *Ambulatory Pediatrics for Nurses*. New York: McGraw-Hill, 1975.

Caghan, S. B. "The Adolescent and Nutrition." *Am J Nurs* 75:1728–1731, October 1975.

Committee on Adolescence, Group for Advancement of Psychiatry. *Normal Adolescence*. New York: Charles Scribner's Sons, 1968.

Committee on Standards of Child Health Care, American Academy of Pediatrics. *Standards of Child Health Care,* 3rd ed. Evanston, Ill.: American Academy of Pediatrics, 1977.

Dansky, K. H. "Assessing Children's Nutrition." *Am J Nurs* **77**:1610–1611, October 1977.

Fraiberg, S. *Every Child's Birthright.* New York: Basic Books, 1977.

Fraiberg, S. *The Magic Years.* New York: Charles Scribner's Sons, 1959.

Freidman, A. S. and D. B. Freidman. "Parenting: A Developmental Process." *Pediatric Annals* 6:10–22, September 1977.

Giuffra, M. J. "Demystifying Adolescent Behavior." *Am J Nurs* 75:1724–1727, October 1975.

Green, M. and R. J. Haggerty. *Ambulatory Pediatrics II.* Philadelphia: Saunders, 1977.

Kempe, C. H., et al. *Current Pediatric Diagnosis and Treatment.* Los Altos, Calif.: Lange Medical Publications, 1976.

Pearson, G. A. "Nutrition in the Middle Years of Childhood." *Am J Maternal Child Nursing* 2:378–384, November–December 1977.

Waechter, E. H. and F. G. Blake. *Nursing Care of Children,* 9th ed. Philadelphia: Lippincott, 1976.

White, B. *The First Three Years of Life.* Englewood Cliffs, N.J.: Prentice-Hall, 1975.

4

Assessment of the Newborn

The immediate newborn period, while a time of joy and excitement for most parents, is also a period fraught with anxieties and concerns. Parents are in the process of identifying and examining their infant and adjusting their prenatal images and fantasies to the reality of the actual infant. They need reassurance that the baby is "all right" and explanations of the normal variations that are transient and nonpathologic. Nurse practitioners are key figures in assisting parents through this initial phase of adjustment. This chapter presents information on assessment and early care of the newborn and includes several specific tools for assessing the term infant and the premature infant.

ASSESSMENT

Early Assessment Tools

APGAR SCORE

This is an evaluation of the newborn infant using Apgar's (1955) five-factor score. Commonly used in all delivery rooms at birth, this score is valuable in identifying those infants who are at special risk, need prompt diagnosis and treatment, and need careful watching. It is based on five signs which are evaluated at 1 minute and again at 5 minutes after birth. The five signs are given in Table 1 in acronym form for ease of use and for committing to memory.

Five signs of Apgar score. These are:

1. Appearance. This may also be described as color. All babies are cyanotic or pale at birth but change to pink within 1 to 3 minutes. Even with prompt onset of respiration and good circulation, the hands, feet, and presenting parts may remain cyanotic for more than a day. Persistent cyanosis of other parts indicates a need for prompt diagnosis and treatment.

2. Pulse. This is also described as heart rate. A heart rate under 100 is a danger signal.

3. Grimace. This may also be described as reflex irritability. Absence of reflex irritability is evidence of a depressed nervous system. It can be tested by slapping the feet tangentially. This should cause the infant to cry or make some motion.

4. Activity. This may also be described as muscle tone. Poor muscle tone is a danger signal. A flaccid baby is usually in shock or narcotized.

5. Respiration. Spontaneous respiration should be well established within 1 minute. Absence of breath sounds or inadequate respirations are indications for immediate assistance.

Scoring. At 1 and again at 5 minutes after the complete birth of the infant, the signs are evaluated and a score of 0, 1, or 2 assigned to each. A score of 10 at 1 minute reflects the best possible condition. An infant scoring 0–3 will probably need resuscitation. An infant scoring 4–8 may need only a few whiffs of oxygen.

CLINICAL ASSESSMENT OF GESTATIONAL AGE (DUBOWITZ SCALE)

This is a scoring system for gestational age (Dubowitz, 1970), based on 10 neurologic and 11 "external" criteria, which is most reliably and effectively used during the first 5 days of life. The scoring

Table 1
Apgar Score

Signs		0	Scoring 1	2
Appearance	Color	Blue, pale	Body pink Extremities blue	All pink
Pulse	Heart rate	Absent	Slow Below 100	Over 100
Grimace	Reflex irritability, response to stimuli on sole of foot	None	Some grimace	Cry
Activity	Muscle tone	Limp	Some flexion of extremities	Active motion
Respiration		None	Slow, irregular	Good, strong cry

Source: Reprinted by permission from the NEW YORK STATE JOURNAL OF MEDICINE, copyright by the Medical Society of the State of New York, Apgar, V., "Role of Anesthesiologist in Reducing Neonatal Mortality," *N Y State J Med* 55:2365–2368, August 1955.

system is more objective and reproducible than trying to guess gestational age on the presence or absence of individual signs. The criteria used are easily defined, and the scoring system can be readily learned in about 10 minutes with a little practice.

Indications for use. The scale may be used to assess infants in these instances:

1. Premature or SGA infants to determine problems which may occur
2. LGA infants to guard against misjudgment of gestational age
3. Dehydrated infants to discriminate the malnourished child
4. Full-term infants to assess condition or as a teaching tool to parents

External criteria. The 11 external criteria and their scoring scale are presented in Table 2.

Neurologic criteria. These are used in conjunction with Figure 1 for scoring purposes.

1. Posture. Observed with infant quiet and in supine position. Score 0: Arms and legs extended; 1: beginning of flexion of hips and knees, arms extended; 2: stronger flexion of legs, arms extended; 3: arms slightly flexed, legs flexed and abducted; 4: full flexion of arms and legs.
2. Square window. The hand is flexed on the forearm between the thumb and index finger of the examiner. Enough pressure is applied to get as full a flexion as possible, and the angle between the hypothenar eminence and the ventral aspect of the forearm is measured and graded according to diagram. (Care is taken not to rotate the infant's wrist while doing this maneuver.)
3. Ankle dorsiflexion. The foot is dorsiflexed onto the anterior aspect of the leg, with the examiner's thumb on the sole of the foot and the other fingers behind the leg. Enough pressure is applied to get as full flexion as possible, and the angle between the dorsum of the foot and the anterior aspect of the leg is measured.
4. Arm recoil. With the infant in the supine position the

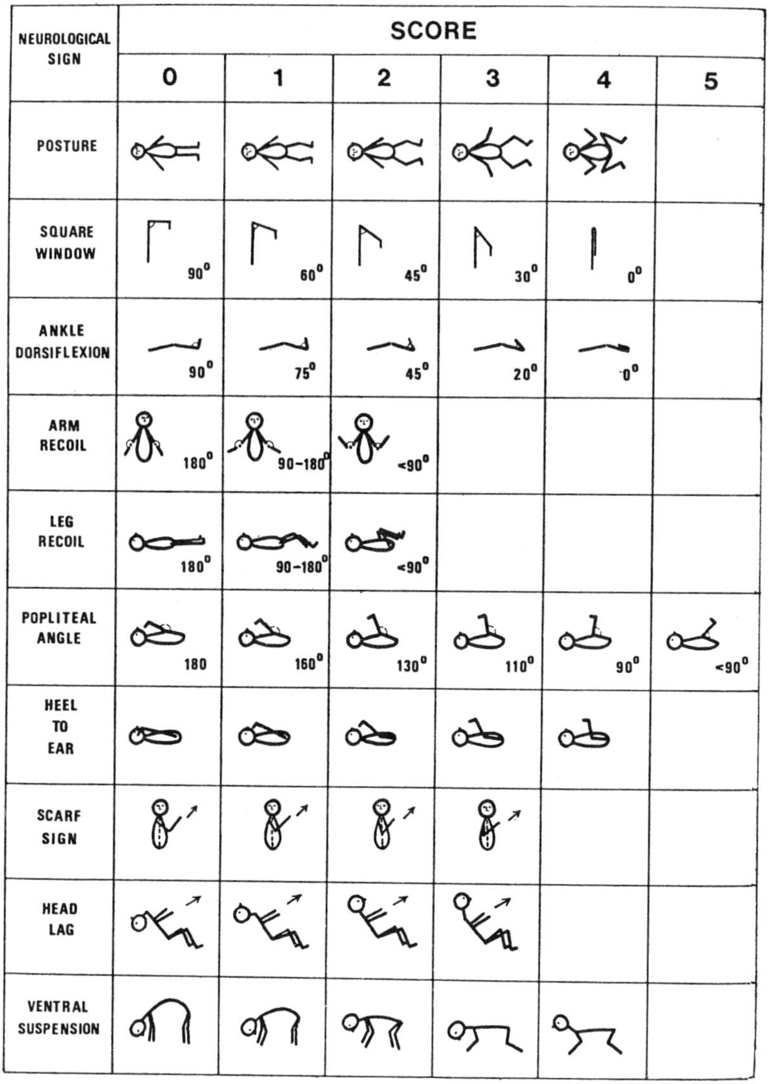

NEUROLOGICAL SIGN	SCORE					
	0	1	2	3	4	5
POSTURE						
SQUARE WINDOW	90°	60°	45°	30°	0°	
ANKLE DORSIFLEXION	90°	75°	45°	20°	0°	
ARM RECOIL	180°	90–180°	<90°			
LEG RECOIL	180°	90–180°	<90°			
POPLITEAL ANGLE	180	160°	130°	110°	90°	<90°
HEEL TO EAR						
SCARF SIGN						
HEAD LAG						
VENTRAL SUSPENSION						

Figure 1. Scoring system for neurologic signs. These signs are used together with neurologic criteria. (Reproduced with permission from L. M. S. Dubowitz, V. Dubowitz, and C. Goldberg, "Clinical Assessment of Gestational Age in the Newborn Infant," *J Pediatr* 77:1–10, July 1970.)

Table 2
Scoring System for External Criteria

External Sign	Score[a]				
	0	1	2	3	4
Edema	Obvious edema of hands and feet; pitting over tibia	No obvious edema of hands and feet; pitting over tibia	No edema		
Skin texture	Very thin, gelatinous	Thin and smooth	Smooth; medium thickness; rash or superficial peeling	Slight thickening; superficial cracking and peeling, especially of hands and feet	Thick and parchmentlike; superficial or deep cracking
Skin color	Dark red	Uniformly pink	Pale pink; variable over body	Pale; only pink over ears, lips, palms, or soles	
Skin opacity (trunk)	Numerous veins and venules seen, especially over abdomen	Veins and tributaries seen	A few large vessels clearly seen over abdomen	A few large vessels seen indistinctly over abdomen	No blood vessels seen
Lanugo (over back)	No lanugo	Abundant; long and thick over whole back	Hair thinning, especially over lower back.	Small amount of lanugo and bald areas.	At least half of back devoid of lanugo
Plantar creases	No skin creases	Faint red marks over anterior half of sole	Definite red marks over > anterior half; indentations over < anterior third	Indentations over > anterior third	Definite deep indentations over > anterior third

External Sign	Score[a]				
	0	1	2	3	4
Nipple formation	Nipple barely visible, no areola	Nipple well-defined; areola smooth and flat, diameter < 0.75 cm	Areola stippled, edge not raised; diameter < 0.75 cm	Areola stippled, edge raised; diameter > 0.75 cm	
Breast size	No breast tissue palpable	Breast tissue on one or both sides < 0.5 cm diameter	Breast tissue on both sides; one or both 0.5 to 1.0 cm	Breast tissue both sides; one or both > 1 cm	
Ear form	Pinna flat and shapeless, little or no incurving of edge	Incurving of part of edge of pinna	Partial incurving whole of upper pinna	Well-defined incurving whole of upper pinna	
Ear firmness	Pinna soft, easily folded, no recoil	Pinna soft, easily folded, slow recoil	Cartilage to edge of pinna, but soft in places, ready recoil	Pinna firm, cartilage to edge; instant recoil	
Genitals Male	Neither testis in scrotum	At least one testis high in scrotum	At least one testis right down		
Female (with hips half abducted)	Labia majora widely separated, labia minora protruding	Labia majora almost cover labia minora	Labia majora completely cover labia minora		

Source: Reprinted with permission from L. M. S. Dubowitz, V. Dubowitz, and C. Goldberg, "Clinical Assessment of Gestational Age in the Newborn Infant," *J Pediatr* 77:1–10, July 1970.
[a]If score differs on two sides, take the mean.

forearms are first flexed for 5 seconds, then fully extended by pulling on the hands, and then released. The sign is fully positive if the arms return briskly to full flexion (Score 2). If the arms return to incomplete flexion or the response is sluggish it is graded as Score 1. If they remain extended or are only followed by random movements the score is 0.

5. Leg recoil. With the infant supine, the hips and knees are fully flexed for 5 seconds, then extended by traction on the feet, and released. A maximal response is one of full flexion of the hips and knees (Score 2). A partial flexion scores 1, and minimal or no movement scores 0.

6. Popliteal angle. With the infant supine and the pelvis flat on the examining couch, the thigh is held in the knee-chest position by the examiner's left index finger and thumb supporting the knee. The leg is then extended by gentle pressure from the examiner's right index finger behind the ankle, and the popliteal angle is measured.

7. Heel-to-ear maneuver. With the baby supine, draw the baby's foot as near to the head as it will go without forcing it. Observe the distance between the foot and the head as well as the degree of extension at the knee. Grade according to diagram. Note that the knee is left free and may draw down alongside the abdomen.

8. Scarf sign. With the baby supine, take the infant's hand and try to put it around the neck and as far posteriorly as possible around the opposite shoulder. Assist this maneuver by lifting the elbow across the body. See how far the elbow will go across and grade according to illustrations. Score 0: Elbow reaches opposite axillary line; 1: Elbow between midline and opposite axillary line; 2: Elbow reaches midline; 3: Elbow will not reach midline.

9. Head lag. With the baby lying supine, grasp the hands (or the arms, if a very small infant) and pull him slowly toward the sitting position. Observe the position of the head in relation to the trunk and grade accordingly. In a small infant the head may initially be supported by one hand. Score 0: Complete lag; 1: Partial head control; 2: Able to maintain head in line with body; 3: Brings head anterior to body.

10. Ventral suspension. The infant is suspended in the prone position, with examiner's hand under the infant's chest (one hand in a small infant, two in a large infant). Observe the degree of extension of the back and the amount of flexion of the arms and legs. Also note the relation of the head to the trunk. Grade according to diagrams.

If score differs on the two sides, take the mean.

Scoring. The steps for establishing gestational age are as follows:

1. The external criteria are scored as shown in Table 2.
2. The neurologic criteria are scored as described in the preceding section and in Figure 1.
3. When the scores are obtained for both categories (see Table 3), they are added together and computed using the formula given in Figure 2. The resulting gestational age is then recorded on the graph.

Table 3
Total Scores for Neurologic and External Criteria

Neurologic Criteria		External Criteria	
Criterion	Score	Criterion	Score
Posture	0–4	Edema	0–2
Square window	0–4	Skin texture	0–4
Ankle dorsiflexion	0–4	Skin color	0–3
Arm recoil	0–2	Skin opacity	0–4
Leg recoil	0–2	Lanugo	0–4
Popliteal angle	0–5	Plantar creases	0–4
Heel to ear	0–4	Nipple formation	0–3
Scarf sign	0–3	Breast size	0–3
Head lag	0–3	Ear form	0–3
Ventral suspension	0–4	Ear firmness	0–3
		Genitals	0–2
Total	0–35	Total	0–35

Source: Reprinted with permission from L. M. S. Dubowitz, V. Dubowitz, and C. Goldberg, "Clinical Assessment of Gestational Age in the Newborn Infant." *J Pediatr* 77:1–10, July 1970.

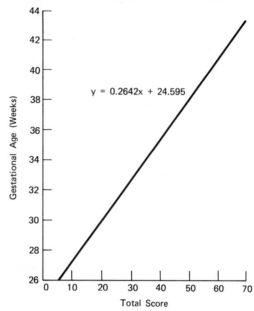

Figure 2. Graph for reading gestational age from total score obtained on the gestational age scale. Formula for obtaining gestational age score is shown above with "x" as the total score and "y" as the gestational age score. (Reproduced with permission from L. M. S. Dubowitz, V. Dubowitz, and C. Goldberg, "Clinical Assessment of Gestational Age in the Newborn Infant," *J Pediatr* 77:1–10, July 1970.)

DANGER SIGNS IN THE NEWBORN

In assessing a newborn any of the signs listed below should be considered for reevaluation or referral:

- Positive family history (e.g. diabetic mother, toxemia)
- Complications of gestation and delivery
- Abnormal position of the baby
- Atypical intrauterine growth
- Any congenital malformation (e.g., asymmetry of chest)
- Rapid or difficult respirations
- Rapid, slow, or irregular pulse

- Abnormal cry
- Cough
- Cyanosis
- Low Apgar score
- Sweating
- Excess salivation
- Diarrhea
- Vomiting of bile
- No meconium stool (for 48 hours)
- Delayed or inadequate voiding
- Abdominal distention
- Cord odor or exudate
- Bleeding from circumcision or cord
- Single umbilical artery
- Full fontanelle (hydrocephalus)
- Small head for size
- Convulsions, twitching, excessive irritability
- Lethargy
- Fever or hypothermia
- Paralysis
- Jaundice
- Pallor
- Petechiae
- Change in behavior or condition ("not looking right")

Signs indicating poor prognosis at birth. These signs are as follows:

- Complete immobility
- Opisthotonus
- Absence of sucking reflex
- Absence of blink reflex
- Absence of Moro reflex
- Absence of muscle tone
- Absence of incurvation reflex

Signs of dehydration. These signs of dehydration may be observed at any stage of infancy. They are:

- Weight loss
- Dry skin with poor turgor (tenting)
- Dry, cracked lips and dry, coated tongue and mouth
- Sunken and dry eyes
- Sparse or concentrated urine
- Weak cry
- Sunken anterior fontanel

DERMAL ICTERUS INDEX

The prevention of bilirubin encephalopathy requires careful recognition of hyperbilirubinemia in the newborn. See also Chapter 20.

Definition. In newborn infants, progressive hyperbilirubinemia is accompanied by a caudad advancement of dermal icterus which begins at the face and proceeds to the trunk, the extremities, and finally the palms and soles. In 1969, Kramer noted that there is a positive relationship between the concentration of serum bilirubin and the caudad progression of dermal icterus which suggests that simple inspection of the skin of the newborn infant provides useful information about the actual bilirubin level. See Table 4 and Figure 3. Additional findings by Kramer include the following:

1. Dermal icterus is not discernible at serum bilirubin levels of less than 4 mg/dl. At higher bilirubin concentrations a predictable direct relationship between bilirubin levels and the cephalo-pedal progress of dermal icterus has been noted.
2. The cephalo-pedal progression of dermal icterus was noted to continue only as long as the concentration of serum bilirubin increased.
3. The point of most distal skin icterus remains unchanged as serum bilirubin levels remain at a fixed level.
4. The dermal staining always fades gradually in all affected skin areas at the same time as the serum bilirubin concentration begins to fall from its peak level.

Table 4
Indirect Serum Bilirubin Concentration
and Its Relationship to the Progression
of Dermal Icterus

Dermal Zone	Full-Term Infants Bilirubin (mg/100 ml) Range	Infants of low birth weight Bilirubin (mg/100 ml) Range
1	4.3–7.8	4.1–7.5
2	5.4–12.2	5.6–12.1
3	8.1–16.5	7.1–14.8
4	11.1–18.3	9.3–18.4
5	15	10.5

Source: Reprinted with permission from L. I. Kramer, "Advancement of Dermal Icterus in the Jaundiced Newborn," *Amer J Dis Child* 188:454–458, September 1969. Copyright 1969, American Medical Association.

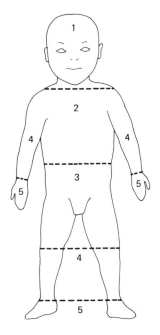

Figure 3. Dermal zones of progressive cephalo-pedal icterus. 1: Head and neck; 2: Trunk to umbilicus; 3: Groin, including upper thighs; 4: Knees to ankles and elbows to wrist; 5: Hands and feet, including palms and soles. (Reproduced with permission from L. I. Kramer, "Advancement of Dermal Icterus in the Jaundiced Newborn," *Am J Dis Child* 188:454–458, September 1969. Copyright 1969, American Medical Association.)

5. Some infants of low birth weight show a more rapid progression of skin icterus than do full-term infants, and the variation in the pattern of skin staining in some low-birth-weight infants reduces the usefulness of determining serum bilirubin levels by dermal inspection.

Comments. This dermal zone method of inspection is not meant to replace laboratory determinations. This method depends on the inspection of the undressed infant under blue-white fluorescent lighting. The mechanism for the cephalo-pedal progression of dermal icterus in newborn infants with rising levels of serum bilirubin is not understood.

Temperature Control in Infancy

BODY TEMPERATURE CONTROL

This is a function of heat production and of heat loss. Heat production in the newborn is unreliable. The demands of relatively great surface area, the immaturity of sweating and shivering mechanisms (lack of development of the heat-regulating center in the diencephalon), the probable disadvantages of delicate skin, and meager subcutaneous fat are all handicaps to controlling both rate and amount of heat loss.

SHIVERING AND BODY ACTIVITY

These tend to increase heat production. Vasoconstriction of the surface vessels tends to conserve heat, and perspiration and surface vasodilation tend to reverse the action by disseminating heat.

SWEATING

In infants, sweating normally begins after 1 month of age. Under 1 year of age and under normal circumstances sweating may be profuse and is usually due to exercise, crying, eating, or an overly warm atmosphere.

MAINTENANCE OF NORMAL BODY TEMPERATURE

A normal infant's temperature should be 36.4° to 37°C (97.5° to 98.6°F). Axillary temperature is 96° to 99°F. The room temperature should be maintained at 74° to 76°F for the newborn. Body heat can be maintained with the swaddling of one soft blanket. Although care should be taken to avoid chilling and a subsequent drop in body temperature, it is now suggested that infants who are protected from chilling at all times may be less able to respond to cold stress later.

TEMPERATURE CONTROL IN PREMATURITY

Premature infants over 1000 gm are kept at an optimal incubator temperature that will maintain an axillary temperature of the infant at approximately 36°C (96.8°F). This is usually an air temperature of approximately 31.7°C (89°F). Humidity is maintained between 60 and 70%. If an incubator is not available, these conditions of temperature and humidity can be attained by the use of blankets and warm water bottles and by controlling the temperature and humidity of the room. Prematures can be moved to areas of less heat and humidity only when the gradual change to the new environment is not accompanied by a significant change of temperature, color, or activity. The removal may be only a day or 2 after birth for some infants or at more than a month of age for the less mature ones. Small-for-gestational-age (SGA) infants with less subcutaneous fat should be kept warmer than larger infants.

MANAGEMENT

Care of the Newborn

FEEDING METHODS

See Chapter 7, Feeding in Infancy and Childhood and Breast Feeding.

IMPORTANT EARLY NEEDS

Among these needs are the need to suck and a feeling of being loved and cared for which includes:

1. The need to have a strong attachment to one or more persons
2. The need to know that someone will answer a cry
3. The need to have bodily contact and to be held and gently stimulated

For more information see Chapter 8, Psychological Needs of Infancy.

SAFETY NEEDS

See Chapter 9, Accident Prevention and Safety.

SLEEPING NEEDS

See Chapter 8, Sleeping Patterns.

PHYSICAL CARE OF THE NEWBORN

Bathing the newborn. Unless otherwise indicated these procedures should be followed:

1. The entire body is bathed daily, especially in deep folds and creases, with warm water and a mild soap. Neutragena soap is recommended.
2. Oils and lotions are not recommended for use on the skin. They tend to interfere with normal skin secretions and may cause rash in the newborn. Dryness of the skin at this age is not an abnormal condition. See Chapter 15, General Care of the Skin.
3. Powder in small amounts may be used in the diaper area only. See Chapter 15, Lotions, Powders. Powder should be applied by hand.
4. Daily shampooing using mild shampoos is recommended to aid in the prevention of cradle cap. See Chapter 24, Cradle Cap.

5. At bath time or whenever necessary the eyes may be wiped using cotton balls and warm water, wiping from the inner canthus to the outer and changing to a clean cotton ball for each eye. Abnormal amounts of tearing or yellow mucous discharge from the eyes should be assessed for the cause.

6. No special attention should be given the nose beyond removing obvious mucous plugs as they appear at the nares. This is done with a clean washcloth or cotton ball. Yellow nasal discharge should be assessed for the cause.

7. Cleaning the ears is done only with a clean washcloth and only on that area which can be easily reached. The ears should not be cleaned with the aid of Q-tips. Wax (cerumen) lubricates the ear canals, insulates them against temperature extremes, repels insects, keeps water and soap out, and helps to prevent itching.

Care of the umbilical cord. Once or twice daily the cord should be gently lifted and rubbing alcohol applied to its base to facilitate drying. Any discharge or bleeding should be assessed for the cause.

Care of the genitalia. See also Chapter 23, The Genitalia.

FEMALE. The female genitalia are wiped clean using cotton balls or a washcloth. No excess pressure is necessary; some waxy material may remain. Slight bloody or white mucous discharge is normal. Yellow discharge or frank bleeding should be assessed for the cause.

MALE. Normal bathing of the penis is recommended. It is not necessary to push or to retract the foreskin.

Care of the circumcision. Gentle bathing with warm water and a washcloth is recommended. Emersion in a basin or small tub may be done being careful not to wet the umbilical cord. Vaseline is not used since this causes maceration and delays healing. The plastic bell may remain attached by a threadlike tissue which will release in time. Excess swelling, redness, yellow discharge, or bleeding should be assessed for the cause.

Dressing the newborn. The infant can be kept warmly snug in a cotton receiving blanket. A loose shirt and diapers should be sufficient clothing. An additional blanket may be used with weather changes. The extremities of the newborn are normally somewhat blue and cold because of immaturity of the small blood vessels in these areas.

COMMON CLINICAL PROBLEMS

Common Conditions of the Newborn

This area consists of a variety of conditions of the skin and other organs found in the newborn assessment, a large number of which are within normal limits or are normal variants. Many of the conditions are transitory and most of them are nonpathogenic. Included here are the most commonly encountered conditions.

BEDNAR'S APHTHAE

Assessment.   These are ulcers which may be seen on the hard palate posteriorly. Usually bilateral, they are thought to be due to vigorous sucking.

Management.   None is necessary beyond explanation to the parents.

BRACHIAL PALSY

Assessment.   This is paralysis of the upper arm with or without paralysis of the forearm and hand. It is caused by an injury to the brachial plexus when traction is exerted on the head during delivery of the shoulder. The child has a characteristic position of adduction and internal rotation of the arm with pronation of the forearm. The biceps reflex and the Moro reflex are absent on the affected side. Differentiation must be made from fractures of the clavicle, fracture and injuries to the humerus, and cerebral injury.

Management. If the condition is due to edema and hemorrhage, a return of function will occur within a few months. If it is due to laceration permanent damage may result. Splinting to prevent deformity and necessary physiotherapy are indicated.

CAFE-AU-LAIT SPOTS

Assessment. These are light to dark brown pigmented areas of the skin of various sizes.

Management. One or two patches may be within normal limits; however, five to seven or more may indicate fibromas or neurofibromatosis and a referral is made to a neurologist.

CAPUT SUCCEDANEUM

Assessment. This is clear fluid trapped under the scalp but on top of the pericranium and is not confined to one bone. It is ill defined, pits on pressure, and is not fluctuant. This sometimes occurs with an elongated head and may indicate a long delivery. It is caused by the head pressing on the pelvic outlet in the last period of labor. This fluid disappears in about a week.

Management. Beyond explanation to the parents none is necessary.

CEPHALOHEMATOMA

Assessment. This is a soft, fluctuant, well-outlined mass of blood trapped beneath the pericranium and confined to one bone. Possibly due to birth trauma, it occurs commonly. It is sometimes not noted until the second postpartum day. A ridge may be felt around the hematoma for as long as 6 months.

Management. If the cephalohematoma crosses the midline, referral should be made for further assessment. Infants with large hematomas should receive additional iron in their diet. See Chapter 6, Iron Requirements in Infancy.

CIRCUMORAL CYANOSIS

Assessment. This is pallor which occurs around the mouth that may be displayed by an infant when crying or cold during the first few days of life.

Management. None is necessary beyond explanation to the parents.

CRANIOTABES

Assessment. This is softening of the outer layer of the scalp and may be seen in premature infants. It is felt upon examination as a ping-pong ball sensation as the scalp is pressed with the fingers behind and above the ears. It may indicate a pathologic condition: rickets, syphilis, hypervitaminosis A, or hydrocephaly.

Management. Reassessment of the cause and referral are indicated with the presence of craniotabes.

CYANOSIS

Assessment. This develops when the hemoglobin is reduced by 5 gm/dl. The newborn usually has high hemoglobin levels, therefore, cyanosis occurs more easily and with less relative oxygen unsaturation than in the older child. Normally, by 4 hours of age cyanosis will show less in hands and feet. Pathologically it may be caused by pulmonary disease, congenital heart disease, central nervous system disorders, or hypoglycemia. It is sometimes confused with ecchymosis. Pressure on the cyanotic area will blanch the skin temporarily. The ecchymotic area remains blue with pressure.

Management. Continued cyanosis should be reassessed for the cause and referral is indicated.

DESQUAMATION

Assessment. This is dryness and peeling of the skin. It occurs normally in the newborn and is felt to denote postmaturity.

Management.   It clears with no special attention generally after a few tub baths.

ECCHYMOSIS

Assessment.   These marks are evidence of blood under the skin usually due to bruising or birth injuries. See this chapter, Cyanosis.

Management.   They disappear as the blood is reabsorbed.

EPSTEIN'S PEARLS

Assessment.   These are small epithelial cysts occurring along both sides of the median of the hard palate or along the alveolar ridge.

Management.   They are not pathologic and disappear with time.

ERYTHEMA TOXICUM NEONATORUM

Assessment.   This is a rash consisting of small maculo-papular lesions that develops in the first few days of life. It resembles varicella or "flea-bites." Of unknown origin, it is transitory and may disappear within 8 hours.

Management.   None is necessary beyond explanations to the parent.

FACIAL NERVE PALSY

Assessment.   Usually the paralysis is peripheral and results from pressure over the facial nerve in utero during labor or from forceps during delivery. Movement on only one side of the face is noted and the mouth is drawn to that side. Sometimes the eye on the affected side cannot close and the nasolabial fold is absent. Prognosis depends on whether the nerve is intact or whether the nerve fibers are torn. Improvement will occur within a few weeks in the former case.

Management. Care of the exposed eye is essential. Frequent irrigations with normal saline solution are recommended. Referral to a neurologist is indicated if severe nerve damage is suspected.

FONTANELLES

Assessment. Both anterior and posterior fontanelles must be assessed.

ANTERIOR. This is the unossified membranous space in the skull at the junction of the sagittal, coronal, and frontal sutures or the junction between the frontal and parietal bones. It may be small or absent at birth, then enlarges to an average of 2.5 by 2.5 cm, closing between 9 and 19 months. Early closure is not a reason for concern so long as the head growth continues normally. Tenseness or bulging of the anterior fontanelle may be an indication of a pathologic condition. This is best noted if the infant is in a sitting position.

POSTERIOR. This is the junction of the lambdoidal and the sagittal sutures or the parietal and the occipital bones. Often not palpable at birth, it averages 1 by 1 cm and closes approximately by the second month. There are additional fontanelles located over the mastoid and the sphenoid areas.

FRENULUM (TONGUE-TIE)

Assessment. This is the thin mucous membrane that attaches the tongue to the floor of the oral cavity. It is also called frenulum linguae.

Management. A referral to the appropriate specialist is recommended only if the frenulum keeps the tongue from reaching the gum line.

HARLEQUIN COLORING

Assessment. This is a condition in which half of the newborn's body appears red while the other half appears pale. It may possibly be due to poorly developed vasomotor reflexes. It is transitory, usually occurring when the infant cries lustily.

Management. This is not significant and needs only an explanation to parents.

HEMANGIOMAS (STRAWBERRY MARKS)

Assessment. These are evenly rounded formations of immature blood vessels from 1 to 10 cm or more in transverse measurement. They may be present at birth but more often begin to appear in the first or second month of life. Hemangiomas tend to enlarge diffusely and sometimes rapidly. With large or multiple hemangiomas it must be considered clinically that one or more additional hemangiomas may be present in some internal structure. They should be noted for size and shape.

Management. The hemangiomas may reach their maximum size in a few months and slowly start to shrink sometime between 6 and 18 months. For very large ones the process may take 5 years or longer. Referral to the appropriate specialist is recommended if the hemangioma interferes with normal bodily function.

JAUNDICE

Assessment. Jaundice is a deposit, in the skin, of unconjugated bilirubin which has built up in the blood stream. The skin color may range from yellow to orange to sometimes greenish tones.

Management. See this chapter, Dermal Icterus Index, and Chapter 20, Jaundice in the Newborn.

LANUGO DISTRIBUTION

Assessment. This is the first fine hair to cover the body during fetal life. It is usually found over the shoulders, back, and sacral areas. This hair generally disappears before or shortly after birth.

Management. Parents may need reassurance that it will soon disappear.

LARYNGEAL STRIDOR (CROWING)

Assessment. Congenital laryngeal stridor is a noisy, crowing respiratory sound. Common in the neonatal period and during the first year of life, it may be due to a "flabby" epiglottis. The condition is seldom serious, and the symptoms become less severe, generally disappearing by 1 year.

Management. Severe crowing with dyspnea and inspiratory retractions should be further assessed for malformations of the larynx.

MILIA

Assessment. These are white pinpoint-sized lesions usually found over the bridge of the nose, the chin, or the cheeks. They are due to retained sebum generally disappearing after the first few weeks of life.

Management. No treatment is necessary.

MOLDING (FACIAL ASYMMETRY)

Assessment. This is a result of overriding of the sutures at birth due to intrauterine molding or molding during delivery because the bones are soft and pliable. Flattening of part of the head or face may occur in an infant who lies in only one position or who has unusually soft bones. If present at birth, it generally disappears in a few days.

Management. If the flattened occiput is due to a static position in the crib, it is recommended that the infant's position in the crib be reversed daily. The infant will turn toward the light thereby giving equal pressure to the bones on both sides of the head.

MONGOLIAN SPOTS AND OTHER BLUE NEVI

Assessment. These are massive aggregations of melanin-rich dark cells which give the affected area a purple-black or blue-black color. They are usually found over the sacrum and coccygeal area of over 50 percent of the newborns of Black, Chicano, and Asiatic-Indian origin. They have no clinical significance. They are distributed through the deep layers of the skin tissues and cannot be disposed of by radiotherapy, freezing, or chemical caustics. They are not malignant; most of them disappear with time.

Management. Nevi may be distinguished from ecchymosis by their distribution. They may be concealed by cosmetic covering later in life if desired.

MOTTLING

Assessment. This is an overall red and white coloration of the skin that generally occurs in fair children who are chilled.

Management. No treatment is necessary.

PETECHIAE

Assessment. These are tiny, reddish-purple, sharply circumscribed lesions found in the superficial layer of the epidermis. They may be due to birth injury or can be a sign of severe systemic disease such as sepsis, erythroblastosis fetalis, hemorrhagic disease, or thrombocytopenic purpura meningococcemia.

Management. Petechiae should be assessed immediately for the cause.

PSEUDOSTRABISMUS

Assessment. This is due to the epicanthal folds (vertical folds of the skin covering the inner canthus of the eye) which makes the eye appear "crossed."

Management. True strabismus is ruled out with the light reflex test. The beam of light should normally be reflected in the same position in each eye. (See Chapter 16, The Eye.)

PTOSIS

Assessment. This is drooping of the upper eyelid usually due to a congenital underdevelopment of the lid muscles. It may also be an acquired deformity. If acquired, it may be due to an interference with the cranial nerve as a result of meningitis or encephalitis.

Management. Acquired ptosis needs immediate assessment and referral to the appropriate clinic or physician.

QUIVERING CHIN

Assessment. This is a nonspecific response of the central nervous system after a difficult birth or as a concomitant of various perinatal problems. In the absence of additional factors the tremor may be regarded as insignificant.

Management. No treatment is necessary.

SCLERAL HEMORRHAGES

Assessment. These are slight hemorrhages which are noted on the sclerae sometimes occurring as a result of a difficult delivery. These hemorrhages are usually of no clinical significance and disappear within a few weeks after delivery.

Management. They should be noted on the record and followed until they resolve.

"SETTING-SUN SIGN"

Assessment. In this condition the sclerae are exposed above the iris when the eyes are open normally. It is normal in full-term infants and in many premature infants but may also be found in association with an enlarging head circumference (e.g., hydrocephalus).

Management. It should be noted and followed along with careful measurements of head size.

"SNORTING"

Assessment. This is a nasal sound made by some infants on respiration. It has no significance and may be due simply to thickened nasal mucus.

Management. Parents need reassurance since they may fear that the infant is having difficulty breathing.

SUCKING TUBERCLE

Assessment. This may be found in the middle of the upper lip of some infants whether they are bottle- or breast-fed. It is caused by friction and strength of sucking. It appears as small blisters, broken skin, or as a small callus.

Management. No treatment is necessary. It will heal spontaneously after weaning.

SUTURES

Assessment. The cranium is composed of eight bones joined together by immovable sutures which are spaces between the skull bones. The coronal suture extends from ear to ear across the top of the skull. The sagittal suture divides the parietal bones running at right angles to the coronal suture. The lambdoidal suture separates the parietal bones from the occipital bones. Sutures are frequently palpable at birth and are felt as prominent ridges from the overriding of their edges during the birth process.

Management. Sutures generally flatten by 6 months of age. See this chapter, Molding and Fontanelles.

TELANGIECTASIAS (CAPILLARY HEMANGIOMAS, NEVUS FLAMMEUS, PORT-WINE STAIN)

Assessment. These are irregular, blotchy, pink capillary lesions of the skin. They may be superficially or deeply involved in the dermis. They are found frequently at the back of the neck, the base of the neck, the base of the nose, the center of the forehead, and on the eyelids. They tend to disappear by 2 years of age after gradually fading.

Management. Parents need reassurance and support.

UMBILICAL GRANULOMA

Assessment. This is umbilical tissue which persists after the cord has dried and fallen off. It is sometimes white and glistening, or it may be pink to red in color.

Management. Umbilical granulomas can be removed by an application of silver nitrate followed by a wash of normal saline solution. Large ones with peduncles may be tied off.

UMBILICAL HERNIA

Assessment. This is seen as an opening of the aponeurosis of the obliquus externus abdominis muscle felt under the skin at the umbilical area. The size should be judged by the actual palpated opening. Most hernias decrease by the end of the first year; referral should be made if it has not decreased by that time.

Management. Explanations to the parents of the cause and aiding them in palpation of the opening are necessary. The size of the hernia is not judged by its appearance when the infant cries. A coin should not be taped to the abdomen since it may interfere with the closure and cause maceration of the skin.

VAGINAL DISCHARGE

Assessment. A bloody discharge called pseudomenstruation may be due to absorption of maternal hormones. This is not usually observed beyond the first month of age. White mucous discharge is a normal discharge. Yellow mucous discharge is an indication of a pathologic condition.

Management. Assessment should be made for the cause if the discharge is yellow.

VERNIX CASEOSA

Assessment. This is a cheesy, white material covering the entire body of the newborn, sometimes occurring only in the skin folds or nail beds. Yellow discoloration of the vernix is an indication of intrauterine distress or a pathologic state.

Management. Normal vernix is presently left on the skin for protection. Indications of a pathologic condition should be assessed for the cause.

Prematurity

ASSESSMENT

History. A complete prenatal and natal history is taken including length of time the infant spent in the hospital, how the family managed, how the baby was fed, and all treatments and medications received.

Definitions. There are several designations for infants based on gestation and weight. They are as follows:

1. *Premature* (preterm) infant is one born before the end of the thirty-seventh week of gestation, regardless of birth weight. The majority of infants who weigh less than 2500 gm (5 lb 8 oz), and almost all infants below 500 gm are prematurely born.

2. *Term* infant is one born between the beginning of the thirty-eighth week and the completion of the forty-first week.

3. *Postmature* infant is one born at the onset of the forty-second week or any time thereafter.

4. *Low-birth-weight* (LBW) infants are designated as follows:

    • Infants whose rates of intrauterine growth are normal at birth, even though they are small because they are delivered before the end of the thirty-seventh week, are termed *appropriately grown for gestational age* (AGA).

    • Infants whose rates of intrauterine growth are slow, who are delivered at or later than term, and are small are termed *small-for-dates* or *small for gestational age* (SGA).

    • Infants whose rates of growth in utero are retarded, and who, in addition, are delivered prematurely are termed *small-for-dates* and *premature*.

5. *High-birth-weight* infant. An infant who weighs 4000 gm or more is considered high birth weight. Infants are considered *large for gestational age* (LGA) at any weight when they fall above the ninetieth percentile on the intrauterine growth curves.

Determination of gestational age.   Methods of eliciting this information are listed below:

1. History of pregnancy. Count the weeks that have elapsed from the first day of the last menstrual period (LMP). This is valid in 75 to 85 percent of clients. First maternal perception of fetal heartbeat is at approximately 20 weeks; first perception of fetal movement is approximately 16 weeks.

2. Prenatal tests. Analysis of the amniotic fluid may determine, among other things: bilirubin levels, creatinine levels, and the lecithin-sphingomyelin ratio which is helpful in determining gestational age. Also used is cellular examination for fat-laden cells.

3. Postnatal examination. Clinical assessment of gestational age (Dubowitz scale) is commonly used. See this chapter, Clinical Assessment of Gestational Age.

Factors disposing to prematurity. These factors are:

- Chronic hypertensive disease
- Toxemia
- Placenta previa
- Abruptio placenta
- Cervical incompetence
- Low socioeconomic status, including poor nutrition, chronic infection, fatigue, and generally poor personal and environmental hygiene
- Absence of prenatal care
- Multiple pregnancies
- History of previous premature delivery
- Age (highest incidence is age under 20)
- Order of birth (highest incidence is in first pregnancies)

Mortality and morbidity. Eighty to ninety percent of prematures are at risk in the first year due to anorexia, birth injuries, hyaline membrane disease, bronchopneumonia, septicemia, and other infections. Because of improved methods of delivering intensive care the survival rate for infants over 2000 gm is 95 percent, for infants weighing 1500 to 2000 gm it is 70 percent, and for infants 1000 to 1500 gm it is 60 percent. For infants weighing less than 1000 gm the outlook is not good.

Principal causes of morbidity include hemorrhage, kernicterus, retrolental fibroplasia, anemia, and infection.

MANAGEMENT

The management of prematures is directed at follow-up care of the infant according to the problems which may have been associated with the prematurity, at working with the family to improve relationships if necessary, and at gaining an awareness of the developmental and other factors associated with prematurity.

Follow-up care. For the infant close to 2500 gm (5 lbs 8 oz) who will leave the hospital 5 to 6 days postnatally, the weight should be checked weekly or biweekly for assurance of gain, and the family should be in close contact with the care facility for the first month. This infant's care should not be different from that of a full-term infant. It is preferred that no special attention be given to the prematurity.

Infants of lower birth weight and who have had prolonged illnesses with hospitalization need these extra attentions in follow-up care:

1. More frequent visits are necessary for careful physical and neurologic assessment and follow-up of earlier problems.

2. Length, weight, and head circumference are taken at each visit. Deviations and lags are observed and recorded.

3. Developmental screening tests are done at routine times. Determining the developmental level of the infant is done by subtracting the number of weeks of prematurity from the infant's chronologic age.

4. Added help is offered with nutrition. See Chapter 6, Nutritional Needs of Low-Birth-Weight Infants. Breast-feeding is important for its special nutritional and immunologic factors and its effects on maternal-infant relationships. For some infants with a poor sucking reflex there is a unique device which allows the infant to nurse at breast at the same time delivering milk contained in a plastic bag via a tube attached to the nipple. For further information write or call Lact-Aid, Box 6861 Dept. KA, Denver, CO, 80206.

5. The treatment of the skin of the premature does not differ essentially from that of the mature infant. Maceration is the most common factor which may cause disruption of the protective barrier of the stratum corneum. Sometimes there is depigmentation following as simple a procedure as applying or removing adhesive tape. Explanations to the parents should be made to reassure them that the marks will disappear in time.

6. The environment of the premature may need to be considered. Because of their lack of adipose tissue prematures need to be kept warmer until weight has been restored to normal levels. See this chapter, Temperature Control in Infancy. These infants may also enjoy a bright, noisy environment for a time following lengthy hospitalization, particularly if most of the time was spent in the intensive care nursery.

7. Incidence of illnesses should be discussed. Because gamma globulin levels are lower, the resistance to upper respiratory infections and diarrhea is low. (See this chapter, Sepsis in the Newborn.) Infants, while they may go out, should be kept away from large groups or from persons with obvious infections. Colic may appear when the infant has reached an age approximately 2 weeks beyond the expected date of delivery.

Referrals. These should be made at appropriate times for the following reasons:

1. A circumcision which may have been deferred at birth may need to be scheduled.

2. Early dental assessment may be required. Stimmler (1973) suggests that structural defects occur in the primary dentition of all children who have suffered from low calcium levels for even a few days. It occurs 12 months following the appearance of the teeth as enamel hyperplasia.

3. Hearing assessment may be necessary. Causes of hearing loss in the premature may occur from incubator noises, high bilirubin levels, or from drugs such as kanamycin, gentamicin sulfate, and furosemide.

4. Ophthalmologic examination is done before the infant leaves the hospital and again at 4 to 6 months by an ophthalmologist to rule out retrolental fibroplasia; early signs may be observed at this time.

Counseling. This includes offering support and reassurance to the family that their child is normal. The parents should be given opportunities to express their feelings and attention should be given the following:

1. Mother-infant relationship. Early separation interferes with the development of normal mothering skills, attitudes, and relationships. Mothers need to be taught that this lack of response is not a reflection of poor mothering so future relationships between mother and infant are not jeopardized. See Chapter 5, Assessment of Parent-Child Interaction.

2. "Prematurity neuroses." Parents need to be cautioned against overprotectiveness of the premature. Brown and Bakeman

(1977) suggest that mothers of prematures compensate for the inactivity of their infants and continue to do so even when this is no longer adaptive, and that prematures, therefore, have less opportunity to regulate their own activity patterns. The over-protective feeling may also be fostered by the excessive caution-ary advice given the parents by medical personnel.

3. Community resources. The local community should be as-sessed for sources available to aid the family such as house-keeping help, visiting nurses, developmental disabilities agency, hearing and vision screening, La Leche League, an-other family with a premature infant as a role model or even a "premature club."

Sepsis in the Newborn

ASSESSMENT

Sepsis refers to a bacterial infection involving the blood stream; it may also often involve the meninges. Neonates up to 1 month of age are particularly susceptible to sepsis and will have infections from organisms other than those of major significance in older age groups. The reasons that the newborn is at special risk for infec-tions include exposure to contaminated nursery equipment; un-recognized infections in other newborns, personnel, and/or par-ents; their immune system is not fully developed, and they lack effective phagocytosis. The sites vulnerable to entry of infection are the nasopharynx, the umbilicus, and the skin. Infections may spread rapidly with few signs and symptoms. All infections in the neonate are approached as potentially serious. See Chapter 29, Bacterial Meningitis.

Etiology. Gram-negative bacilli are relatively common etiologic agents of septicemia and meningitis in the first 2 months of life. In a few instances such infection is due to a strain of organisms of unusual virulence against which the infant has acquired no immu-nity. Most often, however, the infection would appear to be due to inoculation of the infant with a massive dose of organisms of rela-tively low virulence. Staphylococcal infections occur less than in the past. Group B-beta-hemolytic streptococci have been a more recent cause.

INFECTIONS OF THE UNBORN INFANT. These come from the mother's vaginal flora, from infected amniotic membranes, when the membranes rupture many hours before birth, or from urinary tract infections. The routes of these invasions are the umbilicus, the respiratory tract, or the skin. The organisms are *E. coli, Klebsiella,* or paracolon bacilli; rarely, *Pseudomonas.*

INFECTIONS AFTER DELIVERY. These come from contaminated nursery equipment, especially water in bottle warmers, humidifiers, oxygen sources, isolettes, and from procedures and treatments involving catheters and resuscitation equipment. The routes of these invasions are the nasopharynx, the umbilicus, and the skin. The organisms are the above-mentioned enteric organisms but more commonly are soil and water bacteria such as *Pseudomonas, Proteus, Alcaligenes,* and *Flavobacterium.*

INFECTIONS OF PREMATURE INFANTS. Sepsis is magnified in the preterm infant. A localized infection may cause rapid development of sepsis and meningitis. Most instances of infection occur in premature infants who have had an idiopathic respiratory syndrome. The antibiotics used for the respiratory disease are ineffective against the bacteria which inhabit water and nursery equipment.

Clinical findings. Signs and symptoms of sepsis in the newborn are subtle and may be difficult to define. See also this chapter, Danger Signs in the Newborn. If meningitis is present, stiff neck and pain on flexion of the neck are less common in the neonate. Signs and symptoms are:

1. The anterior fontanelle may be full and lack normal pulsations or it may be tense and bulging
2. Hypothermia may occur
3. Lethargy, anorexia, apneic attacks, or seizures may occur
4. Diarrhea, vomiting, or spitting up may occur or the infant may be feeding poorly with a weak suck

5. Petechiae, a shrill cry, and abdominal distention may be present
6. Jaundice and an enlarged liver may occur on the fourth to the eighth day

Laboratory procedures. Cultures are taken of the blood, urine, spinal fluid, skin lesions, and area about the umbilicus.

Prognosis. The case fatality is high, meningitis being responsible for 60 to 75 percent. Up to 85 percent of the survivors suffer serious consequences such as subdural effusion, hydrocephalus, brain abscess, and intellectual impairment.

MANAGEMENT

This is directed at immediate antibiotic therapy. Sepsis is managed collaboratively with a physician.

Medication. An antibiotic effective against environmental gram-negative bacteria should be administered immediately without waiting for the results of the cultures.

Prevention. Environmental sources must be searched for the identical bacteria.

Counseling. Added support is given the parents of an infant who is treated for neonatal sepsis following those guidelines outlined for prematurity. See this chapter, Prematurity Counseling.

References

Alexander, M. A. and M. S. Brown. *Pediatric Physical Diagnosis for Nurses.* New York: McGraw-Hill, 1974.

Apgar, V. "Role of Anesthesiologist in Reducing Neonatal Mortality." *NY State J Med* 55:2365–2368, August 1955.

Avery, G. B., editor. *Neonatology.* Philadelphia: Lippincott, 1977.

Barness, L. E. *Pediatric Physical Diagnosis.* Chicago: Year Book Medical Publishers, 1972.

Beckwith, L. "Premature Birth and Caregiver-Infant Interaction." *Ped Research* 11:374, April 1977.

Brazelton, T. B. *Infants and Mothers.* New York: Delacorte, 1969.

Brown, J. V. and R. Bakeman. "Behavioral Dialogues Between Mothers and Infants; The Effects of Prematurity." *Ped Research* 11:375, April 1977.

Dubowitz, L., V. Dubowitz, and C. Goldberg. "Clinical Assessment of Gestational Age in the Newborn Infant." *J Pediatr* 77:1–10, July 1970.

Erickson, M. L. *Assessment and Management of Developmental Changes in Children.* St. Louis: Mosby, 1976.

Graef, J. W. and T. E. Cone, editors. *Manual of Pediatric Therapeutics.* Boston: Little, Brown, 1974.

Jacobs, A. H., and R. L. Cahn. "Birthmarks." *Pediatric Annals* 5:6–28, December 1976.

Korones, S. B. *High-Risk Newborn Infants,* 2nd ed. St. Louis: Mosby, 1976.

Kramer, L. I. "Advancement of Dermal Icterus in the Jaundiced Newborn." *Am J Dis Child* 188:454–458, September 1969.

Rudolph, A. M., editor. *Pediatrics,* 16th ed. New York: Appleton-Century-Crofts, 1977.

Shinefield, H. R. "Neonatal Septicemia in the Premature." *Pediatric Annals* 1:12–20, November 1972.

Silverman, W. and J. C. Sinclair. "Temperature Regulation in the Newborn Infant." *N Engl J Med* 274:92–94, January 1966.

Stimmler, L., G. Snodgrass, and E. Jaffe. "Dental Defects Associated with Neonatal Symptomatic Hypocalcaemia." *Arch Dis Child* 48:217–220, March 1973.

Waechter, E. H. and F. G. Blake. *Nursing Care of Children,* 9th ed. Philadelphia: Lippincott, 1976.

White, B. *The First Three Years of Life.* Englewood Cliffs, N.J.: Prentice-Hall, 1975.

5

Assessment of Parent-Child Interaction

Although the deleterious effects of maternal deprivation have been known for over 30 years, application of this knowledge has developed slowly. Institutional environments were the first targets of concern and much progress has been made in modifying the hospital setting to reduce the impact of separation. It is only in recent years that the nature of the parent-child relationship has become a major focus of pediatric primary care.

There is no longer any doubt that interaction with a mother figure, with resulting attachment, is essential for the healthy development (physical, emotional, social, and cognitive) of the infant. What has recently become clear is that infants living at home in intact families can also experience insufficient interaction with a mother figure. As reports of failure to thrive, neglect, and child abuse have increased, more attention has been paid to studying the process of attachment and the factors influencing that process. (It is acknowledged that an increasing number of fathers are deeply involved in interaction with their infants and, in fact, the term "parenting" is coming into more frequent use, but for purposes of this chapter, the mother will be the primary reference point.)

Practitioners working with parents and children in primary care settings must be knowledgeable about attachment; must recognize that each mother or parent-infant relationship is unique

151

and a function of the individual characteristics of parent, infant, and their environment; and must be able to assess interaction accurately and objectively to predict successful, at-risk, or disturbed situations. With such understanding we enhance our value as supportive figures to parents and contribute more effectively to optimum development. It is safe to say that "all therapeutic and preventive components of well-child care ultimately relate to the nature of the parent-child relationship" (Lamper, 1974, p. 72).

This chapter reviews the theory of attachment, presents data to be used in assessing parent-child interaction, and discusses implications for management. Information on failure to thrive and child abuse is found in Chapters 32 and 33.

THEORETICAL CONSIDERATIONS

The relationship between a mother and her newborn infant used to be examined and analyzed mainly in terms of the mother. New mothers were evaluated on their qualities of mothering and motherliness, which are described as follows:

- *Mothering* refers to the many active and practical attitudes necessary to take care of the offspring and to guide its maturation and primary learning.

- *Motherliness* is the characteristic quality of a woman's personality which supplies the emotional energy for maintaining the tasks of mothering. It is the capacity of the mother to receive from her child; her ability to be continuously gratified by this exchange and to use this gratification unconsciously in her emotional maturation (Benedek, 1956).

More current research and study have broadened our knowledge and have identified a wide range of variables which influence the mother-child relationship. Of major importance is recognition that the characteristics of the infant contribute significantly and reciprocally to the development of the mother-infant bond.

Terms

A new terminology has emerged to describe the processes through which positive family relationships develop.

ATTACHMENT

Attachment is the term used to describe the unique emotional relationship between mother and infant. It has been defined by Ainsworth (1970, p. 50) as "an affectional tie that one person or animal forms between himself and another specific one—a tie that binds them together in space and endures over time."

ATTACHMENT BEHAVIORS

For attachment to occur both mother and infant must demonstrate behaviors which elicit reciprocal and complementary behaviors from each other. These are termed attachment behaviors.

Maternal attachment behavior. This is defined as "the degree to which a mother is attentive to and maintains physical contact with her infant" (Leifer, 1972, p. 1205).

Infant attachment behavior. This is that behavior which promotes proximity to or contact with the mother figure (Bowlby, 1969). Bowlby postulates that an infant's attachment to his mother is a product of the activity of a number of behavioral systems that have proximity to the mother as a predictable outcome. Sucking, clinging, following, crying, and smiling are initial behaviors of the infant that contribute to attachment. However, between the ages of about 9 to 18 months these simpler behavioral systems "become incorporated into far more sophisticated goal-corrected systems . . . so organized and activated that a child tends to be maintained in proximity to his mother" (Bowlby, 1969, p. 180).

Classes of Infant Behaviors Mediating Attachment

Attachment serves many important functions, the cardinal advantage being protection of the infant. This protection provides the infant with a sense of security that allows for exploration of the environment. Such exploration is viewed as highly related to later cognitive development. Those behaviors which assist the infant in achieving these goals are as follows:

1. Orientational behaviors. To keep informed of the mother's whereabouts, the infant orients to her, tracking her movements visually and aurally.
2. Signalling behaviors. These behaviors stimulate the mother to come into closer proximity or contact with the infant (e.g., crying, smiling, babbling, calling, and raising arms to her) (Bell, 1972).
3. Active behaviors. These are behaviors through which an infant achieves proximity or maintains contact once it has been attained (e.g., clinging, approaching, following, climbing).

Phases in Development of Attachment

Attachment develops in phases described as follows:

Phase 1: Orientation and signals without discrimination of figure
   Behaviors: During the first few weeks the infant responds to anyone in the vicinity by orienting, tracking with the eyes, grasping, smiling, reaching, and by ceasing to cry on hearing a voice or seeing a face.

Phase 2: Orientation and signals directed toward one or more discriminated figures
   Behaviors: The infant behaves as in Phase 1 but in a more marked fashion to the mother than to others. The infant displays differential behavior to the mother's voice; stops crying differentially according to who provides comfort; cries differentially when the mother leaves; smiles and vo-

calizes differentially; and maintains a differential visual-motor orientation toward the mother.

Phase 3: Maintenance of proximity to a discriminated figure by means of locomotion as well as by signals

Behaviors: When able to crawl and move about, the infant shows differential behaviors such as approaching, following, climbing upon, exploring, and clinging to the mother and uses the mother as a secure base from which to explore and as a safe haven to which to return.

Phase 4: Formation of a reciprocal relationship

Behaviors: By about 4 years of age, when the child's cognitive and judgment abilities improve, the child can predict the mother's movements, infer what her goals are (e.g., to remain close or to leave) and can initiate behavior to attempt to change her goals to fit his/her own (Bowlby, 1969; Ainsworth, 1969).

FACTORS AFFECTING MOTHER-INFANT INTERACTION AND DEVELOPMENT OF ATTACHMENT

The mother-infant dyad is a reciprocal relationship with each member contributing to interaction or to lack of interaction. In addition to the characteristics of both mother and infant, environmental factors also influence the interaction and the development of attachment. The following factors are known to affect relationships between mothers and infants and, depending on the context, will exert either positive or negative influence.

Maternal Factors

PAST EXPERIENCES

These include the following:

1. Own experience being mothered; relationship with own mother

2. Genetic and cultural background
3. Incorporation of cultural values and expectations
4. Skill in interpersonal interaction
5. Relationships and experiences with family members, including mate
6. Parity
7. Experiences with previous pregnancies and infants
8. Self-concept, self-image, and level of psychosexual maturity

EXPERIENCES WITH CURRENT PREGNANCY

These include the following:

1. Planned or unplanned pregnancy
2. Acceptance of pregnancy
3. Perception of fetus as a separate individual
4. Fantasies about newborn
5. Age of the mother
6. Health of the mother; physical and emotional reserves
7. Fears and worries about fetus, labor, and delivery
8. Actual labor and delivery, length of labor, amount of pain

NEONATAL PERIOD

Factors during this period include the following:

1. Mother's perception of labor and delivery
2. Physical comfort
3. Hormonal levels
4. Comparison of fantasized infant and real infant
5. Ability to identify and to accept infant as an individual
6. Ability to perceive infant's cues
7. Feeling of competence to care for infant

Infant Factors

Factors in the infant that influence attachment include the following:

1. Size
2. Sex
3. Gestational age
4. General health
5. Presence or absence of visible blemishes
6. Activity level
7. Perceptual and sensory capacity:
   - Ability to receive stimuli
   - Ability to attend to stimuli
   - Ability to discriminate stimuli
   - Ability to respond to stimuli
8. Sensory sensitivity (low or high sensory threshold)
9. Infant-state:*
   - Sleep patterns
   - Alert levels
   - Crying behaviors
10. Regularity of infant-state: sleep-wakefulness-hunger cycles
11. Arousal and calming characteristics (ease of pacification)
12. Ability to initiate interaction and elicit mothering
13. Reactions to mother's ministrations

External Factors

Other factors influencing attachment include:

1. Economic status
2. Housing

---

*Infant-state: levels of tension or perceptual arousal reflecting both need and availability for contact with the external environment (Clark and Affonso, 1976, p. 553).

3. Father's response to mother and infant
4. Support from husband, family, peers, and culture
5. Family goals
6. Siblings
7. Societal and cultural values
8. Other responsibilities (job, home, children)
9. Course of labor, delivery, and immediate postpartum period
10. Behavior and attitudes of hospital staff
11. Hospital policies
12. Time of initial contact with infant
13. Multiple births

The Acquaintance Process

There is a process that occurs at the beginning of all interpersonal relationships and that forms the basis of subsequent interpersonal behavior (Kennedy, 1973). It consists of three steps:

1. The acquisition of information about the other individual
2. The assessment of the other's attitude in relation to oneself
3. The continuous collection of data to validate or to negate initial impressions (Newcomb, 1961)

Mothers and infants experience this process which begins while the baby is in utero and continues after delivery. It is important that the mother acquires valid and sufficient information about the infant, and that the assessment of the data be accurate and positive. Otherwise, problematic relationships might develop. Additionally, all the factors listed above can influence this process.

Many new, inexperienced, uncertain, or ambivalent mothers will need assistance in this initial identification or claiming process to assess accurately their infants' characteristics, cues, and response patterns. The more a mother recognizes and responds to the cues that the infant presents about its needs, the more likely is a sense of attachment and competence to be developed in both.

BEHAVIORAL OBSERVATIONS

Accurate assessment is based on objective data, not intuition. This section presents information about maternal and infant behaviors that can be observed to assess and to predict the development of attachment.

Maternal Behaviors

PRENATAL PERIOD

Observations during this period include:

1. Expressions of attitude about changing body image (e.g., pride, discomfort, embarrassment, shame)
2. Verbalizations about fetus

   - Is fetus discussed as a separate individual?
   - Does mother wonder what the baby will be like?
   - Is mother thinking about a name for the baby?
   - Is the fetus referred to by sex?

3. Response to quickening
4. Preparations for baby

   - Purchase of baby supplies
   - Home arrangements for baby
   - Decision on feeding method
   - Interest in learning about infant care

5. Degree of anxiety and fear about labor and delivery
6. Desire for knowledge about labor and delivery
7. Degree of emotional lability

INTRAPARTAL PERIOD

Observations during this period include:

1. Spontaneous verbalizations and response at moment of delivery

2. Attempts to see and to touch baby
3. Questions asked about condition, appearance, and behavior of baby
4. Reactions to sex of baby

POSTPARTAL PERIOD

Claiming and identification behaviors to be observed include:

1. Touch. Touch has several aspects as follows:
   Proximal contact:

   • Does the mother touch the infant?
   • How much does she touch the infant?
   • Does she begin by touching the infant's extremities with her fingertips and soon proceed to massaging and encompassing the infant's trunk with her full hand (Kennell, 1971)?

   Ventral contact:

   • Does she hold and enfold the infant close to her body?

   Affectionate contact (not associated with feeding):

   • Does she kiss the infant?
   • Does she fondle, cuddle, rock, pat, or caress the infant?

2. Distal contact

   • Does she talk to the infant?
   • What does she say to the infant?
   • Does she express love?
   • Are any special designations used (e.g., "he," "it," "angel," "bad girl," "sour puss")?
   • Does she look, sing, laugh, or smile at the infant?

3. Eye contact

   • Does she attempt eye-to-eye contact with the baby?

- How often?
- Does she use the "en face" position?*

Note: Visual contact and use of the "en face" position are considered *cardinal* attachment behaviors.

4. Individualization of infant

- Does she identify the infant's individual characteristics and personality?
- Does she identify particular features of the infant with herself or with other family members? If so, in a positive or negative way?

5. Caretaking

- How does she respond to the infant's behavior (e.g., cry, yawn, sleep, cough) (Clark, 1976)?
- How is the infant held for feeding? What is the feeding procedure?
- Is the mother aware of the infant's reactions while dressing and undressing?
- Is the mother able to comfort and to protect the infant?
- Does mother reluctantly relinquish the infant to the nurse?

PERIOD OF HEALTH SUPERVISION

Observations during early infancy include the following:

- How does the mother hold the baby (e.g., close to her, protecting baby's head, awkwardly)?
- Does she hold the baby or place it on the exam table?
- How often does she glance at the baby?
- What does she do when the baby cries? How quickly does she respond?
- Does she comfort the baby without being told? How does she comfort the baby?

---

*"En face" position: the mother's face in such a position that her eyes and those of the infant meet fully in the same vertical plane of rotation (Klaus, 1970, p. 1023).

- What does she do during the physical exam (e.g., stay by the baby without being told, back away, ignore procedure)?
- What does she do during the immunization procedure? What is her facial expression? Does she comfort the baby after the procedure?
- How does the mother react when given a compliment about the baby? Where does she look? Facial expression? What does she say (e.g., positive comment, negative comment, change the subject, no response) (Levy, 1964)?

Infant Behaviors

Babies show a series of behavior patterns that are essential for establishing mother-infant interaction. The extent to which the infant himself takes the initiative in seeking interaction is surprising.

INITIAL BEHAVIORS

Initial behaviors to be observed include the following:

1. Rooting
2. Sucking
3. Grasping
4. Clinging
5. Regular changes between sleep, wakefulness and activity, and crying
6. Smiling and babbling
7. Normal activity level
8. Responds to ministrations by calming
9. Visual alertness (fixes object and briefly tracks*)
10. Responds to sensory stimuli with pleasure or displeasure
11. Quiets when presented with mother's face, voice, touch
12. Responds to feeding (sucks eagerly, cuddles, smiles, and sleeps after feeding)

---

*The newborn has ability to attend and to follow during the first hour of life (Klaus, 1972).

LATER INFANT BEHAVIORS

See this chapter, Phases in Development of Attachment.

Descriptions of High and Low Attachment

Conditions of high and low attachment have been described (Lamper, 1974). Examples are provided to demonstrate the range of behaviors that must be assessed before making such evaluations.

HIGH ATTACHMENT

At 28 to 32 days after birth the mother:

1. Is preoccupied and vigilant about the baby
2. Provides appropriate visual, auditory, and tactile stimuli during caretaking activities
3. Is successful at eliciting responses from the baby
4. Fondles the baby and looks at the baby "en face"

At 8 months of age:

1. Mother often takes the baby out with her
2. Mother avoids even brief separations
3. Mother comments on positive features of the baby
4. Mother not observed to physically reject or mistreat the child
5. Baby actively tries to approach the mother after separation
6. Baby seeks contact and initiates interaction
7. Baby is more interested in the mother than in a stranger

LOW ATTACHMENT

At 28 to 32 days after birth the mother:

1. Has limited proximity, contact, and communication with the baby
2. Does not respond to the baby's cry but is likely to let the baby "cry it out"

3. Enjoys leaving the baby with someone else
4. Is detached during the physical exam
5. Is less attentive during feeding

At 8 months of age:

1. Mother rarely takes the baby out with her
2. Mother openly finds fault with the baby
3. Mother comments on negative features of the baby
4. Mother uses physical punishment inappropriately
5. Mother rejects the baby's efforts to establish contact with her
6. Mother interrupts the baby's on-going activities
7. Infant has little tendency to approach or to contact the mother after separation but may ignore or turn away from her
8. Infant responds to strangers as to the mother
9. Infant may prefer objects to people

DISORDERS IN MATERNAL ATTACHMENT

There are many variables related to the strength and security of attachment and many individual differences in the rate of development of attachment, the ways a child manifests attachment, and the figures to whom attachments are made. Nonetheless, knowledge and experience point to certain observations, signs, symptoms, and environmental factors that predispose to or indicate disturbances in mother-infant relationships. Information (adapted from Green, 1975, and Barbero, 1975) is presented here on predisposing factors to and early manifestations of mothering disabilities.

Predisposing Factors

PAST EVENTS

Events in the mother's past that predispose to mothering disabilities include:

1. Poor relationship between the mother and her own mother

2. Emotional deprivation, rejection, lack of affection in the mother's childhood
3. Long-term emotional disturbance or medical illness in the mother's childhood
4. Loss of parent figures early in the mother's life
5. Death or illness in prior children (unresolved grief)
6. Repeated pregnancies and children at short intervals
7. Previous abortions
8. Marital discord or separation

PREGNANCY

Predisposing factors during pregnancy include:

1. Strongly unwanted pregnancy
2. Attempts to obtain or to induce an abortion
3. Protracted emotional or physical illness
4. Deaths or major illness of key family members
5. Highly unrealistic views of motherhood (e.g., "sheer bliss")
6. Out-of-wedlock pregnancy
7. Geographic move late in pregnancy
8. Lack of social supports

PERINATAL EVENTS

Predisposing factors during the perinatal period include:

1. Complications of parturition. Maternal affectional ties may be easily disturbed in the immediate newborn period by such minor problems as poor feeding, slight hyperbilirubinemia, or mild respiratory distress.
2. Acute illness of the mother or infant
3. Congenital defects
4. Prematurity
5. Multiple births
6. Difficult labor and delivery, unplanned obstetrical interventions, use of medications

7. Prolonged separation of the infant from the mother; institutional disruptions
8. Maternal depression in the first year
9. Husband psychologically or physically absent
10. Level of infant activity
11. Social isolation
12. Financial stresses
13. Failure of the infant to meet parental expectations
14. Mental illness, alcoholism, drug abuse

Manifestations of Maladaptation of Mothers to Their Infants*

Many mothers may exhibit one or more of these behaviors at different times and for different reasons and are not "maladapted" mothers. However, if constellations of these behaviors exist and persist over time, they may be indicative of maladaptive mothering. Such behaviors are exhibited by mothers who:

1. See their infants as ugly or unattractive
2. Perceive the odor of their infants as revolting
3. Disgusted by drooling of infants
4. Disgusted by sucking sounds of infants
5. Upset by vomiting, but seem fascinated by it
6. Revolted by any of infant's body fluids that touch them or that they touch
7. Annoyed at having to clean up infant's stools
8. Preoccupied by odor, consistency, and number of stools
9. Let infant's head dangle without support or concern
10. Hold infants away from their own bodies

---

*List adapted with permission from M. G. Morris, "Maternal Claiming-Identification Processes: Their Meaning for Mother-Infant Mental Health." In A. Clark, et al. *Parent-Child Relationships: The Role of the Nurse.* Paper presented at a Continuing Education Program for Nurses' Workshop, College of Nursing and University Extension Division, Rutgers, The State University of New Jersey, 1968.

11. Pick up infant without warning by a touch or by speech
12. Juggle and play with infant roughly after feeding even though the infant often vomits at this behavior
13. Think infant's natural motor activity is unnatural
14. Worry about infant's relaxation following feeding
15. Avoid eye contact with infants or stare fixedly into their eyes
16. Do not coo or talk to their infants
17. Think that their infants do not love them
18. Consider that their infants expose them as unlovable, unloving parents
19. Think of their infants as judging them and their efforts as an adult would
20. Perceive their infant's natural dependent needs as dangerous
21. Fears of infant's death appear at mild diarrhea or minor cold
22. Convinced that their infant has some defect, in spite of repeated physical examinations which prove negative
23. Constantly demand reassurance that no defect or disease exists and cannot believe relieving facts when they are given
24. Demand that feared defect be found and relieved
25. Cannot find in their infants any physical or psychologic attribute which they value in themselves (probably the most diagnostic of these signs and readily elicited)
26. Cannot discriminate between infant signs signaling hunger or fatigue, need for soothing or stimulating speech, comforting body contact, or for eye contact
27. Develop inappropriate responses to infant needs:

   - Over- or under-feed
   - Over- or under-hold
   - Tickle or bounce the baby when he is fatigued
   - Talk too much, too little, and at the wrong time
   - Force eye contact or refuse it
   - Leave infant in room alone
   - Leave infant in noisy room and ignore infant

28. Develop paradoxical attitudes and behaviors. Example: Bitterly insist that infant cannot be pleased, no matter what is

done, but continue to demand more and better methods for pleasing infant.

29. Express serious concern about "bad" behavior of infant and "spoiling" the baby
30. Fail to select a name for the baby or select "impossible" names
31. Unable to give a good history; cannot report what has been going on with baby

Manifestations of Mothering Disabilities in Infants

Infants who are involved in disturbed parent-child interactions exhibit behaviors (adapted from Green, 1975) which include:

1. Feeding problems (anorexia, refusal of solids)
2. Recurrent vomiting or rumination
3. Developmental delay
4. Failure to gain weight
5. Recurrent diarrhea
6. Irritability or excessive crying
7. Listlessness or lethargy
8. Sleep disturbances
9. Unusual visual alertness ("radar gaze")
10. Decreased cuddliness
11. Baby not physically well cared for
12. Undiscriminating attachment
13. Minimal vocalization

Failures in Attachment

The most extreme manifestations of attachment disorders are represented by the conditions of severe failure to thrive and child abuse. See Chapter 32, Failure to Thrive, and Chapter 33, Child Abuse. Characteristics of "potential" abuse situations are known (Helfer, 1975) and should be assessed to prevent such severe distortions of parenting behavior.

PARENTAL CHARACTERISTICS

Parental characteristics include:

1. Neglect or abuse during parent's early childhood resulting in a missing "mothering imprint"
2. Extreme personal and social isolation as exemplified by the absence of friends and supportive relationships
3. Poor marital relationship
4. Low self-esteem
5. Parent-child role reversal. Parents see the child as the source of their emotional support and gratification.

CHILD FACTORS

Factors in the child include the child who:

1. Is seen as different or difficult by parents
2. Does not respond in the manner expected by parents
3. Was born prematurely or by cesarean section. These children have abuse rates much higher than those of general population.

PRECIPITATING EVENT OR CRISIS

Abuse situations in a family at risk can occur in the presence of any stress or combination of stresses, major or minor.

ASSESSMENT TOOLS

Care providers must be alert to the behaviors described in the preceding sections and must be able to systematically observe interactions to collect the most reliable data possible. Observation of behavior for purposes of evaluating interaction is a complex and difficult task and should be performed only by professionals with

Table 1

Tool 1. Categories of Adaptive and Maladaptive Mothering Behaviors

Adaptive	*Maladaptive*
1. Feeding Behaviors	1. Feeding Behaviors
Offers appropriate amounts and/or types of food to infant.	Provides inadequate types or amounts of food for infant.
Holds infant in comfortable position during feeding.	Does not hold infant, or holds in uncomfortable position during feeding.
Burps baby during and/or after feeding.	Does not burp infant.
Prepares food appropriately.	Prepare food inappropriately.
Offers food at comfortable pace for infant.	Offers food at pace too rapid or slow for infant's comfort.
2. Infant Stimulation	2. Infant Stimulation
Provides appropriate verbal stimulation for infant during visit.	Provides no or only aggressive verbal stimulation for infant during visit.
Provides tactile stimulation for infant at times other than during feeding or moving infant away from danger.	Does not provide tactile stimulation or only that of aggressive handling of infant.
Provides age-appropriate toys.	No evidence of age-appropriate toys.
Interacts with infant in a way that provides for infant's satisfaction.	Frustrates infant during interactions.
3. Infant Rest	3. Infant Rest
Provides quiet or relaxed environment for infant's rest, including scheduled rest periods.	Does not provide quiet environment or consistent schedule for rest periods.
Ensures that infant's needs for food, warmth, and/or dryness are met before sleep.	Does not attend to infant's needs for food, warmth, and/or dryness before sleep.

170

4. Perception
   Demonstrates realistic perception of infant's condition in accordance with medical and/or nursing diagnosis.
   Has realistic expectations of infant.
   Recognizes infant's unfolding skills or behavior.
   Shows realistic perception of own mothering behavior.

5. Initiative
   Shows initiative in attempts to manage infant's problems, including actively seeking information about infants.

6. Recreation
   Provides positive outlets for own recreation or relaxation.

7. Interaction with Other Children
   Demonstrates positive interaction with other children in home.

8. Mothering Role
   Expresses satisfaction with mothering.

4. Perception
   Shows unrealistic perception of infant's condition.
   Demonstrates unrealistic expectations of infant.
   Has no awareness of infant's development.
   Shows unrealistic perception of own mothering.

5. Initiative
   Shows no initiative in attempts to meet infant's needs or to manage problems. Does not follow through with plans.

6. Recreation
   Does not provide positive outlets for own recreation or relaxation.

7. Interaction with Other Children
   Demonstrates hostile-aggressive interaction with other children in home.

8. Mothering Role
   Expresses dissatisfaction with mothering.

Source: Copyright March/April 1976, the American Journal of Nursing Company. Reproduced with permission from MCN, The American Journal of Maternal Child Nursing Vol. 1, No. 2.

training and skill in this area. When at-risk or maladaptive interaction is observed or suspected, the most effective approach to intervention is via consultation and joint planning with those qualified members of the health team.

Several tools and instruments have been developed to assist in more objective and systematic assessment. A sample of available tools is presented here.

The Harrison Tools

Characteristics of adaptive and maladaptive behaviors of mothers (Table 1) and infants (Table 2) have been developed by Harrison (1976). Guidelines for use of these tools are as follows:

1. Purpose: The tools were designed to measure changes in mother and infant behaviors during the course of intervention.
2. When to use: The tools should be used for initial baseline assessment and then at intervals to measure change.
3. How to use: Harrison stresses the value of direct observation in the home setting since the mothering behaviors observed at home are more likely characteristic of the mother's general behavior.

The Neonatal Perception Inventory (NPI)

Broussard and Hartner (1971) have developed two simple questionnaires for mothers that determine the mother's concept of what an "average" baby's behavior is like and then her assessment of what her own baby is like. Guidelines for use of the NPI are as follows:

1. Purpose: This screening instrument can be used in identifying infants at risk for subsequent emotional disorders.
2. When to use: The Neonatal Perception Inventory I (see Table 3) is administered on the first or second postpartum day. The Neonatal Perception Inventory II (see Table 4) is administered when the infant is 1 month of age.
3. Instructions for administering the Neonatal Perception Inventory:

Table 2

Tool 2. Categories of Adaptive and Maladaptive Infant Behaviors

Adaptive	Maladaptive
1. Sleeping Behavior Receives adequate sleep for normal growth—at least 16 hours per day—without restless sleep patterns or prolonged crying at nap or bedtime after other needs have been met.	1. Sleeping Behavior Receives inadequate sleep for normal growth—less than 16 hours per day. Shows restless sleep patterns and/or prolonged crying at nap or bedtime.
2. Feeding Behavior Actively seeks food offered. Effectively sucks and swallows food. Demonstrates pleasurable relief after eating.	2. Feeding Behavior Resists food offered. Does not suck effectively. Remains fussy after adequate amount of feeding—no pleasurable relief.
3. Response to Environment Demonstrates active response to environment by exploring or reaching-out behavior.	3. Response to Environment Seems apathetic to environment.
4. Vocalizing Demonstrates vocalizations when alert, if developmentally ready.	4. Vocalizing Makes infrequent or no vocalizations during visit although developmentally ready.
5. Smiling Demonstrates smiling behavior if older than two months.	5. Smiling Does not demonstrate smiling behavior during visit.
6. Cuddling Cuddles when held.	6. Cuddling Resists being held or stiffens when held.

Source: Copyright March/April 1976, the American Journal of Nursing Company. Reproduced with permission from MCN, The American Journal of Maternal Child Nursing Vol. 1, No. 2.

Table 3
Neonatal Perception Inventory I

AVERAGE BABY

Although this is your first baby, you probably have some ideas of what most little babies are like. Please check the blank you think best describes the AVERAGE baby.

How much crying do you think the average baby does?

| a great deal | a good bit | moderate amount | very little | none |

How much trouble do you think the average baby has in feeding?

| a great deal | a good bit | moderate amount | very little | none |

How much spitting up or vomiting do you think the average baby does?

| a great deal | a good bit | moderate amount | very little | none |

How much difficulty do you think the average baby has in sleeping?

| a great deal | a good bit | moderate amount | very little | none |

How much difficulty does the average baby have with bowel movements?

| a great deal | a good bit | moderate amount | very little | none |

How much trouble do you think the average baby has in settling down to a predictable pattern of eating and sleeping?

| a great deal | a good bit | moderate amount | very little | none |

Table 3 (*Continued*)

YOUR BABY

While it is not possible to know for certain what your baby will be like, you probably have some ideas of what your baby will be like. Please check the blank that you *think* best describes what *your* baby will be like.

How much crying do you think your baby will do?

| a great deal | a good bit | moderate amount | very little | none |

How much trouble do you think your baby will have feeding?

| a great deal | a good bit | moderate amount | very little | none |

How much spitting up or vomiting do you think your baby will do?

| a great deal | a good bit | moderate amount | very little | none |

How much difficulty do you think your baby will have sleeping?

| a great deal | a good bit | moderate amount | very little | none |

How much difficulty do you expect your baby to have with bowel movements?

| a great deal | a good bit | moderate amount | very little | none |

How much trouble do you think the average baby has in settling down to a predictable pattern of eating and sleeping?

| a great deal | a good bit | moderate amount | very little | none |

Source: Reprinted with permission from E. R. Broussard and M. S. S. Hartner, "Further Considerations Regarding Maternal Perception of the First Born." In J. Hellmuth, editor, *Exceptional Infant: Studies in Abnormalities Vol. 2,* (New York: Brunner/Mazel, Inc.), 1971, pp. 442–447.

Table 4
Neonatal Perception Inventory II

AVERAGE BABY

Although this is your first baby, you probably have some ideas of what most little babies are like. Please check the blank you think best describes the AVERAGE baby.

How much crying do you think the average baby does?

| a great deal | a good bit | moderate amount | very little | none |

How much trouble do you think the average baby has in feeding?

| a great deal | a good bit | moderate amount | very little | none |

How much spitting up or vomiting do you think the average baby does?

| a great deal | a good bit | moderate amount | very little | none |

How much difficulty do you think the average baby has in sleeping?

| a great deal | a good bit | moderate amount | very little | none |

How much difficulty does the average baby have with bowel movements?

| a great deal | a good bit | moderate amount | very little | none |

How much trouble do you think the average baby has in settling down to a predictable pattern of eating and sleeping?

| a great deal | a good bit | moderate amount | very little | none |

Table 4 (*Continued*)

YOUR BABY

You have had a chance to live with your baby for a month now. Please check the blank you think best describes your baby.

How much crying has your baby done?

| a great deal | a good bit | moderate amount | very little | none |

How much trouble has your baby had feeding?

| a great deal | a good bit | moderate amount | very little | none |

How much spitting up or vomiting has your baby done?

| a great deal | a good bit | moderate amount | very little | none |

How much difficulty has your baby had in sleeping?

| a great deal | a good bit | moderate amount | very little | none |

How much difficulty has your baby had with bowel movements?

| a great deal | a good bit | moderate amount | very little | none |

How much trouble has your baby had in settling down to a predictable pattern of eating and sleeping?

| a great deal | a good bit | moderate amount | very little | none |

Source: Reprinted with permission from E. R. Broussard and M. S. S. Hartner, "Further Considerations Regarding Maternal Perception of the First Born." In J. Hellmuth, editor, *Exceptional Infant: Studies in Abnormalities Vol. 2,* (New York: Brunner/Mazel, Inc., 1971), pp. 442–447.

The Neonatal Perception Inventory is easily and quickly administered by telling the mother:

"We are interested in learning more about the experiences of mothers and their babies during the first few weeks after delivery. The more we can learn about mothers and their babies, the better we will be able to help other mothers with their babies. We would appreciate it if you would help us to help other mothers by answering a few questions."

The procedures are identical for administering the Average Baby form of the NPI on the first or second postpartum day and the NPI at one month of age. The mother is handed the Average Baby form while the individual administering the Inventory says: "Although this is your first baby, you probably have some ideas of what most little babies are like. Will you please check the blank you think *best describes what* most little babies are like."

The tester waits until the mother has completed the Average Baby form and takes it from the mother and then hands the mother the Your Baby form.*

The procedure for administering the Your Baby forms of the NPI is the same at Time I and Time II. However, the instructions given to the mother vary slightly to take into account the time factor. At Time I the tester tells the mother: "While it is not possible to know for certain what your baby will be like, you probably have some ideas of what your baby will be like. Please check the blank that you think *best describes what* your *baby will be like."*

At Time II, she says:

"You have had a chance to live with your baby for a month now. Please check the blank you think best describes your baby."

Method of Scoring

The Average Baby Perception form elicits the mother's concept of the average baby's behavior. The Your Baby Perception form elicits her rating of her own baby. Each of these instruments consists of six single item scales. Values of 1-5 are assigned to each of these scales for each of the inventories. The blank signified none *is valued as* 1 and a great deal *has a value of 5. The lower values on the scale represent the more desirable behavior.*

The six scales are totaled with no attempt at weighting the scales for

---

"*The tester remains with the mother during the entire administration procedure."

each of the inventories separately. Thus a total score is obtained for the Average Baby and a total score is obtained for the Your Baby.

The total score of the Your Baby Perception form is then subtracted from the Average Baby Perception form. The discrepancy constitutes the Neonatal Perception Inventory score.*

The inventories have shown both construct and criterion validity.

The Degree of Bother Inventory

The Degree of Bother Inventory (Broussard, 1971) is another easy-to-administer questionnaire useful in assessing infant behavior that is of concern to mothers. Guidelines for use of this tool are as follows:

1. Purpose: The tool (see Table 5) is used to assess problems of infant behavior. It is important to note that "since the threshold of parental annoyance varies widely according to a parent's emotional orientation to a child, the ultimate decision as to what constitutes a problem for a specific mother varies among mothers" (Broussard, 1971, p. 435).

2. When to use: The tool is administered when the infant is 1 month of age.

3. How to use: After the mother fills out the inventory the score is calculated by assigning values of 1 to 4 to each of the six items on the inventory and totaling the values. A score of 24 indicates that the mother is easily annoyed by her infant; a score of six indicates that the mother is not bothered or annoyed at all by her infant.

"*Example: Given a total Average Baby score of 17 and a total Your Baby score of 19, the Neonatal Perception Inventory score is −2. One-month-old infants rated by their mothers as better than average (+ score) are considered at Low-Risk. Those infants not rated better than average (− or 0 score) are at High-Risk for subsequent development of emotional difficulty." (Reprinted with permission from E. R. Broussard and M. S. S. Hartner, "Further Considerations Regarding Maternal Perception of the First Born." In J. Hellmuth, editor, *Exceptional Infant: Studies in Abnormalities Vol. 2,* (New York: Brunner/Mazel, Inc., 1971), pp. 442–447.

Table 5
Degree of Bother Inventory

Listed below are some of the things that have sometimes bothered other mothers in caring for their babies. We would like to know if you were bothered about any of these. Please place a check in the blank that best describes how much you were bothered by your baby's behavior in regard to these.

Crying	a great deal	somewhat	very little	none
Spitting up or Vomiting	a great deal	somewhat	very little	none
Sleeping	a great deal	somewhat	very little	none
Feeding	a great deal	somewhat	very little	none
Elimination	a great deal	somewhat	very little	none
Lack of a predict- able schedule	a great deal	somewhat	very little	none
Other: (Specify)	a great deal	somewhat	very little	none
....	a great deal	somewhat	very little	none
....	a great deal	somewhat	very little	none
....	a great deal	somewhat	very little	none

Source: Reprinted with permission from E. R. Broussard and M. S. S. Hartner, "Further Considerations Regarding Maternal Perception of the First Born." In J. Hellmuth, editor, *Exceptional Infant: Studies in Abnormalities Vol. 2,* New York: Brunner/Mazel, Inc., 1971, pp. 442–447.

The Brazelton Neonatal Behavioral Assessment Scale

It is possible to evaluate some of the integrative processes and determine subtle behavioral responses of the neonate (Brazelton, 1973a). General guidelines for the use of the Brazelton Scale are as follows:

1. Purpose: The Brazelton Scale tests and documents the infant's use of state behavior (state of consciousness), the infant's response to various kinds of stimulation, and how the infant affects the environment. It can be used to alert professionals and parents to the potential individual strengths of the neonate.

    "The behavior exam tests for neurological adequacy with 20 reflex measures and for 26 behavioral responses to environmental stimuli, including the kind of interpersonal stimuli which mothers use in their handling of the infant as they attempt to help him adapt to the new world" (Brazelton, 1973, p. 370).

    In the exam, a graded series of procedures (including talking, hand on abdomen, restraint, holding, and rocking) are designed to soothe and alert the infant. The infant's responsiveness to animate stimuli (e.g., rattle, bell, red ball, white light, temperature change) is assessed. Estimates of vigor, attentional excitement, motor activity and tone, and automatic responsiveness are assessed as the infant changes state. Over a period of several days the exam outlines:

    A. The initial period of alertness immediately after delivery
    B. The period of depression and disorganization which follows and lasts for 24 to 48 hours in infants with uncomplicated deliveries and no medication effects
    C. The curve of recovery to optimal function. This third period may be the best single predictor of individual potential function and basic CNS intactness and organization (Brazelton, 1973a).

2. When to use:
    A. Repeated exams on any 2 or 3 days in the first 10 days after delivery

    B. During pediatric examinations throughout the neonatal period

3. How to use: Special training is required for use of the full scale and several teaching films are available to assist with training. Such films are:

    A. The Brazelton Neonatal Assessment Scale: An Introduction

    B. The Brazelton Neonatal Assessment Scale: Variations in Normal Behavior

    C. Self-Scoring Examination

       Films may be obtained from E.D.C. Distribution Center, 39 Chapel Street, Newton, MA 02160

Modified forms of the scale have been developed and used by nurses to assist mothers and infants toward healthy attachment (Clark and Affonso, 1976).

Other Tools

Several other instruments designed to assess various aspects of parent-child interaction are described and evaluated in the article by Cowan (1976).

MANAGEMENT IMPLICATIONS

The primary objective for application of information in this chapter should be the prevention of parenting disabilities and attachment problems. Assessments revealing potential risk situations call for early and active intervention (see Chapters 32 and 33). However, all parents deserve the benefits of knowledgeable and sensitive support as they begin to adapt to their new infants.

General Guidelines

1. Assessment and supportive measures should begin during the prenatal period.
2. Parents can develop and improve parenting capabilities.
3. Expectant parent classes, rooming-in, and other programs can strengthen preparation for parenthood.
4. Careful observations in the very first minutes of mother-newborn interaction can provide helpful data.
5. Allowing mothers to nurse their infants on the delivery table can facilitate attachment.
6. Mothers need time to form attachments. In the early transition period mothers need time for recovery, and expecting too much too soon can result in anxiety and guilt.
7. When premature or sick infants are separated from parents, every effort must be made to provide contact.
8. Active nursing support is essential as new mothers learn to feed and care for their new infants. Mothers should not be left alone. Institutional disruptions should be minimized.
9. The skilled professional should assist the mother in observing and assessing her infant's characteristics, behaviors, and response patterns to provide accurate data to the mother.
10. Mothers need to be aware that the infant contributes to interaction. Often mothers think the source of difficulties is exclusively in their handling of the baby.
11. Early discharge should be avoided if there are problems in the mother-infant acquaintance period.
12. A home visit during the first week of age provides critical feedback and support to new parents.
13. The first well-baby visit should be scheduled by 2 weeks of age.
14. The focus of the well-baby visits must be on the parents as well as the infant.
15. Mothers must be allowed to verbalize their feelings, positive and negative, related to the baby.
16. Parents must be assisted to understand the meaning of the infant's behavior.

17. Nurse practitioners must be alert to signs of disturbance in parent and/or infant.
18. Nurse practitioners must be available to parents on a 24-hour basis.

References

Ainsworth, M. D. S. "The Development of Infant-Mother Interaction Among the Ganda." In B. M. Foss, editor, *Determinants of Infant Behavior II.* New York: Wiley, 1963. Pp. 67–112.

Ainsworth, M. D. S. "Object Relations, Dependency, and Attachment: A Theoretical Review of the Infant-Mother Relationship." *Child Dev* 40:969–1026, December 1969.

Ainsworth, M. D. S. and S. M. Bell. "Attachment, Exploration, and Separation: Illustrated by the Behavior of One-Year Olds in a Strange Situation." *Child Dev* 41:49–65, March 1970.

Barbero, G. "Failure to Thrive." In M. H. Klaus, T. Leger, and M. A. Trause, editors, *Maternal Attachment and Mothering Disorders: A Round Table.* New Brunswick, N.J.: Johnson and Johnson Baby Products Co., 1975. Pp. 9–12.

Bell, S. M. and M. D. S. Ainsworth. "Infant Crying and Maternal Responsiveness." *Child Dev* 43:1171–1190, December 1972.

Benedek, T. "Psychobiological Aspects of Mothering." *Am J Orthopsychiatry* 26:272–278, April 1956.

Binzley, V. "State: Overlooked Factor in Newborn Nursing." *Am J Nurs* 77:102–103, January 1977.

Bishop, B. "A Guide to Assessing Parenting Capabilities." *Am J Nurs* 76:1784–1787, November 1976.

Bowlby, J. *Attachment and Loss. Volume 1. Attachment.* New York: Basic Books, 1969.

Brazelton, T. B. "Assessment of the Infant at Risk." *Clin Obstet Gynecol* 16:361–375, March 1973.

Brazelton, T. B. *Neonatal Behavioral Assessment Scale.* Clinics in Developmental Medicine Series, Volume 50. Philadelphia: Lippincott, 1973a.

Broussard, E. R. and M. S. S. Hartner. "Further Considerations Regarding Maternal Perception of the First Born." In J. Hellmuth, editor, *Exceptional Infant: Studies in Abnormalities, Vol. 2.* New York: Brunner/Mazel, 1971. Pp. 432–449.

Clark, A. L. "Recognizing Discord between Mother and Child and Changing It to Harmony." *Am J Maternal Child Nursing* 1:100–106, March–April 1976.

Clark, A. L. and D. D. Affonso. *Childbearing: A Nursing Perspective.* Philadelphia: Davis, 1976.

Clark, A. and D. D. Affonso. "Infant Behavior and Maternal Attachment: Two Sides of the Coin." *Am J Maternal Child Nursing* 1:94–99, March–April 1976a.

Cowan, D. B., J. C. Bouchard, and M. M. Suarez. "Child Health Screening for the Nurse Practitioner." *Nurse Practitioner* 1:109–120, January–February 1976.

Durand, B. "Failure to Thrive in a Child with Down's Syndrome: A Clinical Nursing Study." *Nurs Res* 24:272–286, July–August 1975.

Green, M. "A Developmental Approach to Symptoms Based on Age Groups." *Pediatr Clin North Am* 22:571–582, August 1975.

Harrison, L. L. "Nursing Intervention with the Failure-to-Thrive Family." *Am J Maternal Child Nursing* 1:111–116, March–April 1976.

Helfer, Ray E. "Relationship between Lack of Bonding and Child Abuse and Neglect." In M. H. Klaus, T. Leger, and M. A. Trause, editors, *Maternal Attachment and Mothering Disorders: A Round Table.* New Brunswick, N.J.: Johnson and Johnson Baby Products Co., 1975. Pp. 21–26.

Kennedy, J. C. The High-Risk Maternal-Infant Acquaintance Process." *Nurs Clin North Am* 8:549–556, September 1973.

Kennell, J. H. and M. H. Klaus. "Care of the Mother of the High-Risk Infant." *Clin Obstet Gynecol* 14:926–954, September 1971.

Klaus, M. H. and J. H. Kennell. "Mothers Separated from Their Newborn Infants." *Pediatr Clin of North Am* 17:1015–1037, November 1970.

Klaus, M. H., et al. "Maternal Attachment: Importance of the First Post-Partum Days." *N Engl J Med* 286:460–463, 1972.

Lamper, C. "Facilitating Attachment through Well-Baby Care." In J. E. Hall and B. R. Weaver, editors, *Nursing of Families in Crisis.* Philadelphia: Lippincott, 1974. Pp. 72–83.

Leifer, A. J., et al. "Effects of Mother-Infant Separation on Maternal Attachment Behavior." *Child Dev* 43:1203–1218, December 1972.

Levy, D. M. *Attitude Study.* Bureau of Child Health, Infant and Preschool Division, New York City Department of Health, 1964, unpublished.

Morris, M. G. "Maternal Claiming-Identification Processes: Their Meaning for Mother-Infant Mental Health." In A. Clark, et al., *Parent-Child Relationships: The Role of the Nurse.* New Brunswick, N.J.: Rutgers University, 1968.

Newcomb, T. *The Acquaintance Process.* New York: Holt, Rinehart and Winston, 1961.

Porter, Cornelia P. "Maladaptive Mothering Patterns: Nursing Intervention." In *ANA Clinical Sessions: Detroit 1972.* New York: Appleton-Century-Crofts, 1973. Pp. 87–102.

Robertson, J. "Mothering As an Influence on Early Development: A Study of Well-Baby Clinic Records." *Psychoanal Study Child* 17:245–264, 1962.

Thoman, E. B. "Development of Synchrony in Mother-Infant Interaction in Feeding and Other Situations." *Fed Proc* 34:1587–1592, June 1975.

6

Nutrition in Infancy and Childhood

The influence of nutrition on growth and development in infancy and childhood is well known and as knowledge accumulates it becomes more evident that nutrition affects most facets of an individual's well-being throughout life.

Parents often lack basic information on nutrition or are confused by the plethora of data, opinions, and material (professional and commercial) aimed at them and at their children. At the same time, there are increasing numbers of parents who have extensive and sophisticated knowledge about nutrition. It is essential, therefore, for the nurse practitioner to be competent in the area of proper nutrition for infants and children.

Nutrition does not occur in a vacuum. Parents bring with them a whole nutritional past including habits and attitudes toward food which have been influenced by culture, education, and socioeconomic factors and which result in a wide range of variability in infant feeding practices. Approaches to infant feeding are discussed in Chapter 7.

Acceptance and knowledge of the many individual styles, methods, and approaches to infant feeding are important aspects of the role of the pediatric care provider. However, the primary concern in nutrition counseling must be that of meeting the known nutritional requirements of the infant and child. Reinforcement of the parent's own efforts is mandatory, but when nutritional practices are based on unsound knowledge then counseling and education must be geared toward providing parents with the information and support necessary to meet the normal nutritional needs of their children. Nutrition education is one of the best preventive health-care measures available.

This chapter presents information on normal nutritional requirements for infants and children, a review of essential nutrients, guidelines for assessing nutritional status, practical information for parent counseling, and brief discussions of some common nutritional problems. Nutritional needs during pregnancy are briefly presented since the nurse practitioner is often a source of advice and counsel for pregnant women.

NUTRITIONAL REQUIREMENTS

The science of nutrition continues to expand, and new and revised data continue to emerge in relation to nutrients and amounts considered essential for optimal growth, development, and health. It is important to recognize that the recommendations made are based on available data and change frequently.

Definitions

- Requirement. The *requirement* of an individual for a specific nutrient is defined as the "least amount of that nutrient that will promote an optimal state of health" (Fomon, 1974, p. 109). Since requirements are expressed in minimal terms, and since these values are estimated and cannot with certainty be used under all circumstances and sets of conditions, they are not used as recommended intakes.
- Recommended Daily Dietary Allowances (RDAs). These values are the levels of intake of essential nutrients considered, in the judgment of the Food and Nutrition Board of the National Academy of Science—National Research Council, to be adequate to meet the known nutritional needs of almost every healthy person. See Table 1. The estimates are intended for

Table 1
Recommended Daily Dietary Allowances[a]
Designed for the maintenance of good nutrition of practically all healthy people in the U.S.A.

	Age (years)	Weight (kg)	Weight (lbs)	Height (cm)	Height (in)	Energy (kcal)[b]	Protein (g)	Vitamin A Activity (re)[c]	Vitamin A Activity (iu)	Vitamin D (iu)	Vitamin E Activity[e] (iu)
Infants	0.0–0.5	6	14	60	24	kg × 117	kg × 2.2	420[d]	1,400	400	4
	0.5–1.0	9	20	71	28	kg × 108	kg × 2.0	400	2,000	400	5
Children	1–3	13	28	86	34	1,300	23	400	2,000	400	7
	4–6	20	44	110	44	1,800	30	500	2,500	400	9
	7–10	30	66	135	54	2,400	36	700	3,300	400	10
Males	11–14	44	97	158	63	2,800	44	1,000	5,000	400	12
	15–18	61	134	172	69	3,000	54	1,000	5,000	400	15
	19–22	67	147	172	69	3,000	54	1,000	5,000	400	15
	23–50	70	154	172	69	2,700	56	1,000	5,000		15
	51+	70	154	172	69	2,400	56	1,000	5,000		15
Females	11–14	44	97	155	62	2,400	44	800	4,000	400	12
	15–18	54	119	162	65	2,100	48	800	4,000	400	12
	19–22	58	128	162	65	2,100	46	800	4,000	400	12
	23–50	58	128	162	65	2,000	46	800	4,000		12
	51+	58	128	162	65	1,800	46	800	4,000		12
Pregnant						+300	+30	1,000	5,000	400	15
Lactating						+500	+20	1,200	6,000	400	15

[a]The allowances are intended to provide for individual variations among most normal persons as they live in the United States under usual environmental stresses. Diets should be based on a variety of common foods in order to provide other nutrients for which human requirements have been less well defined.

[b]Kilojoules (kJ) = 4.2 × kcal.

[c]Retinol equivalents.

[d]Assumed to be all as retinol in milk during the first six months of life. All subsequent intakes are assumed to be half as retinol and half as β-carotene when calculated from international units. As retinol equivalents, three fourths are as retinol and one fourth as β-carotene.

[e]Total vitamin E activity, estimated to be 80 percent as α-tocopherol and 20 percent other tocopherols.

Continued on next page

Table 1 (Continued)

	Age (years)	Weight (kg)	Weight (lbs)	Height (cm)	Height (in)	Water-Soluble Vitamins Ascorbic Acid (mg)	Folacin[f] (μg)	Niacin[g] (mg)	Riboflavin (mg)	Thiamin (mg)	Vitamin B_6 (mg)	Vitamin B_{12} (μg)
Infants	0.0–0.5	6	14	60	24	35	50	5	0.4	0.3	0.3	0.3
	0.5–1.0	9	20	71	28	35	50	8	0.6	0.5	0.4	0.3
Children	1–3	13	28	86	34	40	100	9	0.8	0.7	0.6	1.0
	4–6	20	44	110	44	40	200	12	1.1	0.9	0.9	1.5
	7–10	30	66	135	54	40	300	16	1.2	1.2	1.2	2.0
Males	11–14	44	97	158	63	45	400	18	1.5	1.4	1.6	3.0
	15–18	61	134	172	69	45	400	20	1.8	1.5	2.0	3.0
	19–22	67	147	172	69	45	400	20	1.8	1.5	2.0	3.0
	23–50	70	154	172	69	45	400	18	1.6	1.4	2.0	3.0
	51+	70	154	172	69	45	400	16	1.5	1.2	2.0	3.0
Females	11–14	44	97	155	62	45	400	16	1.3	1.2	1.6	3.0
	15–18	54	119	162	65	45	400	14	1.4	1.1	2.0	3.0
	19–22	58	128	162	65	45	400	14	1.4	1.1	2.0	3.0
	23–50	58	128	162	65	45	400	13	1.2	1.0	2.0	3.0
	51+	58	128	162	65	45	400	12	1.1	1.0	2.0	3.0
Pregnant						60	800	+2	+0.3	+0.3	2.5	4.0
Lactating						80	600	+4	+0.5	+0.3	2.5	4.0

[f] The folacin allowances refer to dietary sources as determined by *Lactobacillus casei* assay. Pure forms of folacin may be effective in doses less than one fourth of the recommended dietary allowance.

[g] Although allowances are expressed as niacin, it is recognized that on the average 1 mg of niacin is derived from each 60 mg of dietary tryptophan.

	Age (years)	Weight (kg)	Weight (lbs)	Height (cm)	Height (in)	Calcium (mg)	Phosphorus (mg)	Iodine (μg)	Iron (mg)	Magnesium (mg)	Zinc (mg)
Infants	0.0–0.5	6	14	60	24	360	240	35	10	60	3
	0.5–1.0	9	20	71	28	540	400	45	15	70	5
Children	1–3	13	28	86	34	800	800	60	15	150	10
	4–6	20	44	110	44	800	800	80	10	200	10
	7–10	30	66	135	54	800	800	110	10	250	10
Males	11–14	44	97	158	63	1,200	1,200	130	18	350	15
	15–18	61	134	172	69	1,200	1,200	150	18	400	15
	19–22	67	147	172	69	800	800	140	10	350	15
	23–50	70	154	172	69	800	800	130	10	350	15
	51+	70	154	172	69	800	800	110	10	350	15
Females	11–14	44	97	155	62	1,200	1,200	115	18	300	15
	15–18	54	119	162	65	1,200	1,200	115	18	300	15
	19–22	58	128	162	65	800	800	100	18	300	15
	23–50	58	128	162	65	800	800	100	18	300	15
	51+	58	128	162	65	800	800	80	10	300	15
Pregnant						1,200	1,200	125	18+[h]	450	20
Lactating						1,200	1,200	150	18	450	25

Source: Food and Nutrition Board, National Academy of Sciences–National Research Council, Revised 1974.

[h]This increased requirement cannot be met by ordinary diets; therefore, the use of supplemental iron is recommended.

general use and are based on the needs of "average" individuals living in temperate environments and expending "average" amounts of energy. These *advisable intakes* are generally higher than the *requirements* and represent amounts of nutrients that are safe and present no hazard. The RDAs do not allow for persons depleted of specific nutrients due to illness or deficiency states.

Essential Nutrients

ENERGY (CALORIES)

Requirements. The energy needs of children vary at different ages and under various circumstances. Energy requirements (see Table 1) depend on energy expenditures due to:

- Basal metabolism
- Body activity
- Growth
- Specific dynamic action of food (i.e., the increased heat production following ingestion of food)
- Fecal loss

Distribution of calories. In addition to total requirements, the distribution of calories must be considered so foods chosen will contain all the other dietary essentials. Diets are generally calculated to provide calories as follows:

Normal full-term infant:	Protein	6–8 percent
	Fat	30–55 percent
	Carbohydrate	approx. 50 percent
Adult:	Protein	10–15 percent
	Fat	35–45 percent
	Carbohydrate	50–60 percent

Sources of calories. Calories are provided as follows:

Protein   1 gm yields 4 calories
Fat   1 gm yields 9 calories
Carbohydrate   1 gm yields 4 calories

WATER

Requirements. Water requirements vary with energy produced or calories metabolized (e.g., greater need in hot weather). Water balance is affected by fluid intake, protein and mineral content of the diet, renal solute load, metabolic rate, respiratory rate, and body temperature. Table 2 presents daily fluid requirements for children and adults under normal conditions.

Deficiency. Effects of deficiency include thirst, dehydration, high specific gravity of urine, loss of kidney function, death.

Excess. Effects of excess include abdominal discomfort, headache, cramps, water intoxication, convulsions, edema, circulatory collapse.

Table 2
Daily Fluid Requirements

Age	ml/kg
1–3 days	60–100
4–10 days	125–150
3 months	140–165
6 months	130–155
9 months	125–145
1–3 years	115–135
4–6 years	90–110
7–9 years	70–90
10–12 years	60–85
13–15 years	50–65
Adult	40–50

Source: Reprinted with permission from J. W. Graef and T. F. Cone, *Manual of Pediatric Therapeutics*, (Boston: Little, Brown, 1974), p. 89.

PROTEIN

Definitions. Important definitions related to proteins are as follows:

- *Proteins* constitute a group of complex nitrogenous compounds that contain amino acids as their basic structural units, and that are essential for growth and repair of all animal tissue.
- *Essential amino acids* are those that cannot be synthesized by the body to meet the demands for normal growth. They must be obtained from outside sources and must be present simultaneously and in sufficient quantity in the body.
- The *quantity* of protein in a given food is estimated by measuring the amount of nitrogen in that food. The RDAs (Table 1) represent baseline values for quantity of protein.
- The *quality* of protein is related to its ability to supply all essential amino acids in sufficient amounts to meet requirements for maintenance and growth.
- *Complete protein* is any protein containing sufficient amounts of the essential amino acids. Most animal protein is complete protein.
- *Incomplete protein* is a protein lacking one or more essential amino acids or supplying too little of an essential amino acid. Most plant protein is incomplete protein.

Deficiency. Protein deficiency results in lassitude, abdominal enlargement, edema, depletion of plasma proteins, negative nitrogen balance, kwashiorkor, marasmus.

Excess. Excessive protein intake is primarily of concern in those disorders which involve defects in amino acid and protein metabolism (e.g., phenylketonuria).

Distribution of calories. The percentage of calories per day that should be protein is:

Infants   6–8 percent
Childhood   10–15 percent

Sources of protein. The best sources of protein include:

1. Complete protein: egg yolk, milk, liver, kidneys, meat, fish, poultry, soybean, wheat germ, brewer's yeast, garbanzo beans, cottage cheese
2. Incomplete protein: whole grains, nuts, seeds, legumes, lentils (Lappe, 1975)

FAT

Definitions. Important definitions related to fats are as follows:

- *Fats* are organic compounds that function in the body chiefly to provide energy, to protect body organs, to maintain body temperature, enable absorption of the fat-soluble vitamins (A, D, E, K), and to provide essential fatty acids necessary for health and growth.
- *Essential fatty acids* are those that cannot be synthesized by the body and must be obtained from outside sources. They are necessary for growth and skin integrity. Essential fatty acids also act as precursors of *prostaglandins* which function on the vascular system to help regulate blood flow and may also be important in mediating inflammatory reactions and in regulating gastric secretions and release of pituitary hormones. The two essential fatty acids are linoleic and arachidonic.
- *Unsaturated fatty acids* contain one or more "unfilled links" between the carbon atoms where other substances can be added and can react with the fatty acid. They are better absorbed than saturated fatty acids. There are two types:
  1. *Monounsaturated fatty acids* are those with one reactive double-bond linkage.
  2. *Polyunsaturated fatty acids* are those with two or more double-bond linkages.
- *Saturated fatty acids* do not contain any open double-bond linkages. They are stable and characteristically firm at room temperature and less easily absorbed by the body.
- *Phospholipids* are waxlike substances essential for cell membrane structure and important in absorption and transport of fatty

acids. They are produced in the liver. *Lecithin* is the most well-known phospholipid and is important because it appears to be capable of breaking down fat and cholesterol into tiny particles which can readily pass into tissues.

- *Cholesterol* is an organic compound whose functions in infancy appear to be:
    1. To participate in the process of myelinization
    2. To permit synthesis of steroid hormones and bile acids
    3. To develop regulatory mechanisms for cholesterol metabolism in adult life (Fomon, 1974, p. 174)

Deficiency. Deficient fat intake results in a lack of satiety, weight loss, and skin problems if essential fatty acids are not provided.

Excess. Excessive fat intake causes obesity. Other concerns related to fat intake are atherosclerosis and hyperlipidemia.

ATHEROSCLEROSIS. It appears that the "fatty streak," the earliest lesion of atherosclerosis, may be found in the arteries of preschool children. Some authorities (McGill, 1974) think that fatty streaks do not necessarily lead to atherosclerosis. Others conjecture that gradual progression of the atherosclerosis lesion occurs from middle or late childhood through adult life. Since the effect of severe cholesterol restriction in infancy may interfere with the functions of cholesterol and may prove harmful, the most reasonable recommendation under the limits of current knowledge is that of moderate restriction of cholesterol intake of all children beyond infancy.

TYPE II HYPERLIPOPROTEINEMIA (FAMILIAL HYPERCHOLESTEROLEMIA). This inherited condition is characterized by increased cholesterol levels, and its consequences include tendon xanthomas (see Chapter 15, Xanthoma) and premature (before age 50) ischemic heart disease. Screening for cholesterol and triglyceride levels should be performed on any child if there is a family history of hyperlipidemia, premature vascular disease, sudden death, or xanthomas in a parent or grandparent, or if the child has xanthomas, unexplained abdominal pain, or is overweight. Those with serum cholesterol levels above 200 mg/dl or triglyceride levels above 120 mg/dl are placed under medical supervision (Rudolph, 1977, p. 737). High intakes of saturated fats and cholesterol are avoided.

Distribution of calories. The percentage of calories per day that should be fat is:

Infants	30–55 percent
Childhood and adolescence	30–45 percent

The percentage of calories per day that should be linoleic acid is 1–3 percent. [*Note:* human milk contains 6–9 percent of total calories as linoleic acid.]

Sources of fat. Common sources of fat are as follows:

1. Unsaturated fatty acids:

   - Monounsaturated: olive oil, peanut oil, human milk, cow milk
   - Polyunsaturated: corn oil, soy oil, safflower oil, sesame oil, fish oils

2. Saturated fatty acids: most animal fats (e.g., milk, butter, egg yolk, bacon, meat, cheese)
3. Essential fatty acids: natural vegetable oils (e.g., corn, soybean, cottonseed, safflower, sesame, sunflower), eggs, milk, poultry
4. Phospholipids (lecithin): natural oils, egg yolk, liver
5. Cholesterol: animal fats

CARBOHYDRATE

Definitions. Important definitions related to carbohydrates are as follows:

- *Carbohydrates* constitute a group of chemical compounds including sugars, starches, and cellulose. They function to provide energy, to store energy in the liver in the form of glycogen, and to provide roughage.

- Carbohydrates are classified as:
  1. *Monosaccharide.* A simple sugar (e.g., glucose, fructose) which is most readily utilized by the body
  2. *Disaccharide.* A sugar that contains two monosaccharides (e.g., lactose, sucrose, maltose)
  3. *Polysaccharide.* A complex sugar that contains many monosaccharides (e.g., starch, cellulose)

Deficiency. Lack of sufficient carbohydrate can result in ketosis, weight loss.

Excess. Carbohydrates taken in excess contribute to obesity. Sucrose is thought to be the chief cause of dental caries. Deficiencies in specific digestive enzymes will cause corresponding malabsorption of the specific carbohydrate (e.g., galactosemia, lactose intolerance).

LACTOSE INTOLERANCE. Lactose intolerance is thought to occur in several situations: in the breast-fed infant, following severe diarrhea, and in congenital form. For a full discussion refer to Chapter 21, Malabsorption: Disaccharide Deficiency.

In the breast-fed infant the high lactose content of human breast milk (37 percent of calories) may explain the characteristic frequent, loose, runny "breast milk stools" of the infant as the lactose intake may be greater than the ability of the lactase enzyme to digest it completely. By 4 to 6 weeks of age lactose can be normally digested.

Distribution of calories. Minimum requirements for carbohydrate are not really known. However, infants receiving primarily human milk or milk-based formulas usually receive 35 to 55 percent of their daily calories from carbohydrate, chiefly in the form of lactose.

Sources of carbohydrate. Sources of carbohydrate are as follows:

1. Monosaccharides: honey, molasses, dates, figs, fruits, and vegetables

2. Disaccharides: Lactose— milk, ice cream, yogurt
   Sucrose—sugar beets, sugar cane, ripe fruits, jellies, cakes, candy, commercially prepared baby foods
   Maltose—corn syrup
3. Polysaccharides: corn syrup hydrolysates (dextri-maltose), grains and grain products, legumes, tuber and root vegetables

VITAMINS

Definitions. Important definitions related to vitamins are as follows:

- *Vitamins* are organic substances, occurring naturally in plant and animal tissue, that are necessary in small amounts for the control of metabolic processes, for normal growth, and for maintenance of health. They are classified as either fat-soluble or water-soluble.
- *Fat-soluble vitamins* (A, D, E, K). These are more stable to heat and less likely to be lost in cooking and processing. They are not excreted in the urine so excesses are stored in the body and may result in toxicity.
- *Water-soluble vitamins* (C, B_1—thiamin, B_2—riboflavin, niacin, B_6—pyridoxine, B_{12}, folacin). Excesses of these vitamins are excreted in the urine so toxicity is decreased. Deficiencies develop more rapidly.

Functions, deficiency, excess, and sources. The functions, symptoms of deficiency or excess, and sources of the vitamins are presented in Table 3.

Advisable intakes. Official recommendations for vitamin intake are found in Table 1. Many parents are reading popular literature regarding nutrition and frequently need guidance to accurately and/or safely interpret the recommendations published in such sources. Two of the most widely read sources of nutrition information are by Adelle Davis: *Let's Eat Right to Keep Fit* and *Let's Have Healthy Children.* See this chapter, References. The amounts of vitamins recommended for infants and children by Davis are ques-

Table 3
Vitamins: Functions, Symptoms of Deficiency and Excess, and Sources

Vitamin	Function	Deficiency or Excess	Sources
Vitamin A (retinol)	Essential for growth, development and maintenance of normal vision, maintenance of epithelial tissue, tooth development	*Deficiency:* impaired vision including night blindness; dry and scaly skin; problems in respiratory, digestive, and GU membranes; failure to thrive; impaired tooth development *Excess:* anorexia, irritability, increased ICP, headache, nausea and vomiting, desquamation of the skin, changes in long bones *Toxic dose:* 18,500 IU of vitamin A given daily for over 1 month. Aqueous suspensions of vitamin A are more easily absorbed, thus toxicity develops with lower doses and in shorter time. The American Academy of Pediatrics recommends *against* the use of vitamin A preparations containing more than 6000 IU per dose.	Carotene, a precursor of vitamin A, is found in carrots, squash, cantaloupe, apricots, yams, all green vegetables (especially chard, kale, and spinach). Vitamin A: dairy products especially egg yolk, liver, fish liver oils, yellow vegetables, green leafy vegetables, fortified margarine

			Note: excessive intake of carotene may result in carotenemia which is not harmful.
Vitamin D	Needed to promote growth; necessary for the absorption of calcium and phorphorus; bone and tooth mineralization	*Deficiency:* rickets, poor growth, poor tooth development, muscular weakness *Excess:* vomiting and diarrhea, symptoms of hypercalcemia, failure to thrive, calcification of soft tissues, renal disorders, cardiac myopathy *Toxic dose:* more than 1800–3000 IU per day. Doses over 1000 IU per day should be avoided.	Fish liver oils, fatty fish (sardines, salmon), fortified milk, sunlight *Note:* Ultraviolet light acting on skin oils produces vitamin D but it is advised not to depend on this source, especially in infancy. 30–60 minutes of exposure per day is needed to provide sufficient Vitamin D.
Vitamin E (tocopherol)	Required for intact muscles, normal reproduction, resistance to hemolysis. Considered essential for human infant. Needed to prevent unsaturated fatty acids from being destroyed in the body. *Note:* As intake of polyunsaturated fatty acids increases, Vitamin E intake must increase.	*Deficiency:* red cell hemolysis, weakness and degeneration of skeletal muscle *Excess:* unknown	Wheat germ, oils of grains, human milk, nuts and seeds, salad oils, margarine, stone-ground whole grain cereals and breads, green leafy vegetables *Note:* Vitamin E cannot be absorbed without fat. Therefore infants on skim milk will not absorb sufficient Vitamin E.

Continued on next page

Table 3 (Continued)

Vitamin	Function	Deficiency or Excess	Sources
Vitamin K	Necessary for normal clotting of blood via formation of prothrombin	*Deficiency*: coagulation problems, hemorrhage *Excess*: unknown	Milk, cabbage, spinach, lettuce, yogurt, pork, liver
Vitamin C (ascorbic acid)	Needed for normal development of collagen (connective tissue) and normal body metabolism; protection from infection (mechanism poorly understood)	*Deficiency*: delayed healing, petechial hemorrhages, irritability, fatigue, swelling of joints and gums, scurvy *Excess*: no harmful effects known; excreted in urine	Citrus fruits, guava, bell pepper, rose hips, cantaloupe, kale, broccoli, strawberries, green vegetables, human milk, tomatoes *Note*: Vitamin C is destroyed by food processing, storage, and heating. Thus vitamin C content of whole cow milk is reduced to negligible amounts by pasteurization, storage, and heating. This applies also to commercially prepared strained baby fruits and vegetables.
Vitamin B_1 (thiamine)	Required for carbohydrate metabolism; promotes appetite	*Deficiency*: fatigue, depression, insomnia, neuritis, headache, beriberi, cardiac problems *Excess*: no harmful effects known; unneeded amounts excreted in urine	Pork, liver, wheat germ, rice polish, brewer's yeast, whole grain cereals, legumes, nuts, milk

Vitamin	Function	Deficiency/Excess	Sources
Vitamin B_2 (riboflavin)	Required for normal energy metabolism; part of several metabolic enzymes; normal tissue function.	*Deficiency*: cheilosis (cracks and splits in tissue of mouth and lips), photophobia, blood-shot eyes and other visual symptoms, skin problems *Excess*: no harmful effects known; excreted in the urine	Liver, yeast, dairy products, cooked leafy vegetables, legumes
Niacin (nicotinic acid)	Required for cellular metabolism	*Deficiency*: pellagra, psychological changes (depression, tension, insomnia), skin problems, diarrhea *Excess*: no harmful effects known; excreted in the urine	Can be synthesized in the body from the amino acid tryptophan; brewer's yeast, liver, wheat germ, kidney, cereal grains, nuts, legumes, poultry
Vitamin B_6 (pyridoxine)	Serves as coenzyme in metabolism of protein, fat, and carbohydrate	*Deficiency*: seizures, irritability, headache; mouth, lip, and tongue soreness; seborrheic dermatitis, anemia *Excess*: no harmful effects known; excreted in the urine	Brewer's yeast, blackstrap molasses, wheat germ, liver, kidney, soybeans, bananas *Note*: B_6 is sensitive to heating, processing, and storage.
Vitamin B_{12} (cobalamin)	Required in protein metabolism, folacin metabolism; essential for normal cell function, especially bone marrow cells	*Deficiency*: pernicious anemia, megaloblastic anemia *Excess*: no harmful effects known; excreted in the urine.	*Only* in animal foods: liver, organ meats, milk, eggs, cheese, meat, fish, human milk

Continued on next page

Table 3 (Continued)

Vitamin	Function	Deficiency or Excess	Sources
Folacin (folic acid)	Serves as coenzyme in protein metabolism; essential for formation of nucleoproteins which in turn are required for normal erythrocyte maturation; normal growth and reproduction	*Deficiency*: megaloblastic anemia, GI disturbances, and diarrhea *Excess*: no harmful effects known; excreted in the urine	Liver, yeast, leafy green vegetables, human milk, cow milk, dried legumes, nuts *Note*: Goat milk does *not* have sufficient folacin for the human infant
Other B-complex vitamins: Pantothenic acid and biotin	Serve as coenzymes in metabolism of protein, fat, and carbohydrate	*Deficiency*: fatigue, headache, sleep disturbances, personality changes, muscle cramps. *Note*: deficiency very rare because they are so widely distributed in most foods *Excess*: no harmful effect known; excreted in the urine	Exists in all cells of living tissue; especially rich sources are yeast, liver, eggs, wheat germ, nuts, and peas Considered as "questionable" vitamins since they have not yet been proven as essential nutrients for normal persons (Rudolph, 1977, p. 194).
Choline	Serves in metabolism and catabolism; is an essential component of phospholipids (especially lecithin); vital in lipid metabolism; a constituent of acetylcholine which plays a role in normal nerve function	*Deficiency*: has not been definitively established *Excess*: no harmful effects known; excreted in the urine	Foods that contain phospholipids, i.e., egg yolk, whole grains, legumes, meats, wheat germ

Table 4
Vitamin Intake for Infants Recommended by Adelle Davis

Vitamin	*Recommended Intake*
Vitamin A	5000 IU/day (up to 10,000 IU)
Vitamin D	1800 IU/day
Vitamin E	600–1600 units daily (no age specified)
Vitamin C Vitamin B$_1$ Vitamin B$_2$ Niacin	Five times the Recommended Daily Allowances of the Food and Nutrition Board of the National Academy of Sciences (see Table 1)

Source: Adapted from Adelle Davis, *Let's Eat Right to Keep Fit,* rev. ed., (New York: Harcourt, Brace, Jovanovich, 1970) and Adelle Davis, *Let's Have Healthy Children,* (New York: Harcourt, Brace and World, Inc., 1959).

tionable and, in the case of the fat-soluble vitamins, potentially harmful. See Table 4. Care providers have a responsibility to inform parents of the consequences of excessive intakes of the fat-soluble vitamins (Table 3). The United States Congress has considered legislation requiring a prescription for large-dose preparations of Vitamins A and D.

MINERALS AND TRACE ELEMENTS

Definitions.   Minerals and trace elements are naturally occurring, inorganic substances, several of which are nutritionally important.

Functions, deficiency, excess, and sources.   Table 5 presents information on functions, symptoms of deficiency and excess, and sources of the most important minerals and trace elements.

Advisable intakes.   The actual minimum requirements for most of the minerals and trace elements are not known and, with the exception of iron and fluoride, are not of practical concern since they are found in adequate amounts in normal diets. See Table 1 for the RDAs for calcium, phosphorus, iodine, iron, magnesium, and zinc. RDAs for fluoride have not been established, although recommendations by professional groups have been made. See Chapter

Table 5
Minerals: Functions, Symptoms of Deficiency and Excess, and Sources

Mineral	Function	Deficiency or Excess	Sources
Calcium	99% of calcium in the body is used in structure of bones and teeth; necessary for blood coagulation; aids in transmission of nerve impulses; lactation; muscle contractility; myocardial function *Note:* Vitamin D necessary for calcium absorption	*Deficiency:* bone demineralization, tooth demineralization, irritability, tetany, rickets, growth retardation, hypocalcemia *Excess:* unknown	Milk, buttermilk, cheddar cheese, canned salmon, mustard and turnip greens, soybeans, blackstrap molasses, cream of wheat, figs, dates, egg yolk, clams, oysters *Note:* one quart of milk will provide approximately 1000 mg of calcium.
Chloride	Formation of hydrochloric acid, maintenance of acid-base balance, electrolyte balance; maintenance of normal irritability of nervous tissue and contractility of muscle tissue.	*Deficiency:* alkalosis, dehydration *Excess:* unknown	Table salt, meat, eggs, dairy products
Fluoride	Necessary for maximal resistance to dental caries.	*Deficiency:* dental caries *Excess:* mottling of tooth enamel, fluorosis. More than 4 mg/day will cause teeth to mottle. See Chapter 17, The Mouth and Teeth.	Most reliable source is fluoridated water—at a level of 0.5–1.0 ppm; fluoride drops or tablets. Seafood is highest food source. Some fish have 6–12 mg/kg, but most is not bio-available; thus diet alone cannot supply sufficient fluoride.

Iodine	Constituent of thyroid hormone, thyroxine; control of basal metabolic rate	*Deficiency:* goiter, cretinism *Excess:* depression of thyroid	Iodized salt, fish, seaweed
Iron	Essential component of hemoglobin for the transport of oxygen to all tissues	*Deficiency:* anemia, low iron stores *Excess:* hemosiderosis, cardiovascular collapse See Chapter 20, Iron Deficiency Anemia.	Liver, kidneys, beef heart, brewer's yeast, wheat germ, lean meats, greens, dried fruits, egg yolk, enriched cereals, and grains See Tables 10 and 11 for additional dietary sources of iron
Magnesium	Needed for structure of bones and teeth; utilization of fats and carbohydrates; enzyme systems; neuromuscular irritability; regulation of body temperature	*Deficiency:* irritability, muscle weakness, tetany, behavioral disturbances *Excess:* none from dietary intake	Nuts, soybeans, cooked whole grains, green leafy vegetables, milk, cocoa, shellfish *Note:* magnesium intake is related to calcium intake. The more calcium in the diet, the more magnesium needed.
Phosphorus	80% of body phosphorus is used for structure of bones and teeth; necessary for normal blood pH; constituent of nucleic acids and nucleoproteins; component of phospholipids which promote fat metabolism and cell permeability *Note:* Vitamin D necessary for phosphorus absorption	*Deficiency:* stunting of growth, poor quality of bones and teeth, muscle weakness *Excess:* possibility of tetany in newborns on formula with low Ca : P ratio	Liver, yeast, lecithin, wheat germ, dairy products, egg yolk, nuts, cereal grains, meat, fish, dates, raisins

Continued on next page

Table 5 (Continued)

Mineral	Function	Deficiency or Excess	Sources
Potassium	Necessary for muscle contraction, nerve impulse conduction, fluid balance, heart rhythm	*Deficiency*: muscle weakness, anorexia, nausea, abdominal distention, nervous irritability, tachycardia, drowsiness *Excess*: heart block	Meats, poultry, fish, fruits, vegetables, whole grain cereals
Sodium	Maintenance of acid-base balance, electrolyte balance, maintenance of normal irritability of nervous tissue, contractility of muscle tissue	*Deficiency*: dehydration, anorexia, nausea, diarrhea, muscle cramps *Excess*: edema	Table salt, soy sauce, baking powder, cheese, milk, eggs, shellfish, meat, seasonings, and preservatives
Zinc	Essential constituent of several enzymes, important for skin keratinization and muscle growth	*Deficiency*: anorexia, retarded growth, delayed sexual maturation, impaired wound healing, intestinal malabsorption *Excess*: relatively nontoxic	Widely distributed; liver, seafood

17, Fluoride. Advisable daily intakes of sodium, potassium, and chloride (Fomon, 1974, p. 269) in early childhood are:

	Sodium (mEq)	Chloride (mEq)	Potassium (mEq)
Birth to 4 months	8	7	7
4 months to 12 months	6	6	6
12 months to 24 months	6	7	6
24 months to 36 months	8	10	8

MATERNAL NUTRITION

Nutrition During Pregnancy

Normal physiologic processes are greatly altered during pregnancy and additional demands are imposed on the maternal organism. The objectives of nutrition during pregnancy are to:

1. Provide for normal maternal maintenance requirements
2. Provide for growth and development of the fetus
3. Reduce the incidence of complications of pregnancy.

RECOMMENDED DAILY DIETARY ALLOWANCES

The RDAs during pregnancy for women of different age groups are listed in Table 1. The pregnant woman needs more calories, protein, vitamins, and minerals than the nonpregnant woman. For most women on well-balanced diets these increases can usually be met by means of increased caloric intake using the Daily Food Guide as presented in Table 6. Supplements are unnecessary except for iron and folic acid. If a careful nutrition history reveals dietary inadequacies, appropriate measures must be taken. Other adjustments must be made on an individual basis considering age, body size, physical status, climate, and cultural factors.

Table 6
Daily Food Guide

	Number of Servings		
Food Group	Non-pregnant Woman	Pregnant Woman	Lactating Woman
Protein foods			
animal[a]	2	2	2
vegetable[b]	2	2	2
Milk and milk products	2	4	5
Breads and cereals	4	4	4
Vitamin C rich fruits and vegetables	1	1	1
Dark green vegetables	1	1	1
Other fruits and vegetables	1	1	1

Source: Maternal and Child Health Branch, California Department of Health, June 1977.
[a]1 serving is 2 oz (60g).
[b]Should include at least 1 serving of legumes.

SUPPLEMENTATION

Iron. Iron is necessary during pregnancy to maintain normal hemoglobin levels and reserves in the mother, to furnish iron requirements to the fetus, and to provide the fetus with sufficient iron stores to be utilized after birth. Six to seven milligrams of elemental iron (usable iron) must be absorbed daily to meet these requirements. Diets consumed by American women rarely contain sufficient absorbable iron to meet these needs. Usually pregnant women ingest 13 to 14 mg of dietary iron per day, most of which is not absorbed. See Absorption of Iron, this chapter.

Recommendation. The Committee on Maternal Nutrition of the National Academy of Sciences (1970) recommends iron supplementation during the second and third trimesters. Ferrous iron, 30 to 60 mg daily, is the recommended dose.

Folic acid. There is evidence that pregnancy is associated with an increased, although small, risk of megaloblastic anemia due to folate deficiency. Other evidence suggests that folate deficiency may predispose toward spontaneous abortion and hemorrhage (Committee on Maternal Nutrition, 1970).

> Recommendation. A daily supplement of 200 to 400 μg of folic acid is recommended throughout the course of pregnancy. This should easily prevent folic acid deficiency in ·practically all women.

WEIGHT GAIN

Limitation of maternal weight gain during pregnancy by limitation of calories has been recognized as potentially hazardous to the fetus. Limiting the weight gain of normal pregnant women to 10 to 14 pounds is not justified. The average acceptable weight gain for a favorable outcome is approximately 11 to 12 kg or 24 to 27 pounds.

SODIUM RESTRICTION

Sodium restriction and/or prescription of diuretics were formerly employed to prevent preeclampsia. This practice is now recognized as potentially hazardous. To meet the increased need for sodium during pregnancy and to avoid sodium deficit, no sodium restrictions are advised. The use of diuretics is also discouraged.

Nutrition During Lactation

RECOMMENDED DAILY DIETARY ALLOWANCES

A mother's diet may be quite varied without affecting the composition or volume of breast milk as long as good nutrition is maintained according to the RDA's listed in Table 1 and the Daily Food Guide in Table 6. If the diet is deficient, there may be decreased quantity of milk, but the quality will remain constant as long as the mother's body stores can supply the missing nutrients.

LACTATION NUTRITION GUIDELINES

Key factors to include in nutrition counseling during lactation are:

- Follow the Daily Food Guide (Table 6)
- Do not restrict calories
- Drink 2 to 3 quarts of fluid daily
- Take 30 to 60 mg of ferrous iron daily
- Avoid oral contraceptives for 6 weeks post partum

INFANT NUTRITION

This section presents data on the nutritional aspects of breast milk, commonly used infant formulas, iron nutrition during infancy, solid foods, and recommended vitamin and mineral supplementation during infancy.

Breast Milk

COMPOSITION

Colostrum. This is the initial milk secreted during the first 5 to 10 days after birth. Colostrum differs from mature breast milk in that it is:

1. Lower in energy value
2. Higher in protein
3. Higher in sodium, potassium, and chloride

Colostrum is high in antibodies, especially IgA, which may provide protection from enteric infections particularly enteropathic *E. coli.* It also facilitates the elimination of meconium from the GI tract.

Mature milk. Table 7 summarizes and compares the composition of mature human milk and whole cow milk. Significant differences exist and include the following:

- Protein and minerals. Cow milk is higher in these constituents because the growth rate of the calf is twice as rapid as the growth rate of the human infant. Thus, cow milk has a higher renal solute load which may tax the infant's kidney function.
- Casein. The casein content of cow milk is twice as high as in breast milk. This results in formation of a large and difficult-to-digest mass of curds in the infant stomach unless cow milk is acidified and heated.
- Fat. The fat of human milk is more easily absorbed than the butterfat of cow milk. Butterfat contains more saturated fatty acids.
- Cholesterol. Human milk is high in cholesterol. See this chapter, Cholesterol.
- Carbohydrate. The lactose content of cow milk is lower than breast milk. Extra sugar is usually added to cow milk formulas.
- Vitamins. Both human milk and cow milk contain *adequate* amounts of Vitamin A and the B complex vitamins and *inadequate* amounts of Vitamin D. Human milk will contain adequate Vitamin C if the maternal diet is adequate in Vitamin-C-containing foods. Cow milk is inadequate in Vitamin C.
- Iron. Both human milk and cow milk contain small amounts of iron. The iron in breast milk is well absorbed and may be sufficient during the first 4 to 6 months. See this chapter, Iron Nutrition in Infancy. The iron in cow milk is not well absorbed and is inadequate without supplementation.
- Fluoride. Both human milk and cow milk are inadequate in fluoride content.
- Antibodies. Mature human milk protects against enteritis and respiratory infections during the first year of life due to the presence of immunoglobulins, lactoferrin, and bifidus factor.

DISTRIBUTION OF CALORIES

The approximate percentages of calories in mature human milk are:

Protein	6–8 percent
Fat	50–56 percent
Carbohydrate	38–42 percent

Table 7
Composition of Mature Human Milk and Cow Milk

Composition	Human Milk	Cow Milk
Water (ml/100 ml)	87.1	87.2
Energy (kcal/100 ml)	75	66
Total solids (gm/100 ml)	12.9	12.8
Protein (gm/100 ml)	1.1	3.5
Fat (gm/100 ml)	4.5	3.7
Lactose (gm/100 ml)	6.8	4.9
Ash (gm/100 ml)	0.2	0.7
Proteins (% of total protein)		
Casein	40	82
Whey proteins	60	18
Nonprotein nitrogen (mg/100 ml)	32	32
(% of total nitrogen)	15	6
Amino acids (mg/100 ml)		
Essential		
Histidine	22	95
Isoleucine	68	228
Leucine	100	350
Lysine	73	277
Methionine	25	88
Phenylalanine	48	172
Threonine	50	164
Tryptophan	18	49
Valine	70	245
Nonessential		
Arginine	45	129
Alanine	35	75
Aspartic acid	116	166
Cystine	22	32
Glutamic acid	230	680
Glycine	0	11
Proline	80	250
Serine	69	160
Tyrosine	61	179
Fatty acids (% of total fatty acids)		
Essential		
Linoleic	10.6	2.1
Major minerals per liter		
Calcium (mg)	340	1170
Phosphorus (mg)	140	920
Sodium (mEq)	7	22
Potassium (mEq)	13	35
Chloride (mEq)	11	29
Magnesium (mg)	40	120
Sulfur (mg)	140	300

Table 7 (*Continued*)

Composition	Human Milk	Cow Milk
Trace minerals per liter		
Chromium (μg)	–	8–13
Manganese (μg)	7–15	20–40
Copper (μg)	400	300
Zinc (mg)	3–5	3–5
Iodine (μg)	30	47[a]
Selenium (μg)	13–50	5–50
Iron (mg)	0.5	0.5
Vitamins per liter		
Vitamin A (IU)	1898	1025[b]
Thiamin (μg)	160	440
Riboflavin (μg)	360	1750
Niacin (μg)	1470	940
Pyridoxine (μg)	100	640
Pantothenate (mg)	1.84	3.46
Folacin (μg)	52	55
B_{12} (μg)	0.3	4
Vitamin C (mg)	43	11[c]
Vitamin D (IU)	22	14[d]
Vitamin E (mg)	1.8	0.4
Vitamin K (μg)	15	60

Source: Reprinted with permission from S. J. Fomon, *Infant Nutrition*, 2nd ed., pp. 362–363,
© 1974 by the W. B. Saunders Company, Philadelphia.
[a]Range 10 to 200 μg/liter.
[b]Average value for winter milk; value for summer milk, 1690 IU/liter.
[c]As marketed; value for fresh cow milk 21 mg/liter.
[d]Average value for winter milk; value for summer milk, 33 IU

SUPPLEMENTATION

The infant who is breast-fed needs the following nutritional supplementation:

- Vitamin D. 400 IU/day. This used to be given in the form of cod liver oil but is now given primarily in combination with Vitamins A and C.
- Iron. See this chapter, Iron Nutrition in Infancy.
- Fluoride. See Chapter 17, Fluoride.

HYPERBILIRUBINEMIA

Breast milk jaundice may in some cases be severe, but generally is not a contraindication to breast feeding. See Chapter 20, Breastfeeding Jaundice.

Formulas and Milks

Milks from various species and in many different forms have been employed successfully in infant feeding. Commercially prepared formulas are currently the most popular because of convenience, standardization of ingredients, and fortification with vitamins and minerals.

INFANT FORMULAS

Several types of milk-based and milk-free formulas are used. Since whole cow milk is not a satisfactory food for infants, commercially prepared formulas are attempts to modify milk so they more closely resemble human milk. Table 8 analyzes commonly used infant formulas with regard to composition, distribution of calories, and supplementation.

FORMS OF COW MILK AND GOAT MILK

Although it is recommended that infants remain on breast milk or iron-fortified infant formula for most of the first year of life, many parents make the switch to some form of fresh cow milk before 6 months of age. It is important to know the composition of available cow milk so adequate nutritional counseling can be provided. Table 9 presents the composition of several forms of cow milk and goat milk. Analysis of these milks reveals several inadequacies related to their use in young infants. These inadequacies are as follows:

- Whole milk. See this chapter, Mature Milk.
- Evaporated milk. Protein content is high if diluted 1:1 with water. See Table 8 for the recipe for evaporated milk formula suitable for infants. Iron and Vitamin C content are inadequate.
- Skim milk. This is not suitable for use in infants under 1 year of age because of:
    1. Insufficient calories due to low fat content
    2. Excessive protein
    3. Insufficient essential fatty acids, Vitamin C, and iron

- "Two Per Cent" or "low fat" milk. This is more suitable than skim milk but still could result in inadequate fat and caloric intake if other foods are not fed. Iron and Vitamin C are inadequate.
- Goat milk. Even though not widely used in the United States, goat milk is a major source of infant nutrition in many parts of the world. The one major deficiency in goat milk is folacin (folic acid), and infants receiving this milk should be given a daily folacin supplement of 50 μg to prevent megaloblastic anemia. Goat milk is also deficient in iron, Vitamin C, and Vitamin D.

OTHER FORMS OF MILK

- Certified milk. Milk which may be raw or pasteurized but has been certified as to cleanliness
- Condensed milk. Milk which has more sugar and less protein than evaporated milk. It should not be used interchangeably with evaporated milk, nor in infant feeding.
- Cultured milk (e.g., buttermilk, acidophilus milk, yogurt). Milk prepared with added lactic acid and which aids in replacing normal bowel flora
- Dry milk. Milk which is a sterile product that can be kept for long periods of time. It is usually made from skim milk since fat particles present storage problems.
- Homogenized milk. Milk which has gone through a process by which fat globules are broken down in size and are more evenly distributed throughout the milk
- Pasteurized milk. Milk which has been sterilized
- Raw milk. Milk which has not been heat treated

MILK SUBSTITUTES

- Filled milks. These are combinations of skim milk solids and nonmilk fat. They may have all the ingredients of regular milk but, if coconut oil is used as the fat, will be deficient in linoleic acid.
- Imitation milk. This consists of water, protein, corn syrup, sucrose, and vegetable oil. It is nutritionally inferior, especially in

Table 8
Analysis of Commonly Used Infant Formulas

Type of Formula	Composition of Formula	Supplementation[a]	Comments
FORMULAS BASED ON COW MILK: 1. Cow Milk with added carbohydrate Evaporated Milk Purevap (Pet)	In these formulas cow protein and cow fat (butterfat) are combined with added lactose or corn sugar. This results in a formula that supplies calories as: Protein 14–16% Fat 36–38% Carbohydrate 46–50% (20 calories per ounce)	Unless added will be deficient in Vitamins C and D and iron	Evaporated milk is the most widely known formula of this type and used to be used extensively in this country. It is still nutritionally sound and an economical approach to infant feeding. Recipe for one day's supply of evaporated milk formula: 13 oz evaporated milk 19 oz water 1½ oz corn syrup Recipe for one individual feeding of evaporated milk formula: 2 oz evaporated milk 3 oz water 2 tsp corn syrup

2. Nonfat cow's milk, vegetable oils, and carbohydrate Enfamil (Mead-Johnson) Similac (Ross) Modilac (Gerber) Bremil (Syntex)	Corn oil, coconut oil, and soy oil are generally used and are well absorbed These formulas provide calories as: Protein 10% Fat 48–50% Carbohydrate 41–43% (20 calories per ounce)	Available with adequate vitamin supplementation Available with or without iron supplementation	*Note:* After 6 months there is no need to add corn syrup since infants are usually on solid foods. Formulas containing butterfat may result in higher fat excretion and occasionally in steatorrhea in young infants. Butterfat also causes a sour odor to vomitus. Available as powder, liquid concentrate, or ready-to-feed Suitable for feeding of full-term and premature infants with no special nutritional requirements
3. Nonfat cow's milk, whey proteins, vegetable oil, and carbohydrate Similac PM 60/40 (Ross) SMA (Wyeth)	These formulas have a protein ratio of whey to casein resembling human milk (60:40). The proteins have also been demineralized so	Available with vitamin and iron supplementation	Special characteristics of these formulas: 1. Low renal solute load in relation to caloric concentration 2. Low sodium content

Continued on next page

Table 8 (Continued)

Type of Formula	Composition of Formula	Supplementation[a]	Comments
	minerals in desired amounts can be deliberately added. This results in mineral concentrations similar to human milk. Calories are supplied as: Protein 9% Fat 48% Carbohydrate 43% (20 calories per ounce)		This makes them desirable for use in infants with renal disease, congenital heart disease, or congestive heart failure, as well as for normal infants.
4. Milk-based formula for older infants Similac Advance (Ross)	This formula is composed of nonfat cow milk and soy-protein isolate, corn oil, and lactose as carbohydrate with calories supplied as follows: Protein 26% Fat 27% Carbohydrate 47% (16 calories per ounce)	Fully supplemented with vitamins and iron	Key features of this formula: 1. Low caloric concentration 2. Low percentage of calories as fat 3. Low in saturated fat 4. Rich in iron (18 mg/liter) 5. High percentage of calories as protein It is designed to be used when infants switch from infant formula to other

	forms of cow milk. The age at which an infant switches from infant formula is important here since the infant under 6 months of age would be receiving more calories from protein and fewer calories from fat than those amounts advised. Other foods in the diet must be considered in terms of fat content since most commercially prepared baby foods are high in protein and carbohydrate but low in fat.		Suitable for use in feeding infants and children with celiac disease, cystic fibrosis, diarrhea, or other conditions involving steatorrhea or *Continued on next page*
5. Special milk-based formulas			
Probana (Mead-Johnson)	Probana is high in protein, high in carbohydrate, and low in fat. Carbohydrate is from simple sugars and banana powder.	Supplemented with vitamins but does *not* contain iron	

Table 8 (*Continued*)

Type of Formula	Composition of Formula	Supplementation[a]	Comments
	It supplies calories as: Protein 27% Fat 14% Carbohydrate 51%		poor fat absorption. Renal solute load is high. Watch for dehydration.
Lonolac (Mead-Johnson)	The special feature of this formula is its very low sodium content. It contains 1 mEq sodium per liter.	Not supplemented. Need to add Vitamins C and D and iron	Designed for use in infants with congestive heart failure. The low sodium content makes it unsuitable for long-term use.
MILK-FREE FORMULAS: 1. Soy-based formulas Isomil (Ross) Prosobee (Mead-Johnson) Nursoy (Wyeth) Neo-Mull-Soy (Syntex) I-Soyalac (Loma Linda) Mull-Soy (Syntex)	These formulas provide protein in the form of soy-isolate or soy flour, fat as vegetable oils, and carbohydrate as sucrose or corn sugar. Soy-isolate formulas provide calories as: Protein 12–15% Fat 45–48% Carbohydrate 39–40% (20 calories per ounce)	Most of these formulas have been supplemented with calcium, iodine, vitamins, and iron. Labels on individual products should be checked for adequacy of supplementation.	Suitable for use in feeding milk-sensitive infants

CHO-Free Formula Base (Syntex)	This is a soy-isolate protein, soy oil, and essentially carbohydrate-free formula. (12 calories per ounce)	Supplemented with adequate vitamins and iron	For short-term use in feeding infants and children with intolerance to disaccharides or other complex sugars; may be used in management of galactosemia. Must be supplemented with carbohydrate (glucose) or else will result in a ketogenic diet
2. Nonsoy, milk-free formulas.			
Meat-Base Formula (Gerber)	The protein comes from beef heart, the fat is both animal and vegetable, and the carbohydrate content is low.	Supplemented with calcium, vitamins, and iron	A nutritionally adequate formula for infants and children intolerant to cow and goat milk.
Nutramigen (Mead-Johnson)	The protein is in hydrolyzed form specially processed to remove allergenic substances. The fat is highly refined corn oil and the carbohydrate is from sugar and tapioca starch.	Fully supplemented with vitamins and iron	Suitable for use in infants and children allergic or intolerant to ordinary food proteins. Provides lactose-free feedings in galactosemia.

Continued on next page

Table 8 (*Continued*)

Type of Formula	Composition of Formula	Supplementation[a]	Comments
	Calories provided as: Protein 13% Fat 35% Carbohydrate 52%		
Lofenalac (Mead-Johnson)	The protein has been treated to remove most of the phenylalanine Calories provided as: Protein 13% Fat 35% Carbohydrate 52%	Vitamins, minerals, and iron are added	For use as basic food in low-phenylalanine management of infants and children with phenylketonuria; provides essential nutrients without the high phenylalanine content present in natural food proteins
Portagen (Mead-Johnson)	This formula is essentially lactose free and also uses medium chain triglycerides which are	Fully supplemented with vitamins and iron	For use in the management of children with impaired fat absorption, pancreatic and liver disease

more easily digested and absorbed than conventional food fat. Calories provided as:

Protein	14%
Fat	42%
Carbohydrate	44%

Pregestimil (Mead-Johnson)

Contains protein hydrolysate, medium chain triglycerides, and carbohydrate as glucose. Calories provided as:

Protein	13%
Fat	36%
Carbohydrate	51%

Fully supplemented with vitamins and iron

Useful in the management of infants and children with severe gastrointestinal abnormalities in which absorption of several nutrients is impaired

---

[a]Fluoride supplementation. Currently marketed milks and formulas have variable fluoride. Need for fluoride supplementation must be evaluated based on the amount of water subsequently added to the milk or formula, the amount of water consumed on its own, and the level of fluoride in the community water supply. Due to difficulties in determining amounts of fluoride an infant is getting, current recommendations are to avoid supplementation during the first 6 months (Fomon, 1974). See Chapter 17, Fluoride.

Table 9

Composition of Several Forms of Cow Milk and of Fresh Fluid Goat Milk

	Cow Milk				Goat Milk (Fresh Fluid)
	Whole Milk	Evaporated Diluted 1:1 With Water	Fresh Fluid Skim Milk	"Two Per Cent"	
Energy (kcal/100 ml)	66	68.5	36	59	67
Major constituents (gm/100 ml)					
Protein	3.5	3.5	3.6	4.2	3.2
Fat	3.7	3.8	0.1	2.0	4.0
Carbohydrate	4.9	4.8	5.1	6.0	4.6
Caloric distribution (% of calories)					
Protein	22	19	40	28	19
Fat	48	50	3	31	53
Carbohydrate	30	31	57	41	28

Minerals/liter					
Calcium (mg)	1170	1260	1210	1430	1290
Phosphorus (mg)	920	1025	950	1120	1060
Sodium (mEq)	22	26	23	27	15
Potassium (mEq)	35	39	37	45	46
Iron (mg)	0.5	0.5	trace	1	1
Vitamins/liter					
Vitamin A (IU)	1025	1850	90	800	2074
Thiamin (µg)	440	280	400	400	400
Riboflavin (µg)	1750	1900	1700	2100	1840
Niacin (mg)	940	1.0	0.9	1.0	1.9
Pyridoxine (µg)	640	370	450	—	70
Pantothenate (mg)	3.46	3.5	3.6	—	3.4
Folacin (µg)	55	55	55	55	6
Vitamin C (mg)	11	5.5	19	10	15
Vitamin D (IU)	400	400	—	400	24
Vitamin E (IU)	0.4	1.3	—	—	—

Source: Adapted with permission from S. J. Fomon, *Infant Nutrition*, 2nd ed., p. 372, © 1974 by the W. B. Saunders Company, Philadelphia.

protein, calcium, and phosphorus, and usually lacks vitamin supplementation. Although inexpensive it should not be used as the chief source of milk (Brown, 1975; Fomon, 1974).

Iron Nutrition in Infancy

IRON STORES AT BIRTH

The normal birth weight infant of a well-nourished mother is born with adequate stores of iron to meet body needs for hemoglobin production up to 4 to 6 months of age. After this time body stores must be re-supplied to ensure proper blood formation and to prevent iron deficiency anemia (see Chapter 20, Iron Deficiency Anemia).

In small and preterm infants, neonatal iron stores will be depleted after about 2 months of age.

IRON REQUIREMENTS

The normal healthy infant at birth has approximately 135 mg of iron stored in body tissues. At 1 year of age the infant should have 270 mg of iron since the red blood cell mass doubles during the first year. Thus, another 135 mg of iron must be absorbed from exogenous sources during the first year. This breaks down to 0.3 mg of iron absorbed per day. Additional but smaller amounts are required for production of other iron compounds and to account for dermal losses (Rudolph, 1977).

ADVISABLE INTAKES

The RDAs (see Table 1) for iron intake in infancy are:

Age	Amount
0 to 6 months	10 mg/day
6 mo. to 3 yr.	15 mg/day

These are amounts that, considering the various rates of absorption from different sources of iron, are sufficient to meet known requirements.

ABSORPTION OF IRON

Absorption of iron varies with age, state of health, form of iron ingested, source of iron, amount of iron, and the interaction of iron with other dietary components and with intestinal secretions (e.g., iron absorption is enhanced in the presence of ascorbic acid and amino acids).

Form of iron. Absorption occurs in the small intestine in the *ferrous* form. Other forms must be broken down to the ferrous form. The absorption of different forms of iron is as follows:

Good Absorption	*Poor Absorption*
Heme iron (animal)	Vegetable iron (inorganic)
Ferrous iron including:	Ferric iron including:
Ferrous sulfate	Ferric cholinate
Ferrous succinate	Ferric orthophosphate
Ferrous lactate	Sodium iron pyrophosphate
Ferrous fumarate	Reduced iron of large
Ferrous gluconate	particle size
Reduced iron of small	
particle size	
(electrolytic iron	
powder)	

Rate of absorption. It is generally assumed that from 1 to 20 percent (an average of 10 percent) of ingested iron is absorbed. Vegetable iron (e.g., rice, spinach, beans, corn, wheat, soy beans) is in the lower range of 1 to 10 percent; animal products are in the upper range of 10 to 20 percent. Human breast milk has a small amount of iron (approximately 0.5 to 1.5 mg/liter) but it is well absorbed at approximately 50 percent. Cow milk has a similar amount of iron but is absorbed at a rate of 10 percent. Iron-fortified formulas and cereals have iron absorption rates of about 5 percent.

IRON SUPPLEMENTATION IN INFANCY

To provide sound nutrition and to prevent iron deficiency anemia it is recommended that all infants receive iron supplementation from one or more sources during the first year of life. The level of supplementation suggested by the American Academy of Pediatrics (Committee on Nutrition, 1976, p. 765), is as follows:

Term infants	1 mg/kg/day
Preterm infants	2 mg/kg/day up to 15 mg/day

Sources of iron should be introduced not later than 4 months in full-term infants (see below for breast-fed infants) and not later than 2 months in preterm and low-birth-weight infants.

Breast-fed infants. Since breast milk contains up to 1.5 mg of iron per liter which is absorbed at a rate of 50 percent, many breast-fed infants will absorb 0.75 mg of iron per day, more than enough to meet requirements (see this chapter, Iron Requirements). Therefore, the infant who is exclusively breast-fed does not need other exogenous sources of iron until its birth weight triples (McMillan, 1976, p. 689). When breast-feeding is discontinued before 6 months of age, an iron-fortified formula and iron-fortified cereal should be given.

SOURCES OF IRON

Iron content of some infant foods and major sources of iron are listed in Tables 10 and 11. In early infancy when the variety of foods ingested is limited the chief sources of dietary iron supplementation are iron-fortified formulas and dry infant cereals.

Iron-fortified formulas. These are adequately fortified with absorbable iron (approximately 12 mg/liter) and should be used as long as possible during the first year of life. When infants are switched to fresh cow's milk during the first year there is a high incidence of enteric blood loss which can contribute to iron deficiency.

Infant cereals. Dry infant cereals are currently fortified with re-

Table 10
Iron Content of Selected Foods Fed to Infants in the United States

Food	Elemental Iron	
	(mg/100 gm of food)	(mg/100 kcal)
Milk or formula		
Human milk	0.05	0.07
Cow milk	0.05	0.07
Iron-fortified formula	0.9–1.3	1.2–1.8
Formula unfortified with iron	<0.05	<0.05
Infant cereals		
Iron-fortified (dry) mixed with milk[a]	7–14	7–14
Wet-packed cereal-fruit	1–6	1.3–7.5
Strained and junior foods		
Meats		
Liver and a few others	4–6	4–6
Most meats	1–2	1–2
Egg yolks	2–3	1.0–1.5
"Dinners"		
High meat	<1	<1
Vegetable-meat	<0.5	<0.5
Vegetables[b]	<0.5	<0.5
Fruits[b]	<0.5	<0.5

Source: Reprinted with permission from S. J. Fomon, *Infant Nutrition*, 2nd ed, p. 314, © 1974 by the W. B. Saunders Company, Philadelphia.
[a] Assuming that one part by weight of dry cereal is mixed with six parts of milk
[b] A few varieties of vegetables and fruits provide 1 to 2 mg of iron/100 gm (1 to 3 mg/100 kcal).

duced iron of small particle size which is well absorbed. Three to six tablespoons of dry cereal served twice a day will provide sufficient iron to meet most infants' needs. This form of cereal is also recommended for use during the second year of life.

Medicinal iron.   See Chapter 20, Iron Deficiency Anemia.

Solid Foods

Infants receiving breast milk or formula with appropriate vitamin and mineral supplements do not need additional foods before 6 months of age. No nutritional or psychologic advantages accrue to

Table 11
Typical Foods as Sources of Iron

Food	Size of Serving	Iron, in Milligrams per Avg. Serving	Iron, in Milligrams per 100 Grams of Food
Liver			
Lamb, broiled	2 slices (75 gm)	13.4	17.9
Beef, fried	2 slices (75 gm)	6.6	8.8
Chicken, cooked	¼ cup (50 gm)	4.3	8.8
Meats (lean or med. fat)			
Beef, round, cooked	1 lg. hamburger (85 gm)	3.0	3.5
rib roast, cooked	3 slices (100 gm)	2.6	2.6
Pork, chop, cooked	1 med. lg. chop (80 gm)	2.5	3.1
Lamb, shoulder chop	1 chop, cooked (90 gm)	1.6	1.8
Baked beans, canned with			
pork and molasses	½ cup (130 gm)	3.0	2.3
pork and tomato	½ cup (130 gm)	2.3	1.8
Fruits, dried (uncooked)			
Apricots	4 halves, (30 gm)	1.7	5.5
Prunes	4–5 medium, (30 gm)	1.2	3.9
Figs	2 small (30 gm)	0.9	3.0
Raisins	2 tbsp (20 gm)	0.6	3.5
Legumes			
Soy beans, dry	½ cup scant, cooked (30 gm dry)	2.5	8.4
Peanut butter	2 tbsp scant (30 gm)	0.6	2.0
Lima beans, fresh	½ cup, cooked (80 gm)	2.0	2.5
Peas, fresh, green	½ cup, cooked (80 gm)	1.4	1.8

Molasses, med.	1 tbsp (20 gm)	1.2	6.0
Eggs, whole	1 med. (50 gm)	1.2	2.3
Leafy vegetables			
Spinach	½ cup, cooked (90 gm)	2.0	2.2
Beet greens	½ cup, cooked (100 gm)	1.9	1.9
Chard	½ cup, cooked (100 gm)	1.8	1.8
Kale (leaves only)	½ cup, cooked (55 gm)	0.9	1.6
Turnip greens	½ cup, cooked (75 gm)	0.8	1.1
Vegetables			
Potatoes, sweet	1 med., baked (110 gm)	1.0	0.9
white	1 med., baked (100 gm)	0.7	0.7
Broccoli	⅔ cup (100 gm)	0.8	0.8
Brussels sprouts	5–6 med. (70 gm)	0.8	1.1
Cauliflower	¾ cup, cooked (100 gm)	0.7	0.7
Carrots	⅔ cup, diced, cooked (100 gm)	0.6	0.6
String beans	¾ cup, cooked (100 gm)	0.6	0.6
Beets	2, 2-in. diam. (100 gm)	0.5	0.5
Bread			
White, enriched	1 slice	0.6	2.5
Whole-wheat	1 slice	0.5	2.3
White, unenriched	1 slice	0.2	0.7
Cereals, whole grain (oats, corn, wheat, rice)	See label on package—range from 0.2 to 0.7 mg unenriched, up to 10 mg enriched, per serving.		
Fresh fruits and fruit vegetables	100 gm serving, mostly	0.3–0.6	
Milk, whole, fluid, cow's	½ pint, or 8 oz glass (244 gm)	0.10	0.04
Human	½ pint, or 8 oz (244 gm)	0.24	0.1

Source: Reprinted with permission from L. J. Bogert, et al., *Nutrition and Physical Fitness,* (Philadelphia: Saunders, © 1973), p. 269.

infants started on solids during this period. In addition, the cost per unit of calories is considerably more for commercially prepared baby foods than for most milks and formulas. The possibility also exists that early introduction of solids might contribute to habits of overfeeding and later overeating. Constipation can occur if solid food intake is high. Another factor involves the possibility of food allergy since foreign proteins in foods can become antigens due to the lack of sufficient IgA production in the infant under 6 to 7 months. Nonetheless, surveys of current infant feeding practices in the United States reveal that most infants are receiving commercially prepared strained foods by 4 weeks of age.

From a developmental perspective, infants by 5 to 6 months of age are interested in chewing, picking up food, and putting everything available into their mouths. Many parents and professionals feel it is appropriate to introduce solids during this period to satisfy these developmental needs.

NUTRITIONAL CONSIDERATIONS

The trend toward early introduction of solid foods will not be easily or quickly reversed. Nurse practitioners provide education and support for parents based on current knowledge but must also accept parents who, for a wide variety of reasons (family tradition, peer pressure, competition with neighbors, and others) insist on early feeding of solids. Parents must not be made to feel guilty about their feeding practices. Information that may help parents to make informed decisions follows.

Distribution of calories. When solid foods are introduced it is possible that marked variation in caloric distribution will occur. See Table 12. Generally speaking, solid baby foods are rich sources of carbohydrate, moderate sources of protein, and poor sources of fat. When infants are fed solids and also switched to whole cow milk, 2% milk, or skim milk, protein calories will be very high (an expensive and inefficient method of providing calories) and, in the case of skim milk, fat calories will be very low. See Table 9. Diets that provide excess amounts of protein, sodium, and other solutes can be a hazard for the infant because they create a large solute load which the infant cannot efficiently excrete unless body fluid reserves are drawn upon. If the infant then becomes febrile,

Table 12
Caloric Density and Distribution of Calories in Strained Foods Relative to Human Milk and Infant Formula

Food	kcal/ 100 gm	Percentage of Calories From		
		Protein	Fat	Carbohydrate
Egg yolks	192	21	76	3
Meats	106	53	46	1
Desserts and puddings	96	4	7	89
Fruits	85	2	2	96
High-meat dinners	84	29	47	24
Human milk	75	8	50	42
Infant formula	67	9	48	43
Fruit juices	65	2	2	96
Creamed vegetables	63	13	13	74
Soups and dinners	58	16	28	56
Plain vegetables	45	14	6	80

Source: Adapted from T. A. Anderson, "Are Infants Getting the Right Foods?" in *Year ONE: Nutrition, Growth, Health,* (Columbus, Ohio: Ross Laboratories, 1975), p. 19.

tachypneic, or develops diarrhea, the increased water lost via the skin, lungs, and intestines may not be adequately met from body fluid reserves and the potential exists for hypernatremia or dehydration.

Commercially prepared infant foods

COMPOSITION. The composition and nutritional quality of commercially prepared infant foods vary widely and without knowledge of the facts or understanding of how to read labels, parents can unknowingly purchase nutritionally inferior products. Some examples are as follows:

1. Iron content of infant cereals. Dry cereal preparations (rice, barley, oatmeal, high-protein) contain from 72 to 80 mg of iron per 100 gm of cereal. By contrast, the wet-pack cereals with fruit, often purchased because parents think they will be more appealing to the infant, contain only 0.2 to 5.3 mg of iron per 100 gm (Fomon, 1974, pp. 410–411).

2. Combination dinners. In the combination meat and vegetable dinners the label is the key to nutritional ingredients. Gerber's *Beef* with *Vegetables* contains 6.1 gm of protein per 100 gm, while Gerber's *Vegetables* with *Beef* contains 1.6 gm of protein per 100 gm.
3. Single preparations. Single products are usually more nutritional than combinations. For example, plain meats contain from 12 to 15 gm of protein per 100 gm.

Thus, it behooves the nurse practitioner to obtain listings of baby foods and their ingredients to share the facts with parents. Complete listings are available from the major manufacturers (Gerber, Heinz, Beechnut).

RECENT CHANGES. In recent years pressures brought by consumers and professionals have resulted in many changes in the manufacture of strained and junior foods. Some of the more significant changes are:

1. Reduction of excessive sodium content of many infant foods. The amount of sodium chloride has been reduced, and the addition of monosodium glutamate (MSG) has been discontinued.
2. Reduction of sucrose. The amount of sucrose added to fruits, desserts, vegetables, and dinners has been reduced but sucrose-containing fruits and desserts are still sold and purchased widely.
3. Use of more bio-available forms of iron in infant cereals. Electrolytic iron powder (reduced iron of small particle size) is now used in most cereals.

STORAGE AND REFRIGERATION OF COMMERCIAL BABY FOODS. Guidelines are as follows:

1. Formulas. Once a can of liquid ready-to-feed or concentrate has been opened it should be refrigerated, and the unused portion should be discarded after 48 hours.
2. Baby foods. After the first portion has been served, the lid should be replaced on the jar, and the jar should be refrigerated. If jars are being saved for another meal, the food should be taken out of the jar for heating. Once a jar has been opened

the entire contents should be served in 2 to 3 days, or else it should be discarded.

Home preparation of baby foods. Many parents are interested in preparing their own baby foods at home for both economic and nutritional benefits. This practice should be encouraged.

REFERENCES FOR PARENTS. Two inexpensive paperback books for parents are:

1. Castle, S. *The Complete Guide to Preparing Baby Foods at Home.* Garden City, NY: Doubleday, 1973.
2. Kenda, M. E. and P. S. Williams. *The Natural Baby Food Cookbook.* New York: Avon, 959 Eighth Ave., 1972.

DIRECTIONS FOR BLENDER PREPARATION. A good blender can be purchased for approximately $35.00, and a baby-food grinder is available for under $10.00.

1. Scrub all equipment with hot water and soap and rinse well.
2. Prepare food for cooking, removing skin, pits, or seeds. Bring to a full boil and cook until tender.
3. Add 1 cupful food at a time to blender with ¼ cup liquid (cooking liquid). More water may be needed for meat to allow blades to operate; care should be taken, however, to use as little water as possible.

Several methods may be used to prepare feedings for a number of days:

• Freeze pureed food (from blender) in ice-cube trays putting 2 tablespoons in one cube, or using 24 tablespoons for a 12-cube tray. When food is frozen hard the cubes may be stored in a plastic bag in the freezer.
• Place 2 tablespoons of the food in a paper cupcake liner and freeze on a cookie tray. When hard, store as above.
• Wrap 2 tablespoons of the food in a piece of aluminum foil and store in freezer.
• To reheat: Place food in a glass custard cup and heat until very hot in a covered pan of boiling water. Cool before feeding.

BLENDER RECIPES. A sample of recipes is included so nurse practitioners can assist parents who have questions.

Meats

½ cup cubed cooked meat
⅛ teaspoon salt (optional)
2 tablespoons milk, formula, or liquid from boiled meat

Place all ingredients in a blender and mix at high speed until perfectly smooth. To test for smoothness, put a small amount on the palm of your hand. Rub with finger. If any large particles can be felt, process again.

Chicken

½ cup cooked chicken, cut in pieces
½ tablespoon cream or milk
Pinch of salt (optional)

Place ingredients in blender and mix to a smooth pulp. Yield: 1 to 2 servings.

Vegetables

½ cup freshly cooked vegetable
2 tablespoons milk or formula
Dash salt

Put all ingredients in blender. Run at high speed until perfectly smooth. Test for smoothness. Yield: 1 to 2 servings.

Green Beans

½ cup cooked green beans
2 tablespoons milk or water
1 teaspoon butter or margarine
Dash salt (optional)

Place in blender and blend to a smooth pulp.

Tomato
___

1 fresh tomato
⅛ tsp. salt (optional)

Wash tomato thoroughly. Cut into quarters. Place in blender and blend to a smooth pulp.

Fruits
___

¾ cup cooked or canned fruit
½ teaspoon sugar
2 teaspoons liquid from fruit

Put all ingredients in blender. Blend at high speed until perfectly smooth.

Peaches
___

½ fresh peach, sliced
¼ teaspoon sugar (optional)

Peel peach and place in blender. Add sugar. Blend to smooth pulp.

Apricot Creme
___

½ cup apricots
¼ cup apricot juice
1½ cups milk
¼ cup sugar
3 tablespoons cornstarch
2 tablespoons non-fat dry milk solids

1. Blend apricots, juice, and 1 cup milk for 2 minutes at high speed.
2. Add non-fat dry milk solids and blend 2 minutes at low speed.
3. Heat mixture to boiling.

4. Mix sugar and cornstarch. Add ½ cup milk to this to form a paste.
5. Add to heated mixture and cook for 20 minutes.
6. Pour into serving dishes. Yield: 4 cups.

Serving size. At birth the stomach capacity of the infant is 30 to 60 ml (1 to 2 oz); at one month 90 to 150 ml (3 to 5 oz); and by 1 year of age will hold 240 ml (8 oz) of fluid and 1 cup of solids. Small amounts (e.g., a teaspoon) of each new food should be offered and gradually increased as tolerated. After initial introduction the following quantities are suggested as guidelines for serving sizes during the first year:

- Cereal. Up to 6 tablespoons daily in one to two servings. The usual dilution of cereal with milk or formula is one part cereal to six parts milk.
- Juices. Begin with 1 to 2 ounces and increase up to 4 ounces.
- Strained and junior foods. Serve one third to one half of the jar. Jar sizes of commercial foods (Brown, 1975, p. 148) are:

Strained foods: 3¾ to 4½ ounces
Meat and egg yolks: 3½ ounces
Junior foods: 7½ to 7¾ ounces
Junior meats: 3½ ounces
Junior high-meat dinners: 4½ to 4¾ ounces
Juices: 4½ ounces

Nutritional Needs of the Low-Birth-Weight Infant

DEFINITION

The low-birth-weight infant is defined as one with a birth weight less than 2500 gm.

NUTRITIONAL CONSIDERATIONS

The low-birth-weight infant requires a special approach to nutrition in view of the early cessation of transplacental supply of nutrients, immature metabolic systems, and the potential for an unusually rapid growth rate ("catch-up" growth). Specific features of the low-birth-weight infant related to nutrition include:

- Need for increased calories and protein for growth
- Need for increased vitamins and minerals for growth
- Efficient absorption of protein and carbohydrate but decreased absorption of fat (due to liver immaturity). Vegetable oils and human milk fat are relatively well absorbed.
- Loss of fat-soluble vitamins and calcium as a result of fecal fat loss
- Early depletion of iron stores predisposing to iron deficiency sometime after 2 or 3 months of age
- Low body stores of Vitamin E predisposing to Vitamin E deficiency during the first 3 months of life
- Inadequate stores of folic acid during the first 3 to 4 months of life (Dallman, 1974, pp. 750–751)

NUTRITIONAL MANAGEMENT

Early feeding of the low-birth-weight infant should be managed collaboratively with the physician. Nutritional management of the preterm and low-birth-weight infant includes:

- Additional calories. Approximately 110–150 cal/kg/day
- Distribution of calories as:

Protein	11 percent
Fat	50 percent
Carbohydrate	39 percent

- Additional vitamins (A, C, D, the B group) and calcium
- Iron supplementation by 2 to 3 months of age at 2 mg/kg/day. See this chapter, Iron Nutrition in Infancy.
- Vitamin E supplementation during the first 3 months of life. Alpha-tocopherol acetate (Aquasol E) in a dose of 5 to 25 IU/day is recommended. This is a water-soluble form of Vitamin E and is better absorbed. The requirement for Vitamin E increases as the levels of iron and polyunsaturated fats in the diet increase.
- Folic acid supplementation during the first 3 months of life at a dose of 50 μg/day (Dallman, 1974, pp. 750–751).

NUTRITION IN CHILDHOOD AND ADOLESCENCE

The Toddler and Preschool Period

During this period several factors affect nutritional status. Physical growth rate decreases, motor development matures, and cognitive and personality development increase. Although provision of adequate nutrition remains the parents' responsibility, the child affects the process by developing self-feeding skills, food preferences, and individual patterns of food intake. Guidelines for nutrition during this period include the following:

- A balanced diet that meets the RDAs (Table 1) should be offered.
- Food may need to be offered five to seven times a day (Pipes, 1977, p. 125).
- Milk intake need not exceed 16 ounces per day.
- The exact amounts of specific foods to be given cannot be rigidly prescribed and depend on the individual child's appetite. Suggestions are given in Table 13.
- A useful rule of thumb regarding minimal serving sizes for preschoolers is one bite (or teaspoonful) for each year of age of each food served.
- Finger foods should be emphasized. Protein-rich finger foods include peanut butter and crackers, cheese squares, hard-boiled eggs.
- Nuts, bony fish, popcorn should be avoided in the toddler because of the risk of aspiration or impaction.
- During these two periods when appetite slackens and independence needs of the young child further affect eating patterns, the temporary use of vitamin supplements may reassure the concerned parent of nutritional adequacy.
- Preschool children are at risk for iron-deficiency anemia and dental caries. Adequate iron-containing foods must be provided and excessive intake of sweet foods should be avoided.

School Age

The healthy school-age child usually presents few nutritional problems and adapts to family eating patterns. Table 13 gives suggestions for recommended foods and serving sizes for the school-age child. Snacks continue to be a primary source of nutrients, and an increasing amount of nutrition is obtained outside of the home. Assessment of nutritional status is important as undernutrition during this age period can contribute to poor school performance.

Adolescence

Nutritional needs are greatly influenced by this period of physical and emotional adjustment. It is a time when caloric needs increase due to the adolescent growth spurt; when protein, mineral, and vitamin needs reach adult values; and when female adolescents need increased iron coincident with menarche (see Chapter 20, Iron Deficiency Anemia). It is also a period when rebellion against previously acquired family eating habits is common, when activities outside the home increase and snacking becomes a major source of nutrients, and when strivings for self-identity and concerns over body image lead to extreme diets. The RDAs for adolescents are presented in Table 1.

NUTRITIONAL STATUS

A recent study found that adolescents from ages 10 to 16 years had the most unsatisfactory nutritional status of any age group (Torre, 1977, p. 118). Although protein deficiency is not extensive, deficiencies in iron, Vitamin A, calcium, Vitamin C, riboflavin, and thiamin are commonly found. Food sources of these nutrients are found in Tables 3 and 5.

SNACKS

Since adolescents obtain significant amounts of essential nutrients through snacks, suggested snacks include: fresh fruits, fruit juices,

Table 13
Recommended Food Intake for Good Nutrition[a]

Food Group	Servings/Day	Average Size of Servings					
		1 year	*2-3 years*	*4-5 years*	*6-9 years*	*10-12 years*	*13-15 years*
Milk and cheese (1.5 oz cheese = 1 C milk) (C = 1 cup – 8 oz or 240 gm)	4	½ C	½-¾ C	¾ C	¾-1 C	1 C	1 C
Meat group (protein foods)	3 or more						
Egg		1	1	1	1	1	1 or more
Lean meat, fish, poultry (liver once a week)		2 Tbsp	2 Tbsp	4 Tbsp	2-3 oz (4-6 Tbsp)	3-4 oz	4 oz. or more
Peanut butter			1 Tbsp	2 Tbsp	2-3 Tbsp	3 Tbsp	3 Tbsp
Fruits and vegetables	At least 4, including: 1 or more (twice as much tomato as citrus)						
Vitamin C source (citrus fruits, berries, tomato, cabbage, cantaloupe)		⅓ C citrus	½ C	½ C	1 medium orange	1 medium orange	1 medium orange
Vitamin A source (green or yellow fruits and vegetables)	1 or more	2 Tbsp	3 Tbsp	4 Tbsp (¼ C)	¼ C	⅓ C	½ C

Food group							
Other vegetables (potato and legumes, etc.) *or*	2	2 Tbsp	3 Tbsp	4 Tbsp (¼ C)	⅓ C	½ C	¾ C
Other fruits (apple, banana, etc.)		¼ C	⅓ C	½ C	1 medium	1 medium	1 medium
Cereals (whole-grain or enriched)	At least 4						
Bread		½ slice	1 slice	1½ slices	1-2 slices	2 slices	2 slices
Ready-to-eat cereals		½ oz	¾ oz	1 oz	1 oz	1 oz	1 oz
Cooked cereal (including macaroni, spaghetti, rice, etc.)		¼ C	⅓ C	½ C	½ C	¾ C	1 C or more
Fats and carbohydrates	To meet caloric needs						
Butter, margarine, mayonnaise, oils: 1 Tbsp = 100 calories (kcal)		1 Tbsp	1 Tbsp	1 Tbsp	2 Tbsp	2 Tbsp	2-4 Tbsp
Desserts and sweets: 100-calorie portions as follows: ⅓ C pudding or ice cream 2-3" cookies, 1 oz cake, 1⅓ oz pie, 2 tbsp jelly, jam, honey, sugar		1 portion	1½ portions	1½ portions	3 portions	3 portions	3-6 portions

[a]Based on Food Groups and the Average Size of Servings at Different Age Levels

Source: Reprinted with permission from V. C. Vaughan and R. J. McKay, *Nelson Textbook of Pediatrics*, 10th ed., p. 159, © 1975 by the W. B. Saunders Company, Philadelphia.

dried fruits, cheese, milk beverages, peanut butter and crackers, raw vegetables, nuts, leftover meats.

SPECIAL PROBLEMS

Pregnant adolescent. The RDAs for pregnant adolescents are found in Table 1. Iron, calcium, and Vitamin A are the nutrients most often lacking in these young women.

Oral contraceptives. Women taking oral contraceptives need increased amounts of Vitamin B_6 (pyridoxine), Vitamin C, and iron (Torre, 1977, p. 121). See this chapter, Maternal Nutrition.

Athletes. From a minimum of 2300 to 5000 calories per day may be required for individuals involved in very strenuous exercise and optimum distribution of calories is thought to be:

Protein   10–15 percent
Fat   25–35 percent
Carbohydrate   50–65 percent

Extra water and salt are also indicated (Torre, 1977, p. 122).

CULTURAL CONSIDERATIONS

Food preferences and eating patterns are influenced by many factors. Among the most significant factors are ethnic, racial, and cultural influences. It is impossible to identify an absolute diet pattern for any cultural group since no two people eat exactly alike. The information presented in Table 14 is intended to serve as a guide toward better understanding of predominant food choices of selected major cultural and ethnic groups.

Table 14
Acceptable Foods of Some Cultural and Ethnic Groups

Food Group	Mexican-Spanish	Chinese	Japanese	Black	American Indian
MILK	Milk (fresh, dry, evaporated), cheese (Cheddar, Monterey Jack, Parmesan, cottage, Mexican), Flan (very sweet custard), ice cream	Milk, especially flavored (usually in small quantities until taste is developed)	Larger quantities of milk are being consumed by the younger generations	Fresh homogenized milk, buttermilk, evaporated, nonfat dry (limited use in food preparation), ice cream, puddings (bread, rice, chocolate, coconut), cheese (Cheddar, cottage, Longhorn, American)	Fresh milk, evaporated (used in cooking), ice cream, cream pies
MEAT Poultry Eggs Legumes Game Fish and Seafoods	Beef, pork, lamb, chicken, tripe, hot sausage, beef intestines, fish, bologna, frankfurters, eggs, nuts, dry beans (especially pinto), chick peas	Pork, fish and shellfish, duck, chicken, organ meats, eggs, soybeans, nuts, red beans, black beans, split peas, bean curd (Tofu), pork sausage (frequently eaten three times a day; also is lower in fat content than regular sausage)	Pork, beef, fish, shellfish, chicken, soya beans, soya cake, red beans, lima beans, Tofu, eggs, nuts	Pork (fresh and cured—all cuts), organs, chitterlings (pork intestines), beef, lamb, tripe, chicken, turkey, duck, goose, fresh fish, tuna and salmon canned, eggs, nuts, cow peas, blackeyed peas, chick peas, beans: navy, red, and pinto, peanut butter, game: rabbit and venison	Pork, beef, lamb, chicken, duck, turkey, goose, fish (fresh and canned), shellfish, eggs, legumes: red, white or black beans, blackeyed peas, sunflower seeds, California walnuts, acorns, pine nuts, peanut butter, rabbit.

Continued on next page

Table 14 (Continued)

Food Group	Mexican-Spanish	Chinese	Japanese	Black	American Indian
FRUITS AND VEGETABLES					
Good sources of Vit. A	Spinach, wild greens, tomatoes, carrots, green peppers, yellow corn, pumpkin, peaches	Bok choy (Chinese mustard cabbage), many other leafy greens, green peppers, tomatoes	Sweet potatoes, spinach, carrots, tomatoes, yellow squash	Leafy greens (fresh ones preferred: wild greens, spinach, mustard, chard, beet tops, collards), tomatoes, sweet potato, carrots, pumpkin (if available), yellow squash, green peppers, okra	Tomatoes, pumpkin, carrots, yellow squash, leafy greens (dandelion, mustard), watercress
Good sources of Vit. C	Chili pepper (fresh), green peppers, tomatoes, Guava fruit, oranges, lemons, limes, papaya	Bok choy, green pepper, tomatoes (fresh), fruits (usually not eaten frequently) melons, oranges, papaya, watercress	Tomatoes (fresh), oranges, cabbage (raw)	Oranges (and juice), melons, green peppers, tomatoes, lemons, strawberries, collard, chard, mustard, and turnip greens, cabbage (raw)	Turnips (raw), cabbage (raw), oranges, grapefruit, melons, lemons, strawberries, mustard greens, watercress

Fair sources of Vit. C	Cactus leaves, potatoes, cabbage, cactus fruit, Zapote (a fruit), radishes	Leafy greens, Chinese cabbage, celery	Potatoes (in limited amounts), cabbage (cooked)	Potatoes (sweet and white), cabbage (cooked), turnips (cooked), radishes	Cabbage (cooked), potatoes (sweet and white), turnips (cooked)
Others	Summer squash, green peas, green beans, hominy, beets, celery, onions. When income permits: bananas, apples, fruit juices other than grapefruit or orange, fruit cocktail	Peas in pod, okra, summer squash, green beans, white turnips, mushrooms, eggplant, cucumbers, bamboo shoots, soybean sprouts	String beans, radishes, onions, eggplant, cucumber, pickled vegetables (as dessert), mushrooms, celery	Grapes, bananas, peaches, fruit cocktail, pineapples, apples, string beans, mixed vegetables, beets, turnips, canned green peas, onions, corn	Grapes, bananas, peaches, pears, fruit cocktail, apples, pineapple, green peas, green beans, beets, turnips, onions (green and bulb), cucumbers, eggplant, lettuce, corn
BREADS AND CEREALS	Rice, oats, cornmeal, corn flakes, thin spaghetti, noodles, macaroni, sweet breads, tortilla, biscuits	Rice, millet, oats, wheat, rice cakes, noodles, macaroni, refined bread, rice noodles, rice flour	Rice, rice cakes, crackers, refined bread, noodles	Refined breads, hot yeast breads, cornbread, biscuits, pancakes, cream of wheat, oats, grits, rice, cornmeal, flour, corn flakes and other dry cereals, macaroni	Refined bread, whole wheat bread, biscuits, cornbread, pancakes, cream of wheat, oatmeal, rice, dry cereal

VEGETARIAN DIETS

Types of Vegetarian Diets

Definitions of vegetarian diets are as follows:

1. Lacto-ovo-vegetarian diet is an all vegetable diet supplemented with milk, cheese, and eggs.
2. Lacto-vegetarian diet is an all vegetable diet supplemented with only milk and cheese.
3. Pure vegetarian or vegan diet excludes all foods of animal origin.

Nutritional Adequacy

Vegetarian diets can be nutritionally adequate and provide for normal growth and development in children provided they are based on sound nutritional knowledge.

- The protein sources must be varied to supply the essential amino acids. Most plant protein is incomplete protein. Exceptions are: soybeans, garbanzo beans, wheat germ, and brewer's yeast, which are complete proteins. Table 15 presents amino acid composition of selected foods.
- Amino acids in one food can supplement those in another food. For example, wheat is low in lysine but beans are high in lysine; rice is low in methionine but dried beans are high in methionine. Thus, two or more foods containing incomplete protein may be eaten at the same meal and supply complete protein.
- Folacin and Vitamin C sources must be included via a variety of fruits and green leafy vegetables.
- A diet which excludes all animal foods will be deficient in Vitamin B_{12}. Symptoms of B_{12} deficiency are soreness of the mouth and tongue, numbness and tingling of the hands and feet, back pain, pernicious anemia. To prevent B_{12} deficiency the vegetarian diet should include some animal protein such as eggs,

Table 15
Amino Acid Composition of Some Foods[a]

Essential Amino Acids	Cheese Eggs Milk Meat	Corn	Cereal	Legumes	Whole Grains (with germ)	Nuts Seed Oils Soybeans	Sesame and Sunflower Seeds	Peanut Protein	Green Leafy Veg. Leaf Prot.	Gelatin[b]	Yeast
Cystine[c]			−	−			x				
Methionine		x	x	−	x	−	x	−	−	−	x
Isoleucine	x	x		−	x				−	−	
Leucine	x										
Lysine	x		x	x	x	x					
Phenylalanine		−	−	−	−		−	−		−	−
Threonine	x	−	x	−	x		x				x
Tryptophan		−	−		x			−		−	x
Valine	x										

Source: Reprinted by permission from the Journal of Nutrition Education, 2:135–139: Spring 1971. Society for Nutrition Education.

Symbols: x = High amount of amino acid present in that food.
    − = Low amount of amino acid present in that food
    Blank spaces indicate a generally good balance of amino acids present with respect to other amino acids in the food.

[a] Be sure to complement a low amino acid with a food high in that amino acid at the same meal.
[b] Gelatin is not a good source of all essential amino acids.
[c] Not essential but added because hard to get in a vegetarian diet. Methionine and cystine can be compared as one.

cheese, or milk. If the vegetarian will not eat these foods, a B_{12} supplement is advised.
- A form of iodized salt should be used to provide needed iodine.
- Vitamins and minerals will be supplied adequately if good quality protein (including milk products and eggs), vegetables, and fruit (including dark green leafy, deep yellow, and citrus) are supplied regularly. Vegetarian sources of calcium, iron, and zinc are listed in Table 16.

In summary, any vegetarian diet which includes some animal foods (poultry, fish, milk, eggs, or cheese) can be nutritionally sound with careful planning. The strict vegetarian diets must be supplemented with a Vitamin B_{12} preparation and cannot be considered satisfactory for young children.

Sample Vegetarian Diet

A sample vegetarian diet compared to a typical American diet is found in Table 17.

OVERNUTRITION IN INFANCY AND CHILDHOOD

Assessment

Even though there are more well-fed children in the United States today than ever before, the problem of excessive weight gain and obesity must not be ignored when considering infant nutrition. Not only does obesity have serious physical, psychologic, and social consequences for the affected child but it is also well known that obesity predisposes to serious disease states in adulthood. Evidence currently indicates that 80 percent of overweight children will continue to be obese as adults (Rudolph, 1977, p. 254). Since treatment programs for obesity have proven generally ineffective, the prevention of obesity seems to be the most logical approach.

Table 16
Some Vegetarian Sources of Calcium, Iron, and Zinc

	Food	Calcium[a] (mg)	iron[a] (mg)	zinc[a] (mg)
Animal	hamburger, lean, 3 oz	10	3.0	3.8
protein	liver, beef, 2 oz	6	5.0	2.9'
foods	milk, fluid whole, 1 c	288	0.1	0.9
	milk, non-fat dry, ¼ c	219	0.1	0.8
	cheese, cheddar, 1 oz	213	0.3	0.5
	cheese, cottage, ½ c packed	115	0.3	—
Beans,	navy beans, ½ c cooked	48	2.5	0.9
seeds,	mature soybeans, ½ c cooked	37	1.3	—
nuts	sesame seeds, whole, ½ c	1160	10.5	—
	sesame seeds, hulled, ½ c	110	2.4	—
	sunflower seed kernels, ¼ c	36	2.1	—
	almonds, ½ c	166	3.3	—
	soybean milk, 1 c	60	1.5	—
Vegetables	spinach, ½ c cooked	*	2.0	0.8
	beet greens, ½ c cooked	*	1.4	—
	dandelion greens, ½ c cooked	126	1.6	—
	kale, ½ c cooked	74	0.6	—
	mustard greens, ½ c cooked	97	1.3	—
	turnip greens, ½ c cooked	126	0.8	—
	collards, ½ c cooked	144	0.6	—
	broccoli, ½ c cooked	68	0.6	—
	green peas, ½ c cooked	19	1.5	—
	sweet potatoes, 1 sm. (110 gm.)	44	1.0	—
Dried	dried apricots, ¼ c uncooked	25	2.0	—
fruits	dried figs, 1 large, uncooked	26	0.6	—
	prunes, 4 uncooked	14	1.1	—
	raisins, ½ oz. (1½ tbs)	9	0.5	—
Cereals,	rice, brown, ⅔ c cooked	7	0.3	1.1
breads	oatmeal, 1 c cooked	22	1.4	1.2
	oatmeal, dry, ¼ c (18 gm.)	10	0.8	0.7
	wheat bran flakes, 40%, 1 oz	21	1.3	1.0
	wheat germ, ¼ c	18	2.4	3.6
	white bread, enriched, 1 sl	21	0.6	0.2
	whole wheat bread, 1 sl	25	0.8	0.5

Source: Copyright December 1975, the American Journal of Nursing Company. Reproduced from the American Journal of Nursing Vol. 77 No. 12.

[a]RDA for adult male or female for calcium—800 mg.
  RDA for adult male for iron—10 mg; for adult female—18 mg.
  RDA for adult male or female for zinc—15 mg.
*Calcium in spinach and beet greens is present as insoluble calcium oxalate and cannot be absorbed.
—indicates values not reported.
Values for calcium and iron calculated from U.S. Dept. of Agriculture Handbook No. 8, *Composition of Foods*, and U.S. Dept. of Agriculture Home and Garden Bulletin No. 72, *Nutritive Value of Foods*.
Values for soybean milk obtained from U. D. Register and L. M. Sonnenberg, "The Vegetarian Diet." *J Am Dietet Assoc* 62:253–261, Mar 1973.
Values for zinc calculated from E. W. Murphy, B. W. Willis, and B. K. Watt. Provisional Tables on the Zinc Content of Foods. *J Amer Dietet Assoc* 66:345–355, May 1975.

Table 17
Sample Menus: Lacto-Ovo-Vegetarian and Typical American

Lacto-Ovo-Vegetarian	Cal.	Pro. (gm)	Fat (gm)	Carb. (gm)
½ c orange juice	60	1	tr	15
1 c oatmeal, cooked	130	5	2	23
1 tsp honey	22	tr	0	6
1 c skim milk	90	9	tr	12
1 sl whole wheat toast	60	3	1	12
1 tbs peanut butter	95	4	8	3
Hot cereal beverage	0	0	0	0
Total	457	22	11	71
1 c meatless split pea soup sandwich	145	9	3	21
2 sl whole wheat bread	120	6	2	24
1 oz cheddar cheese	115	7	9	1
½ tbs mayonnaise	33	tr	3	1
2 lettuce leaves	10	1	tr	2

Typical American	Cal.	Pro. (gm)	Fat (gm)	Carb. (gm)
½ c orange juice	60	1	tr	15
1 egg, scrambled	110	7	8	1
2 sl bacon	90	5	8	1
1 sl toast	60	3	1	12
1 pat butter	35	tr	4	tr
1 tbs jelly	50	tr	tr	13
1 c coffee				
(1 tbs cream)	30	1	3	1
(1 tsp sugar)	13	0	0	4
Total	448	17	24	47
1 c chicken noodle soup sandwich	220	8	6	33
2 sl white bread	120	6	2	24
2 sl bologna	80	3	7	tr
½ tbs mayonnaise	33	tr	3	1
2 lettuce leaves	10	1	tr	2

Left menu:

raw green pepper, ½ pod	7	tr	tr	2
raw apple	70	tr	tr	18
2 fig bars	100	2	2	22
1 c whole milk	160	9	9	12
Total	760	28	34	103
Spanish soybeans over rice and bulgur	451	18	17	61
spinach and mushroom salad				
1 c raw spinach	13	1	1	2
1 tbs oil in dressing	125	0	14	0
1 c skim milk yogurt	125	8	4	13
1 raw peach	35	1	tr	10
1 c apple juice	120	tr	tr	30
⅓ c mushrooms	9	1	tr	1
Total	878	29	35	117
Grand total	2095	85	74	291
% of total calories		16%	32%	55%

Right menu:

10 potato chips	115	1	8	10
1 choc. chip cookie	50	1	2	7
12 oz soft drink	145	0	0	37
Total	773	20	28	114
3 oz ground beef	245	21	17	0
½ c mashed potatoes	93	2	4	12
½ c green peas	58	5	1	10
iceberg lettuce wedge	15	1	tr	3
1 tbs blue cheese dressing	75	1	8	1
1 slice apple pie	350	3	15	51
1 c coffee				
(1 tbs cream)	30	1	3	1
(1 tsp sugar)	13	0	0	4
Total	879	34	48	82
Grand total	2100	71	100	243
% of total calories		13%	43%	45%

Source: Copyright December 1975, the American Journal of Nursing Company. Reproduced from the American Journal of Nursing Vol. 77 No. 12.

DEFINITION

Children with weights 10 to 20 percent above the mean for their height and age are defined as *markedly overweight;* those with weights greater than 20 percent above the mean are defined as *obese* (Rudolph, 1977, p. 255).

INCIDENCE

No definitive statistics are available, but it has been estimated that approximately 10 to 30 percent of American children are affected by obesity.

INFLUENCING FACTORS

All the following are thought to play a part in the complex etiology of obesity:

- Activity patterns, energy balance, metabolic rate
- Genetic influences
- Number and size of adipocytes. Adipocytes are those cells of adipose tissue capable of storing fat. They increase in number until puberty when adult values are reached. Obese children have increased cell *size,* and those who are already obese by 1 year of age have marked increases in *number* of cells as well.
- Nutritional habits (e.g., overfeeding)
- Psychologic factors
- Quantity of food ingested. This is regulated by caloric requirements for maintenance and growth, attitudes of caretakers, and types of food offered.

OVERFEEDING IN INFANCY

Calorie requirements.   Many recent studies have documented the frequency and extent of overfeeding of infants in our society. Two of these studies revealed the following:

- Sixty-seven percent of infants under 1 month of age making their first visit to a child health clinic were receiving solid foods.

By 2 months of age, 96 percent were receiving solids (Paige, 1975).

- Twenty percent of 130 full-term infants seen at a well-child clinic had been introduced to one or a combination of solid foods by 1 week of age (Paige, 1975).
- All these infants were being fed nutrients in excess of the RDAs.

Attitudes of caretakers. Attitudes with a significant effect on over-feeding include the following:

- The failure of public and professional encouragement and support of breast-feeding is significant. The breast-feeding mother relies on the infant's signals to determine length of feeding and satiety. The mother who is bottle-feeding tends to rely on the amount of formula in the bottle and persists until the bottle is empty. This frequently leads to overfeeding.
- The myth persists that a chubby baby is a healthy baby.
- Early introduction of solids is viewed as a sign of developmental progress or else as a way of relieving family and/or peer pressure.

Types of food offered. (See this chapter, Solid Foods.)

Management

PREVENTION

Attempts at nutritional counseling and education should begin in the prenatal clinic. Points to include in counseling are the following:

- Encourage breast feeding
- If bottle feeding, help parents to learn to interpret infants' cues relative to hunger and satiety
- When giving water avoid adding sweeteners
- Delay introduction of solids
- Encourage home preparation of solid foods

- Avoid the use of commercially prepared mixed dinners, wet-pack cereals, and desserts
- Encourage a range of activity patterns
- Assure parents that one pint of milk a day is adequate for an infant over 1 year of age
- Reinforce positive parent-child interactions other than feeding which provide mutual satisfaction

FOOD ALLERGY

Assessment

Reactions to milk and other foods may result from a wide variety of mechanisms and may be seen as a wide range of signs and symptoms. A full discussion of these factors is beyond the scope of this chapter. See Chapter 28, Allergies. It is possible that the occurrence of food allergies in infants is related to the slow development of IgA barriers, and that after 1 year of age IgA barriers are fully developed, and thus the incidence of food allergies decreases markedly (Rudolph, 1977 p. 367).

COMMON ALLERGENIC FOODS

Certain foods are thought to be commonly allergenic at early ages, and thus parents are advised to avoid them during the early months of life. The most common offenders are:

- Cow milk
- Wheat and corn
- Egg whites
- Chocolate
- Citrus products
- Nuts
- Fish, shellfish

MANIFESTATIONS

Most children develop onset of symptoms within 1 month or more after institution of the antigenic food. Symptoms include diarrhea, rhinitis, abdominal pain, vomiting, allergic skin reactions, and behavioral symptoms (lethargy, irritability, restlessness, moodiness).

HISTORY AND PHYSICAL EXAMINATION

History and physical examination of a child suspected of food allergy include:

- Family history of allergy
- Age of onset of symptoms
- Continuous or intermittent symptoms
- Diet
- Parents' and child's suspicions regarding offending foods
- Infections
- General appearance
- Nutritional status
- Eczema
- Character of feces

Management

INFANTS SENSITIVE TO COW MILK

Elimination of cow milk and milk products from the diet is recommended. See Chapter 28, Milk-Free Diet. Cow milk substitutes, mainly soy formulas, with vitamin and mineral supplementation, have been shown to be very effective and result in normal growth curves. Most children with milk allergy in infancy are able to tolerate cow milk by 3 years of age. Parents should be encouraged to breast-feed for the first 6 months and to limit the introduction of new foods until after 6 months of age when the IgA barrier is close to fully developed.

Table 18

Levels of Nutritional Assessment for Infants and Children

| Level of Approach[a] | History | | Clinical Evaluation | Laboratory Evaluation |
	Dietary	Medical and Socioeconomic		
		Birth to 24 Months		
Minimal	1. Source of iron 2. Vitamin supplement 3. Milk intake (type and amount)	1. Birth weight 2. Length of gestation 3. Serious or chronic illness 4. Use of medicines	1. Body weight and length 2. Gross defects	1. Hematocrit 2. Hemoglobin
Mid-level	1. Semiquantitative a) Iron-cereal, meat, egg yolks, supplement b) Energy nutrients c) Micronutrients—calcium, niacin, riboflavin, vitamin C d) Protein 2. Food intolerances 3. Baby foods—processed commercially; home cooked	1. Family history—diabetes, tuberculosis 2. Maternal—height, prenatal care 3. Infant—immunizations, tuberculin test	1. Head circumference 2. Skin color, pallor, turgor 3. Subcutaneous tissue paucity, excess	1. RBC morphology 2. Serum iron 3. Total iron binding capacity 4. Sickle cell testing

In-depth Level	1. Quantitative 24-hour recall 2. Dietary history	1. Prenatal details 2. Complications of delivery 3. Regular health supervision	1. Cranial bossing 2. Epyphyseal enlargement 3. Costochondral beading 4. Ecchymoses	Same as above, plus vitamin and appropriate enzyme assays; protein and amino acids; hydroxyproline, etc., should be available
		For Ages 2 to 5 Years		
	Determine amount of intake	Probe about pica; Medications	Add height at all levels; add arm circumference at all levels; add triceps skinfolds at in-depth level	Add serum lead at mid-level; add serum micronutrients (vitamins A, C, folate, etc.) at in-depth level
		For Ages 6 to 12 Years		
	Probe about snack foods; determine whether salt intake is excessive	Ask about medications taken; drug abuse	Add blood pressure at mid-level; add description of changes in tongue, skin, eyes for in-depth level	All the above plus BUN

Source: George Christakis, editor, "Nutritional Assessment in Health Programs," Supplement, *Am J Public Health* 68:46, 1973.

[a]It is understood that what is included at a minimal level would also be included or represented at successively more sophisticated levels of approach. However, it may be entirely appropriate to use a minimal level of approach to clinical evaluations and a maximal approach to laboratory evaluations.

Table 19
Nutrition History: Birth to 24 Months

NAME: _____

CLINIC: _____

DATE: _____ AGE: _____

Birth weight: _____ Present weight: _____ Percentile: _____

Birth height: _____ Present height: _____ Percentile: _____

Hemoglobin: _____ Hematocrit: _____

(most recent visit) (most recent visit)

Breast fed: _____ Bottle fed: _____

Any concerns about this method of feeding? _____

BREAST FED

a) For how long is the baby on the breast? _____

b) How much time between feedings? _____

c) Do you supplement breast milk with a bottle? _____

BOTTLE FED

Kind of formula: _____ How is it prepared: _____

Amount of formula taking:

    a) ounces per feeding: _____

    b) number of feedings per day: _____

    c) total milk intake in 24 hours: _____

Do you add anything to the bottle? _____

(let mother respond without suggestions as to kinds of mixtures that might be used)

If yes, what is it?

Cereal: _____ Amount: _____ times per day: _____

Sugar: _____ Amount: _____ times per day: _____

Honey: _____ Amount: _____ times per day: _____

Other: _____ Amount: _____ times per day: _____

If water is offered, do you add anything else? _____

Kind: _____ Amount: _____ times per day: _____

Vitamin supplements:

Kind: _____ Amount: _____ times per day: _____

Solids being given: _____

What do you offer first: milk (bottle or breast) _____ or solids? _____

Commercially prepared baby food: _____ home cooked: _____

Kind: _____ Amount: _____ time of day: _____

Overall feeding schedule: _____

Explore about snack foods: _____

Determine whether salt intake is excessive: _____

Developmental feeding skills: _____

Table 19 *(Continued)*

INITIAL EVALUATION SUMMARY AND RECOMMENDATIONS

Adequacy of diet in terms of nutrients: _____

_____

Anticipatory guidance (counseling needed for future developmental-nutritional needs) _____

_____

Follow-up: _____

_____

_____

Date: _____

Source: Yolanda Gutierrez, M.S., Assistant Clinical Professor, Department of Family Health Care Nursing, University of California, San Francisco.

Table 20
24-Hour Recall

Name: _____
Date and time of interview: _____
Length of interview: _____
Date of recall: _____
Day of the week of recall: _____

         1-M 2-T 3-W 4-Th 5-F 6-Sat 7-Sun

I would like you to tell me everything you (your child) ate and drank from the time you (he) got up in the morning until you (he) went to bed at night and what you (he) ate during the night. Be sure to mention everything you (he) ate or drank at home, at work (school), and away from home. Include snacks and drinks of all kinds and everything else you (he) put in your (his) mouth and swallowed. I also need to know where you (he) ate the food, and now let us begin.

What time did you (he) get up yesterday? _____
Was it the usual time? _____
What was the first time you (he) ate or had anything to drink yesterday morning? (List on the form that follows.)

(Continued)

263

Where did you (he) eat? (List on form that follows.)
Now tell me what you (he) had to eat and how much?
[Occasionally the interviewer will need to ask:
  When did you (he) eat again? Or, is there anything else?
  Did you (he) have anything to eat or drink during the night?]
Was intake unusual in any way? Yes _____ No _____
(If answer is yes) Why? _____
                    In what way? _____
What time did you (he) go to bed last night?
Do(es) you (he) take vitamin or mineral supplements:
  Yes _____ No _____
(If answer is yes) How many per day? _____
                    Per week? _____
What kind? (Insert brand name if known)
Multivitamins _____ Iron _____
Ascorbic Acid _____ Other _____
Vitamins A and D _____

Suggested Form for Recording Food Intake

Time	Where Eaten*	Food	Type and/or Preparation	Amount

*Code:
  H—Home
  R—Restaurant, drug store, or lunch counter
  CL—Carried lunch from home
  CC—Child care center
  OH—Other home (friend, relative, babysitter, etc.)
  S—School, office, plant, or work
  FD—Food dispenser
  SS—Social center, e.g. Senior Citizen, etc.

Source: Screening Children for Nutritional States: Suggestions for Child Health Programs, Washington D.C., U.S. Govt. Printing Office, 1971, p. 13.

CHILDREN WITH OTHER FOOD ALLERGIES

A child suspected of having a food allergy is usually placed on an elimination diet of suspected foods until symptoms completely clear. Later foods are reintroduced slowly (one every 6 to 7 days) in a systematic challenge. Once a food has been identified as the causative antigen, strict avoidance is the only effective treatment. See Chapter 28, Allergies, for a full discussion.

EVALUATION OF NUTRITIONAL STATUS

In identifying potential or real health problems and in planning for optimal health care services, evaluation of the nutritional status of individuals and groups must be undertaken by those involved in child care.

Individual Nutritional Assessment

Data to be collected in performing nutritional assessments include family history, birth history, past and current medical history, nutrition history, physical examination, and laboratory procedures. Table 18 provides a framework for nutritional assessment of infants and children. Additional information includes knowledge of family economic status, cultural background, educational level, and family food patterns.

NUTRITION HISTORY

A convenient form for recording a nutrition history in infants and toddlers is presented in Table 19.

TWENTY-FOUR-HOUR RECALL

Frequently it is difficult for busy parents to remember exactly what a child eats during a 24-hour period. A convenient form for collecting this information is presented in Table 20.

GENERAL CHARACTERISTICS OF GOOD AND POOR NUTRITION

Table 21 outlines physical manifestations of both good and poor nutrition.

Table 21
Characteristics of Good Nutrition and Poor Nutrition

Good Nutrition	*Poor Nutrition*
Well-developed body	Body may be undersized, or show poor development or physical defects
About average weight for height	Usually thin (underweight 10 percent or more), but may be normal or overweight (fat and flabby)
Muscles well developed and firm	Muscles small and flabby
Skin turgid and of healthy color	Skin loose and pale, waxy, or sallow
Good layer subcutaneous fat	Subcutaneous fat usually lacking (or in excess)
Mucous membranes of eyelids and mouth reddish pink	Mucous membranes pale
Hair smooth and glossy	Hair often rough and without luster
Eyes clear	Dark hollows or circles under eyes or puffiness; eyes reddened
Good natured and full of life	Irritable, overactive, fatigues easily or Phlegmatic, listless, fails to concentrate
Appetite good	Appetite poor
General health excellent	Susceptible to infections Lacks endurance and vigor

Source: Reprinted with permission from L. J. Bogert, et al., *Nutrition and Physical Fitness*, (Philadelphia: Saunders, © 1973), p. 419.

Community Screening Programs

When nutritional screening programs are conducted in communities, data in addition to individual and family information must be collected. Such knowledge of the community includes:

- Demographic data
- Socioeconomic and educational levels
- Racial and ethnic groups
- Source of food and water supplies
- Local food customs

References

Adams, C. F. *Nutritive Value of American Foods in Common Units.* Agriculture Handbook No. 456, Agricultural Research Service, U.S. Department of Agriculture, Washington, D.C., 1975.

Anderson, T. A. "Are Infants Getting the Right Foods?" In *Year ONE: Nutrition, Growth, Health.* Columbus, Ohio: Ross Laboratories, 1975.

Bogert, L. J., G. M. Briggs and D. H. Calloway, *Nutrition and Physical Fitness.* Philadelphia: Saunders, 1973.

Brown, M. S. and M. A. Murphy. *Ambulatory Pediatrics for Nurses.* New York: McGraw-Hill, 1975.

Christakis, G. "Nutritional Assessment in Health Programs." *AJPH Supplement* 63, November 1973.

Committee on Maternal Nutrition, Food and Nutrition Board, National Research Council. *Maternal Nutrition and the Course of Pregnancy.* Washington D.C.: National Academy of Sciences, 1970.

Committee on Nutrition, American Academy of Pediatrics. "Fluoride as a Nutrient." *Pediatrics* 49:456–459, March 1972.

Committee on Nutrition, American Academy of Pediatrics. "Iron-Fortified Formulas." *Pediatrics* 47:786, April 1971.

Committee on Nutrition, American Academy of Pediatrics. "Iron Supplementation for Infants." *Pediatrics* 58:765–768, November 1976.

Committee on Nutrition, American Academy of Pediatrics. "Nutritional Needs of Low-Birth-Weight Infants." *Pediatrics* 60:519–527, October 1977.

Dallman, P. R. "Bioavailability of Iron: The Form is More Important than the

Quantity." *Pediatric Basics*, No. 17. Fremont, Michigan: Gerber Products Co., January 1977.

Dallman, P. R. "Iron, Vitamin E, and Folate in the Preterm Infant." *J Pediatr* 85:742–752, December 1974.

Erhard, D. "Nutrition Education for the 'Now' Generation." *Journal of Nutrition Education* 2:135–139, Spring 1971.

Erhard, D. "The New Vegetarians, Part 1, Vegetarianism and its Medical Consequences." *Nutrition Today* 8:4–12, November–December 1973.

Fomon, S. J. *Infant Nutrition*, 2nd ed. Philadelphia: Saunders, 1974.

Food and Nutrition Board, National Research Council. *Recommended Daily Dietary Allowances*, 8th ed. Washington D.C.: National Academy of Sciences, 1974.

Graef, J. W. and T. F. Cone. *Manual of Pediatric Therapeutics*. Boston: Little, Brown, 1974.

Harper, A. E. "Those Pesky RDA's." *Nutrition Today* 9:15, March–April 1974.

Lappe, F. M. *Diet for a Small Planet*, rev. ed. New York: Friends of the Earth/ Ballantine Books Inc., 1975.

Maternal and Child Health Unit. *Nutrition During Pregnancy and Lactation*. California Department of Health, Sacramento, California, 1975.

McGill, H. C., et al. *Developmental Nutrition: Atherosclerosis, No. 9*. Columbus, Ohio: Ross Laboratories, March 1974.

McMillan, J. A., S. A. Landaw, and F. A. Oski. "Iron Sufficiency in Breast-Fed Infants and the Availability of Iron from Human Milk." *Pediatrics* 58:686–691, November 1976.

Paige, D. M. "Avoiding Overnutrition in Infancy." In *Year ONE: Nutrition, Growth, Health*. Columbus, Ohio: Ross Laboratories, 1975.

Pearson, G. A. "Nutrition in the Middle Years of Childhood." *American Journal of Maternal Child Nursing* 2:378–384, November–December 1977.

Pipes, P. L. *Nutrition in Infancy and Childhood*. St. Louis: Mosby, 1977.

Rudolph, A. M., editor. *Pediatrics*, 16th ed. New York: Appleton-Century-Crofts, 1977.

Screening Children for Nutritional Status: Suggestions for Child Health Programs. Maternal and Child Health Service, Health Services and Mental Health Administration, Department of HEW, Rockville MD, PHS Publication #2158, 1971.

Slattery, J. S. "Nutrition for the Normal Healthy Infant." *Am J Maternal Child Nursing* 2:105–112, March–April 1977.

Smith, N. J. *Developmental Nutrition: The Challenge of Obesity, No. 1*. Columbus, Ohio: Ross Laboratories, June 1972.

Smith, N. J., editor. *Iron Nutrition in Infancy: Report of the 62nd Ross Conference on Pediatric Research*. Columbus, Ohio: Ross Laboratories, 1970.

Torre, C. T. "Nutritional Needs of Adolescents." *Am J Maternal Child Nursing* 2:118–127, March–April 1977.

U. S. Department of Agriculture, Home and Garden Bulletin No. 72. *Nutritive Value of Foods*. U.S. Office of Documents, Washington D.C., 1964.

Vaughan, V. C. and R. J. McKay, editors. *Nelson Textbook of Pediatrics*, 10th ed. Philadelphia: Saunders, 1975.

Watt, B. K. and A. L. Merrill. *Composition of Foods: Raw, Processed, Prepared.* Agriculture Handbook #8, U.S. Department of Agriculture, Washington D.C., 1963.

Williams, E. R. "Making Vegetarian Diets Nutritious." *Am J Nurs* 75:2168–2173, December 1975.

7

Feeding in Infancy and Childhood

A positive feeding interaction between a parent and child establishes the basis for a warm, trusting bond. Early parental education and guidance fosters successful feeding experiences and prevents feeding problems. The role of the nurse practitioner is to provide parental guidance in early feeding techniques, to help parents to establish adequate nutritional practices for the child's later growth and development and to understand their own attitudes, feelings and expectations around feeding, and to encourage parental problem solving when feeding questions arise.

This chapter describes the development of feeding behaviors, feeding techniques, and food patterns. Chapter 6, Nutrition in Infancy and Childhood provides nutritional information. Chapter 8 discusses some of the common problems related to feeding.

DEVELOPMENT OF INFANT FEEDING BEHAVIOR

Feeding behavior is a function of motor development. For example, the child's ability to suck, to chew, and to swallow is determined by the acquisition of fine, gross, and oral motor skills; the child's ability to self-feed depends on the motor development of the trunk, arms, and hands.

Developmental Sequence of Feeding Behaviors

Birth to 4 weeks: presence of the rooting and sucking reflexes; tongue moving in an up-and-down motion

10 weeks: recognition of the bottle or breast as the food source

16 weeks: maturation of the sucking pattern with the tongue moving back and forth; ability to draw in lower lip as spoon is removed making spoon feeding easier; ability to clasp hands on the bottle

24 to 28 weeks: beginning of chewing movements and up-and-down jaw movements. Critical or sensitive period for learning to eat solids (Illingworth, 1964). Readiness to finger feed indicated by ability to grasp objects, to put them into the mouth, and to maintain a sitting posture; ability to grasp objects with palm of hand (indicates readiness for finger feeding); ability to obtain the bottle in a sitting posture; messiness and spilling may conflict with parent's interest; awareness of the cup

28 to 32 weeks: maturation of the tongue is more sophisticated in regard to spoon feeding than drinking from a cup; ability to sit alone without support, to reach and grasp objects, and to use fingers to transfer items from one hand to another; around 32 weeks ability to bring head forward to receive spoon as it is presented; increased mobility of the tongue allows increased manipulation of food in mouth before swallowing

36 to 48 weeks: further development of the pincer grasp; ability to manage bottle alone and to rescue it if it gets lost; by 48 weeks the pattern of eating changes from sucking to beginning rotary chewing movements; beginning ability to self-feed; greater tongue mobility allows true drinking action from cup as opposed to sucking action.

15 months: ability to use spoon is poor due to lack of wrist control; ability to manage cup is still difficult, often tilting cup too rapidly

16 to 17 months: ulnar deviation of wrist allows the child to use spoon more effectively and to minimize spilling

18 months: ability to lift elbow as spoon is raised and to flex wrist as the spoon reaches the mouth results in only moderate spilling.

18 to 24 months: ability to tilt cup with finger manipulation; by 24 months refinement of rotary chewing movements achieved. Table 1 summarizes the important developmental landmarks and suggests food for appropriate changes in feeding behavior.

BREAST FEEDING

Anatomy and Physiology of the Breasts

The breast is composed of approximately 15 to 20 milk-producing glands called milk lobes. Each lobe is divided into lobules which contain alveoli. The alveoli are the basic organs of milk production and excretion. They contain the secretory cells which produce the milk, a cavity which collects the milk, and contractile myoepithelial cells which expel milk from the cavity. The milk is expelled into the ductile system (lacteriferous ducts) which takes it to the lacteriferous sinus or reservoir and through the nipple to the infant.

The nursing infant causes stimulation of afferent nerves in the nipple to stimulate the anterior pituitary to release prolactin hormone which causes the secretory cells of the alveoli to initiate milk production. The posterior pituitary releases oxytocin, a hormone which causes milk to be released from the alveoli into the lacteriferous ducts.

Mechanism of Drug Excretion

The excretion of drugs is dependent on the following physio-chemical characteristics:

- The pH gradient between plasma and milk
- The pKa or degree of ionization of the drug (Generally basic drugs are excreted in higher concentrations in milk, and acidic drugs are excreted in lower concentrations.)
- The lipid-water solubility of the drug

Table 1

Developmental Stages of Readiness to Progress in Feeding Behaviors

Developmental Landmarks	Change Indicated	Examples of Appropriate Foods
Tongue laterally transfers food in the mouth Voluntary and independent movements of the tongue and lips Sitting posture can be sustained Beginning of chewing movements (up and down movements of the jaw)	Introduction of soft, mashed table food	Tuna fish; mashed potatoes; well-cooked mashed vegetables; ground meats in gravy and sauces; soft diced fruit such as bananas, peaches, pears; liverwurst; flavored yogurt
Reaches for and grasps objects with scissor grasp Brings hand to mouth	Finger feeding (large pieces of food)	Oven-dried toast, teething biscuits, cheese sticks, peeled Vienna sausage (food should be soluble in the mouth to prevent choking)
Voluntary release (refined digital grasp) Rotary chewing pattern	Finger feeding of smaller pieces of food Introduction of more textured food from family menu	Bits of cottage cheese, dry cereal, peas, small pieces of meat Well-cooked chopped meats and casseroles, cooked vegetables and canned fruit (not mashed), toast, potatoes, macaroni, spaghetti, peeled ripe fruit

Approximates lips to rim of the cup Understands relationship of container and contained	Introduction of cup Beginning self-feeding (messiness should be expected)	Food that when scooped will adhere to the spoon, such as applesauce, cooked cereal, mashed potato, cottage cheese
Increased rotary movements of the jaw Ulnar deviation of wrist develops	More skilled at cup and spoon feeding	Chopped fibrous meats such as roast and steak Gradually introduce raw vegetables and fruit
Walks alone	May seek food and get food independently	Food of high nutrient value should be available
Names food, expresses preferences; prefers unmixed foods Goes on food jags Appetite appears to decrease		Balanced food intake should be offered and child should be permitted to develop food preferences without concern that they will last forever

Source: Reproduced with permission from P. L. Pipes, *Nutrition in Infancy and Childhood*, (St. Louis: C. V. Mosby, 1977).

- The distribution of the drug by body transport mechanisms
- Concentration gradient of diffusable drug between plasma and milk (The more easily a drug can be dialyzed, the greater the concentration it will achieve in breast milk.)

Any drug taken orally or administered parentally and absorbed by the mother will be excreted in her milk. Most drugs achieve insufficient concentration in the milk, but some drugs can achieve high concentrations. Nursing mothers should take medications 15 minutes after nursing or 3 to 4 hours before the next feeding. This allows enough time for most medications to be cleared from the maternal serum and to achieve a relatively low milk concentration. Medications taken 30 to 60 minutes before breast feeding usually achieve peak serum milk concentrations.

The reader is referred to the reference section of this chapter and the following authors: Anderson, Herfindal, and O'Brien, for information concerning specific medications excreted in breast milk and their effect on the nursing infant.

Establishing A Successful Breast Feeding Routine

MATERNAL POSITION

There are several positions that allow for maternal comfort during breast feeding. The woman may lie on her side with one arm under her head and the other arm and hand supporting the breast used for feeding. The infant lies next to the mother. A second position is for the mother to sit up in bed in a semi-Fowler's position or in a chair with a pillow under her arm and resting on her abdomen for support. The infant is held supine in her arms on the pillow.

MATERNAL ANXIETY

The most common deterrent to establishing a successful breast-feeding routine is maternal anxiety. Frequently women feel the cause of their anxiety relates to breast feeding, and in many instances this is not the reason. For example, there may be anxiety over lack of preparation for the maternal role, physical discomfort from delivery and common behaviors of newborns (crying, regurgitation, and passage of flatus). The woman may be anxious because of: fear of rejection by a sleeping newborn, faulty breast-feeding technique, engorgement, and sore nipples.

The reasons for maternal anxiety are assessed. Questions are answered. Encouragement, reassurance, and emotional support are maintained. Support services are initiated including use of family and friends, public health nurse, breast-feeding groups.

COUNSELING

General considerations. Adequate stimulation of the breasts requires feeding every 2 to 4 hours during the day. At night the infant's sleep is not interrupted for feeding. Usually the infant nurses on the first breast for approximately 10 minutes and on the second breast for 10 to 20 minutes. The protein curd of breast milk (lactoalbumin) is easier to digest than the protein curd of cow milk (casein), hence the faster emptying time of the stomach and the more frequent breast feedings. A reduction in breast size is a normal physiologic reaction to the establishment of a smoothly functioning breast routine.

Technique. The nurse practitioner discusses stimulation of the rooting reflex: stroking the side of the infant's cheek closest to the mother's nipple. Newborn development in reference to feeding is reviewed: some infants sleep for the first 2 or 3 days and need to be stimulated to nurse; the infant is not expected to nurse for long periods in the first 3 days but to learn through frequent association the feel of the mother's nipple and where the milk is. The mother's nipple and areolar are washed with water before nursing. The nipple is made more protuberant for easier grasp by the infant by rotating it between the thumb and forefinger. The infant is held in a position most comfortable to the mother. Sleepy newborns are unwrapped from blankets and their feet are gently rubbed. When the infant opens the mouth the nipple and part of the areolar is inserted. It is normal for newborns to suck for a few moments and then to fall asleep. Sucking is re-established by having the mother put her finger under the newborn's chin and gently push it upward. A specific area for sucking is established by having the woman place her index and middle finger around the margin of the areolar. This also establishes an air space for the infant to breathe. To break the suction after nursing the woman places her small finger in the side of the infant's mouth to release the pressure and removes the breast.

Let down reflex. Anxiety effects the release of oxytocin from the posterior pituitary and inhibits milk let down from the acini glands (milk-producing glands). The let down reflex is described by breast feeding women as a "pins and needles" sensation in the breasts occurring before or at the beginning of feeding. However, many women have normally not experienced this sensation. Some authorities recommend oxytocin nasal spray when there is concern that the let down reflex is not functioning properly. Other ways to help release the let down are to obtain adequate maternal rest and nutrition and to reduce the causes of anxiety. Ways to relieve anxiety are to establish a nonchaotic home routine, to drink a liquid before and during breast feeding (warm milk, wine, beer), and to use support systems (public health nurse, empathetic family members, La Leche League).

Use of creams. Lanolin creams are used occasionally during pregnancy to help lubricate dry nipples. They are also used after birth for the same reason. The cream is placed on the areolar and never directly on the nipple so as to not interfere with milk drainage. The cream is wiped off before nursing.

Breast pumps. These devices are used to maintain the milk supply through routine stimulation of the breasts when the woman is not able to nurse herself. There is controversy over using hand and electric pumps. Some authorities feel that the amount of pressure exerted by the pumps is painful and injurious to the lacteriferous ducts. However, if pain is not present when using the pumps they are recommended by the authors.

BOTTLE FEEDING

Formulas

The preparation of formula is reviewed with the parents to identify any mixing errors. The available commercial formulas are reviewed in Chapter 6.

STERILIZATION OF FORMULA

Researchers (Hargrove, 1974; Kendall, 1971) have not found any differences in the incidence of illness or infection in infants fed formulas prepared by the clean technique or by terminal sterilization. The results were found regardless of socioeconomic background or housekeeping methods. In spite of this sterilization of formula is often recommended. For a discussion of sterilization methods the reader is referred to any standard pediatric nursing text.

Clean technique (Pipes, 1977)

1. Wash hands carefully before preparing the formula.
2. Thoroughly wash all equipment to be used during the preparation: cans that contain the milk, bottles, nipples.
3. Cover and refrigerate opened formula cans.
4. Prepare formula immediately before each feeding.
5. Discard any remaining milk not consumed after the formula is heated and the infant is fed.

COUNSELING

Care of equipment. Careful washing of the bottles, nipples, screw rings, and caps with detergent soon after the feeding avoids milk drying in the equipment. Brushes for the bottle and the nipple facilitate cleaning. After the nipples are washed, a toothpick is twisted in each nipple hole to prevent clogging.

Technique of bottle feeding

POSITION. A comfortable chair and position are essential with the baby cradled in the parent's arm. An armchair and a pillow under the elbow are often helpful. Bottle propping is avoided. The bottle is tilted so the milk fills the neck of the bottle to prevent the swallowing of too much air.

NIPPLE. It usually takes about 20 minutes of continuous sucking for an infant to complete an 8-ounce bottle. To prevent a vacuum which collapses the nipple and makes sucking harder, parents are cautioned not to screw the nipple cap too tightly.

Nipple hole.   A test for the right size of the nipple hole is to invert the bottle and to observe the pattern of milk flow from the nipple. If the milk comes out in a fine spray for 1 to 2 seconds and then switches to drops, the nipple hole is correct. If it continues to spray, the nipple hole is too large. If it starts with slow drops, the nipple hole is too small (Spock, 1976). Parents can enlarge nipple holes as follows (Spock, 1976, p. 151):

1. Stick the dull end of a fine (No. 10) needle into a cork for safety reasons
2. Hold the cork and heat the needle point in a flame until it is red hot
3. Stick the needle a short distance into the nipple top
4. Test the milk flow

Clogged nipple holes.   A solution to this problem is to purchase nipples with holes that are "crosscut," which means that a small cross has been cut in the tip of the nipple. The edges of the cut remain together until the baby sucks. Parents can make crosscuts on regular nipples as follows:

1. Pinch the nipple tip to form a narrow ridge
2. Cut across it with a razor blade
3. Repeat the previous two steps pinching the nipple at right angle to the first pinch

This problem can occur if parents mix solid foods with formula, for example, cereal mixed with formula. In this case larger nipple holes will not solve the problem. Parents need to be counseled that the desirable way to serve cereal is with a spoon.

NEED TO FEED

Parents are often overly concerned about the amount of food their child eats. This can result in overfeeding, early introduction of solids, and feeding problems. A feeding problem occurs most often when the child fails to meet the expectations of the parents. The nurse practitioner can effectively prevent feeding difficulties by increasing the parents' awareness of their own expectations of the child's food intake and feeding behavior. The following areas are explored:

- Parental understanding and knowledge of growth and development
- Expectations (parents, relatives, friends)
- Cultural factors

DEVELOPMENT OF FEEDING PATTERNS IN YOUNG CHILDREN

The first 5 years of life are of utmost importance in developing feeding patterns in young children.

Patterns of Food Ingestion

Between the ages of 1 and 2 years normal developmental feeding problems start more frequently than at any other period. Parents especially need guidance at this time because impatience and anger at the problem will perpetuate it and initiate others.

DISINTEREST IN FOOD

Between approximately 1 and 3 years of age the child becomes disinterested in food and the appetite falls off dramatically. Milk intake usually decreases. The disinterest can last from several months to a few years. Food jags are common and the child's tastes and behaviors become unpredictable. Often a favorite food will be rejected for a period of time, or the child may become more interested in playing at meals. Calcium, phosphorus, iron, and vitamin A intake during the preschool years decreases as iron-fortified infant cereals are omitted, milk intake is decreased, and vegetables are disliked. After 3 to 4 years of age there is a steady increase in all nutrient intake.

MEALTIME

Rituals. They are associated with the preparation and service of food. Often the child may demand that the milk be served in the same glass, or that the sandwich be quartered and arranged in a set pattern on the plate.

Evening meal. It is generally the least popular and acceptable meal to children, and it presents the most concern to parents. Preschoolers tend not to eat for the following reasons:

1. Tension at mealtime
2. Fatigue (parents and children)
3. Unrealistic parental expectations
4. Inappropriate size of eating utensils
5. Pattern of being bribed with sweets if food is not eaten
6. Large meal or milk already consumed
7. Parental attention received for dawdling or playing with food

Preparation of Food

The following is a list of suggestions for parents in the preparation of food:

Infancy period. Select and prepare foods that can be manipulated in the mouth without a potential of choking or aspiration. Examples are well-cooked vegetables, canned fruits, well-cooked ground meats or sauces, liverwurst, minced chicken livers, drained tuna fish, custards, puddings.

Preschool period.

1. Prepare simple menus with a variety of colorful foods.
2. Combine dry foods with one or two moist foods, and sharp with mild flavors.
3. Combine soft food, crisp food, and chewy foods.
4. Offer mild flavors, mildly salted foods, strong-flavored raw vegetables.
5. Make foods softer in texture by adding milk to dry, starchy foods.

6. Prepare foods that are easy to eat (thickened soups, finger foods).
7. Cut pieces of food so they are large enough for the fork yet small enough to be eaten.
8. Offer ground meat or frankfurters instead of steak because 2-to-3-year-old children do not grind meat as easily as adults do.
9. Serve at room temperature.
10. Serve portions smaller than you expect child to eat so the child can gain a sense of accomplishment.

Feeding Environment

An environment that is conducive to eating provides positive interactions between parent and child with a minimum of distractions and is physically comfortable for the child. The child should be situated in a sturdy, well-balanced chair with the feet supported. The furniture should fit the child's body contours. The food should be within reach to avoid spilling. The dishes and glasses should be unbreakable, and the glasses should be small enough to allow the child's hands to encircle them.

UTENSILS

A spoon with a round shallow bowl and blunt tip allows the child to push food from a plate. The handle of the spoon should be blunt, short, and easily held in the palm.

A fork with short, blunt tines adapts easily to the child's palm. Sharp tines spear food more easily but may be used as a weapon.

Parental Counseling

Meeting the variable and predictable nutritional needs of a growing child is a time-consuming and often unrewarding job. Parents should be counseled to (Lowenberg, 1977):

1. Observe the child's hunger pattern and identify the time of day when the child takes the new food most easily
2. Be patient, positively reinforcing, and understanding of each attempt with a new feeding process

3. Encourage the infant to self-feed (9 to 12 months) and offer assistance when the infant fatigues
4. Feed individual foods and not mixtures to help the infant learn to appreciate foods for their own textures and tastes
5. Prepare individual foods in as many different ways as possible to enlarge the child's experience
6. Introduce new tastes and textures slowly
7. Serve foods that are well prepared, colorful, tasty, and textured to create a friendly attitude toward the food
8. Provide an emotionally and physically comfortable eating environment
9. Obtain the entire family's cooperation
10. Understand normal behavioral responses, as well as their own expectations and attitudes.

COMMON CLINICAL PROBLEMS

Breast Feeding

INSUFFICIENT BREAST MILK

Assessment. The following are considered:

- Why does the mother feel this way?
- How often is the mother nursing?
- How often are supplements given?
- Is the infant taking both breasts?
- Is the mother anxious?
- How adequate is the mother's nutrition and amount of rest?
- How many wet diapers in 24 hours?
- Is the mother taking any medication that would reduce the milk supply?
- Weighing the infant

Management. The following are discussed:

- Nursing more frequently to enhance milk production but not sooner than every two hours

- Eliminating bottle supplements if possible
- Obtaining a balanced diet for mother
- Drinking a glass of warm milk before and during feeding and/or a glass of wine to help relax the mother
- Reassuring the mother that six to eight wet diapers in 24 hours is evidence of adequate fluid intake
- Explain that breast fed infants gain more slowly in the early weeks.

FREQUENT FEEDINGS

Assessment. The following are considered:

- How often is the mother feeding?
- Is the feeding causing maternal exhaustion and anxiety?
- Are there problems with lack of privacy and feedings in the home?

Management. The following are discussed:

- Normal frequency of breast feeding is usually every 2 to 4 hours.
- Feeding more frequently than every 2 hours will cause the infant to consume only small amounts of milk and hence to be hungry more frequently.
- Breast-fed babies are routinely fed more often than bottle-fed babies.
- Breast milk is easier to digest than cow milk hence the faster emptying of the stomach.
- Early or frequent supplements with formula enhance maternal anxiety that breast feeding is inadequate.
- With frequent feedings every 2 to 4 hours during the day, no formula supplements should be given for the first 2 months.

FUSSY, CRYING INFANT

Assessment. The following are considered:

- How frequently is the infant feeding?
- What is the duration of the feeding?

- How often is the baby burped?
- Is the nursing position comfortable for the mother and the infant?
- Has the mother indented a portion of the breast to allow for an unobstructed airway while the infant is feeding?
- Is the nipple and part of the areolar in the infant's mouth?
- Are there any symptoms of illness?
- Is the home routine chaotic or peaceful?
- Is the mother getting enough rest and eating a balanced diet?

Management.   The following are discussed:

- Usual frequency of feeding: every 2 to 4 hours during the day and letting the infant sleep as long as possible at night
- Frequently burping to eliminate flatus
- Symptomatic relief of crying: wrap tightly in receiving blanket, use of pacifier, rocking infant in chair, ride in car or carriage.
- Eliminating stressful situations in the home
- Obtaining a well-balanced diet and enough rest for the mother

INFANT REFUSING ONE BREAST OR SUPPLEMENTS

Assessment.   The following are considered:

- Is the mother using both breasts at each feeding to allow for equal stimulation?
- After a routine breast feeding pattern has been established how does the infant respond to supplements?

Management.   The following are discussed:

- Continue to offer the rejected breast at each feeding. Start first with the accepted breast and change after a few minutes to the other breast.
- Apply honey to the nipple of the rejected breast.
- Supplements: start with water or apple juice first; many infants will accept this rather than cow milk, initially.

SUBTLE INFLUENCES OF SOCIETY AGAINST BREAST FEEDING

Assessment. The following are considered:

- How does the mother respond to busy hospital routine and pressures: Does she ask questions? Are hospital personnel willing to instruct?
- Is the infant's father and other family members encouraging in their attitude toward breast feeding?
- Is mother aligned with other breast-feeding women?

Management. The following are discussed:

- Aligning the breast-feeding mother with an empathetic professional, with a woman who has breast-fed, or with a member of La Leche League International or other supportive group.
- Arranging a family conference to discuss their feelings about breast feeding and to explain misconceptions
- Obtaining physical rest, adequate nutrition, and psychologic support

SORE NIPPLES

Assessment. The following are considered:

- How many days post partum is the mother?
- Sore nipples usually appear between the fifth and fourteenth day depending on the frequency and duration of nursing.
- Inspection of the nipples ascertains if there is abrasion of the tissue.
- Palpation of the breasts for heat and inspection for erythema helps to rule out the presence of mastitis.

Management. The following are discussed:

- Short feedings during the first 3 days allows the breast tissue to become accustomed to the stimulation.
- Exposing the nipples to the air between feedings
- Using a sun lamp in moderation for cracked nipples
- Manually expressing a small amount of milk before nursing to cause the infant to suck less hard initially to bring down the milk

- Assuming different nursing positions to relieve pressure on various areas of the nipple
- Not using soap or alcohol on the nipples or bras with plastic liners

ENGORGEMENT

Assessment. The following are considered:

- How many days post partum is the mother? (Engorgement is caused by the production of milk usually around the third day.)
- How comfortable or uncomfortable do the breasts feel upon touch? (Engorged breasts are hard and painful to touch.)

Management. The following are discussed:

- Nursing frequently
- Before nursing: application of hot towels to the breasts or a warm shower or tub bath to help stimulate milk flow
- Before nursing: manual expression of breast milk to soften nipple and areolar to allow for easier grasp by the infant

FLAT OR INVERTED NIPPLES

Assessment. The nipples are examined.

Management. The following are discussed:

- For flat nipples during pregnancy perform nipple rolling exercise: nipple is held between thumb and index finger and is gently pulled out and rolled. Exercise is done two times a day starting in the last trimester.
- After birth use of a nipple shield intermittently to establish suction and to allow the nipple to become more protuberant. Constant use will decrease milk production because of the baby's weak sucking response.
- For inverted nipples as early as possible during pregnancy breast shields are worn inside the bra. These shields have an opening at the areolar and nipple site and exert pressure on that area to allow the nipple to become more protuberant. Early

shields were called Woolwich breast shields. Currently Netzy Cups, which produce the same physiologic effect, are used in the United States. If they cannot be obtained locally, write to La Leche League International, Franklin Park, Illinois, 60131.

MASTITIS

Assessment. The following are considered:

- Are symptoms of infection present: extreme tenderness, erythema, heat in the breast tissue?
- Is there maternal fever? Lethargy?

Management. The following are discussed:

- Prevention: massaging plugged milk ducts
- Applying heat to the breasts: wet compresses or a heating pad
- Forcing fluids and physical rest for the mother
- Nursing is continued on the affected breast to allow release of plugged milk ducts
- Using oral antibiotics to decrease the infection. *Staphylococcus* is the most frequent causative organism.

NURSING TWINS

Assessment. The following are considered:

- Mother's motivation to nurse twins
- Amount of help at home

Management. There are two approaches:

- Complete breast feeding: nurse infants at the same time using one breast for each infant or nurse one infant at different times. If one infant is nursed at different times the mother can experiment with the amount of milk available in the breast. If milk production is adequate she can use both breasts for one infant. If there is inadequate time for milk production she should use only one breast to feed infant.
- Breast-feeding combined with supplements: at feeding time nurse one infant and bottle-feed the other. At subsequent

feedings, breast-feed the infant that was bottle-fed last and bottle-feed the infant that had the breast at the last feeding.

PREMATURE INFANT

Assessment. The following are considered:

- How is the infant currently being fed?
- Is the infant's sucking reflex established?
- Is the mother knowledgeable about manual expression of the breast if the infant is gavage fed?

Management. The following are discussed:

- Manual expression of breast if infant is gavage fed
- Use of breast pump
- Other methods of milk stimulation, possibly having husband help
- Frequent expression of breast milk at least every 4 hours is necessary to maintain supply.

HYPERBILIRUBINEMIA

See Chapter 20, Hematopoietic System: Breast-Feeding Jaundice.

WEANING

Assessment. The following are considered:

- How long has the mother been breast-feeding?
- What are the reasons for stopping?

Management. The following are discussed:

- Proceeding slowly: offer one replacement bottle or cup once every week to prevent engorgement
- Wearing a tight bra to help reduce engorgement
- No stimulation to the breasts

Inappropriate Feeding Behavior (dawdling, gorging, stuffing)

ASSESSMENT

This is often an attention-getting device. It may also be an attempt to exert independence. Questions to ask are:

- What initiates the behavior?
- What has the parent done to handle the problem?
- How would the parent describe the feeling milieu at home?
- How much time does the parent spend with the child?

MANAGEMENT

Parents need to recognize that it is the child's choice of whether to eat or to continue with the behavior. The child is positively reinforced for all attempts at appropriate behavior, and ignored for continuing the inappropriate behavior. See Patterns of Food Ingestion. Guidelines for coping with the behavior include:

- Firm limit setting
- Patience
- Rewarding positive behavior

Lack of Appetite

ASSESSMENT

It is a common concern raised by parents of toddlers, and it is also a common indicator of illness. A detailed history of the onset, duration, pattern, and associated symptoms (e.g., nausea, diarrhea, fever) is obtained. In exploring the concern the parent's expectations and meaning of "lack of appetite" are clarified. The nutritional intake (See Chapter 6), feeding environment, pertinent past medical history, development, parent-child relationship, rate of growth, and other physical factors such as fatigue are assessed. Questions to ask include:

- How is the food prepared and served?

- What does the parent do when the child refuses to eat?
- What and when does the child snack (type of food, quantity, time of day, location)?

MANAGEMENT

There are no magic solutions to this problem, and patience is often necessary. If the poor appetite is not related to illness, explanations about normal development and patterns of appetite, ideas about food preparation, ways to enhance the feeding environment, and showing the child's growth chart may help. See this chapter, Disinterest in Food, Preparation of Food, and Parental Counseling. Parents may need help in exploring their own discomforts with the poor appetite and in anticipating ways to prevent continuing resistance.

If a nutritional deficiency is identified, parents are counseled on foods to prepare. Supplemental vitamins or minerals may also be prescribed. If an obvious cause is not identified and there are associated physical signs and symptoms such as failing to thrive, further medical and laboratory investigation is indicated.

Refusal of a New Food

ASSESSMENT

This is a common problem. A description of the behavior that is interpreted as rejection is necessary. For example, inexperienced parents commonly misinterpret tongue thrusting in the infant as food rejection. In the older child refusal may be an attempt at independence and autonomy. Questions to ask are:

- How is the food prepared and served?
- What is the child's behavior when the food is served?
- What is the parent's response when the food is served?
- Does the parent like the new food?

MANAGEMENT

Patience and persistence are necessary. Often familiarity with the new food will increase the likelihood of acceptance; however, children will show food preferences just as adults, and it may be that the child dislikes the taste or texture. Pressuring the child to eat the food may set the stage for future resistance. See Patterns of Food Ingestion. The following suggestions are recommended:

1. Introduce the new food calmly and be prepared for its rejection.
2. If rejected, serve the food again several days later prepared differently if possible.
3. Serve the new food with a favorite food.
4. Introduce it when the child is hungry.
5. Compliment the child after trying even a bite.

Refusal of Specific Food Groups

ASSESSMENT

It is not uncommon for a child who likes a specific food group, such as vegetables, to suddenly reject them for several weeks or months. If the child is not pressured, the food group will usually resume favor. Questions to ask are:

- How is the food prepared and served?
- What has the child's previous experience been with the food?
- What does the parent do when the child refuses the food?
- What is the child's response?
- Does the parent like the specific food group?

MANAGEMENT

This is often a passing stage. It is important not to pressure the child to eat the food group because it may set the stage for future resistance. The parent may need guidance in preparing the food for the child or in selecting another food within the same food group that provides the same nutritive value. For example, vegetables can be served raw in strips and slices or lightly cooked, or if food dislike is for squash, parents can offer carrots. See Patterns of Food Ingestion and Preparation of Food.

References

Anderson, P. O. "Drugs and Breast Feeding." *Drug Intelligence and Clinical Pharmacy* 11:208–223, April 1977.

Applebaum, R. M. "The Modern Management of Successful Breast Feeding." *Pediatr Clin North Am* 17:203–225, February 1970.

Committee on Nutrition, American Academy of Pediatrics. "Commentary on Breast Feeding and Infant Formulas, Including Proposed Standards for Formulas." *Pediatrics* 57:276–285, February 1976.

Eiger, M. and S. Olds. *The Complete Book of Breastfeeding.* New York: Bantam Books, 1973.

Fraiberg, S. H. *The Magic Years.* New York: Charles Scribner's Sons, 1959.

Haire, D. "Checklist for Counseling Breastfeeding Mothers." *International Childbirth Education Association*, 1971.

Haire, D. "Instructions for Nursing Your Baby." *International Childbirth Education Association*, 1971.

Hargrove, C. B., et al. "Formula Preparation and Infant Illness." *Clin Pediatr* 13:1057–1059, 1974.

Herfindal, E. T. *Clinical Pharmacy and Therapeutics.* Baltimore: Williams and Wilkins, 1975.

Illingworth, R. S. and J. Lister. "The Critical or Sensitive Period with Special Reference to Certain Feeding Problems in Infants and Children." *J Pediatr* 65:839–848, 1964.

Jelliffe, B. D. and E. F. Jelliffe. "Current Concepts in Nutrition, Breast is Best: Modern Meanings." *N Engl J Med* 297:912–915, October 27, 1977.

Kendall, W., V. C. Vaughan, and A. Kusakcioglu. "A Study of Preparation of Infant Formulas." *Am J Dis Child* 122:215–219, 1971.

La Leche League, *The Womanly Art of Breast Feeding.* Franklin Park, Ill.: La Leche League International, 1963.

Lowenberg, M. E. "The Development of Food Patterns in Young Children." In P. L. Pipes, *Nutrition in Infancy and Childhood.* St. Louis: Mosby, 1977. Pp. 85–100.

O'Brien, T. E. "Excretion of Drugs in Human Milk." *Amer J Hosp Pharm* 31:844–854, September 1974.

Peterson, L. W. "Operant Approach to Observation and Recording." *N.O.* 15:28, 1967.

Pipes, P. L. *Nutrition in Infancy and Childhood.* St. Louis: Mosby, 1977.

Spock, B. *Baby and Child Care.* New York: Hawthorn Books, 1976.

8

Common Problems of Infancy and Early Childhood

This chapter concentrates on defining and dealing with common problems and the factors that lead to them. It also includes the psychologic needs of infancy, the differences in personality and temperament of children, and a brief tool for teaching basic developmental concepts.

In their own words parents "worry about" many aspects of early parenting. They need reassurance about their role and need to understand the external and internal forces exerted upon them as parents. To better prepare parents for their role, nurse practitioners must be empathetic to the problems of parenting and must have a sound knowledge of the emotional and social development of children. Teaching parents to appreciate and to gratify their infant's early needs and to understand normal developmental behavior may help to avoid many of the most common problems and may keep more serious problems from developing. The use of parenting groups or classes has been extremely helpful in educating parents in this area.

Definition of a Common Problem

A common problem may be defined as behavior of the infant or child that disturbs parental expectations, evokes anxieties and insecurities, and causes emotionally charged reactions. In the early parental experience these reactions may produce a "negative atmosphere or aura" that is disturbing to the infant, and that possibly may contribute to tension that causes the infant to react "negatively," for example, unexplained and prolonged crying.

Many common problems may be classified as:

1. Developmental disorders. These are due to the inevitable and characteristic conflicts associated with the successive stages of psychologic development. They are usually transitory and, within certain limits, are to be regarded as part of normal development, such as obstinacy, negativism, or temper tantrums in the toddler years. The intensity and duration of the symptoms vary with the severity of the environmental situation. Treatment usually consists of working with the parents to help them to perceive and to change those attitudes or reactions which are felt to be threatening to the relationship between parent and child.

2. Situational disorders. These stem from abnormal environmental situations with which a child is unable to cope at a given age. Any of the problems that occur as developmental disorders may also be seen in situational disorders. The latter is suspected if symptoms are severe, persistent, and especially, clearly defined. Treatment consists mainly in alleviation of the disturbed environmental situation. Parents will need to become more understanding to elicit a change in the child's behavior. Older children can be talked to with the aim of increasing their understanding, easing their anxiety, and giving emotional support. Some examples of situational disorders are colic, feeding and sleeping problems, breath holding, and excessive masturbation.

CONTRIBUTING FACTORS

Among these factors are:

1. Unrealistic parental expectations of a child's behavior for his/her age. Expectations that are too advanced or below normal

for his/her age are obviously a handicap for the child and tend to produce conflicts in the parent-child relationship.
2. Lack of parenting experience and insufficient parental knowledge of the infant's psychologic and physical needs, temperament of the child, and the normal developmental aspects of child behavior
3. Unrealistic expectations of the parenting role
4. The emotional impact on the young parent as bonding and attachment occur with realization of the ever-present need for giving full attention to a helpless infant
5. The age, sex, and temperament of the child as well as what is going on in the family
6. Parental over-concern with regard to the management of minor problems

General Management

To be effective, the management of common problems is directed toward:

1. Prevention. This may be accomplished through early and continued education at parenting groups or classes and by ongoing provision of emotional support by the nurse practitioner.
2. Alleviation of the immediate situation. See the individual problem in this chapter.
3. Identification of the source of the problem. This may be accomplished by careful history taking and interviewing and by additional counseling sessions with the family.
4. Assistance from appropriate specialists as needed. This may be a physician, a psychologist, or a psychiatric social worker.

FACTORS TO CONSIDER

Factors that are considered in the management of common problems are the needs of the child, the needs of the parents, and the individual characteristics of each family that influence the behavior of the family.

Needs of the child. The child's self-image is critical to future development. To assure self-esteem a child needs:

1. Thoughtful and adaptive care. Praise, reassurance, companionship, and intellectual stimulation are essential.
2. Consistent and fair treatment
3. Rights as an individual and acknowledgment as a member of the family
4. Management from a base of affection and intelligent concern. Limits set by the parents should be reasonable and consistent.
5. A feeling of protection from external dangers as well as from his/her own impulses

Needs of the parents. How parents feel about themselves is probably the most important determinant of their child's maturation and development. To feel "good" they need:

1. To understand themselves better to develop a healthy self-image which will aid them in raising their children
2. To examine their feelings and expectations of parenthood, of each other as parents, and of their child's behavior
3. To be allowed to develop as parents
4. To have their concerns recognized and to be given attentive and considerate professional care
5. To understand the differences in children
6. To appreciate that they haven't necessarily been wrong in their treatment of childrearing
7. To understand developmental stages of infancy and childhood for better understanding of the underlying causes of problems (See Table 1.)
8. To establish mutual agreement on methods of childrearing and on the handling of problems.

Individual characteristics of families. The most important include:

1. Expectations of the child's behavior by the parents
2. The structure of the family, the sex of the child, and whether the child is an only child, a twin, a stepchild, an adopted child, or an illegitimate child

Table 1
Tool for Teaching Parents Basic Developmental Concepts and Appropriate Parenting

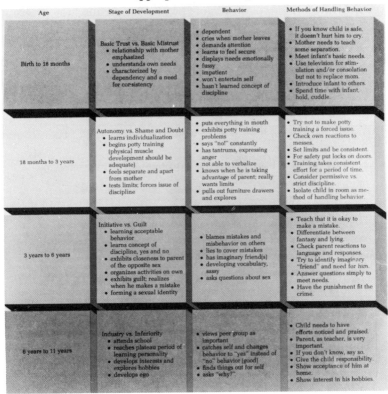

Age	Stage of Development	Behavior	Methods of Handling Behavior
Birth to 18 months	Basic Trust vs. Basic Mistrust • relationship with mother emphasized • understands own needs • characterized by dependency and a need for consistency	• dependent • cries when mother leaves • demands attention • learns to feel secure • displays needs emotionally • fussy • impatient • won't entertain self • hasn't learned concept of discipline	• If you know child is safe, it doesn't hurt him to cry. • Mother needs to teach some separation. • Meet infant's basic needs. • Use television for stimulation and/or consolation but not to replace mom. • Introduce infant to others. • Spend time with infant, hold, cuddle.
18 months to 3 years	Autonomy vs. Shame and Doubt • learns individualization • begins potty training (physical muscle development should be adequate) • feels separate and apart from mother • tests limits; forces issue of discipline	• puts everything in mouth • exhibits potty training problems • says "no!" constantly • has tantrums, expressing anger • not able to verbalize • knows when he is taking advantage of parent; really wants limits • pulls out furniture drawers and explores	• Try not to make potty training a forced issue. • Check own reactions to messes. • Set limits and be consistent. • For safety put locks on doors. • Training takes consistent effort for a period of time. • Consider permissive vs. strict discipline. • Isolate child in room as method of handling behavior.
3 years to 6 years	Initiative vs. Guilt • learning acceptable behavior • learns concept of discipline, yes and no • exhibits closeness to parent of the opposite sex • organizes activities on own • exhibits guilt; realizes when he makes a mistake • forming a sexual identity	• blames mistakes and misbehavior on others • lies to cover mistakes • has imaginary friend(s) • developing vocabulary, sassy • asks questions about sex	• Teach that it is okay to make a mistake. • Differentiate between fantasy and lying. • Check parent reactions to language and responses. • Try to identify imaginary "friend" and need for him. • Answer questions simply to meet needs. • Have the punishment fit the crime.
6 years to 11 years	Industry vs. Inferiority • attends school • reaches plateau period of learning personality • develops interests and explores hobbies • develops ego	• views peer group as important • catches self and changes behavior to "yes" instead of "no" behavior (good) • finds things out for self • asks "why?"	• Child needs to have efforts noticed and praised. • Parent, as teacher, is very important. • If you don't know, say so. • Give the child responsibility. • Show acceptance of him at home. • Show interest in his hobbies.

3. The size of the family, the presence of relatives in the home, established values and customs, and race and nationality
4. Whether a child is quick or slow to learn; whether the child is physically healthy or unhealthy
5. The socioeconomic position of the family
6. The marital situation in the home

OBTAINING THE HISTORY

Information about the family. This may best be obtained by directing the questions at the factors involved in creating the problem and at the factors that influence the behavior of the family. See preceding sections.

Information about the child. To help in handling behavioral problems it is necessary to find out more about the child, such as:

- Where does the child fit in the family?
- What are the child's habits of eating, sleeping, playing, and using spare time?
- How is the child disciplined or punished and by whom?
- What is the nature of contact with other children?
- How many are in the family and how is the child treated by the various members?
- What is going on in the family, such as a newborn, geographic move, divorce, and/or the death of a family member?
- Are parents in agreement about methods of handling problems?

Questions common to most problems. These include:

- How is the problem defined in the parent's own words?
- How long has the problem existed?
- What has the parent done so far to deal with it?
- Why does the parent consider it to be a problem?
- What are the parent's expectations of the child?

Psychologic Needs of Infancy

These are instinctive needs upon which the child's subsequent emotional and social adjustments are based. The infant whose psychologic needs are not fulfilled is definitely handicapped in personality growth and in early capacity to trust and to respond to others. The denial of fulfillment of their needs causes some children to develop such common problems as excessive thumbsucking, head-banging, and other forms of tensional outlet. In severe cases of unfulfilled needs, marasmus can occur which exhibits as "wasting away," infantile atrophy, or debility.

IMPORTANT EARLY NEEDS

Early mothering and sucking are the most important needs of the newborn followed by the needs of feeding, sleeping, and help in the development of specific skills.

Early mothering. Infants need a strong attachment to one person; one who can be trusted to answer their cries and to give them a feeling of security, of well-being, and of being loved and cared for. This is a continuance of the closeness of the prenatal state with the additional factor of touch or positive contact. The more nearly it imitates the condition before birth the more successful it is. The infant needs periods of close contact with the mother which include being held, rocked, carried about; being sung and spoken to; and being fondled and caressed. From being held and allowed to suck freely and frequently, the infant receives reflex stimulation which primes breathing mechanisms into action, and which finally enables the whole respiratory process to become organized under the control of the nervous system.

MOTHERING ATTITUDE. A positive attitude of mothering is extremely important. Early mothering needs are best met by a parent without hesitation, without a feeling of duty, without a feeling of sacrifice. The mother (or mother-figure) should have a feeling of following her maternal instincts, of being good to herself, and of caring for her "inner child." These feelings bolster the positive attitude, creating a "positive atmosphere or aura" for the infant, the benefits of which will last throughout the child's lifetime. To accomplish this for her child the young mother needs help, support, and understanding from her husband, her family, her friends, and from the primary health care provider. She needs space and time from normal activities to accomplish her goals. That is, she should be free from household duties or other commitments as much as possible in the first month. The parents need to reach a mutually agreed upon and compatible philosophy of childrearing to help the mother with her early tasks.

Sucking need. The mouth is the center of the child's universe, the avenue through which hunger and thirst are assuaged. Babies feel with their mouths; it is fundamentally an organ of touch. In the first 6 months sucking is the most satisfying absorbing activity performed by the infant. It assists the infant to breathe, and it increases the amount of blood sent to the brain probably contributing to its development. Tension, which is very evident in early infancy (a fact not well understood), can be relieved by sucking and comfort is restored. Satisfying this need does not develop a dependency, rather, denying this need may contribute to its continuous occurrence in later years, such as thumbsucking beyond the age of 3 or 4 years.

AMOUNT OF SUCKING. Infants need a minimum of 2 hours a day, including feeding time, for oral exercise; more time is needed by immature or premature infants. Sucking needs are fulfilled by breast feeding, bottle feeding, and by allowing the infant to suck on a pacifier which may be held in the infant's mouth if necessary. See this chapter, Use of the Pacifier. Some infants are able to suck their thumbs at birth, but most infants cannot until approximately 3 months of age.

LESSENING OF THE SUCKING NEED. Sucking reaches a maximum intensity about the fourth month and, if it has been fully exercised and the child has received good early mothering, the urgency tends to diminish as the child begins to vocalize, to bite, and to grasp. (Parents can look for cues at this time for eliminating the use of the pacifier.)

Overfeeding can develop as a result of misinterpretation of the infant's needs. When infants cry they may be signaling a need to suck separate from a need to eat. For information regarding the needs of feeding see Chapter 7, Feeding in Infancy and Childhood.

Differences in Temperament and Personality

The term temperament designates the behavioral style of the individual irrespective of the content, level of ability, or motivation of the particular activity. The child's temperament influences the behavior and attitudes of peers, siblings, parents, and teachers. In the first few months of life the basic foundation of a child's personality and temperament is being formed. During this time newborns have quick changes of moods; their behavior is fragmented. Each child has a different personality and temperament, and parents need to be aware of the differences as part of understanding the child's behavior. Thomas et al (1977) in a study of different personalities found that children show distinct individuality of temperament in the first weeks of life independent of the parent's handling or personality style. The environment heightens, diminishes, or modifies behavior, but the basic temperament is the child's own.

"EASY" CHILDREN

Forty percent of the children studied by Thomas were termed "easy," exhibiting these characteristics:

1. Positiveness of mood
2. Regularity of body functions
3. Low or moderate intensity of reaction, adaptability, and positiveness in a new situation

"SLOW-TO-WARM-UP" CHILDREN

This category included 15 percent of the children studied, who were characterized by:

1. Low activity level
2. A tendency to withdraw on first exposure to new stimuli
3. Slow adaptability
4. Somewhat negative mood
5. A low intensity of reaction to situations

"DIFFICULT" CHILDREN

This category included 10 percent of the children studied who were characterized by:

1. Irregularity in body functions

2. Intensity in reactions
3. Withdrawal in the face of new stimuli
4. Slow adaptation to change in the environment
5. Negative mood

Thirty-five percent of the children showed a mixture of traits.

APPLICATIONS TO CHILD CARE

Using these criteria parents can be taught to provide child care which includes these objectives:

- To respond flexibly to the individual requirements of each child
- To view their children with more objectivity
- To provide firm, steady, and consistent care
- To create a positive, relaxed atmosphere in which the child may grow
- To understand that certain features of their child's development and actions are not due to something they did or did not do
- To learn to emphasize the positive aspects of their child's temperament

COMMON CLINICAL PROBLEMS

Parental Concerns of Infancy

BURPING

Assessment. In infancy swallowed air bubbles are trapped in the stomach as infants feed. It occurs more in bottle-fed infants. Although a minor problem, the correct method of burping an infant can help to relieve the stomach of air and to alleviate pain and crying. If crying occurs during a feeding, air should be suspected.

Management. Babies need to be burped frequently, at least before, during, after, or in between feedings if crying occurs. The most satisfactory position for burping is an upright one. The baby sits on the parent's knees. The baby's back is held straight and upright with one hand, while the other hand grasps the baby's distal arm. The baby rests forward against the same wrist which holds the distal arm. The back may be gently rubbed. It should not be slapped or patted. If the baby doesn't burp after a few minutes try again in 10 to 15 minutes if the infant is still awake.

COLIC

Assessment. Colic is defined as unexplained bouts of crying, sometimes accompanied by abdominal distention, spasms, and/or passing of gas. It generally occurs at the same time of the day, usually at the busiest period of the day. It may be caused by feeding problems, maternal anxiety, or allergy to milk. It is aggravated by tension in the household. The infant is not ill; something, possibly immaturity of the digestive system, causes hyperactivity of the bowels. It generally lasts for 3 months. Coincidentally the digestive system is more mature and the infant is able to satisfy sucking need with the thumb. Colic is one of the most trying of the common problems along with crying, its chief symptom. See this chapter, Crying, and Gas.

HISTORY.   The same history is taken as that for "crying."

Management. This is directed at trying to find the source of the problem and at giving support to the parents. There is almost always a reason. Suggestions for helping with suspected colic are as follows:

- Review the basic infant needs. See this chapter, Psychological Needs of Infancy.
- Review feeding methods carefully
- Keep a record of the time during the day that it occurs. Soothe the child before the crying spell is expected.
- Wrap the infant warmly, including booties
- Walk or rock the infant or take him/her for a ride in a car

- Rest the infant with his/her abdomen on a warm and/or hard surface, such as the parent's knees or shoulder
- Try infant on a soy milk formula if bottle fed
- Give whiskey 10–20 gtts in warm water 30 minutes before expected crying spell
- Change the household routine to produce a quieter environment (if possible) if the colicky spells occur during a very active time
- Advise a mild sedative only in extreme cases
- Offer reassurance to the parents that the infant is not ill, and that they are giving good care
- Emphasize that it definitely will go away

CONSTIPATION IN INFANCY

Assessment. The consistency of stools (hard, pebbly, rocklike) defines constipation in infancy. It is not related to the frequency of bowel movements, straining, grunting, or the number of days between movements.

STOOL PATTERNS OF INFANCY. These are generally as follows:

Breast-fed infant. This infant has many stools per day (sometimes one after each feeding) in the first month or 2 progressing to one stool a day or even many days (4 or 5 days) in the later months before solid foods are introduced to the diet. The stool resembles pale, yellow curds unless iron is given which makes the stool darker. It is watery and it is explosive in nature; there is no unpleasant odor. A green stool in the neonate who is not taking iron may denote that the infant is not receiving enough milk.

Bottle-fed infant. This infant has two to four stools per day in the first month progressing to one to three stools or less per day in the later months. The color may be varied shades of green, brown, or yellow depending on the formula and on whether iron or solid food are taken. The color is not important in a well child. The stool is soft and may have an unpleasant odor.

HISTORY. Ascertain the consistency, color, and frequency of the stools and if accompanied by any mucus or blood. Review the infant's diet. Ask how the parents feel about regular toileting and what their concept is of constipation.

Management. This is directed at educating the parents about normal stool patterns and relieving the cause if the child is constipated. Treatment and guidance include the following:

- The infant may need more liquids in the diet. Offer water between meals.
- The infant may have been introduced to solid foods too soon, or they are being increased too quickly. Discontinue them temporarily until constipation clears up. Begin again with smaller amounts increasing them very slowly depending on the stool consistency.
- Dark Karo syrup, 1 tsp in 2 to 3 oz of water, may be given.
- Fruit may be given; pureed prunes up to 3 tablespoons may be helpful.
- The parents need reassurance that the child is not ill. Discuss with them their attitude and expectations of toileting habits and discourage the use of stool softeners, laxatives, or enemas.

CRYING

Assessment. Periodic crying for unexplained reasons in the neonatal period continues to be one of the most frustrating of the common problems. Crying in the newborn period may assume a definite pattern early. It may be associated with unexplainable tension. It may begin and end at approximately the same time every day (see this chapter, Colic) or it may spread to other hours upsetting the household and provoking feelings of inadequacy and incompetency. The parent may think that the infant is in pain, is hungry, or will hurt him/her self. Crying, aggravated by household tension, may lead to overfeeding, more crying, and more tension resulting in a cycle that leaves parents and infant frustrated and unrelieved. Conflicting advice of relatives and friends adds to the feelings of insecurity of the most secure parent.

HISTORY.   This should include the following:

- At what time and for how long is the crying spell?
- What is the infant fed, how often, and what methods are used? Is the infant bottle- or breast-fed? If bottle, how is it prepared, is the bottle propped or held, how large are the nipple holes, what kind of nipple is used?
- When and how often is the infant burped?
- What is the stool pattern?
- Are the infant's basic needs of contact and sucking met? Does the infant use a pacifier?
- How do the parents handle the cry?
- What are the parents' expectations of crying? Do they agree on methods of handling the cry?
- What is going on in the house? Does the mother have help? Are there siblings?
- Are there allergies in the family?
- Are there any other symptoms?
- How does the parent feel when the infant's cries cannot be stopped?

Management.   Relieving parental anxiety is the most important aspect of management. Ideally assessment and management of crying of the newborn should not be done by telephone. The parents must be reassured that the infant is not in pain, and physical illness should be ruled out. A careful physical examination should be performed. Keep in mind that the parents are feeling inadequate, and that they need support and understanding; explanations should include the following:

- Babies cry for a reason. It is their only way to communicate. All cries should be answered. Do not let the baby "cry it out." Answering cries leads to better attachment between mother and child.
- A clear explanation of basic infant needs, both psychologic and physical should be given. See this chapter, Psychologic Needs of Infancy. One or two periods of crying for 5 to 10 minutes a day can be a breathing exercise or a release into sleep. If the child cries longer, needs should be reassessed.

- A positive, relaxed approach to infant care is beneficial. At fussy periods try to produce a quiet household; infants sleep more soundly in a quiet environment.
- A definite pattern of crying can be anticipated and modified by early offering of physical comforts, such as swaddling, soothing talk, holding, rocking, and sucking.
- A review of feeding and burping methods should be given. The infant may need extra fluids.
- Reinforcement should be given to the parents that they are doing the correct thing; that crying may be a facet of the child's personality.
- If parents are feeling very stressed and frustrated by the infant's crying, respite care and/or around-the-clock availability of the nurse practitioner may be indicated.

GAS (FLATUS)

Assessment. This is air in the stomach or intestines that causes abdominal distress and/or distention and discomfort, and may be expelled through the anus. The causes are:

- Excessive swallowing of air (hyperaerophasia) which is due to physiologic inability to seal off nasal passages during swallowing. The air may be swallowed while crying, while at breast or bottle, or when sucking the pacifier.
- Overfeeding or underfeeding
- An allergy to milk

HISTORY. Ascertain the length of feeding time, size of nipple holes, type of bottle used, and methods of feeding. Is the child held or is the bottle propped? Does the baby use a pacifier? How and when is the baby burped? What is the stool pattern?

Management. This is directed at locating the cause and, if possible, eliminating it by the following methods:

- Calm the infant and burp when picked up after crying
- Burp the infant frequently during and following the feedings

- Enlarge the nipple holes if necessary to cut down on the feeding time
- Place the baby on the left side to ease the expelling of gas
- Try the infant on soy milk formula for a trial period of 2 to 3 weeks if allergies are familial or suspected
- Reassure the parents that the child will outgrow hyper-aerophasia

HICCOUGHS

Assessment. Hiccoughs are caused by sudden, sharp, involuntary spasms of the diaphragm, perhaps by small amounts of food being regurgitated into the esophagus. They usually occur following a feeding but may occur anytime. They are more distressing to the parents than to the infant who would cry if distressed.

Management. It is not necessary to do anything, but often the hiccoughs will cease if the infant is offered water or a pacifier. The parents can be reassured that the infant is not suffering nor ill.

PACIFIER

Assessment. There are many questions about the use and misuse of pacifiers. Parents misunderstand the infant's need for non-nutritional sucking or use the pacifier beyond the child's need for extra sucking. See this chapter, Psychologic Needs of Infancy, Sucking Needs.

POSITIVE USE OF THE PACIFIER. There are times when the pacifier can and should be used. Parents need to understand the following:

- The pacifier may be used immediately after birth. It helps the infant to develop sucking functions of the mouth and aids in establishing breast feeding; it may be held in the mouth if necessary.
- In infancy the pacifier provides a good method for satisfying the sucking need.

- Bottle-fed infants need extra sucking time. They may be held and cuddled at the same time.
- Pacifiers do not become a habit unless the child sucks beyond infancy, becomes ill, or for some reason does not receive enough mothering.
- Some infants will substitute the thumb before or at about 3 months of age.
- Parents can watch for clues to eliminate the use of the pacifier between 3 and 4 months when the infant becomes more active and there is a diminishing need to suck. Stimulation suitable to the age may be substituted.

NEGATIVE USE OF THE PACIFIER.   Prevention of inappropriate use of the pacifier may be accomplished by stressing the following:

- It should not replace holding and/or stimulation.
- It should not be used constantly without first answering other infant needs.
- The child can suck any type of pacifier, but it is better if the pacifier nipple is similar to the other nipples being used, for example, the Nuk nipple comes also as a pacifier.
- Parents should try to discontinue the use of the pacifier beyond 4 to 5 months since a habit may form and may be difficult to overcome. It is preferable that the child suck his/her thumb beyond this time as the thumb may not be used as frequently as when the pacifier is offered by the mother.

SPOILING

Assessment.   Spoiling may occur if basic needs are not gratified in early infancy. The child continues to need them satisfied beyond a normal time limit thereby developing as a demanding, undisciplined child. Overgratification of needs in later infancy and toddler age caused by anxiety, hesitancy, and ambivalence of the parents in setting limits also results in a demanding, undisciplined child. It is felt that a child cannot be "spoiled" under 6 months of age, the age when all of the infant needs should have been satisfied. See this chapter, Crying, and Psychologic Needs of Infancy.

HISTORY. Ascertain what the parents mean by "spoiling" and how the child is disciplined and by whom. Do the parents agree on methods of disciplining?

Management. For concerns regarding "spoiling," counseling should include the following:

- During early infancy needs must be gratified.
- Gradually a child is able to handle frustrations for longer periods of time, generally at about 6 to 9 months.
- At this time it may be difficult to draw an arbitrary line between indulgence and restriction; it must be gentle and gradual.
- Parents who find it difficult to manage a particularly demanding child should spell each other or secure the help of a babysitter.
- A relaxed, calm approach should be tried.
- It is helpful to attend parenting classes to share concerns of "spoiling" with other parents.

SEPARATION ANXIETY

Assessment. This is a gradual process of differentiation of the infant's body from the mother's body. Usually occurring at about 9 to 10 months of age, it signals the beginning of a new attachment to the mother. The infant has not yet learned that when mother goes away she will return.

Management. Peek-a-boo games will help the child to cope with the parent's leaving. A child needs at least 30 minutes to 1 hour to become acquainted with a new person. Parents should not "sneak out" to avoid a scene. It is best for the infant and young child to know that their parents leave and return.

STRANGER ANXIETY

Assessment. This is anxiety which is provoked by a strange human face beginning at about 6 to 8 months of age and gradually vanishing over the next year. It is interpreted as indicating that the child has developed a good schema of the mother's face. A stranger is a discrepancy in this schema that the child cannot handle.

Management. An infant will exhibit less stranger anxiety if held by the mother in the presence of strangers, and if they all spend time together before the baby is left alone with the stranger (e.g., a new babysitter).

Problems Related to Feeding

OVERFEEDING VERSUS UNDERFEEDING IN INFANCY

Assessment. Some mothers find it a problem to determine whether or not a proper amount of milk or solid food is being given to the infant.

HISTORY. Obtain a detailed diet history to include the amounts of milk and solid food and by what methods and how frequently the infant is fed. Obtain the infant's birth weight and present weight. Obtain a description of the stools and how frequently the infant urinates.

Management. This is directed at educating the parents regarding nutritional needs. They need to be aware of basic foods and how to determine the amounts necessary for optimum growth. See Chapter 6. They also need to understand the following:

- Some infants will eat more than they require if food is offered whenever they cry. Explain the infant's needs for non-nutritive sucking and contact.
- "Too loose" a demand feeding schedule may be confusing to the parent. Try to adjust the schedule to a reasonable amount of time between feedings.
- Water may be offered between feedings since the infant may be thirsty. This postpones the next feeding.
- If the infant is gaining weight, the infant is not underfed.
- True constipation, green stools, or scant urine with a strong odor should be reported to the health facility.

REFUSAL OF SOLIDS

Assessment. Parents sometimes feel that once solid foods are introduced the child should eat on schedule; that they must be forced to eat what has been suggested at the health facility. A problem is created for some mothers when the child refuses the offered food.

HISTORY. Ascertain the age of the child, diet history including snacks and foods which the child enjoys, and how the parents feel about the refusal of food.

Management. The management is different for infants and toddlers.

INFANTS. Discuss with the parents the following:

- There is no reason for solids in an infant's diet before 4 to 6 months of age. At this time the child needs to chew and to pick up food and has an added need for iron-containing foods.
- Digestion starts with salivation which occurs at 3 to 4 months.
- Infants enjoy picking up food and feeding themselves at about 6 months of age.
- Solid food feeding is not necessarily related to sleeping through the night.
- Tongue thrusting is a normal phenomenon not a refusal of food. It disappears sooner in some babies than in others.
- An infant may resist food if there is a feeling of being forced.
- Solids may be stopped except for the ones enjoyed by the infant.
- Fruits and cereals or other foods may be mixed together or added to the milk in extreme cases.

Discuss with parents their feelings about feeding and messiness. Suggest a calm and relaxed approach.

TODDLERS. Much of toddlers' refusal of food is determined by their age and the parental attitude. Parents need to understand the following:

- As children grow and become more active they lose interest in food or may refuse to eat as a form of negativism. Parents should resist giving food instead of offering stimulation or taking time to answer other needs of the child.

- Small amounts of food can be offered frequently in place of three meals. There is no reason why the same foods cannot be eaten day after day as long as the nutritional needs are met.
- If possible less milk per day should be offered and non-nutritive snacks should be avoided.
- If milk is refused, powdered milk can be added to solid foods and calcium can be obtained in puddings, yogurt, cheese, ice cream, or via a calcium supplement.
- It should be a pleasure to eat, not a chore; fingers are as good as spoons.

Discuss with the parents their feelings toward food refusal, messiness, and reassure them that the child will grow and stay well.

"SPITTING-UP" (REGURGITATION)

Assessment. "Spitting-up" commonly occurs following a feeding. The causes may be air swallowed along with food, possible inability to relax the esophageal sphincter until later, possible overfeeding, or an allergy to cow milk. Persistent regurgitation tends to be outgrown when the child enters the sitting stage of development.

HISTORY. Obtain a diet history. Determine how the infant is burped, if the entire feeding is brought up, if it is projectile in nature, if it contains mucus or blood, if the infant is gaining weight, if the baby is always hungry, and how long it has been going on.

Management. This is directed at defining the problem and at giving parental support. Parents need to understand the following:

- Correct preparation of the formula, proper nipple hole sizes, or a new nipple may be needed.
- Infants need frequent and regular burping.
- Formula may be changed to one without an iron supplement, to an evaporated milk formula, or to a soy milk formula.
- The child may be kept in an upright position for about 30 minutes following a feeding.
- The formula may be thickened slightly with infant rice cereal.

WEANING FROM BREAST TO BOTTLE

Assessment. Weaning from breast to bottle becomes a problem if the parent has ambivalent feelings about weaning or if the infant refuses the bottle.

HISTORY. Ascertain the age of the child and a schedule of feedings. Determine who wants the baby weaned (the mother, the father, or both) and why.

Management. This is directed at helping the parent to make the decision to wean, and at giving support and advice on methods of weaning.

DECISION TO WEAN. When helping a parent to decide when to wean include the following:

- It should be discussed and decided on by both parents
- It is helpful if the mother makes a contract with herself every 3 months while breast feeding as to whether or not to continue
- The mother needs a very positive attitude toward weaning
- The period between 6 to 9 months of age is not the best time to wean because the infant is experiencing separation anxiety and does not react well to major changes.
- The age of 1 year may be a good time to wean since the infant is ready to use a cup and wishes to be more independent. Some children have a continuing need to suck.

ACTIVE WEANING. Start weaning by substituting a bottle for the breast one feeding at a time for a few days at a time; for example, drop the 2 PM feeding first for a few days, then the 10 AM feeding followed by the 6 PM feeding, and finally the 6 AM feeding.

RESISTANCE TO WEANING. These methods may be tried:

- Give water or juices in the bottle before starting to wean until the infant is used to the bottle
- Make sure that the nipple being used is similar in type to the pacifier or one which has been used in the past
- Heat the milk

- Be firm against succumbing to the infant's demands for the breast
- Have someone other than the mother give the bottle
- Keep to a schedule if possible
- Be firm, positive, and patient

WEANING FROM BOTTLE TO CUP

Assessment. Weaning to the cup successfully is often dependent on the physical and emotional development of the child, the family life style, and stresses within the family. It should be attempted gradually when the child is ready, usually at about the age of 1. Dentists believe that the child continues to need sucking until this age to develop the mouth and jaws properly.

HISTORY.   Ascertain the age of the child, who wants to wean, what has been tried, how many bottles are given per day, if the child can use a cup, and how the sucking needs are satisfied.

Management.   This includes support and counseling as follows:

- Children enjoy the accomplishment of using a cup; it is one of their first steps toward independence.
- They may keep one bottle a day until they are ready to give it up. If this bottle is used at bedtime it should contain water only.
- Forcing a child to use a cup may increase the need to suck.
- It is considered to be more detrimental to wean sooner than later.
- Parents should keep a calm, relaxed attitude.

Problems Related to Sleep

Sleep problems are classified as both developmental and/or situational. They generally occur from infancy through the separation anxiety stages of the 2 to 3 year old.

Sleep problems may follow an especially tiring and stressful day or may occur as the result of waking during an illness or teething.

They occur as bedtime problems and as night-waking problems. To manage sleep problems effectively it is necessary to understand normal sleep patterns. See Table 2.

NIGHTMARES

Assessment. These are frightening dreams from which the child awakens with a feeling of suffocation, fear, and helplessness. They may start at about 3 years of age. They occur as a result of increased sexual and aggressive urges and fantasies.

Management. Reassure the parent that these dreams are considered to be normal. Usually the child recalls the dream and is easily placated by recognizing the parent or sitter. The child usually needs comforting before returning to bed.

NIGHT TERRORS

Assessment. These are dreams which fail to wake the child completely so the child does not remember the experience the following day. The child acts excited, calls out, may believe that there are animals or strange people in the room, or may not know who he/she is nor recognize the parents. After a few minutes the child falls back to sleep. These dreams are rare, occurring mainly between the ages of 2 and 4.

Management. The parents need to be reassured. These terrors tend to disappear spontaneously if not too much fuss is made, and if the child is comforted before returning to bed.

SLEEPING PROBLEMS OF INFANCY

Assessment. Some infants have problems with release into sleep and/or wake easily during the night as often as every 3 hours, causing disturbances within the household. It is thought to be the result of separation anxiety. Teething and illness may also cause sleeping problems.

Table 2
Normal Sleep Patterns

Age	Number of hr/24 hr	Comments About Sleeping Habits
Newborn	Low: 10 Average: 16½ High: 23 (7–8 short naps)	No child fits into a routinely pre-prescribed sleep pattern.
8–12 weeks	(2–4 naps)	Release into sleep varies with infants. Some are more tense than others.
2–4 months	Low: 8–10/night High: 11–12/night 2–3 naps/day	Although there is no correlation with solid food intake and sleeping through the night, the parent's attitude may make the difference.
6–12 months	11–12/night 2–3 naps/day	There should be an established routine for bedtime. Baby may wake due to illness, teething, or separation anxiety.
12–18 months	8–12/night 1–2 naps/day	There may be waking problems after the mother returns to work, even after several months.
2–3 years	8–12/night 1 nap/day	There is a need for rituals and consistency at bedtime. Active children may not nap after 2½ years.
3–4 years	8–12/night May take 1 nap/day	Some children will wake with dreams. (One fifth of the night is spent dreaming.) Many children will wake and wander at night. Some children will accept a net over the crib or a locked half-door on the bedroom. The habit of sleeping with parents should be discouraged.
4 years	8–12/night	This is a good time to shift from crib to bed. Some dreaming and waking may result.
4½–5 years	8–12/night	There may be an increase in bad dreams and night terrors. The child may need considerable attention to get back to sleep. The child may enjoy reading at bedtime before lights out. Dreams may be at a low peak.

HISTORY. Ascertain the infant's age, how long the infant sleeps, what the feeding schedule is, what occurs in the household at bedtime, if the child has been ill or teething, if the infant is fed when he/she wakes, how the parents handle the problem, and how they feel about it.

Management. This is directed at counseling the parents regarding gratification of the needs of infancy (see this chapter, Psychologic Needs of Infancy) and normal sleep patterns of infants. They should understand the following:

- The differences in temperament of children. Carey (1972, p. 34) has found that sleep disturbances in infancy with night-waking is significantly correlated with a low sensory threshold.
- Infants will sleep through the night between 2 to 3 months of age. This can be accomplished by a positive parental attitude and an understanding that the baby at this age does not need nourishment during the night.
- Many infants need help releasing into sleep. This can be accomplished by the use of the pacifier, by holding, rocking, or walking the baby to sleep, or by the mere physical presence of the parent.
- A quiet room should be found for the infant to sleep in when the parents can separate the infant from their room.

SLEEPING PROBLEMS OF THE TODDLER

Assessment. Sleeping problems in early childhood are developmental disorders generally due to separation anxiety or to a fear of aggressive impulses. A poor environmental situation has the effect of increasing the child's impulses and fears, thereby causing more severe sleep disturbances. Teething, illness, or television shows of a violent nature can also be causes.

HISTORY. Ascertain at what time and how often the problem occurs, if the child has bedtime rituals and consistent care, and what is happening in the family.

Management. This is directed at reassuring the child and the parents and at alleviation of the existing environmental situation. Parents need to understand the following:

- The normal development of separation anxiety. See this chapter, Table 1 and Separation Anxiety. The child should be assured that the parents will be present upon awakening.

- Sleeping in the parents room at this age or parental overpermissiveness may be associated with sleeping disturbances.

- There is a need for firm, fair, and consistent treatment at bedtime accompanied by regular rituals.

- Boisterous physical activity or stress prior to bedtime should be avoided.

- A night light or soft music may help a child who has difficulty falling asleep.

- A child who cannot sleep should not be nagged or punished.

Common Habits

Many parents feel that well-adjusted children should not have so-called "bad habits" and feel guilty of poor parenting if bad habits exist in their children. These "habits" generally bother the parent more than the child. Most of the habits listed in Table 3 are classified as developmental or situational disorders; they are also called tensional outlets. Most children have one or more of these habits depending on their temperament and the environment. Some of the habits develop into problems if the parent participates in a contest of wills with the child. The habit will usually be outgrown if the parents and caretakers accept them with a calm, relaxed attitude as developmental behaviors. Children should not be nagged or have undue attention called to the habit. Parents can better handle the problem if they ask "why" the child does it, rather than "how can I stop it."

BITING AND HITTING

Assessment. These occur as a result of aggressive impulses at 2 to 3 years of age. They are usually temporary behaviors often occur-

Table 3
Common Childhood Behaviors

Age	Behaviors
1 year	Sucks thumb, smears stools, shakes bed, bangs and rocks, and masturbates
2 years	As above. Has temper tantrums, tears books or wallpaper, tears bed apart, removes clothes, runs around, and has many pre-sleep demands
2½ years	Above behavior in lesser degree. Stutters and has disruptive aggressive attacks such as hitting and biting
3 years	Less of the above behaviors
3½ years	Again an increase in some of the above behaviors. Spits, picks nose, bites fingernails, and whines
4 years	Runs away, kicks, spits, bites nails, grimaces, calls names, boasts, brags, uses silly language, has nightmares and fears, needs to urinate in moments of emotional distress, has "belly" pains and may vomit
5 years	A decrease in some behaviors, blinks eye, shakes head, clears throat, and sniffles
5½–6 years	All the above behaviors and increased clumsiness
7 years	Tries to control behaviors and may have headaches
8 years	Picks at fingers, cries with fatigue, and makes faces
9 years	Stamps feet, fiddles, drops and breaks things, picks at self, growls and mutters

ring when the child is in a difficult social situation. They may occur when the child is tired or hungry. Too much may be expected of the child regarding social behavior.

Management. Besides looking for tense situations and giving support to the parents, they can be advised as follows:

- It is not desirable to bite or to hit the child in retaliation
- The parent may cup the child's chin as he/she is about to bite and gently push upward with a verbal reminder against biting as acceptable behavior
- The parent may find that temporary isolation for the child in a room is helpful. Many children are looking for limits and enjoy the quiet of a room.
- The child probably should not have too many or many different companions at this age

BREATHHOLDING

Assessment. This is usually one of several signals of a disturbing parent-child relationship, possibly characterized by overprotection. It occurs first at about 2 years of age, rarely before 6 months of age; it disappears after 4 years, rarely seen after 6 years. It has a high familial incidence. Two of the causes may be a tense, rigid feeding regime or prematurely enforced regulation of toilet habits. The child precedes the breathholding with a temper tantrum, holds his breath, and becomes blue in the face. Some children lose consciousness and may have tonic or clonic movements. It should be differentiated from epilepsy. See Chapter 25, Breathholding.

Management. This is directed primarily at parent-child guidance and reassurance. Efforts should be made to understand the family situation. Parents should use purposeful neglect to prevent the child from acquiring satisfaction through using breathholding attacks as a means of dominating the family.

HEAD-BANGING, ROCKING, BED-SHAKING

Assessment. A form of self-stimulation, these behaviors may be classified as situational disorders. They occur in infancy usually as a result of undergratification of the basic infant needs. They occur at bedtime and during the night; the pattern is reinforced if the child goes to sleep during the behavior. Some children may show a tendency to turn inward or withdraw from reality.

HISTORY. Ascertain how the infant's cries are handled, if the basic needs have been gratified, how bedtime is handled, if the child is ill or overstimulated, and the family situation.

Management. This is directed at ruling out a hyperactive child and the need for further medical attention. Support is given to the family who needs to understand the following:

- The basic infant needs should be gratified. See this chapter, Psychologic Needs of Infancy.
- The child should not be left to "cry it out" at bedtime. See this chapter, Crying.
- If possible the parent should spend extra time in a relaxed manner with the infant holding, rocking, or patting the child's back while he/she falls asleep.
- Soft music or a night-light in the bedroom may be helpful.

MASTURBATION

Assessment. A normal physiologic reaction, masturbation is exploration of the body accompanying stimulation of sexual feelings. The resulting pleasureful sexual sensation reinforces the tendency to continue. It may start accidentally in the first year; it may be more purposeful and frequent somewhere around 4 years of age. Masturbation occurs most commonly at bedtime when anxiety is increased owing to separation or fear of loss of control of sexual or aggressive impulses. Excessive masturbation may be a symptom of a neurotic or more severe disorder.

Management. Support is given to the parents, and they need to understand the following:

- It is appropriate to censor open masturbation. Allow the child to know that you understand, then ignore the behavior. It may become a problem if too great an importance is accorded the behavior.

- The child may need some setting of limits. See this chapter, Discipline.
- The parent should not take a punitive attitude, install feelings of guilt, or threaten the child's self-esteem.

STUTTERING

Assessment. Primary stuttering is that which occurs in the younger child who is not aware of the problem. Secondary stuttering occurs in an older child after the age of 3 or 4 years when the child becomes aware that the speech is different. It occurs five times more frequently in males than in females. It may start when attention is called to the normal repeating of words as the child begins speech; it may follow a severe trauma; or it may occur as a result of rigid expectations of feeding or toilet training. The words most generally stuttered are long words, words beginning with consonants, first words of a sentence, and adverbs.

Management. Support is given to the parents. They need to understand the following:

- The child needs plenty of sleep, outdoor activity, good, nourishing food, and a stable home environment.
- The child should not be made to feel that the speech is abnormal and should be given many opportunities to speak, such as a telephone set, a daily game to mimic the parents' speech, or talking and reading aloud in unison.
- The parents should encourage the areas in which the child excels.
- A change of environment is frequently helpful, such as a visit to the grandparents.
- Parents need to watch for the trigger mechanisms and try to avoid them.
- The child should be forewarned of ridicule by classmates.
- If stuttering continues by the age of 5 referral should be made to a speech therapist and/or a psychiatrist.

TEMPER TANTRUMS

Assessment. This is classified as a developmental disorder. Temper tantrums usually occur from 18 months to 3 years of age.

This is the age of negativism and independence. Temper tantrums may occur when the child is hungry, tired, or frustrated by a social situation. They may occur because the child's needs are over-gratified and the child now needs to have limits set. See this chapter, Spoiling.

HISTORY. Ascertain the child's age, when the tantrums occur, and how they are being handled.

Management. This is directed at finding the cause of the tantrums and prevention. The parents need to understand the following:

- A child of this age needs limits. Tantrums demonstrate this need. See this chapter, Discipline.
- A record can be kept of when the tantrums occur, the child's state of hunger, and his frustrations at the time. Intervention may then be made before the actual tantrum begins.
- Isolation by removal of the child to a room is helpful.
- The parents should remain calm and unemotional and should examine their own feelings about the tantrum.

Concerns About Toddlers and Preschoolers

Concerns of the parents of this age child are generally developmental in nature. Parents who do not understand the readiness of a child for a specific behavior have ambivalent feelings about handling certain behaviors. They either allow too much freedom or they try to "train" the child before the child is fully developed. Discipline is necessary for a child's well-being and physical and mental growth but it needs to be differentiated from punishment.

DISCIPLINE

Assessment. Discipline is defined as the job of parents to set forth a set of rules for correct and incorrect behavior and for the safety of the child based on the parents' concept of behavior, feelings, and attitudes. It is a setting of limits and controlling of undesirable acts.

It is learning to behave in a manner acceptable to others and training that develops self-control and character.

PERMISSIVENESS. This is defined as refraining from inhibiting the child's individual development. It produces confidence and an increasing capacity to express feelings and thoughts. It is a form of discipline.

OVERPERMISSIVENESS. This is the allowing of undesirable acts or overgratification of needs. Overpermissiveness brings anxiety and increasing demands for privileges that cannot be granted, resulting in "spoiling." In infancy if limits are not set, the child may cry automatically at any slight discomfort or disappointment. In the early school years if children receive censure for everything they do, they learn that they are displeasing and inept. In adolescence if they are not required to be courteous or obedient, they learn to be self-indulgent.

Management. The setting of limits should be done in a manner that preserves the self-respect of both parent and child. Some desirable and undesirable methods of discipline are in the following list:

- Do set examples for love, honesty, unselfishness, and good manners.
- Do be aware that discipline is essential to healthy growth and development of self-discipline
- Do act in a fair, clear, and consistent method; "treat as you would be treated "
- Do agree on methods of discipline
- Do give simple directions; give warnings; bend a little
- Do allow the child to express feelings; be permissive
- Do respect children; praise, approve, and encourage
- Do not expect behavior beyond the ability or development of the child
- Do not argue, threaten, promise, sermonize, or give rude teaching of politeness
- Do not be overpermissive
- Do not push the child to achieve

- Do not be too authoritarian or overstrict. According to Carey (1972, p. 37), as the educational level and socioeconomic status of the parents go down, the use of authoritarian methods increases and is the most prevalent method of discipline.

PUNISHMENT

Assessment. This is defined as the method of controlling behavior when limits are exceeded. A child needs to feel guilty if he misbehaves; the guilt reaction will eventually serve to inhibit the impulse to repeat the act. The degree of guilt feelings should be appropriate to the act. Most punishment is meted out as a result of the parent's loss of temper. Parent's own motives should be questioned.

Management. There are methods of punishment that are more acceptable than others. Some of both are listed below:

- Do agree on methods between parents
- Do allow room for a cooling-off period
- Do respect the feelings of the child
- Isolation to a room at the time of the misdemeanor may be helpful
- A smack on the clothed buttocks of a toddler at the time of the misdemeanor is preferable to more severe methods
- Do not expect behavior beyond the developmental level of the child
- Do not direct anger at the child, but at the situation
- Do not retaliate by hitting
- Do not belittle, be sarcastic, ridicule, humiliate, or shame the child
- Do not send the child to bed or force him to go without food
- Do not deprive the child of parental love

SEPARATION ANXIETY

Assessment. This is a developmental milestone which can reach a peak at 12 to 13 months of age. It is sometimes a cause of sleep disturbances. The process of appearance-disappearance allows the child to acquire an intellectual control over the environment which helps to overcome this anxiety by the age of 18 months.

Management. This age is not suitable for major changes to occur in the child's life, such as weaning, moving, or mother returning to work. The child who wakes at night should be comforted. See this chapter, Sleeping Problems of the Toddler. Reassurance is given to the parents that the child will outgrow this anxiety.

SIBLING RIVALRY (JEALOUSY)

Assessment. This is described as hostile and aggressive behavior exhibited more often in a child who is not much older than the sibling. The closer the age, the more hostile and aggressive the behavior. It occurs in children who are not yet old enough to cope with sharing the mother; they compete for the exclusive love of the parent. Jealousy is sometimes expressed by competitiveness, regression of toilet training, or other appropriate behaviors. See Table 3.

Management. This is directed at reassuring the parents. They need to understand the following:

- Much is dependent on how the parent reacts to the behavior. They need to understand about the child's feeling of displacement.
- The older child needs some time alone with the parent for some part of each day.
- Each child should be treated as an individual; older children may enjoy special privileges.
- It is best to space children at least 3 years apart. The 3 year old is better able to cope with the displacement.
- The older child should be prepared for the advent of a new sibling along with the rest of the family and should be given simple explanations.
- It may be helpful if the older child can visit the hospital to see the mother and baby, and be allowed to help with care of the baby.

- It is wiser to accept jealousy as a fact and to learn to deal with it than to deny its existence.

TOILET TRAINING

Assessment. Toilet training becomes a concern to parents because they do not understand when to start teaching the child toileting habits; they do not understand the child's development; they wish to be finished with soiled diapers and messiness; and they have social pressures from family and friends. To handle toilet training the parents and counselor should explore their expectations and must understand the readiness of the child (see Table 4). Brazelton (1962), in a study done of 1170 children over a span of 10 years, published these statistics:

- 12 percent of the children accomplished bowel training first
- 8 percent of the children accomplished bladder training first
- 80 percent of the children accomplished both simultaneously
- Most of the children were trained by 27 to 29 months of age
- 40 percent of the children were still bedwetting at age 4
- 30 percent of the children were still bedwetting at age 5

Table 4
Physiologic and Psychologic Readiness of Child for Toilet Training

Physiologic	*Psychologic*
Is able to manipulate sphincter muscles: 1½ to 2 years of age	Sense of self-identity: 1 year of age
Is able to manipulate clothing up and down (needs manual dexterity): 1½ to 2 years	Trust relationship with mother, a need to please: 2 years
Can hold a specific amount of urine in the bladder, up to 5 hours: 2½ years	Sense of independence and wish to do for him/herself: 2 years
Can understand simple questions	Express pride in achievement: 2 years
Can ask to be changed by pulling at pants, grunting: 1½ to 2 years	Emotional capacity to withhold any action or to perform it: 2 years
Can understand simple directions: 1½ to 2 years.	

- A 2 year old voids 12 times in 24 hours, about 2 oz per voiding
- 3 to 6 year olds void 7 to 8 times in 24 hours, about 3 oz per voiding

EXPECTATIONS OF PARENTS.   Since these are important to the attitude of the parents toward toilet training, they should be ascertained when counseling is given at the 9 to 12 month health visit. See Chapter 3, Visit at Nine Months. Find out from the parents the following:

- When had they planned to toilet train?
- Do they expect a female child to differ from a male child?
- Do they understand that toilet training involves both bladder and bowels?
- What are their cultural patterns of toilet training? How were they trained?
- How do they feel about cleanliness, messiness, and modesty?
- What are the pressures from family and friends?
- Are they open to different methods of toilet training?

Management.   This is directed at counseling regarding unrealistic expectations, the readiness of the child, explaining the types of toilet training, and discussing problems related to toilet training.

EARLY TOILET TRAINING.   The trend is away from teaching the child toileting habits at the early age of 10 to 15 months, and it should be discouraged. Physiologically the child is not ready. Psychologically the mother is, therefore, this is called "mother-training" and should be attempted only if the mother is strongly motivated. She should recognize that the child can be bowel trained only, that accidents are due to her, not to the child, and that the training should not be stressful; the child should not feel forced. Mainly, the attitude about early toilet-training should be discussed.

TOILET TRAINING AT 18 TO 30 MONTHS.   Toilet training may be started at this age when the time is right; that is, when there are no major changes occurring in the household; when the child shows interest after observing others, such as mothers' sitting, fathers' standing; when nursery school friends are trained; or when the child becomes aware of wet and dirty diapers versus clean and dry ones. Physical and psychologic development of the child indicates that this is the correct age for training, and parents can begin in the following ways:

- The child can be introduced to his/her own potty chair. Allow the child to play with it, sit on it in clothes, and later with diapers off. The mother may put the stool from the diaper into the potty as the child observes.

- If there is no resistance, the child may be put on the potty for not longer than 5 to 10 minutes at the time that elimination is expected. If the child is successful or shows interest, the times may be increased to 2 to 3 a day.

- With continued interest and success, training pants may be introduced. Allow the child to sit on the potty on demand or at spaced times during the day.

- At no time should this be a stressful situation. If the child resists, it is best to forget it for a few weeks at a time and to try again.

- Toilet training can be accomplished readily, or it can occur over a long period of time. At all times the parent should have a positive and relaxed attitude.

"NATURAL" TOILET TRAINING. There is a trend toward allowing children to train themselves. Parents can bring toileting to the child's attention when it is sensed that the child is ready, but the attitude of "allowing the child to handle the situation all by him/herself" is overcautious. The child needs to know that the parent is willing to help; the child needs limits set at this age and enjoys independence and the feeling of accomplishment.

Problems related to toilet training. Some children are not ready at 18 to 30 months, and some parents need support if the training does not progress well. Some of the problems which may occur and their management are listed below:

- A child may play with feces which is disturbing to the parent. Allow the child to play with soft clay or finger paints for the need to smear.

- Boys may have problems with sitting or standing. It is sometimes easier to start the training by sitting. Other boys may enjoy using a large tin can while standing. (They particularly enjoy the noise this makes.)

- Children may have problems using a large toilet. Efforts should be made for child to have a small potty, one which resembles the large one. A portable toilet seat can be taken on excursions. Use a foot-stool for the child to climb on and use as a foot support.

- A newly trained child may regress due to stress in the family such as moving, a new sibling, divorce, death, or starting to school. Put the child back in diapers if this is acceptable, and say as little as possible. Give extra attention to the child and start retraining within a few weeks.

- Children continue to need help in the area of cleanliness. Parents should support the child if he/she wishes to be independent and should recognize that cleanliness is not the main concern.

- Odd words may be used for bowel movement and urination which may cause trouble when the child is not at home. These words should be conveyed to caretakers outside the home.

- Minor problems which may occur during the course of toilet training are messing with food, temporary food dislikes, smearing feces, and constipation or diarrhea.

- A child can learn early to control the environment by controlling his/her bowels. This can lead to attention-getting devices or more serious problems of severe constipation, enuresis, encopresis, diarrhea, or colitis. These conditions need to be handled in collaboration with other professionals. It is imperative to know what is happening in the home and how the toilet training has been handled.

References

Anders, T. F. and P. Weinstein. "Sleep and Its Disorders in Infants and Children." *Pediatrics* 50:312–324, March 1972.

Bettelheim, B. *Dialogues with Mothers.* New York: Avon, 1971.

Brazelton, T. B. "A Child-Oriented Approach to Toilet-Training." *Pediatrics* 29:121–128, January 1962.

Brazelton, T. B. *Infants and Mothers.* New York: Dell, 1967.

Brazelton, T. B. *Toddlers and Mothers.* New York: Dell, 1974.

Browder, J. A. "Needs and Technics for Counseling Parents of Young Children." *Clin Pediatr* 9:599–604, October 1970.

Brown, J. B. "Infant Temperament, A Clue to Childrearing for Parents and Nurses." *Am J Maternal Child Nursing* 2:228–232, July–August 1977.

Carey, W. B. "Clinical Application of Infant Temperament Measurements." *J Pediatr* 81:823–828, October 1972.

Chamberlain, R. "Parenting Styles, Child Behavior and the Pediatrician." *Pediatric Annals* 6:50–63, September 1977.

Chess, S., et al. *Your Child Is A Person.* New York: Viking, 1965.

Erikson, E. *Childhood and Society.* New York: Norton, 1963.

Fraiberg, S. *Every Child's Birthright.* New York: Basic Books, 1977.

Fraiberg, S. *The Magic Years.* New York: Charles Scribner's Sons, 1959.

Freidman, A. S. and D. B. Freidman. "Parenting—A Developmental Process." *Pediatric Annals* 6:10–22, September 1977.

Ginott, H. *Between Parent and Child.* New York: Macmillan, 1965.

Harris, B. G. "Learning About Parenting." *Nursing Outlook* 25:457–462, July 1977.

Ilg, F. L. and L. B. Ames. *Child Behavior.* New York: McKay, 1972.

Korner, A. "Individual Differences at Birth: Implications for Early Experiences and Later Development." *Am J Orthopsychiatry* 41:608–609, August 1971.

McAbee, R. "Rural Parenting Classes: Beginning to Meet the Need." *Am J Maternal Child Nursing* 2:315–319, September–October, 1977.

Murphy, M. A. "Toilet-Training, When and How." *Pediatric Nursing* 1:22–27, November–December 1975.

Parmalee, A. H., W. H. Wenner, and H. Schultz. "Infant Sleep Patterns." *J Pediatr* 65:576–582, October 1964.

Ribble, M. *The Rights of Infants,* 2nd ed. New York: Columbia University Press, 1967.

Salk, L. *What Every Child Would Like His Parents to Know.* New York: McKay, 1972.

Thomas, A. and S. Chess. *Temperament and Development.* New York: Brunner/Mazel, 1977.

Thomas, A. and S. Chess. "Temperament and the Parent-Child Interaction." *Pediatric Annals* 6: 26–45, September 1977a.

Verville, E. *Behavior Problems of Children.* Philadelphia: Saunders, 1967.

White, B. *The First Three Years of Life.* Englewood Cliffs, N.J.: Prentice-Hall, 1975.

9

Accident
Prevention
and Safety

During the first year of life accidents are the sixth leading cause of death surpassed only by anoxia, congenital anomalies, complications of pregnancy, immaturity, and pneumonia. From age 1 to 38 years accidents become the number one cause of death (National Safety Council, 1974).

By practicing appropriate safety measures most accidents can be prevented. The nurse practitioner as a provider of health care with major emphasis on health supervision can make a major contribution in this area. The counseling of parents on the developmental capabilities and activities of the child and on the measures needed to provide a safe environment are an important aspect of routine health care visits.

This chapter focuses on what the child can do during a given age span, the events or accidents that occur, and age-appropriate counseling in reference to accident prevention and safety and equipment.

BIRTH TO 6 MONTHS

Developmental Perspectives

See Chapter 25, The Waechter Developmental Guides. The young infant is helpless and totally dependent and requires absolute protection. The infant moves about by wiggling and squirming, as well as by rolling over, sometimes unexpectedly. The infant's strong natural sucking reflex results in the infant putting anything and everything into the mouth.

EVENTS

The major events in this age group to be aware of, and to work toward the prevention of, are burns and fires, choking due to obstruction of the respiratory tract through inhalation of food or an object, falls, motor vehicle accidents, and strangulation.

COUNSELING

Safety tips pertinent to the event are described below.

Burns and fires. See Chapter 30, Burns.

1. Avoid bathing the infant in a sink or adult tub near hot water faucets. Test the bath water temperature before putting the infant in; it should be comfortable to the touch of your elbow. Keep one hand on the infant at all times during the bath.
2. Avoid handling hot liquids and do not smoke while tending the infant.
3. Install home smoke alarms, one on each level of the home including the basement.
4. Purchase clothing and furniture that are flame resistant. See this chapter, Flammable Fabrics.
5. Shelter the infant from burning sun rays. Apply a sun screen to exposed areas. Expose the infant to the sun slowly. See Chapter 15, Sunburn.

Choking. See Chapter 30, Asphyxiation.

1. Avoid bottle propping.
2. Burp the infant well before putting him/her into the crib. Place the infant on the stomach and turn the infant's head to one side or prop the infant on one side by using a rolled blanket.
3. Examine all toys and rattles. They should be too large for the infant to swallow, free from sharp edges, strings, detachable parts, and toxic paints. See this chapter, Toys.
4. Keep the diaper pins out of infant's reach. Make a habit of pinning the pins to clothing while changing the diapers.
5. Use only pacifiers that have a large shield at the base.

Falls

1. Always keep one hand on the infant while giving care. Securely fasten the dressing table straps when the infant is on it.
2. Keep the crib sides up and properly fastened whenever the infant is in the crib.
3. Never leave the infant on an elevated surface unattended. If it becomes necessary to turn away from the infant for any reason, put the infant in a crib with the sides up, in a playpen, or on the floor.
4. Put the infant seat in the playpen or on the floor when the infant is in it. Always securely strap the infant in the seat.

Motor vehicle accidents

1. Always use an infant car seat appropriately installed. See this chapter, Infant Carriers and Child Car Seats.
2. Keep the car doors locked.
3. Keep the car interior free of litter and loose objects.
4. Never leave the infant unattended in the car.
5. Use safety restraints for all passengers and the driver.

Strangulation

1. Avoid tying anything, including pacifiers, around the infant's neck.

2. Firmly fasten all mobiles above the infant's crib out of reach of the infant.
3. Never tie the infant down.
4. Purchase cribs with slats no more than 2-3/8 inches apart. Line the crib with bumper pads securely fastened.

6 MONTHS TO 1 YEAR

Developmental Perspectives

See Chapter 25, The Waechter Developmental Guides. The growing infant rapidly develops gross motor skills with the fine motor skills developing at a slower pace. The infant continues to put anything and everything into the mouth. Dangerous items become more accessible as the infant crawls, grabs, reaches, and explores. The infant pulls himself/herself up and everything else down and is completely unaware of danger.

EVENTS

The major events include those of the birth-to-6-months range plus events which occur as a result of the increased mobility of the age. The list now includes burns and fires, choking, falls, injuries from pulling objects over, lacerations from the breakage of objects, motor vehicle accidents, poisonings and ingestions, and suffocation.

COUNSELING

In addition to the safety tips mentioned previously under Birth to 6 Months, the following precautions are recommended to parents.

Burns and fires. See Chapter 30, Burns.

1. Keep all hot foods and drinks away from the edges of tables and counters, and turn all pot handles inward on the stove.

2. Keep all matches and lighters out of child's reach.
3. Keep the kitchen door closed or gated.
4. Never leave the child unattended while a fireplace is burning.
5. Place guards around all open heaters, registers, floor furnaces, and burning fireplaces.
6. Place safety caps on the unused electrical outlets, and eliminate all dangling electrical cords.

Choking. See Chapter 30, Asphyxiation.

1. Do not give the child hard foods such as raw vegetables, candy, peanuts, popcorn, or bones of any kind.
2. Inspect all toys routinely for loose parts, and discard appropriately.
3. Keep the floors, counters, table tops, free from all objects that can be swallowed.

Falls

1. Always use the safety strap when the child is in the high chair or stroller.
2. Buy and use sturdy, stable high chairs or low feeding tables. See High Chairs, this chapter.
3. Keep the car windows by the child closed and the car doors locked.
4. Keep the doors leading to stairs and to the outside locked. Install gates if necessary.

Injuries and lacerations

1. Avoid the use of hanging table cloths.
2. Check the furniture for sharp corners and pad them if indicated.
3. Inspect all toys routinely for breakage, and repair or discard appropriately.
4. Keep items such as sharp objects, scissors, and knives out of the child's reach.

Motor vehicle accidents

1. Check the infant's car seat for appropriateness for age and size. Make the necessary adjustments. Keep the doors locked.

Poisonings and ingestions. See Chapter 30, Poisonings.

1. Avoid giving one child the medicine prescribed for another child. Do not refer to medicine as candy. Read the labels before giving the medicine, and never give medicine in the dark. Keep all medications in a locked cupboard, and replace them to the locked area immediately after use.
2. Discard house plants that are poisonous.
3. Keep syrup of ipecac in the house and understand its use.
4. Lock all insecticides, poisons, plant foods, and harmful cleaning agents in a special cupboard. Keep the area under the sink free of these harmful agents.

Suffocation

1. Remember that accidents are more prevalent during times of stress, fatigue, hunger, and hastiness.
2. Tie all plastic bags in a knot and discard immediately and safely.

1 TO 2 YEARS

Developmental Perspectives

See Chapter 25, The Waechter Developmental Guides. The young toddler is enjoying a very active, curious stage of development. The child is a wizard at climbing and constructing ladders, is packed with energy, and is as quick as a flash. Taking things and toys apart becomes part of play. Putting small items in the mouth, ears, and the nose is not uncommon. The toddler loves water and knows no fear. The toddler seeks autonomy and benefits from consistency in discipline.

EVENTS

The major events are burns and fires, drowning, falls, motor vehicle accidents, poisonings, and ingestions.

COUNSELING

In addition to reviewing the previous safety tips with emphasis on supervised play areas and on play activities using age-appropriate toys, the following precautions are recommended to parents.

Burns and fires. See Chapter 30, Burns.

1. Avoid the use of flowing clothing which is more apt to catch on fire from heating devices.
2. Teach the child the meaning of hot.

Drowning. See Chapter 30, Near Drowning.

1. Continue to supervise bath time.
2. Supervise all swimming even after the child knows how to swim.
3. Teach the child to respect water, and seek professional swimming lessons.

Falls

1. Lock all windows. Open the windows only from the top. Remove from in front of the windows any furniture or other objects that the child could use for a ladder.
2. Permit climbing adventures within the child's capabilities. Provide a soft surface for landing.
3. Remove from the crib bumper pads and large toys that the child could use for a ladder.

Motor vehicle accidents. See this chapter, Infant Carriers and Child Car Seats.

1. Use an appropriate child car seat. The child remains too small for adult seat restraints.
2. Install safety lock adapters on the car doors if they are not built in. These can be purchased at automotive supply stores.

Poisonings and ingestions. See Chapter 30, Poisonings.

1. Keep syrup of ipecac in the house, at the babysitter's, and at the grandparents'. Be certain everyone understands its use.

2. Purchase only medications that are in childproof containers, and keep them in a locked cupboard.

2 TO 3 YEARS

Developmental Perspectives

See Chapter 25, The Waechter Developmental Guides. As the child advances in age so does the scope of the activities performed. The child becomes a great imitator learning from playmates and from adults. The child imitates what is seen and what is heard. The capacity to understand is beginning to develop, but uncertainty as to what is dangerous and why it is so, continues. Curiousness and investigativeness continue to a high degree accompanied by the frustration of restraints. Water fascinates the child, as do big and small animals.

EVENTS

The events remain basically the same as for the 1 to 2 year -old, with motor vehicle accidents the major safety problem. The list continues to be burns and fires, drowning, falls, motor vehicle accidents including children being hit while darting out between parked cars, and poisonings and ingestions.

COUNSELING

The child continues to need protection, but safety practices must be taught to the child. Parents are to be reminded to set a good example for the child to follow; this includes respect for animals at all times. Additional safety tips to review with the parents are listed under each specific event.

Burns and fires. See Chapter 30, Burns. Recheck all furnaces, radiators, and space heaters for safety of operation and protective guards.

Drowning. See Chapter 30, Near Drowning.

1. Continue with swimming lessons and supervised water activities.
2. Never leave the child unattended near any water area including wading pools.

Falls. See Chapter 30, Head Injury.

1. Discourage running in the house.
2. Keep the stairs well lighted and free of clutter.

Motor vehicle accidents

1. Continue to use a special child's car seat. All previous safety tips apply.
2. Keep the child away from unsupervised driveways and streets. Provide a fenced-in play area.
3. Teach the child pedestrian safety. Set a good example.

Poisonings and ingestions. See Chapter 30, Poisonings.

1. Continue to lock all poisons and harmful products including medicines. Do not become lax.
2. Give the house, basement, garage, and garden a good safety check on a routine basis.

3 TO 5 YEARS

Developmental Perspectives

See Chapter 25, The Waechter Developmental Guides. This age sees the child expanding exploration from the house out into the neighborhood. The child is frequently out of sight, playing with peers, and riding tricycles and bicycles. Participation in rough games increases. The child is able to understand safety rules but often forgets them at the height of play.

EVENTS

The major events are burns and fires, drowning, and motor vehicle accidents along with a variety of other events.

COUNSELING

The child in this age group can now benefit from participating in the safety discussion. Some safety tips to review are listed for each event.

Burns and fires. See Chapter 30, Burns.

1. Teach the child what to do if a fire breaks out. Conduct routine household fire drills.
2. Teach the child to roll and to smother clothing if it catches on fire.

Drowning. See Chapter 30, Near Drowning.

1. Continue with swimming lessons and supervised water activities. Have the child swim where lifeguards are on duty.
2. Have the child wear a life jacket if unable to swim and for all water sports.

Motor vehicle accidents

1. Continue to teach pedestrian safety. Look both ways before crossing street and never cross when the light is red.
2. Play to take place in the yard or playground. Never play in the street.
3. Use adult seat belts if the child is over 40 pounds.
4. Use adult shoulder restraints if the child is over 55 inches tall.

Other events

1. Be familiar with the play areas the child frequents, and check on the child's activities often and regularly. Make periodic checks of the neighborhood with particular attention to any construction sites, trash heaps, large holes, and discarded refrigerators.
2. Continue to keep poisons and dangerous substances locked up.

3. Keep bicycles, tricycles, and other play equipment in top condition, and instruct the child in their safe use.
4. Never clean a gun or handle a gun in the presence of a child. Preferably, do not keep guns on the premises.
5. Teach the child safety in using simple tools and household equipment.

5 TO 10 YEARS

Developmental Perspectives

See Chapter 25, The Waechter Developmental Guides. The school age child assumes great responsibility. The child goes to school alone, often using school buses, but also uses public transportation. The child follows peer leaders and will become daring under their pressure. Group activity involvement is important to the child. Increasing participation in sports is seen. Time spent away from home increases and so does the need for assuming greater responsibility for one's well-being.

EVENTS

The major events continue to be burns and fires, drowning, and motor vehicle accidents along with a variety of other events.

COUNSELING

Safety and accident prevention discussion for the school age child needs to be addressed to both the parent and the child. Safety tips to cover for each event are listed below.

Burns and fires. See Chapter 30, Burns.

1. Be aware of the tragedy of fire and learn to respect fire.
2. Douse all campfires and barbecues well with water. Supervision by adults of all campfires is essential.

3. Purchase safe camping gear. Look for fire retardant or fire resistant on the label.

Drowning. See Chapter 30, Near Drowning.

1. Adopt the buddy system for water sports and wear a life jacket while boating and water skiing.
2. Learn to swim under adult supervision, preferably a lifeguard.

Motor vehicle accidents

1. Be a safe pedestrian. Look both ways before crossing the street. Use a crosswalk. Do not cross on a red light.
2. Do not use the street as a playground.
3. Use auto safety restraints at all times, even for short distances. Avoid horse play in the car.

Other events

1. Be certain the child knows his/her name, address, and phone number.
2. Do not keep firearms in one's possession. If they are about, be certain the guns are not loaded. Keep them locked up.
3. Encourage supervised sports and group activities.
4. Know and abide by the bike-riding laws. Wear bright clothing, preferably with fluorescent patches, while biking. Keep bikes in good repair.
5. Learn the proper use of all household gadgets and equipment.
6. Teach the child not to ride with strangers.
7. Teach the child how to contact the police and the fire department.

10 YEARS TO ADULTHOOD

Developmental Perspectives

See Chapter 25, The Waechter Developmental Guides. The pre-adolescent, the adolescent, and the young adult are very independent. Peer pressure is extremely strong. Peer approval regarding behavior is held in higher regard than parental approval. Dares from peers are readily accepted. The need for strenuous physical activity increases. The majority of free time is spent away from home and is unsupervised.

EVENTS

The major events in this age group are drowning, firearm accidents, and motor vehicle accidents.

COUNSELING

In this age group a high percentage of discussion will take place on a one-to-one basis with the child and without the parent. Include the parents whenever possible. Safety measures to discuss for each event are listed below.

Drowning. See Chapter 30, Near Drowning.

1. Know water safety rules. It is never too late to learn to swim. Enroll in lifesaving classes to learn the correct technique.
2. Wear life jackets when participating in boating, water skiing, rafting, or other water sports even if a good swimmer.

Firearms accidents

1. Do not keep loaded guns on the premises.
2. Learn safety handling of firearms if involved in the sport of hunting.

Motor vehicle accidents

1. Emphasize the need for auto restraints for all passengers.
2. Encourage the student to enroll in driver education classes when at the acceptable age.
3. Practice pedestrian safety at all times.

Other events

1. Know and obey all bike-riding laws.
2. Know the dangers of hitchhiking. Do not hitchhike or pick up hitchhikers.

EQUIPMENT

Bicycles

EPIDEMIOLOGY

The U.S. Consumer Product Safety Commission estimates that nearly 400,000 persons suffered bicycle-related injuries requiring emergency room treatment in 1974. The major accidents were as a result of:

1. Loss of control of the bicycle due to: difficulty in braking; riding a bicycle that was too large; riding double on banana seats, rear fenders, handlebars, or on the horizontal top tube on a man's bicycle; stunting while riding; striking a rut, bump, or obstacle.
2. Mechanical and structural problems including brake failure; wobbling or disengagement of the wheel or steering mechanism; difficulty in shifting gears; chain slippage; pedals falling off; or spoke breakage.
3. Entanglement of a person's hands, feet, or clothing in the bicycle.
4. Foot slippage from the pedals.
5. Collision with a car or another bicycle.

SAFETY REGULATIONS

The U.S. Consumer Product Safety Commission is developing safety standards governing the performance and construction of bicycle brakes, wheels, steering system, and frame.

- All uncovered sharp edges and jutting points are to be eliminated.
- Brakes will be required on all sidewalk bicycles with seat height of 22 inches or more.
- Reflectors will be required on the front, back, sides, and pedals to make bicycles visible at night.

TIPS ON BICYCLE PURCHASING

1. Avoid buying bicycles with gear controls, or other protruding attachments, mounted on the top tube of a man's bicycle.
2. Avoid buying bikes with sharp edges and protruding bolts. Check all hand and foot brakes for fast, easy stops without instability or jamming.
3. Check the bicycle for functioning head and tail lights. Attach them if they are not standard equipment.
4. Check the foot pedals for rubber tread. Avoid buying bicycles with slippery, plastic pedals.
5. Check the seat for appropriate adjustment.
6. Choose a bicycle that matches the child's ability and kind of riding the child will be doing.
7. Choose a bicycle to fit the child's present age and size.

TIPS ON BICYCLE RIDING AND MAINTENANCE

1. Assemble the bicycle according to the instructions or have it assembled by a bicycle shop professional.
2. Adjust the seat to the proper height. The rider's feet should touch the ground on both sides.
3. Do not ride double or show off while riding.
4. Do not ride in inclement weather when the brakes may be less reliable.
5. Do not wear loose clothing that may get tangled in the bicycle parts. Use leg clips or bands on the pant legs.
6. Keep the bicycle in a sheltered area to avoid rust and moisture damage.
7. Keep tires inflated to a recommended pressure.
8. Observe all traffic laws. Ride in designated bicycle lanes.
9. Set up and adhere to a regular maintenance program. Periodically check wheel alignment and correct all misalignment; clean and oil all moving parts being careful not to get oil on the rubber parts; replace all broken and nonfunctioning parts; use reflectors that are at least 2 inches in diameter.
10. Use alternative routes rather than ride through busy intersections and heavy or high-speed traffic.

11. Wear rubber-soled shoes for riding. Never ride barefoot or when wearing loose sandals.

Cribs

EPIDEMIOLOGY

The U.S. Consumer Product Commission estimates that 150 to 200 infants die every year in the United States from crib accidents. Another 40,000 infants are injured seriously enough to require medical treatment.

SAFETY REGULATIONS

As of February 1, 1974, a new safety regulation went into effect relating to the design and manufacture of cribs. Important aspects of this regulation are:

1. Any metal hardware used on the crib must be safe and without rough edges.
2. Crib slats must be no more than 2-3/8 inches apart.
3. Locks and latches on the dropside must be safe and secure from accidental release or from release by the infant.
4. There must be strict warnings on the crib carton, in the assembly instructions, and on the headboard advising you to use only a mattress that fits snugly and properly.

TIPS ON PURCHASING SECOND-HAND CRIBS

1. Buy a crib with as narrow a space between slats as possible, preferably no farther apart than 2-3/8 inches. Carry a tape measure with you when you shop.
2. Buy a crib with as large a distance as possible between the top of the side rail and the mattress. The sides, when lowered, should be at least 4 inches above the mattress.
3. Buy a crib without ornamental balls, bells, and teething rails.
4. Check the crib latches and locks. Be certain they cannot be easily tripped.

5. Check the mattress fit. It must be snug. If more than two fingers fit between the mattress and the crib, the mattress is too small.
6. Check the overall condition of the crib. Be certain all the slats, nuts, bolts, and other fasteners are in place and functioning.
7. Check the paint condition of the crib. If in doubt as to the type of paint used, remove the old paint, sand the surface, and repaint with nontoxic paint.

SAFETY-PROOFING THE CRIB IN USE

1. Fit the crib with bumper guards that go around the entire crib. Secure the bumper guards in at least six places using ties or snaps.
2. Leave bumper guards in place until the child can pull up to standing and use them as a ladder.
3. Set the mattress in the lowest position as soon as the child can pull up to standing.
4. Stop use of the crib when the child's height reaches three-quarters of the height of the side rails.

Flammable Fabrics

EPIDEMIOLOGY

Current statistical data are difficult to locate; however, the U.S. Government estimates that annually 750 to 1250 fatalities and 37,000 to 50,000 injuries occur to children under the age of 10 from fabric fires.

SAFETY REGULATIONS

The U.S. Flammable Fabrics Act was passed by Congress in 1953 and amended in 1954 and 1967. The 1967 amendment gave the Secretary of Commerce the authority to issue flammability standards for all wearing apparel including gloves, hats, and footwear as well as fabrics used in interior furnishings, bedding, draperies, upholstery, and related materials.

The U.S. Department of Commerce established a separate, more stringent test method standard for fabrics used for sleepwear in the size range 0 to 6x. Under this standard, DOC FF 3-71, effective July 29, 1972, 0 to 6x sleepwear fabric must be essentially flame resistant. This means that the fabric must not support combustion after removal of the flame source. This flame resistance must persist through the useful service life of the garment, or through 50 launderings.

Various states have legislation governing flammable fabrics. It is important that everyone be familiar with his/her specific state laws. Strong consumer participation is needed in demanding better flammable fabric standards, more specific, clearer, labeling of articles, and very clear laundering instructions to preserve the flame resistance.

Currently there is serious concern regarding the potential cancer-causing properties of some chemicals being used. Studies are being conducted and it is recommended that everyone keep abreast of the findings and purchase accordingly.

TIPS ON PURCHASING (OGLESBAY, 1969)

1. Avoid loose-fitting garments that swing away from the body. They can easily catch on fire from momentary contact with a burning fireplace, floor heater, other space heater, or open burner. Flame spread increases as the amount of air surrounding the clothing increases.

2. Avoid napped surfaces with loose fibers that create air space between them. These ignite rapidly and the flame spread is rapid.

3. Keep in mind that flammability is largely determined by fabric structure or weave. Generally, heavier fabrics have higher flame resistance, are slower burning, and are less apt to ignite from momentary contact. Cotton and rayon generally burn the fastest. Synthetics usually burn less fast; however, they may melt and cause body burns. Animal hair, pure silk, wool, and protein fabrics are more flame retardant. Chemically treated cellulose fibers and inherently flame-retardant fibers such as the modacrylic are the least fire hazardous.

High Chairs

EPIDEMIOLOGY

The U.S. Product Safety Commission estimates that high-chair-related accidents are responsible for 7000 injuries per year that are serious enough to require treatment in a hospital emergency room.

SAFETY REGULATIONS

Currently no specific safety standards are in effect. The American Society for Testing and Materials is working closely with the manufacturers in the development of voluntary standards.

TIPS ON PURCHASING HIGH CHAIRS AND THEIR USE (CONSUMER REPORTS, 1975)

1. Be certain that assembly, use, and maintenance instructions come with the chair. Follow them exactly.
2. Be certain the chair is comfortable for the child, is equipped with adjustable foot rests, and has a padded seat and a high padded back.
3. Be certain the chair is stable and well balanced. The chair should not tip with an active child in it; other children in the house should not be able to tip it over; and any folding high chair must have locks that prevent the chair from collapsing while the child is in it.
4. Be certain that the tray is durable and chip and splinter proof, that the distance from the seat back to the tray can be adjusted, that it is adequate in size and shape to provide support to the child's arms and is made of material that is easily cleaned, and that it is equipped with latches that hold it securely in position.
5. Be certain the chair has an adjustable harness or safety belt that holds the child securely. The restraint should be easy to apply and should prevent the child from slipping and from standing up in the chair. Both a waist and a crotch restraint are recommended.

6. Do not place the chair with the child in it near a stove, electrical appliances, or stairs.
7. Never leave the child unattended in the high chair.

Infant Carriers and Child Car Seats (Consumer Reports, 1974)

EPIDEMIOLOGY

The National Safety Council figures show that in 1974, 1100 children, birth through 4 years, were killed while passengers in motor vehicles and 66,000 were injured. The use of proper infant carriers and child car seats could sharply reduce these figures.

SAFETY REGULATIONS

The Federal Motor Vehicle Safety Standard #213 became effective in April 1971. This standard provides a bare minimum in safety specifications. Much stronger regulations are needed. Health professionals and consumers should demand stringent regulations governing the manufacturing of infant carriers and child car seats.

TIPS ON PURCHASING AND USE

General Guidelines

1. Read and understand all installation and use instructions before purchasing.
2. Be certain that proper installation is possible in your automobile. High back seat restraints often require installation of a top tether which must be securely bolted to a sturdy metal panel to prevent the seat from lurching forward. Some child car seats should not be used in low back auto seats and some should not be used in high back bucket seats. Know your automobile and choose appropriately.
3. Choose another model if installation is too complicated to use the device each time.

4. Choose only those devices specifically designed for automobile use.

5. Place the infant carrier or car seat in the safest part of the automobile. Generally speaking, the center of the seat is safer than the sides and the back seat is safer than the front. Infant carriers, for instance, are designed to face the back of the seat, *never forward.* The type of car must be considered as well as the need for the driver to turn around often to check on the child, thus taking eyes off the road and possibly causing an accident.

6. See the pamphlet "Don't Risk Your Child's Life!" published by the Physicians for Automotive Safety, for a discussion of the crash-tested car seats available. Where to buy and how to use these car seats is described in the pamphlet, which is frequently updated. For copies of the pamphlet (25 cents each), write to: Physicians for Automotive Safety, 50 Union Avenue, Irvington, New Jersey 07111. The car seats, which are made by certain automobile manufacturers, are available at dealers or in department and juvenile specialty stores.

7. See the March 1975 issue of *Consumer Reports* for their list of the top five models and also the April 1978 issue, the article called "CU Answers Readers' Questions on Car Safety Restraints for Children."

Infant Carriers

1. Choose an infant carrier that is equipped with restraining straps that allow the infant to be cradled in a semireclining position.

2. Position the infant carrier facing the rear. Strap to the seat of the car by using the adult seat belts.

3. Protect the infant by using an infant carrier until the infant's development is such that the infant can sit up and hold his/her head erect, about 6 months of age. Some infant carriers can be converted into a child car seat, thus saving an extra purchase.

Child car seats

1. Keep in mind that car seats can be purchased with an impact shield and/or a harness depending on the model. Safety experts

prefer the shield, particularly for children under the age of 2 or 3. The impact shield offers protection by distributing the force of the impact over a large area of the body; however, the shield has a tendency to block the child's view and may contribute to the child's restlessness. The conventional car seat utilizes the harness to restrain the child. This harness must fit properly and be adjustable to allow for sloping, underdeveloped shoulders and the wearing of heavy, bulky clothing.

2. Protect the child by using a car seat until the child attains the age of 4 years and 40 pounds. A bolster cushion may be needed to position the child properly so the lap belt fits across the child's hips at a 45° angle and does not ride up across the child's abdomen.

3. Use adult shoulder straps only if they cross the child's chest and not the face or neck. This is usually possible after the attainment of 55 inches in height.

Toys

EPIDEMIOLOGY

The U.S. Consumer Product Safety Commission estimates that in 1974, 150,000 persons received hospital emergency room treatment for injuries associated with toys. According to a survey sponsored by the National Safety Council, age 5 appears to be the most vulnerable single year for children to receive toy or play injuries. Park and playground equipment such as merry-go-rounds, swings, and jungle gyms account for most injuries to the 2- to 7-year-old child.

SAFETY REGULATIONS

The Child Protection and Toy Safety Act of 1969, effective as of January 1970, authorizes the Food and Drug Administration to remove and to keep from the market toys and other children's products with electrical, mechanical, and thermal hazards.

The U.S. Consumer Product Safety Commission has the authority under the Federal Hazardous Substance Act as amended to ban hazardous toys from sale. The regulations provide that toys having the following characteristics are banned hazardous substances:

1. Any doll, stuffed animal, or similar toy having parts that could become exposed and cause cuts, punctures, or other similar injuries.
2. Any toy with noise-making parts that could be removed by a child and swallowed or inhaled.
3. Baby bouncers and similar articles that support very young children while sitting, walking, or bouncing, which could cause injury to the child such as pinching, cutting, or bruising.
4. Caps intended for use with toy guns or toy guns that cause noise above a certain level.
5. Lawn darts and other pointed items intended for outdoor use that could cause puncture wounds, unless they have included appropriate cautionary language, adequate directions, and warning for safe use, and are not sold by toy stores or stores dealing primarily in toys and other children's articles.
6. Toys known as clacker balls which could break off or fracture and thereby cause injury.
7. Toy rattles containing rigid wires, sharp points, or loose small objects that could become exposed and cause cuts, punctures, or other injuries.

On September 3, 1973, a safety regulation for electrically operated toys went into effect. This regulation:

1. Requires electrical toys to bear warning labels stating that they are not recommended for children under a certain age. For any toy that contains a heating element, the manufacturer may not indicate that the toy is recommended for children under the age of 8 years.
2. Requires reliable electrical construction
3. Specifies maximum temperature for electrical toys

Currently the Commission is developing new regulations that will provide more comprehensive safety standards for all toys and offer special protection for children under the age of 8 years.

To report a product hazard or product-related injury, write to: U.S. Product Safety Commission, Washington DC 20207. In the continental United States you may call the toll-free Safety Hot Line: 800-638-2666. Maryland residents only call 800-492-2937.

TIPS ON TOY PURCHASING AND USE

Playground equipment

1. Anchor all playground equipment firmly to the ground.
2. Be certain all spaces between moving parts are wide enough not to catch or to pinch fingers or toes.
3. Be certain swing sets are strong and have seats with smooth, rolled edges. Swings should be separated a safe distance from each other and be supported by strong chains without open-ended S hooks.
4. Check the equipment frequently for wear and tear, and tighten all bolts and lubricate the joints.
5. Cover all protruding bolt ends with protective plastic caps. Round off any sharp, exposed edges.
6. Report any defective public playground equipment to the appropriate department.

Toys in general

1. Avoid toys that produce extremely loud noises that can damage hearing, as well as toys that have propelled objects that can injure eyes.
2. Check the toy chest for safety. Be certain it has adequate ventilation, has no automatic locking device, has a lightweight lid, and that the hinging action does not present a strong possibility for pinching or squeezing the child's hands or fingers.
3. Choose toys appropriate for the child's age and ability. Consider younger siblings who will have access to the toys intended for older children.
4. Instruct the child in the proper use of the toy.
5. Read the instructions for use before giving the toy to the child.
6. Teach the child proper toy care. Insist that the child put the toys away so they do not get broken and so no one else trips or falls on them.

7. Watch out for toys that have sharp edges, small parts, or sharp points.
8. THINK, TEACH, AND BUY TOY SAFETY.

Tricycles

EPIDEMIOLOGY

The U.S. Consumer Product Safety Commission estimates that approximately 11,000 persons each year sustain tricycle-related injuries serious enough to require hospital emergency room treatment. The major accidents were as a result of:

1. Entanglement in the tricycle's moving parts
2. Inability to stop the tricycle, usually because tricycles are designed without brakes
3. Instability which causes a tricycle to tip over, often at the time of a sharp turn or when speeding up
4. Poor construction or design including breakage while in use, sharp edges, or points
5. Striking obstacles and colliding with other tricycles

TIPS ON TRICYCLE PURCHASING

1. Avoid tricycles with sharp edges, particularly on or along the fenders.
2. Look for pedals and handgrips that have rough surfaces or tread to prevent the child's hands and feet from slipping.
3. Match the size of the child to the size of the tricycle. If the child is too large for the tricycle, it will be unstable. If the child is too small, it may be difficult to control the tricycle.
4. Purchase a stable tricycle. Low-slung tricycles with seats close to the ground offer more stability. Widely spaced wheels provide more stability.

TIPS ON TRICYCLE RIDING AND MAINTENANCE

1. Caution a child against riding double. Carrying a passenger on a tricycle greatly increases its instability.

2. Cover any sharp edges and protrusions with heavy, waterproof tape.
3. Do not leave the tricycle outdoors overnight where moisture can cause rust and weaken the metal parts.
4. Keep the tricycle in good condition. Check it regularly for missing or damaged pedals and handgrips, loose handlebars and seats, broken parts, and other defects. Repair immediately.
5. Teach the child to avoid sharp turns, and to make all turns at low speeds, and not to ride down steps or over curbs or sewer grates.
6. Teach the child about the danger of riding down hill. A tricycle can pick up so much speed that it becomes almost impossible to stop without brakes.
7. Teach the child safe riding habits and check on the child frequently.

Resource Information

Resource information can be obtained from these sources:
1. Bureau of Product Safety, Food and Drug Administration
   U.S. Department of Health, Education, and Welfare
   5401 Westbard Avenue
   Bethesda, MD 20016
2. Children's Bureau
   U.S. Department of Health, Education, and Welfare
   Office of Child Development
   Washington DC 20201

References

Bureau of Product Safety, Food and Drug Administration. "Toy Safety." Department of Health, Education, and Welfare, 1972.
Children's Bureau. "Safe Toys for Your Child." Publication No. 473. U.S. Department of Health, Education, and Welfare, 1971.
Children's Bureau. "Young Children and Accidents in the Home." U.S. Department of Health, Education, and Welfare, 1972.

Consumer Reports. "Car Safety Restraints for Children." 42:314–317, June 1977.

Consumer Reports. "Infant Carriers and Child Restraints." 40:150–154, March 1975.

Consumer Reports. "High Chairs: Safety, Comfort, Convenience." 40:158–163, March 1975.

Dietrich, H. F. "Accident Prevention in Childhood is Your Problem Too." *Pediatr Clin North Am* 1:759–769, 1954.

Matheny, A. P., A. M. Brown, and R. S. Wilson. "Assessment of Children's Behavioral Characteristics: A Tool in Accident Prevention." *Clin Pediatr* 11:437–439, August 1972.

McDonald, Q. H. "Safety of Infants in Automobiles." *Pediatrics* 52:463–464, 1973.

National Safety Council. *Accident Facts.* Chicago, Ill., 1974.

Oglesbay, Floyd B. "The Flammable Fabrics Problem." *Pediatrics,* Supplement 44:827–832, November 1969.

Physicians for Automotive Safety. *Don't Risk Your Child's Life.* Irvington, N.J., 1976.

U.S. Consumer Product Safety Commission. "Fact Sheet No. 10: Bicycles." Washington D.C., May 1974.

U.S. Consumer Product Safety Commission. "Fact Sheet No. 15: Tricycles." Washington D.C., September 1974.

U.S. Consumer Product Safety Commission. "Fact Sheet No. 43: Crib Safety—Keep Them On The Safe Side." Washington D.C., June 1974.

U.S. Consumer Product Safety Commission. "Fact Sheet No. 47: Toys." Washington D.C., November 1974.

U.S. Department of Commerce, National Bureau of Standards. "United States and Canadian Fabric Flammability Standards." N. B. S., Technical Note 742, October 1972.

Young, C. "Playing Safe in Toyland." Food and Drug Administration Papers. March 1971.

10

Health Care of
the Adolescent

Adolescent development encompasses many changes: physiologic, psychologic, economic, social, and legal. Society has recognized the rapid developmental period of adolescence by providing constitutional rights for minors and by lowering the age for some legal responsibilities. Adolescents have also become increasingly verbal in expressing their own feelings about themselves and about their future.

Adolescents are facing problems their parents never dealt with: increasing sexual freedom and its consequences, the uncertainty of future careers in a shrinking job market, and diffuse role models of parents and peers because of rapid social change.

To provide realistic care, the nurse practitioner recognizes society's attitude toward adolescence and understands the developmental tasks that adolescents must deal with to become mature, independent adults.

HORMONAL ACTIVITY DURING ADOLESCENCE

Sequence of Pubertal Phenomena*

In females, puberty takes the following sequence:

1. Initial enlargement of breasts
2. Appearance of straight, pigmented pubic hair
3. Maximum physical growth
4. Appearance of kinky pubic hair
5. Menstruation
6. Growth of axillary hair

In males, puberty takes the following sequence:

1. Beginning growth of the testes
2. Straight, pigmented pubic hair
3. Beginning enlargement of the penis
4. Early voice changes
5. First nocturnal ejaculation
6. Kinky pubic hair
7. Age of maximum growth
8. Growth of axillary hair
9. Marked voice changes
10. Development of facial beard

Hypothalamus

This gland controls the secretions of the posterior pituitary through nerve fibers that originate in the hypothalamus. The secretions of the anterior pituitary are controlled through small pep-

*Reprinted from *Normal Adolescence: Its Dynamics and Impact*, by the Group for the Advancement of Psychiatry with the permission of Charles Scribner's Sons. Copyright © 1968 Group for the Advancement of Psychiatry.

tide hormones called hypothalamic releasing and inhibitory factors. For each type of anterior pituitary hormone there is a corresponding hypothalamic releasing factor, and for some hormones there is also a corresponding inhibitory factor. The most important factors are:

- Corticotropin releasing factor—causes the release of corticotropin
- Follicle-stimulating hormone releasing factor—causes release of follicle stimulating hormone
- Luteinizing hormone releasing factor—causes release of luteinizing hormone
- Growth hormone releasing factor—causes release of growth hormone
- Prolactin inhibitory factor—causes inhibition of prolactin secretion

Anterior Pituitary

This gland controls the secretion of the follicle-stimulating hormone (FSH) and the luteinizing hormone (LH). It is regulated by the hypothalamic gonadotropic releasing hormone.

FOLLICLE-STIMULATING HORMONE

This hormone increases the growth of the ovaries and the ovarian follicles in the female and helps with sperm maturation and development of the seminiferous tubules of the testes in the male.

LUTEINIZING HORMONE

This hormone acts synergistically with FSH to promote growth of the ovarian follicle to eject the mature ovum during the menstrual cycle. It also changes the follicular cells of the ovary into lutein cells or the corpus luteum which secretes estrogen and progesterone.

Estrogen. Estradiol is the major estrogenic secretion from the ovaries, and it is responsible for the development of secondary sexual characteristics. The following changes result:

- Protein. There is a slight increase in total body protein resulting in increased height and weight. This is achieved because of the growth-producing effect of estrogen on the sex organs and other body tissues.
- Skeletal. There is an increased growth rate of bones resulting in increased height; also causes early uniting of the epiphysis of the long bones, thus ending the growth process; broadens the pelvic bones.
- Sexual organs. There is an increase in the size of the uterus, fallopian tubes, and vagina; increased deposits of adipose tissue on the mons pubis and labia majora; enlargement of the labia minora; development of endometrium during the proliferatory and secretory phase of the menstrual cycle.
- Breasts. There is an increase in fat deposits, growth of ductile system, and development of the nipple.
- Skin. There is an increased secretion of the sebaceous glands often resulting in acne; increase in adipose tissue in the buttocks, hips, and thighs; skin texture becomes more soft, smooth, and vascular.
- Hair. There is an increased hair distribution in the axillae and pubic region with triangular distribution of pubic hair, and in the female, development of the hair line on the head which is uninterrupted from temple to temple. See Figures 1 and 2.

Progesterone.   This hormone is secreted by the ovary through the corpus luteum and is active during the secretory phase of the menstrual cycle. During pregnancy progesterone is secreted in large quantities by the placenta. Progesterone is responsible for the following changes:

- Uterus. Prepares uterus for implantation of the fertilized egg; during pregnancy decreases the frequency of uterine contractions
- Fallopian tubes. Promotes secretory changes in the mucosal lining which are necessary for the nutrition of the fertilized dividing ovum
- Breasts. Development of milk lobules and alveoli (milk-

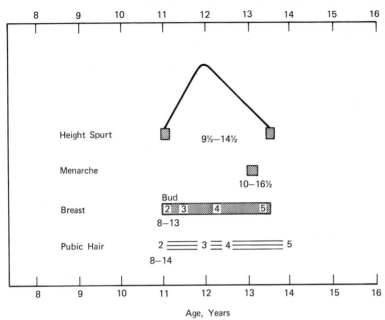

Figure 1 Sequence of events at adolescence in girls. An average girl is represented: the range of ages within which each event charted may begin and end is given by the figures placed directly below its start and finish. (Reprinted with permission from J. M. Tanner, *Growth at Adolescence*, 2nd ed., Oxford, England: Blackwell Scientific Publications, Ltd., 1962.)

producing cells) during pregnancy resulting in enlargement of breasts

INTERSTITIAL CELL STIMULATING HORMONE (LUTEINIZING HORMONE)

This hormone helps in the formation of the Leydig cells in the testes which stimulate production of testosterone and a small quantity of estrogen. The action of estrogen is unknown.

Testosterone. This hormone along with FSH is responsible for spermatogenesis. It is also responsible for the development of secondary sexual characteristics in the male and the following changes:

- Protein. There is an increase in the rate of protein formation in the cells resulting in increased height, weight, and strength.
- Skeletal. There is an increased growth rate of bones resulting in increased height; also causes early uniting of the epiphysis of the long bones thus ending the growth process.
- Muscular. There is an acceleration of muscle size and mass causing increased strength and broadening of the shoulder and thoracic cage.
- Sexual organs. There is an increase in size of the penis, scrotum, and testicles.
- Skin. There is an increased thickness of skin over the entire body and increased secretion of the sebaceous glands often resulting in acne.
- Hair. There is an increased hair growth in the axillae, pubis, face, chest, and extremities.
- Voice. There is an enlargement of the larynx and vocal cords resulting in a deeper voice and the characteristic "Adam's apple."
- Libido. There is an increase in sexual assertiveness and desire. See Figures 1 and 2.

LACTOGENIC HORMONE (PROLACTIN)

This hormone is responsible for the production of breast milk.

GROWTH HORMONE

This hormone is responsible along with estrogen and testosterone for the growth spurt. In females this occurs between 9 and 14 years of age. In males, the growth spurt occurs between 11 and 16 years of age. See Figure 3 for increments in the height of early and late maturing boys and girls.

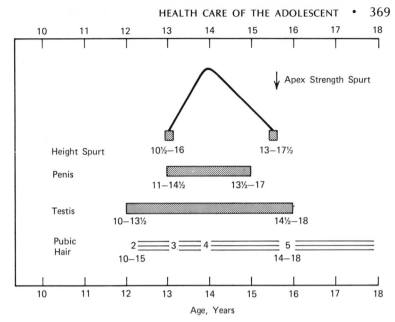

Figúre 2   Diagram of sequence of events at adolescence in boys. An average boy is represented: the range of ages within which each event charted may begin and end is given by the figures placed directly below its start and finish. (Reprinted with permission from J. M. Tanner, *Growth at Adolescence*, 2nd ed., Oxford, England: Blackwell Scientific Publications, Ltd., 1962.)

Adrenals

The term androgen refers to male sex hormones. The adrenal gland secretes approximately five different androgens. The masculinizing activity of these hormones is slight, and they do not cause significant masculine characteristics even in women.

TESTOSTERONE

This adrenal secretion helps in the early development of male sexual organs thereby promoting maturity and an increase in size of the penis, scrotum, and testes.

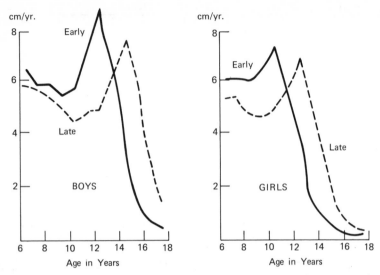

Figure 3 Increments in the height of early and late maturing boys and girls. (Reprinted with permission from H. S. Mitchell, et al, *Nutrition in Health and Disease,* 16th ed., Philadelphia: Lippincott, 1976; presented originally by H. S. Mitchell et al. at the International Congress of Nutrition, Hamburg, Germany, August 8, 1966.

ESTROGEN, PROGESTERONE

The quantity produced by the adrenal gland is too small to exert an effect on the body.

THE MENSTRUAL CYCLE

Menstruation is the result of the cyclic production of estrogen and progesterone by the gonadotropic hormones. It occurs in three phases.

Proliferation of the Endometrium

After menstruation occurs the cells of the endometrium begin to grow rapidly and to increase in thickness due to estrogen secretion. This occurs in the first half of the menstrual cycle.

Secretory Changes of the Endometrium

Progesterone and estrogen are secreted by the corpus luteum of the ovaries. These hormones produce a highly secretory endometrium that provides optimal conditions for implantation of the fertilized ovum. This occurs in the second half of the menstrual cycle.

Menstruation

The sudden decrease in the production of estrogen and progesterone causes desquamation and bleeding of the endometrial layer. This occurs just before the end of the monthly cycle.

HEALTH ASSESSMENT

The following history and physical assessment is presented as it relates to the adolescent. This material is used in addition to the general history and physical examination which is presented in Chapter 1, Child Health Assessment, Tables 1 and 2.

Health History

PRESENTING PROBLEM AS DISCUSSED BY CLIENT AND PARENTS

PAST HISTORY

1. Pregnancy: history of diethylstilbestrol use

SOCIAL HISTORY

1. Behavior: adjustment at home, school, with parents, siblings, and peers
2. Client and parental concerns in reference to the above

SCHOOL EXPERIENCE

1. Grade, name of school
2. Success in school: performance in math, reading, spelling, grades in subjects
3. Favorite subject, most difficult subject, best subject
4. Attitude toward school
5. Have client write: name of school, present subjects, and a sentence in reference to why she/he is here
6. School/work goals for the future

OUTSIDE INTERESTS

1. Work
2. Social
3. Hobbies/activities

PEER RELATIONSHIPS

1. Loner vs many friends
2. Number of friends
3. Relationship with siblings
4. Dating activity

MOOD STATE

Describe client as she/he appears (example: anxious, withdrawn)

SEX

1. Information appropriate for age
2. Sexual activity

3. Knowledge of contraceptive methods
4. Knowledge of symptoms of venereal disease, prevention, and treatment

ATTITUDES

1. Smoking
2. Substance usage: alcohol, prescription and nonprescription drugs

BODY WORRIES

1. Height, weight
2. Skin

REVIEW OF SYSTEMS

1. General health as described by client
2. Dietary history
3. Skin: acne
4. HEENT: headaches, squint
5. Dentition: last dental visit
6. Heart
7. Lungs
8. Gastrointestinal: abdominal pain, weight loss or gain
9. Genitourinary: enuresis, dysuria, urinary tract infection
10. Ortho: joint or back pain
11. Neuro: seizures, emotional problems
12. Menstruation: age of onset, LMP, regularity, frequency, duration, dysmenorrhea, premenstrual tension, client's emotional preparation for menarche, erroneous beliefs, feelings of being frightened

Physical Assessment

See also Chapter 1, Child Health Assessment, Table 2.

1. Height, weight, heart rate, respiration rate, and blood pressure

Table 1
Developmental Stages of Secondary Sex Characteristics

Stage	Female Breast Development	Male Genital Development	Male and Female Pubic Hair Development
1	Pre-adolescent: elevation of papilla only	Pre-adolescent: testes, scrotum, and penis are about the same size and proportion as in early childhood	Pre-adolescent: no pubic hair
2	Breast bud stage: elevation of breast and papilla as small mound. Enlargement of areolar diameter	Enlargement of scrotum and testes; skin of the scrotum reddens and changes in texture; little or no enlargement of penis	Sparse growth of long, slightly pigmented downy hair, straight or only slightly curled, appearing chiefly at the base of the penis or along the labia
3	Further enlargement and elevation of breast and areolar with no separation of their contours	Enlargement of penis, which occurs at first mainly in length; further growth of testes and scrotum	Hair darker, coarser, and more curled; spreads sparsely over the junction of the pubes
4	Projection of the areola and papilla to form a secondary mound above the level of the breast.	Increased size of penis with growth in breadth and development of glans; further enlargement of testes and scrotum; increased darkening of scrotal skin	Hair adult in type but area covered is still considerably smaller than in the adult; no spread to the medial surface of the thighs
5	Mature stage: projection of papilla only due to recession of the areola to the general contour of the breast	Genitalia adult in size and shape	Adult in quantity and type

Source: Reprinted with permission from J. M. Tanner, *Growth at Adolescence*, 2nd ed., (Oxford, England: Blackwell Scientific Publications, 1962).

2. Skin: acne, scars, icterus
3. Eyes: funduscopic
4. Dentition: caries, occlusion, periodontal disease
5. Neck: thyroid
6. Chest: females: breast development, Tanner stage (see Table 1), masses; males: gynecomastia
7. Back: scoliosis or lordosis
8. Genitalia: Tanner stage (see Table 1)
9. Pelvis: perineum, vagina, cervix (describe presence of ectopy, erosion), uterus (describe location, size, consistency), adnexa, adenosis with DES exposure.

Laboratory

CBC; UA; rubella titer; VDRL; Pap smear, cervical gonorrhea culture, if sexually active; sickle cell screening, if indicated.

Screening

1. Visual acuity
2. Audiogram
3. Tuberculin test

Recording of Visit

The problem list is updated as necessary. Plans, health education, and expectant client outcomes are specified.

Ambulatory Health Maintenance Visit

THE ENVIRONMENT

Adolescent appointments are scheduled on different days from well-baby or young-child visits whenever possible. The environmental milieu provides age-appropriate reading material, and the general overall impression should indicate that adolescents are a part of the client population.

The preceding statements promote the concept of the exclusiveness and individuality of the client and provide subtle influences that the client is valued for his or her own self-worth and individuality.

PROCEDURE FOR VISITS

Interview the client first and the parents afterwards. Exceptions to the above: interview the client and the parents together if the client desires that the parent be present, is extremely anxious, immature, mentally retarded, or has a learning or speech disability. The role of the nurse practitioner is defined to the client. The practitioner is the client's provider. The client is free to discuss with the practitioner anything he or she wishes. The procedure for future visits is defined including goals for treatment, approximate number of visits, review of client's progress, and the need for a verbal or written contract.

The nurse practitioner while being interested in the family's concerns, is primarily the client's advocate. This situation encourages a relationship in which the client can assume responsibility in managing his/her own health care.

CONFIDENTIALITY

All matters discussed with the client are confidential except in situations where the client's actions are threatening to self or society, for example, suicide, homicide.

INTERVIEWING

The attitude of the nurse practitioner is one of friendliness and concern. Nonverbal cues such as body position, use of hands, facial expression, and movements alert the nurse practitioner to the adolescent's degree of comfort. The practitioner is aware of the client's reluctance to answer personal questions until rapport has been established. The practitioner maintains a degree of professionalism by not taking sides in any conflict or agreeing with the adolescent unconditionally.

Adolescents will not verbalize thoughts completely until they are comfortable with and feel they can trust the nurse practitioner. The adolescent sees the practitioner as a person who views the problems and situations objectively and does not want the practitioner to function as a peer.

NONCOMMUNICATIVE ADOLESCENT

The nurse practitioner discusses the presenting complaint. If the adolescent is unable to add information in this area, the practitioner discusses what the adolescent thinks the parent's reasons are for the visit. A review of systems occasionally elicits some worries of the client. A discussion of the client's interests about school, hobbies, social activities, and sports occasionally initiates responses. The nurse practitioner discusses feelings in response to the adolescent's nonverbal behavior, "I bet you would rather be somewhere else right now."

The nurse practitioner also recognizes the fact that the client does not wish to verbalize and respects this by keeping the visits short. A discussion of the visit routine helps to alleviate some anxiety about the unexpected.

DOMINEERING PARENTS

This situation can occasionally be avoided by seeing the clients and parents separately. If this is impracticable, parents are counseled separately to ascertain their anxiety in reference to the adolescent. It is important to allow the adolescent to take some direction for the visit. This helps to develop capabilities for coping with situations and problems without parental consultation.

LEGAL ASPECTS OF HEALTH CARE

The judicial system recognizes the constitutional rights of minors such as due process of law when charged with a criminal act, the right to free speech, and in certain instances the right to self-consent. In the past decade legislation has been passed concerning treatment of venereal disease, substance abuse, contraception, and abortion. All 50 states and the District of Columbia have legislation pertaining to various aspects of obtaining health care without parental permission. The state statutes are extremely variable as to age at which minors can seek health care on their own and what type of health care services can be offered. The reader is referred to Resources in this chapter for further information.

Historic Development of Legal Rights

1800

Minors were under the complete authority of adults and had no personal rights. They were not guaranteed an education, had no protection under law against adult abuse, and were placed in adult prisons under criminal law for criminal offenses.

1899

The first juvenile court was established where minors were not punished under criminal proceedings. Instead attempts were made to rehabilitate offenders.

1920 TO 1930

Laws were passed to guarantee a minor an education until 16 years of age and work was prohibited before the age of 14. A minor below the age of 7 was not judged responsible for a criminal act, and those between the ages of 7 and 16 were provided rehabilitation through the juvenile courts and training schools.

THE MATURE MINOR RULE, 1950

This law provides legal sanction for certain activities of minors such as driving a car, buying alcohol, enlisting in the armed services, voting, and consenting to marriage, before the majority age of 21. Individual states have various ages at which minors are deemed sufficiently mature. For example: Oregon, 15 years; Arkansas, a female at 16 years; Alabama, 14 years. In reference to health care the mature minor rule states that a minor can effectively consent to medical treatment if the minor understands the nature of the treatment and its benefits and possible consequences.

TINKER VS DES MOINES INDEPENDENT SCHOOL DISTRICT, 1965

In this Supreme Court decision adolescents were guaranteed the right to freedom of speech.

GAULT CASE, 1967

In this Supreme Court decision adolescents were guaranteed due process of law: the right to legal counsel, to remain silent, to cross examine witnesses, and to obtain notice of charges given.

COMPREHENSIVE STATE STATUTES, 1970

Generally these laws define emancipated minors and under what conditions certain medical and surgical procedures may be instituted. They also broadly define other situations where delay or denial of care because of lack of parental permission would increase the risk to the minor's health and life. The first state to enact such a statute was Pennsylvania. It states that any minor 18 and older may consent to any medical or surgical procedures. The age in Alabama is 14, and that statute adds, "mental health care."

PLANNED PARENTHOOD OF CENTRAL MISSOURI VS DANFORTH, 1976

In this Supreme Court decision, a pregnant, single adolescent under 18 desiring an abortion need not obtain parental permission.

CAREY VS. POPULATION SERVICES INTERNATIONAL, 1977

In this Supreme court decision, the right of minors to contraceptive services was affirmed.

Issues in Health Care

EMANCIPATED MINORS

In the case of an emancipated minor seeking health care services the laws of various states generally offer no legal penalties to the health care agency or individual. An emancipated minor is usually defined as having one or some of the following characteristics:

- Away from home with and in some cases without parental consent
- Earning own support
- Married minors
- Minor parents
- Minors in the service
- 15 years or older depending on individual state statutes
- Working minors at home contributing at least half of their support

UNEMANCIPATED MINORS

It is in this area that health professionals have been reluctant to offer health care services to minors. The laws of the individual states are complex in defining an unemancipated minor and under what conditions an unemancipated minor can be treated.

TREATMENT WITHOUT PARENTAL CONSENT

A minor's right to consent to medical care depends on the minor's ability to give informed consent, by understanding the nature of the procedure, the risks involved, and the available alternatives. The minor must also demonstrate sufficient intelligence and maturity. If capable of the above, he/she is said to have reached "the age of majority."

EMERGENCIES

Courts have held that a physician need not wait to obtain parental consent where an emergency endangers the life or health of a minor. Several states have specific definitions on what constitutes an emergency. However, in many states definitions of emergency care are expanding and are stated in broad general terms.

CONFIDENTIALITY

The majority of state laws allow but do not require health personnel to notify parents if they feel the situation indicates it. However, none of the laws addresses itself to the problem of a minor's right to refuse to consent to care recommended by a physician or contracted for by a parent.

COMMON DEVELOPMENTAL PROBLEMS

The Adolescent and Psychologic Problems

The adolescent experiences many psychologic conflicts that are resolved unconsciously. However, some conflicts are manifested through somatic complaints, deviant social behavior, negativism, and in some instances withdrawal from society and depression.

The adolescent's progress toward resolution of these conflicts is achieved by the self through developmental maturation and also through the support of family, peers, and in some instances from professional counseling.

The developmental tasks of adolescence are:

1. Emancipation from parents and other adults
2. Establishment of a realistic, stable, positive self-image
3. Learning to function psychologically and socially in an adult world
4. Acquisition of skills for future economic independence

The following material is presented as a guide and not as definitive answers to these complex problems.

EFFECT OF CHANGING BODY IMAGE

This is the major developmental problem of early adolescence and occurs between the ages of 11 and 14 years.

Adolescent behavior. If the changes occur in a positive manner, the adolescent accepts the body changes as a normal physiologic development toward adulthood and communicates feelings about the process openly with family members and peers.

If the change occurs in a negative manner, the adolescent has negative, fearful, and possibly guilt feelings toward the changing body image and may deny that the change is taking place or displace the feelings through psychosomatic complaints. There is usually noncommunication with family members, avoidance of social activities, and fear of locker-room activity.

Assessment. The nurse practitioner assesses the adolescent's feelings about the body by asking the following:

1. How do you feel about your height, weight, skin, chest?
2. What would you change about your body if you could?
3. What makes you feel good about your body?
4. What don't you like about your body?
5. Who can you talk to about these feelings?

Management. The nurse practitioner helps the adolescent try to resolve the emotional conflict brought on by the body changes by:

1. Accepting the adolescent's feelings and exhibiting an understanding attitude
2. Discussing normal height, weight curves, development of secondary sexual characteristics, normality of early growth spurt for females, and menarche
3. Re-establishing psychological equilibrium by stressing normalcy of feelings, importance of communicating feelings with appropriate individuals, involvement in social activities, and sublimation of depression into constructive outlets: work, sports, hobbies

EROTIC AND ASSERTIVE URGES

This problem occurs in early adolescence between the ages of 11 and 14 years.

Adolescent behavior. There are sexual fantasies often resulting in pleasurable feelings with resultant feelings of guilt and shame. With males there are wet dreams. With both sexes there may be masturbation and/or intercourse and sexual jokes and innuendos. There is usually very little communication with parents and peers about the intensity of feelings. There may be sublimation towards constructive outlets: hobbies, aggressive sports, work, social causes.

Assessment. The nurse practitioner assesses the adolescent's feelings by asking the following:

1. Has the adolescent had a family life course in school?
2. How much time is spent in daydreaming?
3. What fantasies does the adolescent have about boys (girls), kissing? To elicit these personal feelings, it helps to preface the sentence by: "Some people have dreams and fantasies about having sexual contact with a friend. These feelings are very normal at this age. What feelings do you have that are like these and are they worrisome to you?"
4. What type of activities is the adolescent involved in after school?
5. Does the adolescent have close friends?

Management. The nurse practitioner helps the adolescent to try to resolve the conflict by:

1. Encouraging participation in family life course in school
2. Discussing the importance of daydreaming as a therapeutic escape from emotional conflicts
3. Discussing the normalcy of erotic urges and fantasies, wet dreams, and masturbation
4. Discussing the importance of physical activity to lessen the tension of the erotic urges
5. Discussing the importance of communicating with appropriate individuals and thereby validating own feelings

DEPENDENCE VERSUS INDEPENDENCE

This problem occurs in middle adolescence between the ages of 14 17 years.

Adolescent behavior. There is psychologic conflict because of the adolescent's obedience to parental rules which conflict with wishes for being an individual and establishing a separate identity. Behavior ranges from cooperation to rebellion.

There are feelings and periods of confusion, loneliness, isolation, and fear at eventually leaving the family unit. There are feelings of anger at parents for feeling misunderstood. As parents allow more autonomous activities there is a mourning for the loss of family security with feelings of moodiness, crying, and depression. Supportive peer relationships to replace family ties are established.

Assessment. The nurse practitioner assesses:

1. The adolescent's degree of conflict with the family in assuming responsibility for decisions and activities
2. How the adolescent deals with angry feelings toward parents
3. Frequency of feelings of moodiness, isolation, and depression
4. Involvement in peer, social activities
5. Adolescent's future goals in reference to work, school

Management. The nurse practitioner helps the adolescent try to resolve the conflict by:

1. Discussing possible ways to resolve family conflicts and recommending family counseling for severe conflicts
2. Discussing constructive ways to deal with intense feelings: verbal communication, physical exercise
3. Discussing normalcy of feelings of moodiness, isolation, depression, and anger
4. Establishing secure peer relationships
5. Planning for future work: school, job training

IDEALISM

This problem occurs in late adolescence between the ages of 17 and 21 years See this chapter, The Adolescent and the Family: Rebellion Against Family Traditions and Values.

Adolescent behavior. The gradual loosening of parental ties and less preoccupation with own self results in thinking directed toward social issues and ideologies. The adolescent's idealism causes active questioning of societies' and families' values. There is occasional anger at authority figures for lack of interest in improving society. There are feelings of cynicism alternating with renewed idealism.

Assessment. The nurse practitioner assesses:

1. The adolescent's degree of conflict with the family and other authority figures
2. Availability of constructive activities as an outlet for the idealism and to ease feelings of loneliness

Management. The nurse practitioner helps the adolescent try to resolve the conflict by:

1. Discussing the adolescent's feelings about conflicts with the family over idealist issues and ways to resolve the conflicts
2. Discussing personal goals for self-development and social outlets for feelings of loneliness

SEXUALITY

Sexual feelings both conscious and unconscious occur throughout adolescence.

Adolescent behavior. In early adolescence increased hormone production produces physical changes and increased sexual urges and aggressiveness occasionally causing denial and guilt. In middle adolescence the sexual drive is occasionally sublimated through aggressive sports, creative hobbies, humanistic causes, and group activity with the same or opposite sex. Relief from sexual urges is also attained through masturbation and intercourse.

In late adolescence there is occasionally a move from an emphasis on a physical relationship to one of emotional commitment.

Assessment. The nurse practitioner assesses:

1. The adolescent's understanding of the normalcy of body changes and increased sexual urges
2. The use of constructive activities to sublimate sexual drives
3. The adolescent's ability and willingness to discuss feelings about body changes with the appropriate individuals

Management. The nurse practitioner helps the adolescent to try to resolve the conflict by:

1. Discussing the adolescent's knowledge and feelings about menarche, nocturnal seminal emissions, body changes, and increased sexual urges
2. Discussing activities to relieve sexual drives: contact or intramural sports, jogging, household chores, masturbation
3. Discussing adolescent's feelings with appropriate individuals: health professionals, peers, empathetic adult figures
4. Discussing protective measures against pregnancy and venereal disease if sexually active

The Adolescent and the Family

The experiences and pressures of the peer group, school, and the social milieu help adolescents test various methods of asserting their individuality or conformity. But it is within the family unit that adolescents experience a large part of the emotional conflicts that will help to establish their own identity.

However, the nuclear family in some situations has undergone major changes: an increasing divorce rate, rapid role diffusion of parents because of social change, and less emphasis on traditional class values. The result for many adolescents is increased psychologic chaos.

The following material is presented as a guide and not as definitive answers to these complex problems.

MOODINESS AND NONCOMMUNICATION WITH FAMILY MEMBERS

These developmental problems occur throughout early, middle, and late adolescence.

Adolescent behavior. There are mood swings: from nonverbal communication to exultation depending on the degree and type of emotional conflict the adolescent is experiencing and the progress toward resolution. Some major conflicts are fear at establishing an individual identity, developing a mature sexual orientation, feelings of depression and worry over changing body image, and social relationships.

Assessment. The nurse practitioner assesses the degree of conflict or acceptance with other family members in reference to the adolescent's moodiness by asking the following:

1. How often do you need to be alone?
2. How does your family accept this?
3. Who in the family do you talk with when you're feeling good or bad?

Management. The nurse practitioner helps the adolescent to try to resolve the conflict by:

1. Reassuring the adolescent of the normalcy of wanting to be alone, mood swings, fears about social relationships and the future

2. Discussing family conflicts around adolescent's moodiness and possible solutions
3. Discussing the importance of communication with appropriate family members to validate own feelings and to relieve psychologic isolation

REBELLION AGAINST FAMILY TRADITIONS AND VALUES

This problem occurs in middle and late adolescence between the ages of 14 and 21 years.

Adolescent behavior. The adolescent experiences conflict between the traditional culture and beliefs of the family and the values and pressures of peers and society. There are frequent discussions and arguments with family members in reference to their own value systems, religious beliefs, and routine of daily life.

Assessment. The nurse practitioner assesses relationships with family members by asking the following:

1. How do you get along with your family?
2. Who do you feel most comfortable with, least comfortable with?
3. What do you like about your relationship with your family, what do you dislike?

Management. The nurse practitioner helps the adolescent to try to resolve the conflict by:

1. Offering feedback to the client in the form of statements previously expressed by the client ("I hear you saying that . . ."). This helps the adolescent review the statement and possibly examine it closer.
2. Role playing a variety of solutions
3. Availability of peers and health professionals to discuss feelings about family conflicts and therefore to help to validate the adolescent's feelings
4. Helping the adolescent to become aware of his own needs and desires and therefore to become less influenced by the opinions of others

UNSTABLE FAMILY STRUCTURE

Adolescent behavior. Because of family dysfunction the adolescent experiences a lack of appropriate role models for identity and a decreased amount of parental guidance. The adolescent may experience some or all the following: moodiness, loneliness, isolation, feelings of loss, panic, anger, depression, and denial. These feelings may be manifested through psychosomatic complaints, insomnia, social misconduct, or school problems.

Assessment. The nurse practitioner assesses:

1. The family structure: number of members, means of financial support, living arrangements
2. From which family member the adolescent obtains psychologic support
3. The adolescent's worries about the family
4. What type of changes the adolescent wishes within the family

Management. The nurse practitioner helps the adolescent to try to resolve the conflict by:

1. Offering a consistent source of psychologic support through frequent health visits or through referral for therapeutic counseling
2. Discussing the adolescent's strengths as perceived by him/her in helping to cope with the family crisis
3. Discussing involvement in constructive activities: school, hobbies, exercise
4. Investigating sources of adult role models: other available family members and friends, community organizations

The Adolescent and the Peer Group

It is with the peer group that the adolescent accomplishes through trial and error several developmental tasks. There is sublimation of sexual drives through a variety of activities: sports, group social activities, and individual dating. There is discussion of different ideals and feelings in reference to the self and to society. Validation of the adolescent's feelings with peers helps in developing a positive self-image and a mature identity.

While the peer group is generally supportive and accepting of the individual, there are instances when the group becomes a negative force for adolescent development. This is accomplished when peer pressure is put on the individual in reference to sexual promiscuity, substance abuse, and conformity to the group at all costs.

The following material is presented as a guide and not as definitive answers to these complex problems.

CONFORMITY TO THE GROUP

This occurs in early and middle adolescence, between 11 and 17 years.

Adolescent behavior. There is conformity in styles of dress, dancing, music, vocabulary, and social activities. The allegiance to the peer group helps adolescents to challenge adult authority and provides psychologic support and validation for their feelings. Extreme degrees of conformity may conflict with the adolescent's own need for individual identity.

Assessment. The nurse practitioner assesses:

1. The adolescent's participation in peer activities: type of activity, number of friends
2. The adolescent's feelings about the peer group: likes peers, wants more involvement, wants less involvement
3. Pressures of the peer group on the adolescent to conform

Management. The nurse practitioner helps the adolescent to try to resolve the conflict by:

1. Discussing the normalcy of peer allegiance and conformity
2. Discussing ways in which the group conflicts with the adolescent's own goals and how this is resolved by the adolescent

INFERIORITY FEELINGS ABOUT THE DEGREE OF GROUP ACCEPTANCE

This occurs in early and middle adolescence between 11 and 17 years.

Adolescent behavior. There may be feelings of loneliness and depression if the adolescent does not have some involvement in peer social activities. The adolescent may become introverted, a loner, and excessively shy. There is a great need for conformity and popularity within the peer group. This is usually achieved by participation in sports, by excellence in scholastic achievements, and by being involved in own social group.

Assessment. The nurse practitioner assesses the adolescent's feelings about peer participation by asking the following:

1. How do you get along with classmates?
2. What school activities are you involved with?
3. What do you do after school and on weekends?
4. How important is it for you to feel popular?
5. Do you ever feel lonely?
6. Are you dating?

Management. The nurse practitioner helps the adolescent to try to resolve the conflict by:

1. Discussing degree of social involvement with peers
2. Discussing participation in after-school activities: intramural sports, football games, plays, hobbies, dancing
3. Encouraging the client to discuss feelings about self: likes and dislikes, desired changes in self-image
4. Discussing the adolescent's strengths as perceived by the client and the practitioner
5. Discussing feelings about dating

DISAGREEMENTS WITH PEERS

This problem takes place in middle and late adolescence between 14 and 21 years.

Adolescent behavior. With disagreements the adolescent may withdraw from the group, become moody or depressed, or may sublimate feelings through loner activities: reading, television. With peer conformity there is the conflict of also maintaining one's own individuality.

Assessment. The nurse practitioner assesses the adolescent's relationships with peers.

1. How do you get along with your friends?
2. How often are there disagreements?
3. What situations cause disagreements?
4. How do you settle arguments?

Management. The nurse practitioner helps the adolescent to try to resolve the conflict by:

1. Encouraging the adolescent to deal directly with offending peers. This helps to develop an action-oriented approach to problem solving rather than a complaining do-nothing approach.
2. Role playing various approaches to solutions
3. Encouraging use of "I" language when confronting peers

Societal Problems

The developmental tasks of adolescence become more difficult to achieve when adolescents are involved in substance abuse or become parents at an early age. In these situations there is an increased need for a consistently supportive family structure and professional evaluation and counseling. Once the problem is stabilized work continues with the adolescent on achieving a mature, independent identity.

The following material is presented only as a guide and not as definitive answers to these complex problems.

SUBSTANCE ABUSE

This problem occurs throughout adolescence.

Adolescent behavior. There may be infrequent periods of abuse to regular use of drugs or alcohol. The reasons for the abuse are investigated and in many situations are difficult to ascertain. Possible explanations are: conformity to the peer group, feelings of inferiority, need to escape from problems, dismay at personal life style and society's ills, worry over scholastic achievements, inability to be competitive in sports, family instability, economic problems, lack of adult role models, isolation from family and peers, and depression.

Assessment. The nurse practitioner assesses:

1. How the adolescent feels about his/her living situation, personal life style
2. Worries about family, school, peers
3. The adolescent's description of own strengths and weaknesses
4. How the adolescent deals with frustration, anger
5. The adolescent's attitude toward drugs, alcohol
6. Members of family or peer group with abuse problems
7. What individuals the adolescent uses for psychologic support

Management. The nurse practitioner helps the adolescent to try to gain insight into the problem by:

1. Discussing ways the adolescent would like to change living situation, personal life style
2. Discussing worrisome feelings in reference to self, family, school, peers
3. Discussing ways to improve self-esteem: obtaining supportive role models, accomplishing a task
4. Investigating areas of support: adult role models, community, church, school organizations, development of new interests
5. Discussing physical removal from destructive influences

6. Aligning the adolescent with a therapeutic rehabilitation program, if drug, alcohol dependent
7. Offering continued support and counseling

THE PREGNANT ADOLESCENT

Adolescent behavior. Initially there may be feelings of denial, fear, remorse, guilt, anger, and depression. In some instances there are unconscious motivations to become pregnant: as a means to escape from an unpleasant living situation, unrealistic fantasies of being loved by the infant.

If the woman is in early or middle adolescence, she may not be able to view the pregnancy in reference to the effect it will have on her future or to prepare realistically for labor and delivery and the care of the infant, because of concrete thinking processes.

During pregnancy there may be anger and negativism towards the self as evidenced by masochistic behavior: frequent missing of obstetric appointments, noncompliance with medical recommendations, truancy from school.

Assessment. The nurse practitioner assesses the adolescent's:

1. Feelings about being pregnant
2. Feelings about the option of therapeutic abortion
3. Support figures and role models
4. Short-term goals: medical care, school, future relationship with baby's father and other family members

Management. The nurse practitioner helps the adolescent to try to resolve the problem by:

1. Providing pregnancy counseling
2. Acting as a support figure and role model
3. Discussing the importance of support figures in the family or peer group
4. Making appropriate referrals for medical care, social management, health education, school placement

THE ADOLESCENT PARENT

Adolescent behavior. In many situations the adolescent mother assumes the major responsibility for parenting although the maternal grandmother of the infant occasionally assumes large responsibility for the care, also. Adolescent adjustment to parenting is positive when there is constructive and consistent support within the family or residential center. Today more adolescent fathers are willing to participate in the care of the infant.

There may be a desire on the part of the mother to return to school or to work immediately or to remain at home for an indefinite period of time. Along with the demands of parenthood the adolescent continues to work on developmental tasks and continues to struggle with the psychologic conflict of desiring autonomy but being developmentally immature to achieve it.

Assessment. The nurse practitioner assesses the adolescent's:

1. Support figures and role models in the home, residential center, or peer group
2. Knowledge of infant behavior, physical and emotional care
3. Degree of attachment and bonding to the infant
4. Conflicts with family members in reference to routines of infant care and day-care arrangements
5. Relationship with the infant's father
6. Knowledge of family planning methods
7. Short-range goals: personal living arrangements, school, work, provisions for babysitting

Management. The nurse practitioner helps the adolescent parent by:

1. Discussing the importance of consistent support figures
2. Discussing infant behavior and aspects of physical and routine health care
3. Acting as an emotional support figure for the parent and as a role model for parental child interaction
4. Offering appropriate referral services for help with resolving severe family conflicts, obtaining school or work placement

5. Discussing relationship with infant's father and finding solutions to possible conflicts
6. Offering easily accessible family planning services.

Resource Information

For further information regarding a minor's right to health care:
Local:
1. Office of the State Attorney General
2. Department of Public Health
3. Planned Parenthood, Inc.
4. Local government printing office.
National:
1. Government Printing Office, Public Documents Department, Washington DC 20402.
2. Department of Health, Education and Welfare, Public Health Service, Health Services Administration, Bureau of Community Health Services, 5600 Fishers Lane, Room 12 A 33, Rockville, MD 20852.
3. Federal Information Center, Region III Building, GSA, 7th and D Streets SW, Room 5716, Washington DC 20405.
4. Planned Parenthood Federation of America, Inc., 515 Madison Avenue, New York NY 10022.
5. The Alan Guttmacher Institute (The Research and Development Division of Planned Parenthood Federation of America, Inc.), Suite 903, 1666 K St. NW, Washington DC 20006.

References

Barnes, H. U. "Physical Growth and Development During Puberty." *Medical Clin North Am* 59:1305–1317, November 1975.

Brown, F. "Sexual Problems of the Adolescent Girl." *Pediatr Clin North Am* 19:759–764, August 1972.

Brunswick, A. F. "Health Needs of Adolescents: How the Adolescent Sees Them." *Am J Public Health* 59:1730–1745, September 1969.

Committee on Adolescence, Group for the Advancement of Psychiatry. *Normal Adolescence*. New York: Charles Scribner's Sons, 1968.

Daniel, W. A. *The Adolescent Patient*. St. Louis: Mosby, 1970.

Eisenberg, L. "A Developmental Approach to Adolescence." *Children* 12:131–135, July–August 1965.

Erikson, E. *Childhood and Society*. New York: Norton, 1950.

Gallagher, J. R., et al. *Medical Care of the Adolescent*, 3rd ed. New York: Appleton-Century-Crofts, 1976.

Giuffra, M. J. "Demystifying Adolescent Behavior." *Am J Nurs* 75:1724–1727, October 1975.

Guyton, A. C. *Basic Human Physiology: Normal Function and Mechanisms of Disease*, 2nd ed. Philadelphia: Saunders, 1977.

Guyton, A. C. *Textbook of Medical Physiology*. Philadelphia: Saunders, 1976.

Huxall, L. K. "Today's Pill and the Individual Woman." *Am J Maternal Child Nursing* 2:359–363, November–December 1977.

Jekel, J. F., et al. "A Comparison of the Health of Index and Subsequent Babies Born to School-Age Mothers." *Am J Public Health* 65:370–374, April 1975.

Johnson, C. L. "Adolescent Pregnancy: Intervention into the Poverty Cycle." *Adolescence* 9:391–406, Fall 1975.

Leonard, S. W. "How First Time Fathers Feel Toward Their Newborns." *Am J Maternal Child Nursing* 1:361–365, November–December 1976.

Mitchell, H. S., et al. *Nutrition in Health and Disease*, 16th ed. Philadelphia: Lippincott, 1976.

Nadelson, C. "Abortion Counseling: Focus on Adolescent Pregnancy." *Pediatrics* 54:765–769, December 1974.

Parel, E. W. "Danforth and Bellotti: A Breakthrough for Adolescents." *Family Planning Population Reporter* 6:3–5, February 1977.

Reiber, U. D. "Is the Nurturing Role Natural to Fathers?" *Am J Maternal Child Nursing* 1:361–365, November–December 1976.

Reiter, E. O. and A. W. Root. "Hormonal Changes of Adolescence." *Medical Clin North America* 59:1284–1304, November 1975.

Root, A. W. "Endocrinology of Puberty." *J Pediatr* 83:1–19, July 1973.

Tanner, J. M. *Growth at Adolescence*. Oxford, England: Blackwell Scientific Publications, 1962.

11

Family Planning

THE ROLE OF THE NURSE PRACTITIONER IN FAMILY PLANNING

The nurse practitioner because of active association with families becomes an appropriate individual to discuss parental and client needs in the area of contraception. In educating persons about family planning the nurse practitioner is knowledgeable about the various methods, effectiveness rates, contraindications, and side effects. With adequate education and experience the nurse practitioner may provide total contraceptive care or clients may be referred to other agencies or resources.

Health Assessment

CLIENT CONCERNS

Individual concerns are discussed as they are presented by the client.

PRESENT HISTORY

1. Age
2. State of health
3. Name of primary health care provider or agency
4. Medications

5. Currently breast feeding
6. Health problems as perceived bv client

PAST HISTORY

1. Illnesses, surgery, hospitalizations, serious injuries, blood transfusions
2. Specific illnesss: blood clots in the legs or lungs, heart attacks, strokes, angina pectoris, high blood pressure, liver disease, venereal disease
3. Maternal use of diethylstilbestrol during pregnancy
4. Gynecologic surgery
5. Infertility problems and evaluations

FAMILY HISTORY

1. Allergy, anemia, cancer: breast, uterine; diabetes, epilepsy, heart attacks, hypertension, jaundice, severe depression, tuberculosis
2. Oral contraceptive use: acne, gall bladder disease, hyperlipidemia, hyperthyroidism, liver disease, sickle cell anemia, uterine myomata

SOCIAL HISTORY

1. Marital status
2. Living arrangements: type of housing, persons in household
3. Means of support

MENSTRUATION

1. Date of last menses, length, flow, normality, premenstrual tension, dysmenorrhea
2. Date of previous menses
3. Frequency and regularity of periods
4. Age at menarche; client's feelings about menarche
5. Problems with spotting between periods, menorrhagia, metorrhagia, amenorrhea

PREGNANCIES

1. Number of pregnancies, live births, abortions: spontaneous or induced; breech births, cesarean sections
2. Health during pregnancy; complications (gestational diabetes, hypertension, toxemia, vaginal bleeding, anemia, infection) during pregnancy; complications during delivery
3. Current pregnancy status

CONTRACEPTIVE USE

1. Methods, duration of use, side effects
2. Reason for termination
3. Client's degree of knowledge about types and effectiveness rates for contraceptives

SEXUAL

1. Number of episodes of vaginitis, venereal disease, pelvic inflammatory disease, urinary tract infection
2. Treatment and follow-up for #1
3. Frequency of sexual activity, number of partners
4. Accurate knowledge of protection against venereal disease and pregnancy

REVIEW OF SYSTEMS

1. HEENT: headaches, head trauma, allergies, problems with vision, thyroid disease
2. Chest: breast cancer or fibrocystic nodules
3. Cardiac: rheumatic fever, heart murmur
4. Respiratory: frequency of infections, pneumonia, bronchitis
5. Abdomen: ulcers, liver function problems
6. Genitourinary: urinary tract infections
7. Reproductive: pelvic inflammatory disease, venereal disease, malposition of organs
8. Neurologic: paralysis
9. Skin: acne, history of cholasma

PHYSICAL EXAMINATION

1. Weight, height, heart rate, respiration rate, and blood pressure
2. Thyroid palpation
3. Auscultation of the heart
4. Auscultation of the lungs
5. Inspection and palpation of the abdomen
6. Inspection of external genitalia, and internal genitalia using a speculum, and performing bimanual and vaginal-rectal examinations

LABORATORY

1. Pap smear, GC culture
2. VDRL, CBC, rubella titer, urinalysis
3. Glucose tolerance test, lipid profile if indicated

RECORDING OF VISIT

The problem list is identified and updated as necessary. Plans, health education and expectant client outcomes are delineated.

Frequently Used Terms

WOMEN YEARS

The efficacy of birth control methods are stated in terms of 100 women years. Women years are based on 13 cycles per year for one woman or one cycle for 13 women or any combination thereof. Hence 100 women years means 1300 cycles (13 cycles × 1 woman × 100) or (1 cycle × 13 women × 100). For example, the theoretical effectiveness rate of the diaphragm is three pregnancies per 100 women years of use, i.e. three pregnancies out of 1300 cycles.

THEORETICAL EFFECTIVENESS RATE

This term is used to judge the effectiveness of various birth control methods. It indicates the maximum effectiveness rate of a birth control method without taking into account the element of human error. For example, the theoretical effectiveness rate of the diaphragm is three pregnancies per 100 women years.

USE EFFECTIVENESS RATE

This term is used to judge the effectiveness of various birth control methods. It indicates the effectiveness rate of a birth control method taking into account the probability of human error in its use. For example, the use effectiveness rate of the diaphragm is 20 to 25 pregnancies per 100 women years.

Contraceptive Devices

COMBINED PILL

The combined pill contains the hormones estrogen and progesterone. This combination is more effective in reducing the incidence of pregnancy than the mini pill. See Table 1 for brand name and estrogen and progesterone potency of oral contraceptives.

Mechanism of action. The pill is effective in preventing conception because of the following:

ESTROGEN. This hormone inhibits ovulation through suppression of follicle-stimulating hormone (FSH) and leutinizing hormone (LH) via the hypothalamus. High doses of estrogen inhibit implantation of the fertilized ovum after a midcycle exposure.

PROGESTERONE. It is believed that this hormone causes decreased sperm penetration and transport through the creation of a thick, cellular cervical mucus. It also changes the characteristics of the cervical fluid and does not permit capacitation to occur. Capacitation is the release of spermatic enzymes which allow the

Table 1
Hormone Content of Oral Contraceptives

Brand Name, No. of Pills per Pack, and Manufacturer	Estrogen mg/tab	Progestogen mg/tab
Combination		
Norinyl 1+50 (21,28) (Syntex)	mestranol .05	norethindrone 1.0
Ortho-Novum 1+50 (21,28) (Ortho)	mestranol .05	norethindrone 1.0
Ortho-Novum 10 mg (20) (Ortho)	mestranol .06	norethindrone 10.0
Enovid 5 mg (20) (Searle)	mestranol .075	norethynodrel 5.0
Norinyl 1+80 (21,28) (Syntex)	mestranol .08	norethindrone 1.0
Ortho-Novum 1+80 (21,28) (Ortho)	mestranol .08	norethindrone 1.0
Enovid E (20,21) (Searle)	mestranol .10	norethynodrel 2.5
Norinyl 2 mg (20) (Syntex)	mestranol .10	norethindrone 2.0
Ortho-Novum 2 mg (20) (Ortho)	mestranol .10	norethindrone 2.0
Ovulen (20,21,28) (Searle)	mestranol .10	ethynodiol diacetate 1.0
Loestrin 1+20 (28) (Parke Davis)	ethinyl estradiol .02	norethindrone acetate 1.0
Zorane 1+20 (28) (Lederle)	ethinyl estradiol .02	norethindrone acetate 1.0
Loestrin 1.5+30 (28) (Parke Davis)	ethinyl estradiol .03	norethindrone acetate 1.0
Lo/Ovral (21,28) (Wyeth)	ethinyl estradiol .03	norgestrel 0.3
Zorane 1.5+30 (28) (Lederle)	ethinyl estradiol .03	norethindrone acetate 1.5
Brevicon (21,28) (Syntex)	ethinyl estradiol .035	norethindrone 0.5
Modicon (21,28) (Ortho)	ethinyl estradiol .035	norethindrone 0.5
Ovcon −35 (28) (Mead Johnson)	ethinyl estradiol .035	norethindrone 0.4
Demulen (21,28) (Searle)	ethinyl estradiol .05	ethynodiol diacetate 1.0
Norlestrin 1 mg (21,28) (Parke Davis)	ethinyl estradiol .05	norethindrone acetate 1.0
Norlestrin 2.5 mg (21,28) (Parke Davis)	ethinyl estradiol .05	norethindrone acetate 2.5
Ovcon −50 (28) (Mead Johnson)	ethinyl estradiol .05	norethindrone 1.0
Ovral (21,28) (Wyeth)	ethinyl estradiol .05	norgestral 0.5
Zorane 1+50 (28) (Lederle)	ethinyl estradiol .05	norethindrone acetate 1.0
Microdose		
Ovrette (28) (Wyeth)	none	norgestrel .075
Micronor (35) (Ortho)	none	norethindrone .35
Nor - Q.D. (42) (Syntex)	none	norethindrone .35

sperm to penetrate the ovum. It also decreases ovum transport through the fallopian tubes when given prior to fertilization and may inhibit implantation. Ovulation may also be inhibited.

Theoretical effectiveness rate. There is less than one pregnancy per 100 women years.

Use effectiveness rate. There are approximately two to five pregnancies per 100 women years.

Absolute contraindications.* A history is investigated for the following:

- Thromboembolic disorders
- Cerebrovascular accident
- Impaired liver function
- Malignancy of breast or reproductive system
- Pregnancy

Strong relative contraindications.* A history is investigated for the following:

- Migraine headaches
- Hypertension
- Full-term gestation terminated within the past 4 weeks
- Pre-diabetes or diabetes; strong family history of diabetes
- Gallbladder disease
- Postcholecystectomy
- Cholestasis during pregnancy
- Acute phase of mononucleosis
- Sickle cell disease
- Undiagnosed abnormal vaginal bleeding

Other relative contraindications*

- Varicose veins
- Asthma

---

*Used with permission from R. A. Hatcher, et al, *Contraceptive Technology 1976– 1977,* 8th ed., (New York: Irvington Publishers, Inc.).

- Cardiac or renal disease
- Mental retardation
- Chloasma
- Family history of diabetes
- Uterine fibromyomata
- Epilepsy
- Depression
- Client with profile suspicious for subsequent anovulation and infertility problems: late onset of menses and very irregular, painless menses
- Breast-feeding

Other contraindications. These include:

- Angina pectoris
- Age over 40 years
- Hyperlipidemia
- Cigarette smoking

Estrogen excess side effects. These include:

- Breast tenderness
- Chloasma
- Edema of extremities
- Headaches
- Hypertension
- Nausea
- Thrombophlebitis and embolus
- Weight gain

Estrogen deficiency side effects. These include:

- Absence of withdrawal bleeding
- Decreased menstrual flow
- Decreased sex drive
- Early and midcycle breakthrough bleeding
- Hot flashes

- Psychologic irritability
- Uterine prolapse

Progesterone excess side effects. These include:

- Acne
- Alopecia
- Decreased ability of the liver to excrete conjugated bilirubin resulting in cholestatic jaundice and increased incidence of gallbladder disease
- Decreased length of menstrual flow
- Decreased libido
- Fatigue
- Higher incidence of monilial vaginitis

Progesterone deficiency side effects. These include:

- Delayed onset of menses following last pill
- Heavy menstrual flow
- Late breakthrough bleeding

Protocol for initial health visit. Height, weight, and blood pressure measurements are obtained. A complete history is obtained and a partial physical assessment is done. A complete pelvic examination is done. Laboratory screening: see this chapter, Health Assessment.

Protocol for return visits. A blood pressure measurement is obtained. The presence or absence of side effects is discussed, and serious complications from oral contraceptive use are reviewed. The medication regime is reviewed. Return visits are usually every 6 to 12 months. A repeat physical and pelvic examination is done. Pap smears and a GC culture are obtained. Adolescents are routinely seen more frequently, usually every 3 months because of the higher incidence of irregularities of pill use.

Health teaching. The following are discussed:

MEDICATION REGIMEN. The pill is started on the fifth day after the menses begins. For the 21-day pack one pill is taken every day for 21 days, no pills are taken for the next 7 days, and a new package of pills is restarted on the eighth day. For the 28-day pack, one pill is taken every day for 28 days. A new package of pills is started immediately after taking the last pill. In the 28-day pack the last 7 pills of the cycle are placebos. Twenty-eight-day packs are used by women who have difficulty remembering the regimen of the 21-day pill pack. A second backup method of birth control is used on the first cycle of the pill. The pill is taken at the same time every day to keep a continuous level of the drug in the body.

MISSED PILLS. One: take the pill as soon as remembered. Take the next day's pill at the regular time. Two: take two pills as soon as remembered and two pills the next day. Use a second method of birth control until the pack is finished. Three: if three pills are missed, obtain medical consultation.

SIDE EFFECTS. Review side effects: sharp pain in chest, legs (possible blood clots in heart, legs), sudden shortness of breath (possible clots in heart, lungs), severe chest pain or heaviness (possible heart attack), sudden severe headache, dizziness, fainting, inability to articulate, weakness of an extremity (possible cerebral vascular accident), sudden complete or partial loss of vision (possible blood clot), severe depression, jaundice (possible liver obstruction), breast nodules, severe abdominal pain (possible liver tumor).

OTHER CONSIDERATIONS. Absent menses: if pregnancy is not a consideration, continue taking pills for another cycle. Obtain medical consultation if no menses occurs after second cycle. If pregnancy is a possibility obtain a pregnancy test and pelvic examination. Stop pills if positive; if negative, obtain medical consultation. For breakthrough bleeding after the second cycle obtain medical consultation. Self breast examination is taught.

MINI-PILL

This pill contains progesterone only. It is used when there are side effects related to estrogen.

Mechanism of action. The mini-pill causes decreased sperm penetration and transport through the creation of a thick cellular cervical mucus. It also changes the characteristics of the cervical fluid and does not permit capacitation to occur. Capacitation is the release of spermatic enzymes which allow the sperm to penetrate the ovum. It also decreases ovum transport through the fallopian tubes when given prior to fertilization, and may inhibit implantation. Ovulation may also be inhibited.

Theoretical effectiveness rate. There is approximately 1 to 1.5 pregnancies per 100 women years. Pregnancy rates are highest in the first 6 months.

Use effectiveness rate. There are approximately two to four pregnancies per 100 women years.

Contraindications. A history is investigated for the following:

- Undiagnosed, abnormal vaginal bleeding
- Thromboembolic disorders
- Cardiovascular accident
- Impaired liver function
- Malignancy of the breast or reproductive system
- Pregnancy

Side effects. These include:

- Alterations in liver function studies
- Irregular menses (increased, decreased, spotting, amenorrhea)
- Mild headaches
- Possible increase in tubal pregnancies due to decreased ovum transport
- The increased risk of thrombophlebitis has not been established

Protocol for health visits. The same protocol is observed as with the combined pill. A hematocrit is done for excessive bleeding.

Health teaching. The following are discussed:

MEDICATION REGIMEN. The pill is started on the first day of

the menses and is taken continually even when menses occurs. The number of pills per pack varies from 28 to 42. The next pack is started immediately.

MISSED PILLS. One: take the pill as soon as remembered. Two: take two pills as soon as remembered and two pills the next day. Use a second method of birth control until the pack is finished.

SIDE EFFECTS. Menses can be irregular on the mini-pill: spotting between cycles, increased or decreased flow, infrequent menses.

DIETHYLSTILBESTROL (DES)

These pills are used to prevent conception after unprotected midcycle exposure. The pills must be started within 72 hours after exposure and are usually given for 5 days.

Mechanism of action. Prevents implantation of the fertilized ovum by affecting the endometrium.

Effectiveness rate. There is approximately one failure in 1000 treatment cycles.

Contraindications. The presence or past history of breast or genital malignancy is investigated. The client's refusal to consider a therapeutic abortion (TAB) if treatment failure occurs is a contraindication.

Side effects. These include:

- Breast tenderness
- Headache
- Menstrual irregularities
- Nausea, vomiting
- Possible teratogenic effect on the fetus if DES failure occurs

Protocol for health visit. See this chapter, Health Assessment.

Health teaching. Discuss medication regimen and common side effects. Discuss protocol if menstruation does not occur in one month: pregnancy test, if positive, TAB. Discuss reasons for TAB: possible teratogenesis of the fetus, possible future genital carcinoma in females.

INTRAUTERINE DEVICES (IUD)

Mechanism of action. The IUD functions as a foreign body and produces a local sterile inflammatory response by lysis of the blastocyst.

Theoretical effectiveness rate. There are approximately one to five pregnancies per 100 women years.

Use effectiveness rate. There are approximately six pregnancies per 100 women years.

Contraindications. A history is investigated for the following:

- Uterine anomalies
- Vaginitis
- Cervicitis
- Abnormal Pap smear
- Undiagnosed abnormal vaginal bleeding
- Pelvic inflammatory disease
- Pregnancy status
- Severe dysmenorrhea
- Severe anemia
- Ectopic pregnancy

Side effects. These include:

- Anemia secondary to menorrhagia
- Increased dysmenorrhea
- Increased incidence of tubal pregnancy
- Menorrhagia
- Uterine expulsion
- Uterine perforation
- With multiple partners increased susceptibility to salpingitis and pelvic inflammatory disease

Protocol. Height, weight, and blood pressure measurements are obtained. A complete history is obtained and a partial physical assessment is done. A complete pelvic examination is done. Laboratory screening: see this chapter, Health Assessment.

INSERTION. This is done by a qualified individual. The anterior cervix is held in place with a tenaculum. The uterus is probed with a sound for size and the IUD is then inserted. Some clinicians use a local anesthetic injected paracervically to decrease abdominal discomfort. Responses to the insertion vary according to the individual: mild to severe abdominal cramping; occasional vagal nerve response: nausea, vomiting, bradycardia, pallor, clammy skin, dizziness, and fainting. The client sits up slowly after insertion to decrease vagal nerve response.

Types. The following are commonly used IUDs:

LIPPES LOOP. This device can be left in the uterus indefinitely and does not have to be periodically replaced.

COPPER 7. This device is shaped like a number 7 and has fine copper wire wrapped around its stem. The addition of copper wiring enhances its effectiveness. It is contraindicated in clients who are allergic to copper and those with Wilson's Disease: a skin condition thought to be caused by improper copper metabolism. The copper 7 needs to be replaced every 2 years.

SAF-T-COIL. This device has the shortest length and is used in clients with small uteri.

PROGESTASERT. This device contains a small amount of progesterone which is released over a period of 12 months. The hormone enhances the effectiveness of the device. The IUD needs to be replaced yearly.

DIAPHRAGM WITH CREAM OR JELLY

The diaphragm is a flexible rubber dome which is encircled by a metal spring. There are two types: all flex and coil spring. All are equally effective. For some individuals the all-flex diaphragm is easier to insert.

Mechanism of action. The diaphragm is inserted into the vagina before intercourse and covers the cervix. A spermicidal jelly or cream is placed inside the rubber dome and on the rim before insertion. The diaphragm holds the spermicidal agent near the cervical os. Dislodgement although rare may occur during intercourse as a result of frequent insertions of the penis.

Theoretical effectiveness rate. There are approximately three pregnancies per 100 women years.

Use effectiveness rate. There are approximately 15 to 20 pregnancies per 100 women years.

Contraindications. The history is investigated for the following:

• Severe antiverted or retroverted uterus
• Complete uterine prolapse
• Cystocele
• Rectocele
• Acute pelvic inflammation
• Client unacceptance

Side effects. These include:

• Possible allergic reactions to the rubber or spermicidal agents (rare)

Protocol for initial health visit. See this chapter, Health Assessment. In addition the proximal vagina is measured by the index finger from the posterior fornix to the symphysis pubis. This length is then compared with the appropriate circumference of the various sizes of diaphragms.

Health teaching. The client is instructed to use one tablespoonful of cream or jelly on the inside and the rim of the diaphragm. It can be inserted 2 hours before use. To insert, the client squats or stands with one leg raised on a chair. The diaphragm is pinched together at the rim dome side down with one hand. The other hand spreads apart the lips of the vagina. The diaphragm is inserted back into the vagina as far as it will go; the front rim is tucked behind the symphysis pubis bone. The index finger then follows the rim of the diaphragm to make sure it is in place and also feels for the cervix through the dome. An applicatorful of spermicidal jelly or cream is inserted into the vagina before each additional act of intercourse. The diaphragm is left in place for 8 hours after intercourse. Douching is not done before then. To remove, the index finger is hooked under the rim of the diaphragm at the symphysis pubis bone and it is pulled out. It is washed with water, dried, and kept in a container when not in use.

SPERMICIDAL PREPARATIONS

These preparations contain a foam, jelly, or cream which holds the spermicidal agent against the cervical os and a chemical which kills the sperm.

Mechanism of action. Coital movements spread the medium over the cervical os.

Theoretical effectiveness rate. There are approximately three pregnancies in 100 women years.

Use effectiveness rate. There are approximately 30 pregnancies in 100 women years.

Contraindications and side effects. These include:

• Allergy to foam or rubber (rare)

Protocol for health visits. See this chapter, Health Assessment.

Health teaching. The client is instructed to shake the container before use. Two applicatorsful of the medium are inserted back into the vagina just before intercourse. One applicatorful is inserted before each additional intercourse. If douching is desired, the client waits for 8 hours after intercourse. To increase effectiveness it is recommended that a condom be used in conjunction with the foam.

CONDOM

Mechanism of action. Over an erect penis the condom is a barrier to the expulsion of sperm into the vagina. It also reduces the risk of transmitting or receiving venereal disease.

Theoretical effectiveness rate. There are approximately three pregnancies per 100 women years.

Use effectiveness rate. There are approximately 20 to 25 pregnancies per 100 women years.

Contraindications and side effects

• Allergy to rubber (rare)

Protocol for health visits. Routine health history and examination if client has not had one in one year.

Health teaching. The condom is placed on the erect penis before insertion into the vagina. One-half of empty space is left at the tip of the condom to hold the ejaculate. If lubrication is needed when applying the condom, saliva or K-Y jelly is used; Vaseline causes the rubber to deteriorate. When withdrawing, the condom is held at the proximal end to prevent leakage of sperm into the vagina.

RHYTHM

Mechanism of action. The absence of sexual intercourse or the use of another method is practiced during the fertile period (ovulation). To ascertain the period when ovulation occurs the client has accurate knowledge of her shortest and longest menstrual cycle. The fertile period is calculated by subtracting 18 days from her shortest cycle and 11 days from her longest cycle. This provides a range in which she is at risk for pregnancy. This method uses the following assumptions: ovulation occurs 12 to 16 days prior to menstruation; sperm remain viable for 48 hours; ovum will survive for 24 hours. (See Table 2.)

Table 2
How to Calculate the Fertile Period

If Your Shortest Period Has Been:	Your First Fertile (Unsafe) Day Is:[a]	If Your Longest Period Has Been:	Your Last Fertile (Unsafe) Day Is:[a]
21 days	3rd day	21 days	10th day
22 days	4th day	22 days	11th day
23 days	5th day	23 days	12th day
24 days	6th day	24 days	13th day
25 days	7th day	25 days	14th day
26 days	8th day	26 days	15th day
27 days	9th day	27 days	16th day
28 days	10th day	28 days	17th day
29 days	11th day	29 days	18th day
30 days	12th day	30 days	19th day
31 days	13th day	31 days	20th day
32 days	14th day	32 days	21st day
33 days	15th day	33 days	22nd day
34 days	16th day	34 days	23rd day
35 days	17th day	35 days	24th day

Source: Used with permission from R. A. Hatcher, et al, *Contraceptive Technology* 1976–1977, 8th ed. (New York: Irvington Publishers Inc.).
[a]Count the first day of bleeding as "first day."

Theoretical effectiveness rate. There are approximately 15 pregnancies per 100 women years.

Use effectiveness rate. There are approximately 25 to 35 pregnancies per 100 women years.

Contraindications

• Irregular menses
• Client unacceptance

Side effects. None.

Protocol. A routine health history and physical examination is done if client has not had one in 1 year.

Health teaching. The method to calculate the fertile period is reviewed. Abstinence or a second method of birth control is discussed for use during the fertile period. The effectiveness rate is reviewed.

BASAL BODY TEMPERATURE (BBT) METHOD

The basal body temperature is the lowest temperature attained by the body during waking hours. Just before ovulation the BBT drops. In 24 to 48 hours after this time there is a noticeable temperature rise. The temperature remains elevated for 3 days. By charting body temperature before getting out of bed in the AM a woman can determine when she ovulates.

Use effectiveness rate. When used in conjunction with the rhythm method there are approximately 15 to 20 pregnancies per 100 women years.

Contraindications

- Infections
- Irregular sleeping habits
- Tension
- The use of electric blankets may cause elevations in the BBT

Side effects. None.

Health teaching. Temperature is taken orally every morning and is charted. Charts are reviewed with the couples and interpreted for the first 3 months. Couples refrain from intercourse or use another method at the beginning of a drop in the temperature until after it remains elevated for 3 days.

COITUS INTERRUPTUS

Mechanism of action. By withdrawing the penis before ejaculation the male deposits semen away from the vagina.

Theoretical effectiveness rate. There are approximately 15 pregnancies per 100 women years.

Use effectiveness rate. There are approximately 20 to 30 pregnancies per 100 women years.

Contraindications

• Lack of self control
• Lack of ejaculatory control

Side effects. Psychologic frustration at the method

Health teaching. The semen is released away from the woman's genitals. It is possible that some preliminary ejaculatory fluid can be expelled prior to ejaculation without the knowledge of either partner.

References

Ambrose, L. "Misinforming Pregnant Teenagers." *Family Planning Perspectives* 10:51–57, January/February, 1978.

Emans, S. J. and D. P. Goldstein. *Pediatric and Adolescent Gynecology.* Boston: Little, Brown, 1977.

Gillmore, N. *Nurses in Family Planning.* Department of Gynecology and Obstetrics, Emory University, School of Medicine, Atlanta, Georgia.

Gordon, S. *Facts About Sex for Todays Youth.* New York: John Day, 1973.

Hatcher, R. A. et al. *Contraceptive Technology 1976–1977,* 8th ed. New York: Irvington Publishers, Inc., 1976.

Herbst, A. L., et al. "Effects of Maternal DES Ingestion on the Female Genital Tract." *Hospital Practice* 51:57, October 1975.

Johnson, E. *Love and Sex in Plain Language.* Philadelphia: Bantam, 1967.

Katchadourian, H. *Human Sexuality Sense and Nonsense.* San Francisco: Freeman, 1972.

Katchadourian, H. *The Biology of Adolescence.* San Francisco: Freeman, 1977.

Kreutner, A. K. and D. R. Hollingsworth. *Adolescent Obstetrics and Gynecology.* Chicago: Yearbook Medical Publishers, 1978.

Pomeroy, W. B. *Your Child and Sex: A Guide for Parents.* New York: Dell, 1974.

Stycos, M. "Desexing Birth Control." *Family Planning Perspectives* 9:286–292, November/December 1977.

Taylor, D. "A New Way to Teach Teens about Contraceptives." *Am J Maternal Child Nursing* 76:379–383, November/December 1976.

Wear, J. and K. Holmes. *How To Have Intercourse Without Getting Screwed.* Seattle: Madrona Publishers, 1976.

12

Health Education in Primary Care

Health education is a large component of nursing practice. The methods nurses use to teach clients are varied and depend on the following: the nurse's preparation and previous experience with health education, the learning needs of the client, the amount of time and money available for health education, and the administrative policies of the individual health institutions toward client education. Recently more emphasis has been placed on developing specific standards for client teaching to provide written evidence of accountability for nursing actions and to document health education programs for reimbursement from third-party payers.

The emphasis of this chapter is on health education of parents and adolescents. However, the references contain several articles on health teaching for children through formal instruction or play therapy.

GROUP HEALTH EDUCATION

Principles of Teaching and Learning

MOTIVATION

It is important to understand what the client's reasons are for obtaining health information. If the contact was self-initiated the learning will most probably be positive because of the client's interest. When the health educator understands what clients want to learn then education is structured toward satisfying that need.

LEARNING BY PARTS

It is difficult for clients to learn if they are overloaded with many important points in a short period of time. Depending on the length of the session, it is best to introduce a new concept once every 10 minutes or to concentrate on no more than three main points in a 30-minute discussion.

LEARNING BY DOING

Learning occurs faster when the client is periodically engaged in communication with the educator or participates in a task relevant to the discussion during the learning process. Continuous didactic instruction places the client in the position of a passive participant and therefore decreases attention and impedes the learning process.

SPACED REPETITION

Important points are repeated several times throughout the discussion. The use of a chalkboard and other visual aids pertinent to the discussion helps to vary the repetition and offers a variety of stimulation.

REINFORCEMENT

Verbal positive feedback to participants encourages and reinforces the learning process. The educator explains why questions answered by the participants are correct or incorrect or why a particular task was accomplished in a certain way. These answers help to reinforce learning.

Developing Group Teaching Programs

ASSESSING THE NEED

The learning needs of clients are assessed. Ways to assess client interest include: individual consultation, questionnaires, encouraging suggestions, and discussing possible classes that clients might not have considered such as classes for fathers only, care of ill children. To avoid duplication health education resources and current classes in the community are identified.

COLLECTING DATA

Ideas concerning specific health education classes are discussed with nursing peers, supervisors, staff development personnel, and patient education committees. A review of the literature concerning class content is conducted. Nursing colleagues who are interested in offering input are encouraged. Convenient times for the majority of participants are investigated. The availability of an adequate classroom with appropriate visual aids for teaching is investigated. Methods of advertising the class are considered. Ways to initiate and maintain liaison with the community are assessed.

DEVELOPING CONTENT

The health education needs of the clients are reviewed and the main topic or topics are developed. A survey of the literature concerning the proposed topics is conducted. The type of presentation is decided: lecture, discussion, demonstration. The use and type of visual aids are evaluated: charts, poster, films, slides, role playing. The participation of allied health disciplines is assessed: dentist, nutritionist, pharmacist, play therapist, public health nurse. A written description of the course objectives is given to the participants.

DEVELOPING LEARNING OBJECTIVES

The purpose of objectives are:

1. To clarify goals of the program for the client and the educator
2. To create measurable items that are evaluated at the end of the program to assess the client's progress

DEFINING TERMINAL BEHAVIOR

In writing objectives the client's desired behavior at the end of instruction is defined. This behavior is called terminal behavior and describes the conditions under which the behavior is expected to occur. For example, after completion of the course, the client will demonstrate the appropriate technique of breast massage for milk expulsion or the client will be able to list three causes of serious illness in infants.

Terminal behavior is further defined by describing the acceptable level of performance at which the client must accomplish the task. For example, the client will demonstrate the appropriate technique of breast massage two out of three times. The client is given a copy of the objectives which contain the desired terminal behaviors.

DETERMINING THE CLIENT'S LEVEL OF KNOWLEDGE

A pretest is given to the clients to assess their level of knowledge concerning the topic before instruction begins. Pretests are most commonly given in classes that cover several sessions. The pretest uses several types of questions: true, false, multiple choice, completion. Questions relate to content that will be covered in class.

A second method to determine the client's level of knowledge is to discuss with or interview the client on the topics before the program. After the discussion the educator's impressions of the client's knowledge are recorded.

EVALUATION OF THE CLIENT'S KNOWLEDGE AT THE END OF THE PROGRAM

A post-test is given at the end of the program. It contains the same questions that are in the pretest.

If the second method is used, the client is interviewed at the end of the program. The postinterview notes are compared with the educator's notes from the first interview.

EVALUATION OF THE PROGRAM

The following questions are answered based on the objectives:

1. Did the client's behavior at the end of the instruction fulfill the objectives of terminal behavior?
2. Did the client perform under the conditions stated in the objectives?
3. Did the client perform the task within the accepted level of performance?

If the above were not adequately performed by the client, the following are re-evaluated: learning objectives, content of the program, teaching methods.

REVISION OF THE PROGRAM

The program is revised based on data collected from the problem areas in the evaluation.

Individual Communication and Health Teaching

THE OFFICE VISIT

Introduction. The nurse practitioner introduces her/himself in the waiting area or in the examining room. The child is greeted with remarks appropriate to her/his age. Age-appropriate toys are provided for the child so initial conversation with the parents may proceed uninterrupted.

Defining the problem. The nurse practitioner asks the reasons for the visit. This helps clarify some of the family's feelings about the problem. It also helps in assessing the accuracy of the parents' knowledge or general misconceptions about health issues. Open-ended questions help promote a nonjudgmental atmosphere. Questions with the word "feel" generally promote specific client response and do not give clues as to what answers are appropriate.

Maintaining control. To establish and to maintain effective communication the nurse practitioner listens actively to the client's concerns and questions. This involves maintaining control during the visits by: interrupting the client if digressions develop to reestablish the focus, encouraging the expression of mood states ("How do you feel when the baby cries?"), asking for clarification when necessary, maintaining a nonjudgmental attitude, and offering feedback to the client in summary statements ("I hear you saying that . . .").

Content. Throughout the visit individual health teaching is offered in reference to the client's concerns, nutrition, growth and development, immunizations, anticipatory guidance, prevention and treatment of minor illnesses, safety, routine physical fitness, and family planning.

Closure. The nurse practitioner states that the discussion may be continued at another visit if time has expired. She/he reviews and summarizes the essential components of the visit and re-emphasizes important health education points in writing.

Formulating a plan. A plan for the child's or client's health care is formulated by the nurse practitioner and the client. Important health education goals are re-emphasized.

References

Auerbach, A. *Parents Learn Through Discussion.* Child Study Association of America, Inc., 1968.

Fuhrer, L. M. and R. Berstein. "Making Patient Education a Part of Patient Care." *Am J Nurs* 76:1798–1799, November 1976.

Jennings, C. P. and T. F. Jennings. "Containing Costs Through Prospective Reimbursement." *Am J Nurs* 77:1155–1159, July 1977.

Kemp, J. *Instructional Design.* Belmont: Fearon Publishers, 1972.

Mager, R. F. *Preparing Instructional Objectives.* Belmont: Fearon Publishers, 1972.

Nordberg, B. and L. King. "Third Party Payment for Patient Education." *Am J Nurs* 76:1269–1271, August 1976.

Smith, E. C. "Are You Really Communicating?" *Am J Nurs* 77:1966–1968, December 1977.

ASSESSMENT AND MANAGEMENT OF COMMON CLINICAL PROBLEMS

In the course of providing comprehensive primary care services to infants and children, the nurse practitioner frequently identifies or is presented with signs and symptoms of illness or abnormality. Many common conditions of childhood can be safely and appropriately managed by the nurse practitioner who practices in collaboration with a physician. Other conditions require referral for medical management and collaboration for subsequent care.

The decision as to which problems are managed by the nurse practitioner depends on a number of factors and, admittedly, the scope of practice will vary from setting to setting. Those factors to be considered include the nature of the problem, the experience of the nurse practitioner, the availability of physician consultation, the relationship between the nurse practitioner and physician (e.g., amount of time working together, degree of trust established), the setting (e.g., isolated rural practice, university teaching clinic), the use of standing orders, protocols, or standardized procedures, and the legal statutes of the state.

When referral for medical evaluation and management is indicated, the role of the nurse practitioner does not cease. As the primary care provider for the child and family, the nurse practitioner remains the primary resource person for the family and fulfills that role by coordinating services and by providing the teaching, counseling, and support measures which are the hallmark of nursing services.

Part II is designed to provide information necessary to identify abnormalities and to assess specific conditions of infancy and childhood; to present guidelines for referral; to specify the management role of the nurse practitioner with regard to common clinical problems; and to present pertinent information for parent-child teaching and support during and after diagnosis and treatment.

Detailed information on treatment is presented only for those very common illnesses and problems. In-depth information on treatment of less common or more complicated problems should be obtained from recognized pediatric textbooks. Medications are mentioned as they relate to particular conditions, but dosages are not specified since so many variables affect determination of dose (see Chapter 14) and since this function is almost universally viewed as a collaborative one with the physician.

13

Approach to Illness in Childhood

EFFECTS OF THE DISEASE ON THE INDIVIDUAL CHILD

Acute

Many illnesses during childhood are acute in origin. Respiratory infections are extremely common and other acute illnesses include gastroenteritis, otitis media, exanthems, conjunctivitis, viral syndromes, and fevers. Because of the youthful resilience of the child's body, recovery from acute illness is usually very rapid.

Chronic

Chronic illnesses also occur in children although not as frequently as acute infections. Chronicity in illness may have serious consequences for the child. The consequences may be physical, including decelerated growth pattern and restriction of physical activity or psychologic, including a decrease in the child's self-esteem and in his/her sense of security.

Physical

In the infant and young child problems due to immature organ development are common. The infant frequently regurgitates liquids because of a loose stomach-cardiac sphincter. Frequent middle-ear infections in childhood are due to a short and straight eustachian tube which provides easy access to infectious agents from the oropharynx. Infants and children require increased fluids during illness in proportion to their weight because of heavy losses of fluids with diarrhea and vomiting and because of increased demands of the basic metabolic processes during illness. It is common for infants and children to lose weight or to gain weight slowly during and immediately following an illness. This effect is most noticeable during the rapid growth pattern of infancy. Generally children can withstand the rigors of high temperatures better than adults, and they recover more rapidly from acute illness.

Psychologic

When illness develops in children their personal sense of security is decreased. This is due to the illness itself, the child's thoughts about overcoming the effects of the illness, and the possible absence of adequate emotional support from family members. Illness produces a temporary anxiety state and children may no longer feel that obstacles in the environment can be mastered.

Some children consciously or unconsciously rely on somatic complaints to keep from involving themselves in psychologically traumatizing situations.

Chronic illnesses have serious implications for the normal psychologic development of the child. The feeling of being different, of being unable to compete in normal activities, a pervading sense of guilt in seeing the illness as punishment, fear of hospitalization, and estrangement from family all contribute to insecurity, lack of self-esteem, and depression.

Infants exhibit psychologic problems around illness also. There are frequent outbursts of crying and irritability and the need for physical and emotional comfort is increased.

ASSESSMENT OF THE PRESENTING SYMPTOM

Symptoms

Presenting symptoms are variable depending on the infectious agent, the response of the child to the agent, and the child's health status. For some children there may be only a slight decrease in motor activity or appetite, while others may be actively complaining of discomfort or may exhibit symptoms of acute illness.

The most common symptoms of acute illness in children are fever, lethargy, irritability, anorexia, nausea, vomiting, diarrhea, exanthem, rhinorrhea, cough, and discharge from the eyes.

For infants, the nurse practitioner relies on the parents' information and description of behavior and objective symptoms such as fever to ascertain the presence of illness. While an older child can localize pain to an accurate degree, an infant with pain will be irritable or will try to strike randomly at the area of discomfort.

Infants and young children with fevers do not have chills in contrast to older children and adults. Occasionally a febrile convulsion is the parents' first indication that the child has a fever.

As children mature and are exposed to a larger environment through nursery schools, peer play, and other adults outside the family, the incidence of respiratory infections dramatically increases.

History

Important information to obtain in establishing the data base includes:

- Age of the child
- Presence, duration, and severity of symptom(s)
- Sudden or gradual onset
- Past history of similar symptom(s)
- Events surrounding the first appearance of symptom(s)

- Character of symptom(s) if painful: sharp, dull, radiating, burning
- Location of symptom(s)
- History of exposure to illness, allergens, travel
- Symptom(s) increasing or decreasing in severity
- Appearance of child in relation to the symptom(s)
- Activity level of child
- Presence or absence of appetite
- Recent communications or evaluations with health personnel regarding the symptoms
- Treatment measures at home or in the health care facility
- Pertinent negatives
- Parents' knowledge of infections in the community
- Immunization status

The younger the child the more investigation is exerted in finding a cause of illness. If vague symptomatology such as slight irritability or anorexia is present in infancy, sepsis is always considered. Infants and young children cannot respond to sudden loss of fluids and dehydration is a serious complication of illnesses such as prolonged high fevers or gastroenteritis.

Telephone

It is estimated that in pediatric practice the use of the telephone is two times greater than that of other specialties. The reasons are:

- Parents with infants need guidance and reassurance initially with the parenting role
- Counseling about home treatment of minor illnesses
- Explanations of immediate treatment in emergency situations
- Information in reference to specific questions
- Reassurance that the child is not acutely ill

In assessing illness situations presented by phone the goal is to:

- Ascertain why the parent is calling
- Decide if the child's illness can be managed at home or needs referral to the health agency for further evaluation

- Decide if medical consultation is needed to further assess the illness
- Assess the anxiety level of the parents and their ability to manage the illness if home treatment is indicated.

OTHER CONSIDERATIONS

In assessing illness conditions via telephone consider:

- Is the caretaker known to the nurse? This helps the nurse to assess how reliable the caretaker is in interpreting the child's symptoms and managing the illness at home.
- How far from the health agency do the caretakers live? In situations where parental anxiety is high, a visit to the health professional is encouraged.
- What is the age of the child? Newborns and infants are seen in the health care agency for illness because of the danger of serious infections such as sepsis.
- Have the symptoms been present over a long period of time? In particularly complicated histories it is important to ask why the caretaker is calling at this particular time and what help the caretaker feels the health agency can offer.
- What are the support measures at home?
- Does the caretaker have the name and phone number of the health care professional and agency for follow-up phone calls?
- How appropriate is the phone call? If the symptom is relatively mild in relation to the concern, other anxieties or problems in the home are investigated.

DISADVANTAGES

The nurse practitioner is not able to objectively evaluate the child's physical condition, to note the child's response to the environment, and to physically assess the severity of parental statements such as "trouble breathing" and "bad rash" over the telephone.

With parental anxiety the problem can be assessed to some degree over the telephone, but seeing the parent and child in the office affords more opportunity to observe and to discuss the parents' anxiety and its causes and to evaluate the parents' interaction with the child.

An office visit also affords the opportunity to emphasize treatment regimens and instructions to parents both verbally and in writing.

Indications for Referral to the Health Care Agency

- Age. All children under 6 months of age with the following symptoms are referred: fever, lethargy, extreme irritability, anorexia, vomiting, diarrhea, dehydration, chronic feeding problems.
- In situations where a clear history cannot be elicited from the caretakers
- Any condition which indicates that an acute infectious process is present
- Fever of greater than 4 days' duration
- Fluid intake less than 480 cc in 24 hours
- Copious vomiting and diarrhea
- Extreme lethargy and malaise
- Purulent discharge from eyes
- Abdominal or groin distention
- Hives or other exanthems difficult to diagnose over the phone
- Fever of unknown origin
- Extreme parental anxiety
- Parents' asking that child be seen
- Parents' complaining of lack of support with child care
- Emergencies: falls where there is a loss of consciousness, change in behavior, vomiting, asymmetrical movements of extremities; ingestions; burns; auto accidents

When a child is referred to the health care agency, the nurse practitioner, if unable to see the child, establishes and coordinates services between the family and the physician, consults with medical personnel in reference to information obtained over the phone, and continues to assess the child's progress at home and the parents' compliance with treatment regimens after discharge from the health care agency.

Physical Examination

The vital signs are recorded. A weight is obtained if the child's oral intake has decreased or if vomiting and diarrhea are present. The amount of examination done depends on the presenting symptom, how well the child is known to the examiner, and when the last physical was done. See Chapter 1, Child Health Assessment.

Children who are ill need increased emotional and physical support, and it is necessary to proceed slowly with the examination. In some instances, children tolerate examination more comfortably on the parent's lap than on the examining table.

Indications for Laboratory Studies

Depending on the presenting symptoms and the initial physical evaluation the following procedures are performed:

- Urinalysis to rule out infection
- Hematocrit to rule out anemia
- White blood cell count and differential to aid in assessing presence of infection
- Blood culture to rule out systemic infection
- Lumbar puncture to rule out the presence of meningitis, increased intracranial pressure
- Chest X-ray to rule out infection, foreign body
- Blood electrolytes to help evaluate degree of dehydration, metabolic status

MANAGEMENT

Role of the Nurse Practitioner

Illness in itself causes disruption and confusion in family life. The evaluative process of how the family copes with the child's illness starts at the beginning of the visit.

After the diagnosis is established the nurse practitioner instructs parents as to the treatment regimen. Instructions are verbally given and then re-emphasized in writing. Parental questions are answered. Reactions to medications and symptoms of toxicity are discussed. If necessary, temperature taking is reviewed. Parents are instructed as to increased symptoms of illness and where to contact health personnel if necessary.

Role in Collaboration with Medical Personnel

With medical consultation, the nurse practitioner continues to remain the primary health care person for the client and family.

In the event of hospitalization, the nurse practitioner functions within the health care team, contributing past and present history, and plans with the team for current management and for follow-up care. The role of the nurse and physician is one of interdependence and shared responsibility for client care mutually agreeing on goals for future management.

The nurse practitioner maintains close collaboration with social service, nutritionists, pharmacists, and dentists. In this role the nurse practitioner accepts responsibility for assessment, management, and teaching regimens that are initiated in reference to the client's care.

COMMON CLINICAL PROBLEM

Fever

ASSESSMENT

The symptom of fever in infants and children is extremely common. Fever is defined as an elevation in normal body temperature. The amount of fever does not correspond to the severity of the illness, neither does the absence of fever indicate the absence of infection. Fever is a useful defense mechanism which alerts the individual that physiologic changes in the body are occurring in response to a pathologic process. The evaluation and treatment of the underlying cause of the fever is the primary goal.

In infectious processes, it is believed that fever develops because of the release of an endogenous pyrogen from polymorphonuclear leukocytes. The pyrogen eventually reaches the brain causing chemical changes in the hypothalamus with resulting increase in temperature (Stern, 1977).

Normal values. Normal body temperature is between 36.2°C and 37.8°C rectally and 36°C and 37.6°C orally. Normal ranges in body temperature can vary as much as 1.5°, depending on the amount of activity, emotional stress, type of clothing worn, and temperature of the environment. With exercise, temperatures can normally rise as high as 39.4°C by mouth. At rest, however, temperature is usually below 38°C by mouth. Oral readings above this are generally accepted as fever.

Body temperature in older children and adults varies in response to diurnal fluctuations, the lowest peak occurring between 2 and 6 AM and the highest peak between 4 and 7 PM. During infancy and early childhood, temperature fluctuations are more common and diurnal variation in body temperature is absent during the first 2 years of life. If the amount and consistency of a child's temperature is in question, the parents are instructed to take the temperature rectally over a period of 2 days several times a day, with the child resting and wearing light clothes.

Etiology. Most fevers are the result of an acute infectious process with 90 percent being of viral origin (Graef, 1974). More than half of all fevers involve the upper and lower respiratory tract. The remaining majority involve the genitourinary and gastrointestinal systems (Graef, 1974). The most common foci of infection in the respiratory tract are the middle ears, sinuses, oropharynx, adenoids, tonsils, larynx, and lungs.

Some illnesses produce characteristically high fevers: roseola, rubeola, pneumonia, pyelonephritis (Pascoe, 1973). Persistent low-grade fevers may indicate chronic infections: bacterial gastroenteritis, collagen diseases, blood dyscrasias, and tumors (Ziai, 1975). Tachypnea with fever may be indicative of pneumonia.

In newborns who are septic or who have serious infections fever is usually absent or the infant is hypothermic. Symptoms of poor feeding, lethargy, and irritability are more accurate indications of an infectious process than fever measurements at this age.

History. In obtaining information about fever important questions include:

- Age of the child
- Appearance of the child
- Variations in fever during the day
- Activity level and appetite
- Degree of irritability
- Complaints of pain, chills, and other symptoms of illness: rhinorrhea, cough, tachypnea, ear pain, painful voiding
- History of recent immunizations

Questions in reference to exposure include:

- Contact with other children who are sick or well
- Contact with sick adults
- Contact with foreign visitors

Questions in reference to treatment measures at home include:

- Medications given: prescription, over-the-counter
- Specific home remedies: herbal preparations, vaporizer, sponging

Physical examination. In assessing fever as a presenting symptom, a complete physical examination is done. A well-lighted area is important, preferably natural light to ascertain the presence of beginning exanthems. Cerumen is removed from auditory canals for complete visualization of tympanic membranes. The child should be quiet for adequate auscultation of the chest.

Laboratory. If the cause of the fever is found on physical examination, laboratory studies are usually not necessary except to rule out incidental findings such as anemia. If no cause for the fever is found, the following laboratory studies are performed:

- Routine urinalysis and screening culture to rule out urinary tract infection

- White blood cell and differential counts

    1. Neutrophils (polymorphonuclear leukocytes) are increased in bacterial and early phases of viral infections.
    2. Lymphocytes are increased in viral infections.
    3. Monocytes are increased in the recovery phase of acute infections.

- Nasopharyngeal and throat cultures
- TB test
- Chest X-ray
- Lumbar puncture
- Blood culture

MANAGEMENT

Children under 6 months presenting with fever are always seen in the health care agency because of the possibility of sepsis. All other children with fever longer than 3 days' duration are seen for physical assessment and possible laboratory studies. Children with fever greater than 10 days' duration with unknown etiology may be admitted to the hospital for further evaluation.

The general principle for management is to diagnose and to treat the underlying cause. There is controversy as to whether the fever itself should be treated. In discussions against treatment the following arguments are used:

- Loss of an important diagnostic finding may not justify providing physical comfort for the client.
- Fever may be protective for the host.
- Fever is a symptom causing morbidity and encourages rest and possible medical consultation to determine causes rather than medication to reduce it.
- Some data suggest that fever in viral infections may reduce viral replication and therefore should not be treated (Graef, 1974).

Arguments for treatment state:

- Antipyretics make the client more comfortable.
- Fever reduction may reduce the incidence of febrile convulsions; however, there is no actual evidence that this is true.

General measures. For management of fever, general measures include removal of excess clothing, bed rest, and clear fluids by mouth. There is controversy about sponging with tepid water. If this procedure causes chills and shivering, the hypothalamus will respond with increasing the body temperature. However, most authorities recommend sponging for one-half hour every 2 hours with tepid water for fever above 39°C by mouth. Alcohol and ice water are not used for sponging because of the increased incidence of chills and therefore a possible increase in temperature. Ice water enemas are not used because of the possibility of hyponatremia. Sponging or medication is never instituted if the cause of the fever is environmental or mechanical such as vigorous exercise and increased environmental temperature. In these situations, removal of clothing and rest are more effective.

Indications for consultation. Medical consultation is necessary in the following conditions:

- Infants under 6 months of age with fever only
- All children with fever and vague symptomatology: irritability, poor feeding, lethargy
- Fevers longer in duration than 3 to 4 days
- Child appears ill and toxic

Medications. Drugs commonly used in the treatment of fever are: acetylsalicylic acid (aspirin), and para-aminophenol. They are thought to act on the hypothalamus resulting in dilation of the peripheral blood vessels and increased dissipation of body heat.

ASPIRIN. Because of its effectiveness in reducing fever aspirin is frequently prescribed in adults. It also has analgesic and anti-inflammatory properties. It is not commonly used in children because of the possibility of side effects and accidental ingestion. Aspirin is metabolized more slowly in children under 2 years of age which makes them more susceptible to its side effects. For this reason aspirin is used with caution, if at all, in low doses in this age group. Side effects include dizziness, drowsiness, hypersensitivity resulting in asthma, angioneurotic edema, and anaphylaxis. Gastrointestinal disorders are common including heartburn, gastrointestinal bleeding, and ulceration. Large doses of aspirin (3 to 8 gm/day) can cause tinnitus (ringing in the ears), vertigo, and reduction in plasma prothrombin levels.

PARA-AMINOPHENOLS. Para-aminophenols include acetanilid, phenacetin, and acetaminophen. The three are similar in their antipyretic and analgesic properties but acetanilid is no longer used because of the serious side effects of methemoglobin formation. Phenacetin and acetaminophen are similar to the salicylates in their antipyretic effect. When given in combination with salicylates they increase the effectiveness of lowering the body temperature. The anti-inflammatory properties are less than the salicylates, and they are not used in this regard.

ADVANTAGES OF ACETAMINOPHEN. Acetaminophen has several advantages over aspirin:

- Stable in liquid preparations
- Used when allergy to salicylates is evident
- Does not cause gastric bleeding
- Less toxic in infants

A massive overdose of acetaminophen can cause hepatotoxicity.

In the reduction of fever, studies have shown that acetaminophen is more rapid in onset than aspirin but has a slightly shorter duration of action.

COMMERCIAL PREPARATIONS. There are a variety of brand-name children's aspirin tablets. All are chewable and flavored. They contain 1-1/4 grain (81 mg) acetylsalicylic acid. Bayer children's aspirin and St. Joseph aspirin for children are familiar to many parents.

Commercial preparations of acetaminophen include:

- Tylenol: elixir 120 mg acetaminophen in 5 cc; drops 60 mg acetaminophen in 0.6 cc; chewables 120 mg in each tablet; the drops and elixir contain 7 percent alcohol.
- Tempra contains the same preparations as Tylenol but the alcohol content in the drops and elixir is 10 percent.
- Liquipren drops: 120 mg acetaminophen in 2.5 cc (one full dropper), the dropper is also calculated at 1.25 cc; the preparation does not contain alcohol.

SAFETY PRECAUTIONS. As with all medications parents should keep them out of the reach of children and should purchase only those drugs which have safety caps. Medicine should never be called candy. Prolonged use of any drug should not be continued without proper medical supervision.

CALCULATIONS. Aspirin is calculated according to age or weight. For age: 1 grain is given per year of age up to 10 years, repeated not more than once every 4 hours. For weight: 30–60 mg/kg/day mg/kg of body weight in 4 to 6 doses is prescribed depending on the age and severity of illness.

Counseling. Parents are instructed that fever is a symptom of illness, and that the nurse practitioner should be consulted if the child has other increasing symptoms of illness, such as irritability, lethargy, anorexia, and symptoms related to specific organ systems. For general home management of fever parents are instructed to:

• Increase oral fluid intake to prevent dehydration
• Dress the child lightly to maximize heat loss through the skin
• Increase room air circulation
• Sponge with tepid water rubbing the skin briskly to increase blood flow to the surface where it is cooled

If an etiology is found for the fever parents are instructed about specific management.

References

DuBois, E. F. *Fever and Regulation of Body Temperature.* Springfield, Ill.: Thomas, 1948.

Graef, J. W. and T. E. Cone, Jr. *Manual of Pediatric Therapeutics.* Boston: Little, Brown, 1974.

Green, M. and R. Haggerty. *Ambulatory Pediatrics II.* Philadelphia: Saunders, 1977.

Griffenhagen, G. B. and L. L. Hawkins. *Handbook of Non-Prescription Drugs.* Washington DC: American Pharmaceutical Association, 1973.

Marlow, D. R. *Textbook of Pediatric Nursing,* 4th ed. Philadelphia: Saunders, 1973.

Murphy, D. and C. Dineen. "Nursing by Telephone." *Am J Nurs* 75:1137–1139, July 1975.

Pascoe, D. J., et al. *Quick Reference to Pediatric Emergencies*. Philadelphia: Lippincott, 1973.

Porter, D. P. "Without Standing Orders." *Am J Nurs* 73:1559–1561, September 1973.

Smith, J. W. *Manual of Medical Therapeutics*. Boston: Little, Brown, 1969.

Spivak, J. L. and H. V. Barnes. *Manual of Clinical Problems in Internal Medicine*. Boston: Little, Brown, 1974.

Stern, R. C. "Pathophysiologic Basis for Symptomatic Treatment of Fever," *Pediatrics* 59:92–98, January 1977.

Waechter, E. H. and F. G. Blake. *Nursing Care of Children*. Philadelphia: Lippincott, 1976.

Ziai, M. *Pediatrics*. Boston: Little, Brown, 1975.

14

Approach to Medications in Childhood

The use of medications in infants and children raises several issues of concern to health professionals and to parents. Obviously, there is no question about the validity of specific drug therapy in the treatment of many childhood illnesses, and the development of effective therapeutic agents has greatly reduced morbidity and mortality in childhood. Yet, it is clear that medications are frequently prescribed inappropriately and without adequate consideration of benefit, risk, and cost factors. One study reports that "approximately 95 percent of physicians will issue one or more prescriptions to a patient whom they diagnose as having a 'common cold' and almost 60 percent of these prescriptions will be for an antibiotic" (Asnes, 1974, pp. 84–85). Other studies conducted in the pediatric outpatient department of a large medical center revealed that "46 percent of all patients seen in 1972 during the day received at least one prescription. Interestingly, this figure rose to 70 percent during the evening" (Asnes, 1974, p. 81).

In addition, the notion that there is a "pill for every ill" has become widespread in the United States. This attitude is reinforced by massive advertising through communications media and by the availability of hundreds of over-the-counter medications in pharmacies, supermarkets, department stores, and health food stores. It frequently results in parents pressuring the care provider for

445

medications and in parental dissatisfaction if medication is not prescribed. Nurse practitioners are in a position to influence the medication practices, habits, and attitudes of families they see. The guiding philosophy behind the use of medications is based on considerations of benefit and risk.

With adequate teaching and support it is possible to enable parents and children to manage minor symptoms without the use of medications. It is a more time-consuming effort than writing a prescription or suggesting an over-the-counter remedy but a more useful effort in terms of assisting families to develop their own self-care skills and reducing the expensive and potentially dangerous use of inappropriate and ineffective drugs.

Given such a philosophical stance, this chapter will present information on general guidelines for medication use in infants and children and suggestions for assuring that children receive the medications they need when they need them.

ASSESSMENT

Guidelines for Drug Use in Infants and Children

The effective use of medications depends on consideration of a number of factors including the parents, the child, the health professional (physician and/or nurse practitioner), and the drug selected.

PARENTAL FACTORS

- Attitudes. Some parents think that unless medications are prescribed the child has not received sufficient care. On the other hand there are parents who are suspicious and fearful of medications and do not want to medicate their children.
- Reliability. The parents must be reliable to:

  1. Have the prescription filled
  2. Administer the medication

3. Prepare the correct dosage and administer it at the correct time intervals

4. Continue administration of the medication for the full prescribed dose (Asnes, 1974, pp. 82–83)

• Demographic factors. Age, sex, socioeconomic status, educational level, religion, occupation, marital status, and ethnic background per se are not predictive of compliance with prescribed medical regimen but may interact to provide obstacles to implementing recommendations. For example, a study of the reading level of mothers bringing their children to a large urban pediatric emergency room revealed that at least 45 percent could not read beyond the sixth grade level (Wingert, 1969, p. 657). Since most health education materials are written at above eighth grade levels (eighth to thirteenth grade), it is obvious that such information is incomprehensible to almost half of the population studied.

CHILD FACTORS

• Acute or chronic illness. Diseases causing malabsorption or hepatic or renal dysfunction may effect drug absorption, metabolism, and excretion.

• Age. As a general rule in children under 2 years of age, medications should be used only when absolutely necessary. Infants are more susceptible to toxicity (e.g., an overdose of salicylates leads to metabolic acidosis in infants, rarely in adults) and have limited ability to detoxify drugs (e.g., renal and hepatic functions are not fully developed). Signs of toxicity are difficult to identify early since reactions are less predictable and the child cannot communicate specific distress. The margin for error in dosage is very narrow so slight miscalculations assume greater import.

• Allergy. Hypersensitivity reactions to drugs occur in children as well as in adults. History should include information on past drug allergies or adverse drug reactions.

• Genetic characteristics. Some children have genetic characteristics which may influence various stages of drug absorption, metabolism, and excretion. G-6-PD deficiency (hemolytic anemia with primaquin-type drugs) and mongolism (increased response to atropine) are examples.

- Growth and development. The child's level of growth and development influences the form of drug prescribed and the method of administration.

HEALTH PROFESSIONAL FACTORS

- Communication. The ability to communicate in writing and verbally is essential to avoid errors in medication administration.
- Knowledge. "Rational drug therapy involves prescribing the right drug, for the right patient, at the right time, in the right amount, with due consideration for cost" (Asnes, 1974, p. 85). Such practice requires extensive knowledge and demands that practitioners keep their information current. See this chapter, Resource Information.
- Relationship with client. See this chapter, Compliance.

DRUG FACTORS

- Cost. The cost of drugs is increasing and public attention has focused on the high percentage of mark-up included in the price of retail medications. Generic prescribing, rather than designating a proprietary brand, permits the selection of less expensive forms of the same medication. Both types conform to United States Pharmacopeia (U.S.P.) and National Formulary (N.F.) standards for identity, purity, and strength of products. However, there is some concern that this practice does not guarantee that the form selected will have similar biologic and clinical equivalency.
- Drug incompatibilities. The simultaneous use of multiple medications can cause adverse drug reactions. Persons prescribing medications must possess knowledge of the mechanisms of drug interaction.
- Toxicity. All drugs have toxic effects. Thus, the selection of a drug involves choosing the *least* toxic drug that will produce the desired therapeutic effect.

Basic Formulary

It is recommended that prescribers become familiar with a select number of therapeutic agents and use them consistently. In providing primary care to normal children the types of medications necessary to treat *most* conditions are as follows:

- Analgesic-antipyretic; e.g., acetaminophen
- Antibiotic, systemic; e.g., ampicillin
- Antibiotic, topical; e.g., Neosporin
- Antifungal; e.g., nystatin
- Antihistamine; e.g., chlorpheniramine maleate (Chlor-Trimeton), diphenhydramine (Benadryl)
- Decongestant; e.g., pseudoephedrine hydrochloride (Sudafed), phenylephrine hydrochloride (Neo-Synephrine)
- Emetic; e.g., syrup of ipecac
- Iron; e.g., Fer-In-Sol
- Steroid, topical; e.g., triamcinolone
- Vitamin preparation

Over-the-Counter Medications

Millions of people spend billions of dollars yearly for self-prescribed over-the-counter (OTC) drugs. Analgesics, cough and cold preparations, topical preparations, vitamins, and laxatives are the most common varieties purchased. The practice of self-treatment of minor illnesses is not to be discouraged if it is based on adequate knowledge. Unfortunately, though, the use of OTC drugs may be inappropriate, ineffective, and even dangerous, especially in children. Some of the potential problems are listed.

- The tendency exists to abuse such drugs (i.e., take more than the recommended dosage). Consequently, manufacturers cut down on the published recommended dose to the extent that frequently the dose is not pharmacologically effective.

- For infants and young children doses are not recommended, and many parents guess at an approximate dose.
- Most OTC cold preparations contain multiple ingredients, as many as seven different ingredients (e.g., antihistamine, decongestant, analgesic, vitamin, caffeine, alcohol, flavoring), which makes accurate dosage difficult and evaluation of allergic or toxic side effects confusing.
- The numbers of medications available in homes compounds the dangers of accidental poisoning in young children. See Chapter 9, Accident Prevention and Safety, and Chapter 30, Emergencies.

Compliance

When the indications for drug therapy exist and medication is prescribed, the therapeutic effect will be achieved only if the child receives the medication as prescribed. Many factors mitigate against compliance with medication regimens, and in a recent study of 300 children being treated for acute otitis media in an urban medical center clinic it was found that only 7.3 percent (22 children) received the prescribed dose of antibiotic for the full 10-day course (Mattar, 1975). Compliance with a 10-day course of antibiotic has been reported as 66 percent in private practice settings (Charney, 1967).

GENERAL COMPLIANCE

Factors known to influence general compliance with therapeutic regimens include:

- Parents' perception of the severity of the illness
- Degree of incapacity caused by the illness—direct correlation
- Number of medical restrictions imposed—direct correlation
- Complexity and duration of therapy—inverse correlation
- Number of drugs prescribed—inverse correlation (Mattar, 1974)

• Interaction with the caretaker. If the parents are dissatisfied they are less likely to follow recommendations.

COMPLIANCE WITH MEDICATIONS

Factors influencing incomplete administration of medications to children include:

• Difficulties having prescriptions filled (e.g., pharmacy closed, problems with Medicaid reimbursement)
• Difficulties in getting children to take the medication
• Dispensing errors (e.g., less than prescribed amount dispensed, incomplete or erroneous labeling)
• Financial problems
• Inaccurate measuring devices. Household teaspoons hold volumes from 2.5 to 9 ml (Mattar, 1975)
• Inadequate understanding by parents
• Other family stresses (e.g., emotional factors)

MANAGEMENT

Role of the Nurse Practitioner

Administration of medications prescribed by physicians has long been a traditional nursing role, and content in pharmacology is part of basic nursing knowledge. The development of the nurse practitioner role, which involves collaboration with physicians, has resulted in an expansion of the nurses' responsibility in relation to medications. Many nurse practitioners are prescribing medications for some minor illnesses by use of jointly developed protocols and standing orders, and as state prescribing laws are changed, may soon be able to independently prescribe certain medications. Responsibility and accountability for this function will demand increased knowledge of the many factors involved in safe and effective drug use.

Current acceptable practice models available to nurse practitioners include:

- Individual consultation. In settings where the nurse practitioner and physician work in close proximity, the nurse practitioner consults with the physician when medication is indicated, and the physician either writes and signs the prescription or signs it after the nurse practitioner has written it.
- Protocols and standing orders. In some settings, approved standard procedures are used to manage specific clinical entities and the nurse practitioner can implement the procedure independently once the diagnosis has been confirmed.
- Telephone consultation. When distance separates the nurse practitioner and physician, consultation by telephone and physician communication with the local pharmacy is accepted practice. The use by nurse practitioners of pre-signed blank prescription forms is, simply, bad practice.

Additional role functions of the nurse practitioner include parent and child teaching for optimum compliance and advising clients about the appropriate use of OTC drugs and their potential adverse effects.

The Prescription

Medication errors can be reduced by precisely communicating the instructions on the prescription and label. The essential aspects of prescription writing (Asnes, 1974, p. 88; McMillan, 1977, pp. 464–465) include:

1. Date and time written
2. Name of drug. The official generic or trade name must be spelled correctly.
3. Form of drug. Specify capsules, tablets, suspension.
4. Dosage expressed in metric system (e.g., 125 mg/5 ml)
5. Amount of drug to be dispensed. If 125 mg is to be taken 4 times a day for 10 days, and the drug comes as 125 mg/5 ml, then at least 200 ml must be prescribed and dispensed.
6. Route of administration

7. Directions. Specify amount and time of administration. Use exact hours according to a schedule worked out with the family rather than "three times a day." Specify duration of administration (e.g., "for 10 days" or "until bottle empty"). Do not write, "Take as directed."

8. Indication for drug. If the drug is to be taken "as necessary," specify the indication for its use and the maximum amount to be taken in 24 hours.

9. Special precautions or requirements in administration of the drug

10. Refills. Specify the number of refills or "no refills."

11. Label. The name of the drug should be placed on the label.

12. Signature

Improving Compliance

INTERPERSONAL RELATIONSHIPS

The relationship between the family and the care provider is of prime importance in the outcome of a therapeutic plan. Parent cooperation is likely to be enhanced when the provider:

1. Is known to the family; is a continuity figure
2. Is approachable and conveys warmth
3. Communicates interest and concern
4. Elicits the chief concerns and expectations of the parent and child
5. Acknowledges the parent's anxiety and feelings
6. Provides time for open discussion, questions, and explanations

DEVELOPING THE CARE PLAN

Joint development of the care plan is more likely to promote compliance than a unilateral prescription of orders. The care provider who believes that parents are responsible participants in the care of their child will:

1. Obtain information about past illnesses of the child and family and the family's reactions to them

2. Determine how the parents have managed minor illnesses at home
3. Determine what medications are routinely kept in the home and how they are used
4. Reinforce those practices that are appropriate
5. Assess the parents' understanding of the current illness
6. Provide clear information on the illness and rationale for treatment
7. Elicit the parents' ideas on what approaches to treatment will be most effective for the particular child

PARENT TEACHING RELATED TO MEDICATIONS

When medications are prescribed the care provider can improve the probability of safe and effective compliance by:

1. Limiting the number of medications prescribed
2. Providing verbal and written instructions at the parents' level of comprehension
3. Telling parents the name of the medication. Parents have the right to know what drugs are being given, and such information is essential in managing questions by telephone and in assessing emergency situations (e.g., accidental ingestions).
4. Informing parents of the possible consequences if the drug is not administered
5. Informing parents of the side effects, what to do if they appear, when to call, and when to stop the drug
6. Providing a standard measuring device (e.g., a calibrated dropper, standard teaspoon)
7. Planning dosage schedule in accordance with the family's daily routine
8. Providing a chart, calendar, or check list for keeping track of doses given
9. Discussing methods of administering the drug and what to do if the child refuses. An excellent guide to giving oral medications to young children is found in the article by Ormond and Caulfield, 1976. See this chapter, References.

10. Discussing storage and preparation (e.g., shaking, diluting) of drug
11. Instructing parents on disposal or storage of the drug on completion of treatment
12. Reviewing safety measures regarding drugs in the home. See Chapter 9, Accident Prevention and Safety, and Chapter 30, Emergencies.
13. Asking parents to repeat instructions to clarify misunderstandings
14. Encouraging parents to call with any questions or problems
15. Providing a starter dose (sample) if the visit is at night or pharmacies are closed

Resource Information

Drug information is readily available from a variety of sources and the nurse practitioner should select and become familiar with at least one or two reliable references. Manufacturer's inserts also contain information specific to the particular preparation. In some settings the availability of a clinical pharmacist in the pediatric unit has proven very beneficial for staff and families (Levin, 1972).

In addition to medical, nursing, and pharmacology journals and textbooks, some sources of pharmacotherapeutic information are:

1. American Hospital Formulary Service, American Society of Hospital Pharmacists, 4630 Montgomery Avenue, Washington DC 20014.
2. *Drugs of Choice*, W. Modell, editor, C. V. Mosby Co., St. Louis, MO.
3. *Handbook of Nonprescription Drugs*, American Pharmaceutical Association, 2215 Constitution Avenue NW, Washington DC 20037.
4. *Physician's Desk Reference (PDR)*, Medical Economics Company, Oradell, NJ 07649.

References

Aaron, H. and M. M. Lipman, Editors of Consumer Reports. *The Medicine Show.* Mount Vernon, N.Y.: Consumers Union, 1976.

Asnes, R. S. and B. Grebin. "Pharmacotherapeutics: A Rational Approach." *Pediatr Clin North Am* 21:81–94, February 1974.

Brown, M. S. and M. Collar. "Over-the-Counter Drugs for Upper Respiratory Symptoms." *Nurse Practitioner* 2:18–42, January–February 1977.

Charney, E., R. Bynum, et al. "How Well do Patients Take Oral Penicillin? A Collaborative Study in Private Practice." *Pediatrics* 40:188–195, August 1967.

Cohen, S. M. and J. L. Cohen. "Pharmacotherapeutics: Review and Commentary." *Pediatr Clin North Am* 21:95–101, February 1974.

Korsch, B. M., E. H. Gozzi, and V. Francis. "Gaps in Doctor-Patient Communication, 1. Doctor-Patient Interaction and Patient Satisfaction." *Pediatrics* 42:855–871, November 1968.

Levin, R. H. "Clinical Pharmacy Practice in a Pediatric Clinic." *Drug Intelligence and Clinical Pharmacy* 6:171–176, May 1972.

Liberman, P. "A Guide to Help Patients Keep Track of Their Drugs." *Am J Hosp Pharm* 29:507–509, June 1972.

McMillan, J. A., P. I. Nieburg, and F. A. Oski. *The Whole Pediatrician Catalog.* Philadelphia: Saunders, 1977.

Marston, M. V. "Compliance with Medical Regimens: A Review of the Literature." *Nursing Research* 19:312–323, July–August 1970.

Mattar, M. E., James Markello, and S. J. Yaffe, "Inadequacies in the Pharmacologic Management of Ambulatory Children." *J Pediatr* 87:137–141, July 1975.

Mattar, M. E. and S. J. Yaffe. "Compliance of Pediatric Patients with Therapeutic Regimens." *Postgrad Med* 56:181–188, November 1974.

Ormond, E. A. R. and C. Caulfield. "A Practical Guide to Giving Oral Medications to Young Children." *Am J Maternal Child Nursing* 1:320–325, September–October 1976.

Penna, R. P. and C. Kleinfeld, editors. *Handbook of Nonprescription Drugs*, 5th ed. Washington D.C.: American Pharmaceutical Assoc., 1977.

Wingert, W. W., J. P. Grubbs, and D. B. Friedman. "Why Johnny's Parents Don't Read." *Clin Pediatr* 8:655–660, November 1969.

15

The Skin

Diseases of the skin and allergic skin conditions are closely related. Most of the minor or transient skin disorders treated in the health care facility may be seen and managed by the nurse practitioner. Skin disorders need to be distinguished from more severe problems, many of which are of allergic origin, and may need to be referred for further diagnosis and treatment. This chapter will deal with the assessment and management of common skin problems and with health education of parents in reference to general skin care.

ASSESSMENT

Because of the relationship of skin and allergic conditions, components of the history and physical examination necessarily include aspects of both areas. See Chapter 28, Allergies.

History

PRESENT CONCERNS

If the rash is the primary complaint get a good family history, drug history (specifically aspirin), and allergic history. If the rash is a

457

secondary complaint, it is important to describe it accurately since the skin is the mirror of many internal diseases. See Chapter 13, Assessment of Presenting Symptom.

PAST HISTORY

Obtain information about rashes, allergies (see Chapter 28, History), communicable diseases, immunizations, frequency of upper respiratory infections, nutrition in infancy and related feeding problems, "spitting up," colic, and constipation.

FAMILY HISTORY

Obtain information about skin problems and about allergies.

NUTRITION HISTORY

Obtain information about diet, food allergies, and new foods recently added to diet. If the child is being nursed, ask about presence of food allergies in the mother or recent excessive intake of a particular food in her diet.

ALLERGY HISTORY

See Chapter 28, History.

Physical Examination

SKIN

In examining the skin:

- Observe color (normal pigmentation is due to melanin, a dark pigment in the skin), erythema, jaundice, carotenemia, pallor, or flushing.
- Palpate for temperature and state of hydration.

- Observe scars, birth marks, bruises, scratches, bites, swelling, or lumps.
- Observe and palpate texture of the skin to determine if it is smooth, rough, branny, or scaly.
- Observe and describe any rash fully including color, size of lesions, location, and distribution. See this chapter, Commonly Used Terms.

Skin characteristics of yellow-skinned or dark-pigmented children. Characteristics of the skin of these children may be observed as follows:

1. Infants of dark-skinned parents are lightly pigmented at birth but grow progressively darker with age until pigmentation peaks at about 6 to 8 weeks of age.
2. Some dark-skinned children may have normal blue coloring of the lips or gums.
3. Blacks may have brown frecklelike pigmentations of the buccal mucosa.
4. Pallor or paleness can be detected in the nail beds, conjunctivae, oral mucosa, or tongue, which are normally reddish pink.
5. Jaundice, which can be various shades of yellow or green, is best seen by looking at the sclerae or mucous membranes in daylight.
6. Carotenemia, which does not color the sclera, may be noted periorally, on the palmar surfaces of the hands, and on the plantar surfaces of the feet.
7. Rashes that are difficult to visualize may be palpated to aid in assessment.
8. Hypopigmentation or depigmentation in the diaper area may be observed following diaper rash.

Methods and tools. For observation of the skin daylight is best. It may be necessary at times to take the child to a window to better visualize a rash. Additional tools for assessing skin lesions are as follows:

1. White or yellow overhead light or gooseneck lamp, with at least a 60-watt bulb, is the next choice.

2. A magnifying glass can be useful to distinguish tiny eruptions or to identify the parasites of scabies or the lice of pediculosis.
3. A glass slide or magnifying glass can be used for blanching the skin. This is helpful in identification of petechiae, ecchymoses, or underlying jaundice that would otherwise be masked by flushed skin that is suffused with blood.
4. An ultraviolet lamp (Wood's lamp) when used in a darkened room detects some fungi and causes them to appear fluorescent. A greenish color of the lesion is positive for tinea (ringworm).
5. KOH (potassium hydroxide) preparation is used to aid in the diagnosis of fungal infections. Scrapings from the edge of an active lesion are put on a slide; 20 percent KOH is added; the slide is heated gently and then examined under the microscope for the branching filaments (hyphae) of fungus.

EYES

Observe for swelling of the lids, crusty lids or lashes, discharges, conjunctivitis, and dark circles below the eyes.

NOSE

Observe presence and type of mucous discharges, excoriation of nares, color and state of turbinates, and patency.

MOUTH

Observe the buccal mucosa for lesions and state of hydration; the uvula for color and size; the tonsils for condition and color. See Chapter 17, Physical Examination.

LYMPH NODES

Palpate for enlargement or tenderness of cervical, axillary, and inguinal nodes. These can range from pea size to lima bean size.

LUNGS

Auscultate for rhonchi, rales, or wheezes.

Commonly Used Terms

BULLA(AE).   A vesicle larger than 1 cm, a "blister "

CIRCINATE.   Having a sharply circumscribed and somewhat circular margin

CONFLUENT.   A running together, becoming merged in one

DERMATITIS.   A term applied to all types of skin inflammation regardless of etiology; characterized by a combination of cutaneous reactions, such as erythema, oozing, drying, and scaling

DERMATOSIS.   Any disorder of the skin

EMOLLIENT.   Soothing and softening; a soothing medicine

ERYTHEMA.   Any redness of the skin

EXCORIATION.   Mechanical removal of the epidermis leaving the dermis exposed; a scratch or scrape

KERATOSIS.   A fine papular eruption limited to sebaceous orifices giving the skin a rough, grainy texture; often associated with vitamin A deficiency

MACERATION.   A condition of softened, moist, excoriated areas of the skin usually in the intertriginous areas

MACULE.   A flat, colored skin lesion less than 1 cm

MELANIN.   Dark pigment from choroid, hair, and other dark tissues

NODULE.   A moveable, firm mass under the skin

NUMMULAR.   Resembling a pile of coins

PAPULE.   A raised, circumscribed lesion, less than 1 cm, which may be a variety of red colors

PETECHIAE.   Small reddish purple spots in the superficial layers of the skin which do not blanch; formed by effusion of blood

PITYROID.   A branny, rough texture of the skin associated with pityriasis

PUSTULE.   An elevated, sharply circumscribed lesion, less than 1 cm, filled with purulent material

SEBORRHEA. A discharge of sebaceous matter on the skin; an inflammatory process

VESICLE. A small, sharply defined blister, less than 1 cm, filled with clear fluid

VITILIGO. A depigmentation of the skin of unknown origin. Lesions are usually small and nummular.

WHEAL. An elevated white to pinkish ridge, commonly circular. Associated with allergies it is usually pruritic (e.g., mosquito bite).

XANTHOMA. Small yellow plaques or tumors of various sizes occurring as a result of local accumulation of fatty material.

MANAGEMENT

Care of the Diapers

The following method can be used for the proper cleaning of diapers:

1. Soak the dirty diapers in a solution of Borateen or Borax, 1/2 cup to 1 gallon of water.
2. Pre-rinse in the washing machine.
3. Wash in the full cycle using mild soap such as Ivory Flakes, Lux Flakes, or Ivory soap. These soaps are not irritating to the skin. Detergents or softening agents containing strong acids or alkalis can be irritants and should not be used.
4. Rinse diapers two or three times. Vinegar or bleach, 1/4 cup, may be added to the last rinse for acidification of the diapers.
5. Dry diapers in the sun whenever possible.

COST FACTORS OF DIAPER CARE

The approximate costs of the different methods are:

- Home laundry. Twenty-five percent less than the cost of 100 disposable diapers

- Diaper service. About equal to the average cost of disposable diapers
- Disposable diapers. About equal to diaper service

COMMERCIAL DIAPER SERVICE

Positive factors for the employment of a diaper service include:

1. High sterilization standards of services
2. More professional approach to sanitation and conditioning to meet infant skin needs
3. Superior to home management in many cases
4. Ecologically preferred over disposable diapers
5. Cost factor equal to that of disposable diapers

DISPOSABLE DIAPERS

In comparison with cloth diapers the positive factors of disposable diapers include:

1. Better fit
2. More absorbency
3. Ease of transportation
4. No need for pins, plastic or rubber pants, or liners
5. Less complicated to manage for the uninitiated

Negative factors of disposable diapers include:

1. Unsound ecologically
2. Higher cost
3. Potential allergies.

General Care of the Skin

BATHING

Bathing is beneficial to the skin for these reasons:

1. It returns moisture to the skin as it cleans. However, over-

bathing dries the skin because it removes oil from the keratin barrier.

2. It relaxes muscles, relieves soreness, and eases tension.

3. It may help to prevent and to control minor skin problems such as diaper rashes, seborrheic dermatitis, minor bacterial infections, intertrigo, and miliaria. The present lax attitude about daily, or at least necessary, bathing for infants and children is contributing to these problems.

General considerations. Some factors to consider in bathing children are as follows:

• Infants can be bathed and shampooed daily, using warm water and a mild soap, unless they have unusually sensitive skin or are suffering from atopic dermatitis.

• Alkaline soaps can be irritating to the normal acidic skin (pH 4.5 to 5.5) and should be thoroughly rinsed off, being careful to protect the child's eyes at all times.

• Tub-soaking causes maceration of the skin and is not advised for more than 10 to 15 minutes.

• Lotions, creams, and powders are not necessary following a bath unless they are prescribed. In fact, powders in the diaper area and axillae can be very irritating.

• Bubble bath products are drying and irritative to the skin.

• Older children may bathe as frequently as needed at the parents' discretion following the principles stated above.

DRY SKIN

The significant protective barrier of the skin is limited almost entirely to its outermost layer, the dry stratum corneum. In infancy the stratum corneum is very thin, containing about 15 percent water. Dry skin indicates a lack of both water and oil. Fissures and cracks develop which disrupt the protective function of this layer, and scaliness and itchiness may occur.

Cause of dry skin. Dryness and roughness may be due to:

• Too frequent bathing, improper rinsing, or the use of rough, grainy, alkaline soaps

- Cold weather or overexposure to the sun
- Overexposure to air-conditioning
- Contact with woolly clothes or dressing too warmly

Prevention. Preventive measures include:

- Avoiding preceding items to a practical degree
- Soaking in warm water 3 to 5 minutes using superfatted soaps (Basis, Oilatum) and applying a moisturizing lotion
- Using a humidifier or vaporizer, especially at night
- Increasing fluid intake and eating a proper, nutritious diet rich in vitamins A, C, D, and E.
- Getting regular outdoor exercise to stimulate the flow of blood to carry oxygen to the skin.

SOAPS

Most soaps are alkaline (pH 9 to 10) sodium or potassium salts of fatty acids. They emulsify fats with water and help to remove foreign particles from the skin. Their surfactant and alkaline properties may lead to primary irritation of the skin. The skin must be well rinsed to remove them.

Selection of soaps. Soaps are chosen carefully for skin type:

1. Normal skin

    - Mild soaps such as Ivory, Conti, and Castile
    - Neutral soaps (pH of 7.5 or less) such as Dove, Neutragena, or Sayman's

2. Dry skin

    - Less alkaline soaps such as Alpha-Keri and Lubriderm
    - Superfatted soaps (also less alkaline) such as Basis and Oilatum.

3. Sensitive skin

    - Cetaphil lotion (see Chapter 28, Pharmacologic Therapy, Lotions)
    - Lindora—a liquid soap substitute, bubble bath, and shampoo.

• Neutragena. In addition to the soap, Nutragena Hand Cream can be used.

SHAMPOOS

Shampoos are liquid soaps or detergents used for cleansing and/or therapeutic measures and should be well rinsed from the hair. Eyes of children should be well protected during their use.

Shampoos suitable for children. Among these are Earthborn, Head and Shoulders, Wella, and Protein 21. Baby products such as Johnson's Baby Shampoo or Mennen's Baby Shampoo are also used extensively.

Dandruff shampoos. Among these are Sebulex, Ionil, Head and Shoulders, and Fostex Cream. Selenium- and cadmium-containing shampoos are not indicated for use with children. See this chapter, Dandruff.

POWDERS

Powders are soothing and absorb moisture. They increase evaporation, and provide antipruritic and cooling sensations. They are used chiefly for prophylaxis in intertriginous areas. Some authorities think powders are not helpful and their use should not be encouraged.

Common powders. These are:

• Talc. This is the most lubricant but does not absorb water.
• Cornstarch. This is less lubricant and absorbs water but tends to cake and to irritate the skin, providing an excellent medium for growth of bacteria and fungi, especially *Candida albicans*. It is not recommended for use at any time on the skin.
• Zeasorb. This is a medicated powder. It is useful for its water-absorbing capacity and also because it is mildly antibacterial and antifungal. Other commonly used medicated powders are Caldesene and Desitin.

Application of powder. Powder should first be put on the parent's hand and then applied to the child as a fine film which will not cake or form lumps when wet. Powders used improperly may be inhaled causing respiratory problems or may cake in the body creases causing excoriation of the skin.

LOTIONS

Lotions are suspensions of powder in water that usually require shaking before application. They provide a protective, drying, and cooling effect and may act as a vehicle for other agents. The addition of alcohol increases the cooling effect. Available lotions include Cetaphil, Dermabase, Keri, Alpha-Keri, and Lubriderm.

CREAMS (OINTMENTS)

Creams are emollients which soften the skin by retaining water. Ointments are medicinal emollient preparations having a fatty base, usually petrolatum. Ointments or creams that have been scented should not be used on children with sensitive skin because perfumes are irritators.

Characteristics of creams. Besides acting as softening agents creams react in the following ways:

1. The most important characteristic of creams and ointments is their ability to spread evenly over the skin. With the addition of emulsifiers, it is possible to incorporate large amounts of water. When rubbed onto the skin, the water evaporates slowly, producing a cooling effect. Skin cannot be kept soft and flexible without the aid of water.

2. Creams are cosmetically more attractive than ointments because they tend to "vanish" when rubbed into the skin and are less occlusive than ointments.

3. Creams and other emollients, if overused, diminish the protective barrier of the skin by macerating or otherwise injuring the stratum corneum. In addition, emollients often encourage bacterial growth possibly due to their higher pH.

Commonly used creams and ointments. Some useful vanishing creams are Lubriderm cream, Unibase, Keri cream, and Nivea cream. Commonly used ointments are Caldesene, Desitin, Vaseline, and zinc oxide.

Use of petroleum jelly. Although a popular home remedy for years, petroleum jelly (Vaseline) is *not* advised for use in the diaper area to prevent or to treat diaper rash. It is occlusive, prevents air from reaching the skin, and can cause skin maceration which predisposes to yeast infections.

Use of boric acid. Because of the possibility of systemic poisoning boric acid should never be used in ointments or powders.

Nails

The chief function of nails is that of protection.

GROWTH OF NAILS

Nails grow as follows:

- The average rate of growth of fingernails is 0.5 to 1.2 mm/wk. In some generalized skin diseases growth may take 5-1/2 months from matrix to free edge.
- Toenails take 1 to 1-1/2 years to grow from matrix to free edge.
- Absence of nails is rare; it may occur as part of nail-patella syndrome or abnormality of digits.

COMMON PROBLEMS

These include:

1. Nail biting, cuticle biting, and playing with the nails or cuticles. These are common habits which produce considerable damage to the nails.
2. Brittle nails. This may be due to lack of water vapor similar to chapping. Little is known about the cause.

3. Splitting into layers. This may be due to overimmersion in water.
4. White spots. These may have a number of causes, trauma being the most common. The presence or absence of these spots is of no value as an assessment to health.
5. Staining. This is usually caused by external substances.
6. Separation of nail. This may indicate the start of a fungal infection, trauma, atopic dermatitis, or psoriasis.
7. Ingrown toenail. Trauma is the major factor.
8. Toenail deformity. This may be the result of ill-fitting shoes or a congenital deformity.

COMMON CLINICAL PROBLEMS

Early Skin Problems

CRADLE CAP

Assessment. It is a form of seborrheic dermatitis in the newborn usually occurring because the parent is reluctant to scrub over the anterior fontanelle. See this chapter, Seborrheic Dermatitis.

Management. Treatment includes daily shampoo, removal of the "cap," and medication for secondary infection.

MILD CASES. The head is shampooed daily with warm water and mild soap using firm pressure on the scalp. It is rinsed well and patted dry. The cap can be loosened by massaging warm mineral oil or baby oil into the scalp and allowing 15 to 20 minutes to elapse before shampooing. This treatment may need to be repeated for several days. Combing the scalp with a fine comb after applying the oil may be helpful.

SEVERE CASES. The treatment is as follows:

1. Antiseborrheic shampoo is used daily, then two to three times a week. Sebulex or Ionil shampoos may be used.

2. Topical steroids can be helpful. See this chapter, Seborrheic Dermatitis.

3. Antibiotic therapy may be indicated for secondary infection.

Counseling. The parents should be reassured that vigorous rubbing of the infant's scalp will not injure the fragile-appearing skull.

DIAPER DERMATITIS (DIAPER RASH)

General definition. This is a term used for all rashes of infancy that occur in the diaper area. These include rashes caused by:

1. Contact with sensitizing agents
2. Effects of ammonia and/or water (sweat)
3. Fungal infection

To facilitate their recognition and treatment, the assessment and management of these three types will be presented separately immediately following this section. Since preventive measures are key factors in the management of all types of diaper rashes they will be presented here.

General preventive measures. The overall objective is to keep the diaper area dry, clean, and aerated. Measures to accomplish this include the following:

• Thick diapers and absorbent pads are used since they serve as blotters and drain away wetness. Frequent changing of diapers is recommended. Plastic or rubber pants are not recommended since they keep the area wet and warm.

• Buttocks, thighs, and abdomen are cleansed with water after each diaper change. Emphasis must be placed on the need for this cleansing following each diaper·change. Mild soap and water can be used following a bowel movement.

• A thin film of powder may be used to promote dryness. Caldesene powder, an antifungal and antibacterial powder, is recommended. Cornstarch is not recommended for the prevention or treatment of diaper rashes. See this chapter, Powders.

• The diapers can be removed for short periods during the day, while the infant lies on a pad, to expose the area to air.

• The diapers should be well washed. See this chapter, Care of Diapers.

CONTACT DIAPER RASH

Assessment. It is characterized by erythematous patches of maceration found in the intertriginous areas of the groin, buttocks, inguinal region, and sometimes on the abdomen. This rash is also called "irritative" or "infant" diaper rash. It may occur as the result of contact with disposable diapers, soaps, fabric softeners used for washing diapers, plastic or rubber pants, acids of feces and bacteria of urine from infrequent cleansing of the skin, or diarrhea.

Management. The treatment of contact diaper rash includes preventive measures as listed above, the application of healing ointments, and/or sitz baths.

OINTMENTS. The recommended ointments include Caldesene, Desitin, A & D, or zinc oxide. (Zinc oxide can be drying.) These ointments are to be washed off and reapplied at each diaper change.

SITZ BATHS. These baths may be helpful if the rash is extensive and severe. The child is lowered gently into warm water for a few minutes several times a day. After the area is patted dry, the ointments may be applied. If the rash worsens, the baths should be discontinued.

CONTRAINDICATED TREATMENTS. These include:

• Cornstarch application. See this chapter, Powders.
• Vaseline ointment application. See this chapter, Creams.
• Other topical ointments. These are potential sensitizers. Sometimes exacerbation of an eruption can be traced to ointments used in treatment. If topical ointment is used for a severe rash the "use" test should be employed. See Chapter 28, Pharmacologic Therapy, Corticosteroids.

AMMONIACAL DIAPER RASH

Assessment. This is characterized by an erythematous papulovesicular rash sometimes with ulcerating reactions. It is found on the buttocks, thighs, and the abdomen of infants usually over the age of 7 months. It is caused by the irritative effects of ammonia produced by urea-splitting bacteria in the diaper or on the skin. The odor of ammonia is prominent. In the male ulceration of the external urethral meatus can occur. A history of care of the diapers is obtained.

Management. The treatment of ammoniacal rash includes preventive measures and healing ointments. See this chapter, Diaper Dermatitis. It also includes the use of dry heat and the acidification of the urine and the diapers as follows:

1. Dry heat is applied by placing a lamp with a 25-watt bulb about 12 inches from the rash area for 10 to 15 minutes, four times a day. Care must be taken to prevent burning the skin.
2. Acidification of the urine is accomplished by adding 1 to 2 ounces of cranberry juice daily to the diet. More water can be added to the diet to further dilute the urine.
3. Acidification of the diapers is accomplished by adding 1/4 cup of vinegar or bleach to the final rinse water. See this chapter, Care of the Diapers.
4. Neomycin or bacitracin ointments may be used on infected rashes. Neomycin, however, is a leading allergy producer.

FUNGAL DIAPER RASH

Assessment. This is characterized by a smooth, shiny, "fire-engine" red, papular and nummular rash which has well circumscribed borders and occasional satellite lesions appearing in the inguinal creases. The causes of fungal rash include:

• Monilial (*Candida albicans*) infection in the mother's vagina
• Associated oral thrush in the infant
• Prolonged antibiotic therapy which destroys the normal flora

- Use of cornstarch in treatment of contact of ammoniacal diaper rashes. See this chapter, Powders.

Management. The treatment of fungal diaper rash includes preventive measures, keeping the area as dry as possible, and the use of specific medications. For preventive measures see this chapter, Diaper Dermatitis.

MEDICATIONS FOR FUNGAL DIAPER RASH. These are:

1. Caldesene powder. This is the choice in mild cases.
2. Nystatin (Mycostatin) cream or lotion. It is used two to three times a day for 7 to 10 days for severe cases. This treatment may have to be repeated. If the rash persists after treatment, consider atopic dermatitis, cutaneous thrush, or congenital syphilis.

INTERTRIGO

Assessment. Intertrigo is characterized by redness and maceration which occur where the cutaneous surfaces are in opposition, such as the groin, the buttocks, the axillae, and the neck. The raw surface may ooze serous fluid or be complicated by a bacterial infection. It is seen commonly in fat babies. Intertrigo may be caused by the combination of sweating and chafing and may be aggravated by the presence of urine and stools. *Candida albicans* may be a secondary invader.

Management. The treatment is mainly preventive as follows:

1. The child is bathed daily. A protective, drying, antifungal powder such as Caldesene may be used. If the rash worsens, the powder should be discontinued.
2. The affected areas are exposed to the air frequently to permit complete evaporation of moisture.
3. The clothes are kept light and porous.
4. The following should be avoided:

   - Plastic or rubber pants since these hold in moisture and heat

- Ointments, except as prescribed, since they cause further maceration
- Cornstarch since this may contribute to fungal infection. See this chapter, Powders.

MILIARIA (PRICKLY HEAT)

Assessment. Miliaria is inflamed sweat glands. It is characterized by small, erythematous, papular lesions with tiny vesicles or pustules at the center, usually found on the face, the neck, the shoulders, and the chest. It appears suddenly and can subside as quickly with proper treatment. It is extremely common and often causes undue concern to the parents. It is caused by inflamed and obstructed sweat glands often precipitated by excessive body warmth due to hot weather, too much clothing, or overheated homes.

Management. The treatment is mainly preventive as follows:

1. Tepid baths without soap are given as frequently as necessary to cool the child.
2. The skin is dried by patting. Powder is to be used sparingly. Cornstarch is not recommended. See this chapter, Powders.
3. The use of ointments or lotions can aggravate this condition.
4. The child should not be kept overdressed nor kept in overheated rooms.
5. The parents are taught about the sensitivity of the infant's skin due to the immaturity of the temperature control system. Infants do not sweat until 1 month old. See Chapter 4, Temperature Control in Infancy.

SEBORRHEIC DERMATITIS

Assessment. Seborrheic dermatitis is a common skin rash with a predilection for areas well supplied with sebaceous glands. The lesions are usually multiple, discrete, circumscribed oval or nummular patches covered with fine, yellowish, slightly oily scales on an erythematous base. Intertriginous areas of involvement may become macerated, leading to oozing and crusting, and it may resemble atopic dermatitis (see Chapter 28, Table 5). It can be found on the scalp, the eyebrows, behind and in the ears, on the chest, neck, and in the axilla.

Seborrheic dermatitis is due to excessive discharge from the sebaceous glands, but the cause is not really understood. It may be secondarily infected with *Candida albicans.* It appears in infancy between 2 to 12 weeks of age and usually clears spontaneously by 8 to 12 months of age. Examples of seborrheic dermatitis are cradle cap, dandruff, blepharitis, and otitis externa.

Management. Treatment includes skin care and medications as follows:

1. Areas are bathed daily or as often as necessary
2. Greasy ointments should be avoided since they may cause further maceration
3. Hydrocortisone-containing ointments are used if the rash persists
4. Antibiotics may be necessary if the rash becomes infected

Common Communicable Skin Disorders

IMPETIGO

Assessment. This is a condition involving the superficial layers of the skin which is seen as follows:

- It first appears as discolored spots of various sizes and shapes. Then small vesicles or bullae form and break, spreading germ-laden fluid to the surrounding area.
- The weeping lesions rapidly form yellow, honey-colored, seropurulent crusts and scabs; the tissue around them is red.
- The lesions may be on any part of the body but most often are seen on hands, face, or perineum; as a complication of diaper rash; or as a complication of dermatitis.
- The regional lymph nodes may be palpably enlarged.

ETIOLOGY. It typically begins in a dirty scratch or some other superficial lesion. The pathogenic invaders are staphylococci and streptococci. It may be spread by direct contact with infected persons or by insects.

INCUBATION PERIOD. This is from 2 to 10 days.

LABORATORY. Culture is performed on fluid from an intact vesicle or pustule or the base of a lesion after the crust is removed.

DIFFERENTIAL DIAGNOSIS. This includes ringworm, herpes simplex, or other vesicular or ulcerating lesions.

COMPLICATIONS. Acute glomerulonephritis may follow infection if the strain of *Streptococcus* is nephritogenic.

Management. If treatment includes antibiotic therapy, it is managed collaboratively with a physician. Treatment includes:

1. Preventive measures. The child's washcloth, towels, drinking glass, and bed linen are isolated. Hands are washed before and after treatment, and nails are kept short and clean.
2. Topical treatment. Crusts are soaked with warm water compresses 5 to 10 minutes before removing them. Bacitracin or neomycin ointment is rubbed into lesions including the surrounding areas.
3. Antibiotic therapy. If the child has many lesions, this treatment may be indicated.
4. Follow-up. The child should be seen in 3 days if no improvement is evident.

PITYRIASIS ALBA

Assessment. This is characterized by one or more sharply circumscribed, slightly erythematous, scaly, branny, hypopigmented patches of unknown origin on the cheeks, chin, and forehead. The cause is unknown. It most commonly occurs in pigmented skin of children between 3 and 12 years of age. Hypopigmented areas may slowly repigment but in rare instances may be permanent.

Management. It is treated with application of any bland moisturizer and time. It takes 3 to 4 months to fade and always clears at puberty.

PITYRIASIS ROSEA

Assessment. This is a common, mild, inflammatory disorder characterized by round or oval, discrete and confluent, pale pink, slightly scaly macules or rings. It is branny to the touch. It may be itchy and somewhat resembles ringworm. Patches of rash are distributed on the trunk and on the thighs. A "herald spot," a larger, more prominent patch is present and may appear as early as 10 days before the generalized rash.

Pityriasis rosea is thought to be viral in origin, but the cause is not clear. It is usually found in older children and in young adults. The onset of the eruption is sometimes coincident with mild malaise and symptoms of a viral respiratory tract infection. Mildly infectious, moderate outbreaks are not uncommon. Recovery is spontaneous and uncomplicated occurring within 8 to 10 weeks. It leaves no marks or scars.

Management. Treatment involves care of the skin as follows:

1. Calamine lotion or witch hazel applications can be used for pruritus.
2. Tepid baths of colloidal starch (1 cup Linit starch to 1 tub of water) or oatmeal (Aveeno) can be taken. Hot baths are irritative to the condition, causing more pruritus.
3. Sun exposure to the point of mild erythema shortens the course of the disorder. Care must be taken to avoid sunburn.

SCABIES

Assessment. The basic lesions are papules or small nodules, plus secondary inflammation due to skin bacteria, urticaria, or scratch dermatitis. Scabies typically occurs on the genitals and buttocks; between the fingers; and in the folds of wrists, elbows, armpits, and beltline.

ETIOLOGY. Scabies is caused by a parasite, female itch mite, *Cicaris scabiei* or *Sarcoptes scabiei*. It burrows into the stratum corneum of the skin and lays eggs in the tunnel.

CLINICAL PICTURE. The characteristic burrows appear as fine, wavy lines from a few millimeters to a centimeter in length. Barely visible to the naked eye, they are grey to pink in color, and can be identified with a good magnifying glass or by scraping the skin and examining the scrapings under a microscope. Pruritus, the main symptom, is most severe at night. Scabies is highly contagious and is spread through clothing and bedding, as well as by human contact.

Management. All family members should be examined and treated as needed. Treatment includes the following:

1. The scabicide of choice is 1 percent gamma benzene hexachloride (Kwell) lotion or cream. Penetrating to reach the scabietic burrow, it kills the mites, eggs, and larvae. It often works with one application; however, a second or third application may be made at weekly intervals if needed.
2. Clothing should be washed or dry-cleaned as appropriate.
3. After scabicide treatment, the lesions recede slowly.

TINEA CAPITIS (RINGWORM OF THE SCALP)

Assessment. Tinea capitis is a fungal infection which presents as one or more bald patches, 1 to 5 cm in diameter, with mild erythema, grey scaling, and crusting accompanied by broken stumps of hair. It can cause permanent scarring baldness.

ETIOLOGY. Tinea capitis is commonly caused by *Microsporum canis,* which is transmitted by cats and dogs, or *Trichophyton tonsurans,* which is transmitted by humans.

LABORATORY. Procedures are used as follows:

1. Ultraviolet lamp (Wood's lamp) is used to fluoresce *Microsporum* infections. *T. tonsurans* does not fluoresce.
2. Microscopic examination of a hair shaft with KOH will show round spores. See this chapter, Methods and Tools.
3. Microscopic culture will confirm the diagnosis.

Management. The treatment of choice is ultramicrofine griseofulvin. Local remedies add little to the results obtained from griseofulvin alone.

FOLLOW-UP. The child should be seen after 2 weeks of treatment and the patches should be recultured.

PREVENTION. Preventive measures are as follows:

1. Avoid exchange of headgear
2. Treat infected animals and reexamine them
3. Wash scalp after barbershop haircuts

TINEA CORPORIS (RINGWORM OF THE BODY)

Assessment. Tinea corporis is a fungal infection which presents with a small macule and enlarges by peripheral extension with central healing to form slightly scaly, circular lesions, 0.4 to 5 cm in size. One or more lesions may be found on the face, upper extremities, or the trunk. Dry types tend to become scaly. The moist type becomes vesicular or pustular. Pruritus, when it occurs, is mild.

ETIOLOGY. The most common cause is *Microsporum canis,* which is transmitted by cats or dogs.

LABORATORY. Microscopic examination with KOH will show hyphae. See this chapter, Methods and Tools.

Management. Treatment consists of:

1. Tolnaftate 1 percent solution (Tinactin) for weeping lesions
2. Tolnaftate 1 percent cream (Tinactin) rubbed into chronic lesions. The cream may be used also on weeping lesions as the solution stings.

PREVENTION. Preventive measures include:

1. Avoiding contact with infected animals
2. Avoiding exchange of clothing without adequate laundering
3. Avoiding community showers or bathing places

TINEA PEDIS (ATHLETE'S FOOT)

Assessment. This fungal infection is seen as a vesicular or even bullous eruption with maceration of the skin between the toes. It is rare in young children. Foot dermatitis in children usually is contact dermatitis caused by allergy to some component of the shoe or atopic dermatitis.

ETIOLOGY. Tinea pedis is caused by species of *Trichophyton*.

LABORATORY. Microscopic examination with KOH will show hyphae. See this chapter, Methods and Tools.

Management. Treatment includes:

1. General measures

   • Thoroughly drying between the toes after bathing
   • Use of white, cotton socks, which are changed daily or more frequently as necessary
   • Wearing of well-ventilated shoes or sandals with exposure of feet to the air when possible
   • Wearing of rubber or wooden sandals in community shower or bathing places

2. Antifungal agents

   • Tolnaftate 1 percent solution (Tinactin) is gently massaged into lesions twice a day after washing and drying
   • Desenex or Tinactin powder is sprinkled on mild lesions twice a day or is used as a prophylactic measure

Other Common Skin Disorders

ACNE

Assessment. This common skin condition is seen as inflamed papules, pustules, nodules, comedones (blackheads, whiteheads), and reddened scars, or a combination of these, found on the face, the chest, or the back usually in adolescence or young adulthood.

ETIOLOGY. The sebaceous glands in these areas, which are stimulated by the androgenic hormones of puberty and many other factors (e.g., food, emotion, genetic), overproduce sebum. The sebaceous glands become plugged by sebum, debris, and skin scales. These materials combine to form a hard plug in the opening or along the canal of the oil gland, forming comedones. Acne may worsen during menstruation due to the hormonal changes.

SECONDARY INFECTION. Areas become infected when skin bacteria, *Corynebacterium acne* and *Staphylococcus albus*, become trapped in comedones. Seborrheic dermatitis and dandruff can aggravate the condition.

Management. Treatment of acne includes these measures:

1. Thorough cleansing of the skin two to three times a day using warm water and a mild soap (Fostex, Acne-aid, Acnaveen) or a more abrasive soap (Brasivol, Pernox, Ionax). The type of cleanser and frequency of use is adjusted to each client's tolerance to achieve a mild degree of skin drying without gross chapping or irritation.

2. Drying and peeling lotions used during the day or overnight. Only recommended creams or lotions are to be used. Some of these medicated lotions are:

   • Clear gel: Transact
   • Clear lotions: Benoxyl, Komed, Microsyn
   • Tinted lotions: Acnamel, Fostril, Liquimat, Resulin

3. Exposure to sun and wind. Sunscreens may be used.

4. Frequent shampooing of the scalp, daily, if possible.

5. Proper nutritious diet with added liquids. The client may need help in planning the diet. Certain foods may aggravate the condition in different individuals. Clients can avoid those which aggravate their problem.

6. Removal of comedones by exerting gentle pressure over the comedones, using an extractor or an eye dropper.

REFERRAL. Antibiotic therapy both oral and topical, corticosteroids, X-ray therapy, injections, or minor surgery are prescribed by a physician.

COUNSELING. Guidance and emotional support are offered, and mistaken ideas about the relationship of acne to sexual development are explored.

FOLLOW-UP. Frequent follow-up visits are recommended with time allowed for supportive care and help with management of the treatment regimen.

DANDRUFF

Assessment. A form of seborrheic dermatitis, dandruff is a fine, flaky, slightly oily desquamation of the scalp which may spread to the forehead and eyebrows. True dandruff is seldom found in children before adolescence. Generally only a dry scalp with slight scaling is observed in young children.

Management. Two or three shampoos a week using a commercial antiseborrheic shampoo are recommended. Shampoos containing tar are recommended for severe cases. Among shampoos used are:

1. Shampoos containing sulfur and/or salicylic acid (Ionil, Meted, Sebaveen, Sebulex, Vanseb)
2. Shampoos containing antiseptic agents only (Head and Shoulders, Metasep, Zincon)
3. Shampoos containing tar (Ionil-T, Vanseb-T, Sebutone). Shampoo is left on the hair and scalp for 5 to 10 minutes before rinsing well.
4. Topical corticosteroids may be needed in severe cases.

FOLLICULITIS

Assessment. Folliculitis is inflammation and abscess of hair follicles. The lesions consist of pinhead-sized or slightly larger pustules surrounded by a narrow area of erythema. Many pustules are usually present in the same area. It is found usually on the scalp or the extremities. It may be mildly pruritic. It is frequently caused by *Staphylococcus aureus* and is most often secondary to intertrigo or chronic irritation of the skin.

Management. Treatment consists of:

1. Warm compresses of saline, tap water, or Burow's solution several times a day
2. Topical application of Neosporin ointment
3. Systemic antibiotics for cases with fever and complicating cellulitis
4. Referral for recurrent folliculitis

FURUNCULOSIS (BOILS)

Assessment. Furuncles are deep-seated infections of the sebaceous glands or hair follicles which gradually approach the surface and appear red, elevated, and painful. After several days the skin in the center becomes thin and a pustule may form. A "core" of necrotic material along with liquid purulent discharge is evident when the furuncle ruptures or is incised. Furuncles are most often seen on the neck, face, axillae, and buttocks. The fusion of several furuncles produces a carbuncle. Fever and general malaise may be present.

ETIOLOGY.   The cause of furunculosis is frequently *Staphylococcus aureus*. The disease is strongly familial. Bouts in children may continue to recur over several years; the reason is unknown.

COMPLICATIONS.   Complications of furunculosis are spread of the disease and recurrence.

Management.   Treatment consists of:

1. Soaking lesions for 1 hour, not less than four times daily, using warm tap water or saline compresses
2. Continuous compresses until boil comes to a point if spontaneous drainage or resolution does not occur

3. Incision and drainage when boils come to a point, followed by continuous moist compresses for several days
4. Systemic antibiotics for severe furunculosis

Treatment is continued for 7 to 10 days. Referral is made for recurrent furunculosis.

PEDICULOSIS CAPITIS (HEAD LICE)

Assessment. This is louse infestation presenting with severe itching of the scalp, excoriation, secondary infection, and enlargement of occipital and cervical nodes. It is caused by head lice which may appear as "nits" on the hair shaft. They appear as small, round, grey lumps, difficult to see in blonde hair. The area behind the ears and the back of scalp should be examined closely.

Management. The treatment of choice is Kwell shampoo (gamma benzene hexachloride 1 percent). Treatments are repeated in 1 or 2 weeks and hair is rechecked for nits. Nits are removed by soaking hair in diluted vinegar (vinegar and water 1:1) and combing with fine tooth comb daily. Hats, combs, and hair brushes are thoroughly cleaned. Family members must be examined and treated.

PEDICULOSIS CORPORIS (BODY LICE)

Assessment. This louse infestation which presents with intense itching, multiple scratch marks, and excoriation of the skin is very rare. Close examination reveals hemorrhage points (small, red puncta) where lice have extracted blood. It may be complicated by urticaria or superficial bacterial infection. Lesions are most common on the upper back, sides of the trunk, and the upper, outer arms. The insects live in the folds of clothing.

Management. Treatment is as follows:

1. Gamma benzene hexachloride 1 percent (Kwell) cream or lotion is applied to the entire body following a hot, soapy bath or shower. Skin is dried before application. Freshly laundered or

dry-cleaned clothing is used. The medication remains on for 12 to 24 hours and the treatment is repeated.

2. Clothing is thoroughly washed or dry-cleaned.
3. Bed linen and toilets are scrupulously cleaned.
4. Family members are treated as necessary.
5. Scratch dermatitis can be relieved with oral or intramuscular corticosteroids.
6. Topical antibiotic ointment, Bacitracin, can be used for secondary infections.
7. Treatment may be repeated in 4 days if necessary.

PEDICULOSIS PUBIS ("CRABS")

Assessment. This is louse infestation which presents with intense itching of pubic and rectal areas, resulting in excoriation and secondary dermatitis. Small bluish marks may appear on skin of the trunk, the eyebrows, lashes, and axillary area. Origin of the infection is usually venereal. "Crabs" are extremely rare in children.

Management. The treatment of "crabs" is essentially the same as that for body lice. See this chapter, Pediculosis Corporis.

POISON IVY, POISON OAK, POISON SUMAC

Assessment. A contact dermatitis, the lesions can be multiple vesicles, papules, and bullae on an erythematous base, accompanied by intense itching and burning. Lesions appear in linear streaks. Severe, systemic attacks present with swelling and burning pain.

ETIOLOGY. Poison oak, ivy, and sumac dermatitis are caused by an allergen, the oleoresin which is present in the leaves, stems, and roots of the vines. It can result from contact with smoke or burning leaves, contaminated clothes, tools, or the fur of a cat or dog.

CLINICAL PICTURE. Lesions usually appear on exposed areas of skin, face, and extremities but may be found elsewhere. They appear from several hours to a few days after contact and last from 2 to 4 weeks. The severity of the dermatitis depends on the amount of sap that gets on the skin and on the degree of sensitivity of the person. It is not spread from one part of the skin to another by scratching, or from one person to another by skin-to-skin contact, or by contamination by the blister fluid.

Management. Treatment consists of relieving the pruritus and removing oils from the skin as quickly as possible by bathing with mild soap and lots of water. Strong "yellow" soaps are not beneficial and may be irritating to the skin.

Some methods used to relieve itching are:

1. Applications of cool, wet compresses (1 tablet or package of Domeboro to 1 pint of water).
2. Application of menthol- or phenol-containing lotion such as Calamine lotion. Use of preparations containing the "caine" anesthetic are not recommended due to possible sensitivity reaction. Caladryl, which contains Benadryl, an antihistamine, is not recommended.
3. Cool baths using starch colloidal preparation (1 cup of Linit starch to tub of water) or oatmeal baths such as Aveeno. See Chapter 28, Pharmacologic Therapy, Baths.
4. Cleansing and opening of large blisters.

REFERRAL. For severe attacks immediate referral to a physician, preferably a dermatologist, is recommended. Oral or parenteral hydrocortisone or prednisone in sufficient amounts to afford relief of symptoms may be indicated.

PREVENTION. Preventive measures include:

1. Avoidance of offending plants
2. Learning to identify offending plants
3. Destruction of plants by chemical means when possible
4. Wearing rubber gloves when handling exposed clothing or tools
5. Decontamination of clothes, tools

Desensitization "shots" or antipoison pills have not proven to be effective and are not recommended.

SUNBURN

Assessment. The stages of sunburn are described as follows:

1. Mild or first-degree type sunburn consists of erythema, tenderness, and mild pain of sun-exposed areas.
2. More severe sunburn progresses with more redness, pain, swelling, and blisters.
3. Very severe sunburn includes extensive areas of sunburn, inability to tolerate contact with clothing or sheets, and constitutional symptoms of nausea, tachycardia, chills, and fever.

The history is usually adequate to explain the clinical picture. Factors which predispose to sun sensitivity, such as drug administration or systemic illnesses, need to be ruled out.

Complications. The complications of sunburn may include:

1. Fluid and electrolyte loss
2. Systemic toxicity
3. Infection of ruptured bullae
4. Heat exhaustion

Management. A very severely sunburned child should be referred immediately to a physician or to a hospital clinic for supervision of possible complications.

TREATMENT. Mild to severe sunburn is treated as follows:

1. Cold water or saline solution compresses are applied for 20 minutes, three to four times daily or more frequently as needed.
2. Low-strength corticosteroid cream or ointment (Synalar, Kenalog, or Aristocort) are used to reduce inflammation and pain.
3. Skin emollients, such as Alpha-Keri, Domol, Lubriderm, or Nivea, may be used for dry skin.
4. Blisters may be opened after careful cleansing of the skin.
5. Local anesthetic sprays which are effective are Americaine,

Burn Tame, Tega Caine, although these carry the risks of sensitization.

6. Aspirin or acetaminophen in dosage appropriate to age may be given every 4 hours for pain.

PREVENTION. Skin is exposed to ultraviolet rays whether sunny or overcast. Limited and gradual exposure allows the skin to build up protection naturally by moving melanin (which absorbs ultraviolet light and makes one look tan) up to the surface. Black skin, with greater supply of melanin, is best equipped to withstand ultraviolet radiation, followed by brunettes, redheads, blondes, and nontanners who suffer from radiation soonest.

Infancy. The following measures are used to prevent overexposure to the sun in infancy:

1. Attention is given to the color of hair and skin of the child.

2. Infants may sun out-of-doors or indoors near an opened window. Active rays will not penetrate through window glass.

3. Infants should be kept out of the sun when ultraviolet rays are strongest, generally 11 AM to 3 PM.

4. Infants should be positioned with their eyes away from the sun.

5. Exposure to the sun may begin at 2 weeks of age for a few minutes daily and increased until 10 to 15 minutes daily is reached. The child is observed for overexposure or overheating.

6. Hats or sunbonnets should be used if an infant must be exposed for a long period of time. Sunscreens may be used to help protect the skin from ultraviolet rays.

Young children. Young children should be protected from overexposure to the sun while playing out-of-doors. The color of the child's skin should be considered; hats and clothing should be used for protection; and sun screens may be used.

Sun screens. These are recommended to protect the skin from overexposure to the ultraviolet rays. The effective agent which prevents burning is para-aminobenzoic acid (PABA). Lotions and creams which are used for sun-screening purposes should contain PABA. Some of these products are:

1. Pre-sun and Pabanol. These protect against short-wavelength ultraviolet rays. Light tanning is possible.
2. Uval and Solbar. These protect against short-wavelength ultraviolet rays and partially against longer waves. Moisturizing lotions may be applied 10 to 15 minutes following the application of sun-screens since many lotions contain alcohol and tend to be drying to the skin.
3. Zinc oxide ointment is a sun block, effectively preventing the ultraviolet rays from reaching the skin.

VERRUCAE (WARTS)

Assessment. Verrucae are sharply circumscribed and raised clusters of tiny papillomas, greyish in color, and sometimes crusty. They are seen on any part of the body; however, they are more commonly found on hands, and fingers, or sometimes on the ball of the foot (plantar warts). Verrucae are caused by a virus and are benign. They occur in 10 percent of children and young adults and have a tendency to recur. Often there is a spontaneous remission.

Management. If the verrucae are small, they do not need treatment. Referral is made in the following instances:

1. If danger signs of itching, bleeding, or changes in size or color are apparent
2. If treatment by acid or excision is indicated

References

Alexander, M. M. and M. S. Brown. *Pediatric Physical Diagnosis for Nurses.* New York: McGraw-Hill, 1974.

Allen, A. C. *The Skin,* 2nd ed. New York: Grune and Stratton, 1966.

American Medical Association. *The AMA Book of Skin and Hair.* Philadelphia: Lippincott, 1975.

Arndt, K. A. *Manual of Dermatologic Therapeutics.* Boston: Little, Brown, 1974.

Barness, L. A. *Pediatric Physical Diagnosis,* 4th ed. Chicago: Yearbook Medical Publishers, 1972.

Dixon, P. N. "Role of *Candida Albicans* Infection in Napkin Rashes." *Brit Med J* 2:23–27, April 1969.

Feingold, B. F. *Introduction to Clinical Allergy.* Springfield, Ill.: Thomas, 1973.

Gellis, S. S. and B. M. Kagan. *Current Pediatric Therapy.* Philadelphia: Saunders, 1976.

Handbook of Non-Prescription Drugs, 5th ed. Washington: American Pharmaceutical Association, 1977.

Koblenzer, P. J. "Diaper Dermatitis—An Overview." *Clin Pediatr* 12:368–392, July 1973.

Livesey, R. P. "The Contribution of Diaper Service Accreditation to Infant Health Care." *Clin Pediatr* 11:541–543, September 1972.

Moschella, S. L., et al. *Dermatology*, vol. 1. Philadelphia: Saunders, 1975.

Rudolph, A. M., editor. *Pediatrics*, 16th ed. New York: Appleton-Century-Crofts, 1977.

Silver, H. K., C. H. Kempe, and H. B. Bruyn. *Handbook of Pediatrics*, 12th ed. Los Altos, Calif.: Lange Medical Publishers, 1977.

Vaughan, V. C. and R. J. McKay, editors. *Nelson Textbook of Pediatrics*, 10th ed. Philadelphia: Saunders, 1975.

Wolman, I. J., editor. *Clinical Pediatric Handbook II.* Philadelphia: Lippincott, 1974.

16

The Eye

The evaluation of vision and the detection of eye disorders is an integral component of every health supervision visit. The absence of vision has a devastating effect on a person's life, and the impairment of vision causes continuous readjustments in life routines. The role of the nurse practitioner in the assessment and management of eye problems is:

- To evaluate visual acuity for refractive errors
- To detect the presence of amblyopia
- To evaluate with medical consultation the presence of organic eye disease
- To refer to the ophthalmologist those conditions that require further evaluation and management

ASSESSMENT

Ophthalmic Development

Approximately 75 to 80 percent of infants at birth are hyperopic (farsighted) (Kempe, 1976, p. 213). Normal vision of 20/20 is achieved at 4 to 5 years of age.

Newborns exhibit random eye movements because of immature

retinal development and inability to fixate centrally (Ziai, 1975, p. 709). These movements disappear by 3 months of age. A pupillary reaction to a light stimulus is evidence of a functioning retina and optic nerve, but does not rule out cortical blindness. The lacrimal glands are capable of tear production at birth (Vaughan, 1975). See Table 1 for chronology of ophthalmic development.

History

In the newborn, common eye problems include: those related to birth injuries, anatomic asymmetries, lacrimal duct obstruction, and conjunctivitis. In assessing these conditions, questions include: description of symptoms, length of time present, frequency, discharge, tearing of eyes, increased blinking, fever, other symptoms of illness; past history of eye disorders, treatment measures, and recent eye medications.

In assessing visual disturbances, questions include:

1. In infancy: specific concerns of the parents, presence of nystagmus, inability to fixate and to follow a bright object momentarily, and presence of a history of cross eyes

2. In toddlers: presence of cross eyes, inability to ambulate without bumping into objects, frequent blinking, rubbing, squinting, and holding objects near to eyes

3. In school-age children: headaches, eye pain, double vision, blurred words with reading; blinking, rubbing, squinting, when reading or for distant vision; and cross eyes

4. In assessing the presence of organic eye disease: presence of nystagmus, inability to fixate on objects, cross eyes, white pupil, and bulging eye orbit.

Physical Examination

Each eye is always assessed separately to rule out defective vision in one eye that might not be apparent when both eyes are examined together. A condition called suppression amblyopia develops when

Table 1
Chronology of Ophthalmic Development

Age	Level of Development
Birth	Awareness of light and dark; the infant closes his eyelids in bright light
Neonatal	Rudimentary fixation on near objects (3–30 inches)
2 weeks	Transitory fixation, usually monocular at a distance of roughly 3 feet
4 weeks	Follows large conspicuously moving objects
6 weeks	Moving objects evoke binocular fixation briefly
8 weeks	Follows moving objects with jerky eye movements; convergence is beginning to appear
12 weeks	Visual following now a combination of head and eye movements; convergence is improving; enjoys light objects and bright colors
16 weeks	Inspects own hands; fixates immediately on a 1-inch cube brought within 1–2 feet of eye; vision 20/300–20/200 (6/100–6/70)
20 weeks	Accommodative convergence reflexes all organizing; visually pursues lost rattle; shows interest in stimuli more than 3 feet away
24 weeks	Retrieves a dropped 1-inch cube; can maintain voluntary fixation of stationary object even in the presence of competing moving stimulus; hand-eye coordination is appearing
26 weeks	Will fixate on a string
28 weeks	Binocular fixation clearly established
36 weeks	Depth perception is dawning
40 weeks	Marked interest in tiny objects; tilts head backward to gaze up; vision 20/200 (6/70)
52 weeks	Fusion beginning to appear; discriminates simple geometric forms, squares and circles; vision 20/180 (6/60)
12–18 months	Looks at pictures with interest
18 months	Convergence well established; localization in distance crude–runs into objects which he sees
2 years	Accommodation well developed; vision 20/40 (6/12)
3 years	Convergence smooth; fusion improving; vision 20/30 (6/9)
4 years	Vision 20/20 (6/6)

Source: Reproduced with permission from C. H. Kempe, H. K. Silver, and D. O'Brien, editors, *Current Pediatric Diagnosis and Treatment*, 4th ed., (Los Altos, Calif.: Lange), 1976.

a child uses one eye consistently because of conditions such as strabismus or refractive errors. The unused or idle eye develops decreased vision because the brain blots out the interfering double image it is receiving in the poor eye.

EXTERNAL EXAMINATION

Lids. Inspect for ptosis, asymmetry, ability to close, presence of sties (hordeolum/s), tearing, ectropian (rolling out of lids), entropian (rolling in of lids), and epicanthal folds (vertical folds of skin covering the inner canthus).

Eyelashes. Inspect for presence of discharge, inflammation, and lice.

Eyeball. Examine for size, color, prominence, inflammation, and discharge. A sunken eye orbit is an indication of a severely dehydrated or malnourished child.

Conjunctiva. Examine palpebral portion (lines upper and lower eye lids) for inflammation, erythema, edema, and discharge. Bulbar portion (lies over the sclera): examine for erythema and secretions.

Ocular muscles. Examine movement by having the child's eyes follow a bright object in four quadrants of vision: upper, lower, inner, outer.

Cornea. Examine for clouding, enlargement, ulceration, irritation, and injury.

Sclera. Examine for white color. At birth, the sclera is relatively thin and the underlying uvea imparts the blue tone.

Iris. Examine for color and shape. Heterochromia (irises of different colors, bilaterally), can be normal or can be associated with specific syndromes or low-grade infections.

Pupil. Examine for size. Anisocoria (difference in pupil size) can be normal, or it can be associated with CNS disease, and if found on examination, should always be referred. The pupil is examined for color and constriction to light. A white pupillary reflex can indicate retinoblastoma, cataract, detachment of the retina, and abscess in the vitreous humor. The pupil is also examined for involuntary movements such as nystagmus. See Common Clinical Problems, this chapter.

Lens. Examine for cataracts. They can be detected by shining a light into the eye from an angle or by using an ophthalmoscope. If a cataract is present, the reflex will be white instead of red.

FUNDUSCOPIC EXAMINATION

The fundus, the posterior, inner portion of the retina is examined with an ophthalmoscope. The examination is extremely difficult to perform on infants and can only be adequately done with pupillary dilation. Funduscopic examination of the newborn is not routinely done unless there is a specific indication such as congenital nystagmus, impaired vision, or ocular disease.

Funduscopic examination is performed on all children old enough to cooperate by holding their eyes on a distant object. The optic discs are normally round or slightly oval, the margins are normally sharp, and the color is usually creamy pink. Darker pigmentation exists in black races. In papilledema, a symptom of increased intracranial pressure, the discs are swollen and red in color. The physiologic depression is in the center of the optic disc and the optic nerve emanates from this area. The macula is a small circular area in the disc which contains the fovea centralis, the area of the most accurate acuity. The blood vessels in the fundus are the arteries and veins. The veins are slightly wider than the arteries and show a pulsation.

For examination the room is dark. The nurse practitioner looks into the child's right eye with his/her own right eye. The reverse is true for the left eye. The dial on the ophthalmoscope is at +8 at the beginning of the examination. The red reflex is obtained and opacities on the lens are noted. The dial is turned to the smaller plus numbers while the nurse practitioner comes closer to the child's eye.

Screening for Visual Acuity

The nurse practitioner assesses the eyes for presence of organic eye disease, amblyopia, and refractive errors. It is difficult to perform vision screening for refractive errors on children before the age of 3 years because of their inability to cooperate with instructions. In all visual screening it is imperative that each eye be tested separately to rule out amblyopia.

VISUAL ACUITY

Screening for visual acuity is done through the use of the Snellen illiterate "E" chart or the alphabet chart.

PROCEDURE FOR SNELLEN EYE CHART SCREENING

The child wears glasses if they have been prescribed. If the child wears glasses but does not have them at the time of the visit, screening is done at a later date. If glasses are prescribed and are worn infrequently, screening is done, and a note is written on the chart explaining why the glasses aren't worn. The child keeps both eyes open and does not press the cover card against the covered eye.

Ideally one symbol or one line is exposed at a time. The child is instructed to read from left to right. If the child misses a symbol on a line, the line is repeated having the child read from right to left. If the examiner is using the Snellen "E" chart, the child is asked to show with his/her fingers which way the legs of the "E" are pointing. The child is asked to read all the lines including the 20 foot line. The last line on which the child can read three out of four symbols or four out of six symbols is recorded. During the screening the child is observed for blinking, squinting, rubbing, and complaints of eyes hurting.

Visual acuity is recorded as a fraction. The top number is the distance the child stands from the chart. The bottom number is the last line read correctly.

INDICATIONS FOR REFERRAL

If the first screening is unsatisfactory or the visual acuity is 40 or worse, the child is screened at a later date. If the second screening shows continued poor visual acuity, the child is referred to an ophthalmologist. Generally, all children who screen 20/40 or worse are referred to an ophthalmologist. Children who screen 20/30 and complain of eye strain, headaches, and eye pain are also referred.

Common Parental Concerns

Parents frequently ask questions in reference to the eyes and vision during health supervision visits. Frequent questions are (Stern, 1977):

1. *When do eyes maintain color?*
   Opinions vary, from 6 months of age until 1 to 2 years of age.
2. *When does tearing start?*
   There is no reflex tearing until 3 to 4 months of age.
3. *Can infants see at birth?*
   Yes, estimates of visual acuity vary, from 20/100 to 20/50.
4. *What is the best way to test my infant's vision?*
   By observation to see if the infant follows a brightly colored object.
5. *If my child sits close to the television, is there something wrong with vision?*
   No, children love to see large images especially if they are in color. However, if the child complains of poor vision, an eye examination is indicated.
6. *How often should an eye examination be done for children wearing glasses?*
   Yearly.
7. *Can my child wear contact lenses?*
   Yes, if old enough to adequately place them in the eyes.

MANAGEMENT

General Eye Care

There are no specific routines for eye care except wiping away any mucoid discharge with a moist cotton ball when it is apparent in the inner canthus. This commonly occurs during the newborn period. Occasionally, during this period, an eyelash is seen on the cornea. It is removed by the natural bathing mechanism of the lacrimal duct. It is unwise to instill any drops or ointments in the eyes unless prescribed by a physician.

Counseling

The nurse practitioner discusses with parents symptoms of possible eye disorders.

OBSERVATION FOR DEVIATIONS

The frequency and duration of differences in the range of gaze such as inward or outward turning of the eyes are noted by the parents. Symptoms of conjunctivitis are discussed including discharge, erythema, and tearing. Tearing without crying is a symptom of lacrimal duct obstruction. Parents also observe for anatomic differences between the eyes.

SYMPTOMS OF POOR VISUAL ACUITY

In older children complaints of headache and painful eyes indicate a strain on ciliary muscles used in accommodation. Blurred vision for near and far objects, rubbing, squinting, and frequent blinking are also symptoms of inadequate vision.

Medications

For adequate visualization of the inner eye during diagnostic procedures, pupillary dilation is required.

MYDRIATRICS

These medications dilate the pupil without paralyzing the ciliary muscle of accommodation. They are used in refraction and in genèral ophthalmoscopic examinations, especially in infants. They are contraindicated in clients with glaucoma and hypertension because of the side effects of increased intraocular pressure. Pupillary dilation causes photophobia and blurring of near objects. The maximal duration of effect is up to 1 hour and the recovery time depending on the strength of the solution is 3 to 6 hours.

Common mydriatics are phenylephrine (Neo-Synepherine), 2.5 and 10 percent, and eucatrophine hydrochloride (Euphthalmine Hydrochloride), 2 and 5 percent.

CYCLOPLEGICS

These medications dilate the pupil and produce paralysis of accommodation. They are used in refraction and in the treatment of acute inflammations of the iris and ciliary body. Toxic reactions occur and can be fatal especially in children with mongolism and brain damage.

Common cycloplegics are atropine sulfate, 1 percent; scopolamine hydrobromide, 5 percent; and cyclogyl 1 percent.

TOPICAL ANTIBIOTICS

These medications are used in response to a specific causative organism whose sensitivity has been established. When possible antibiotics are used that are seldom employed systemically to decrease the risk of hypersensitivity reactions. Broad-spectrum antibiotics and the sulfa drugs seldom produce sensitivity.

Some common agents are bacitracin (Baciquent), erythromycin (Ilotycin), and sulfisoxazole (Gantrisin).

TOPICAL CORTICOSTEROIDS

These medications are effective in treating allergic blepharitis, conjunctivitis, contact dermatitis of the eyelids, interstitial keratitis, and iritis. However, there are complications from short- and long-term corticosteroid usage: decreased healing of corneal abrasions, aggravation of herpes simplex keratitis, glaucoma, and possible cataract formation. Prolonged use of topical steroids necessitates management by an ophthalmologist.

Weak steroid preparations include: medrysone, 1 percent; hydrocortisone, 1 percent; and prednisolone, 0.125 percent. Strong preparations include: dexamethasone, 0.1 percent; prednisolone, 1 percent; and triamcinolone, 0.1 percent.

SOLUTIONS AND OINTMENTS

The advantages of ointments include: they remain in the eye with tearing, are comfortable with initial instillation, have less absorption into lacrimal passages, and they are used less frequently since contact time is much longer. The disadvantage is that they interfere with vision by producing a film over the eye.

The advantages of solutions include: they do not interfere with vision, and they cause fewer allergic reactions. A disadvantage is that they must be instilled at frequent intervals because they are washed away easily with tearing.

To instill medications in the eye during infancy, two people are needed. One person leans over the infant securing the legs, trunk, and arms with the body and holds the head straight with the hands. The second person retracts the lids with the fingers of one hand and drops the medication into the palpebral conjunctiva with the other hand.

COMMON CLINICAL PROBLEMS

Blepharitis

ASSESSMENT

Blepharitis is a chronic inflammation of the margins of the eyelids. The common types are: seborrheic (nonulcerative), and staphylococcal (ulcerative). Symptoms of seborrheic blepharitis are oily, easily removed scales at the lid margins. This condition is often associated with dandruff of the scalp. In staphylococcal blepharitis, the scales are dry, and hard to remove with occasional ulcers and pustules. In both conditions there is edema, erythema, crusting, and irritation of the lid margins.

MANAGEMENT

For seborrheic blepharitis, dandruff is controlled and if inflammation is present a sulfonamide medication is prescribed. For staphylococcal blepharitis, antibiotic, sulfonamide medication or a steroid combination topical ointment is prescribed.

Counseling. The parents observe for increased symptoms of infection. Instillation of eye medication is reviewed.

Chalazion

ASSESSMENT

Chalazion is a chronic granulomatous inflammation of the tarsal gland which is a modified sebaceous gland located between the skin and the conjunctiva of the upper lid. The cause is not known. Symptoms are slight tenderness, erythema, and a swelling on the conjunctival surface of the lid.

MANAGEMENT

Occasionally the lesion may reabsorb spontaneously after application of warm compresses. Local excision is sometimes necessary.

Counseling. The parents are instructed to apply warm compresses to the lid four times a day. Symptoms of infection are reviewed.

Color Blindness

ASSESSMENT

Etiology. Color blindness is an X-linked recessive trait. Females are carriers because they have one normal and one defective gene for color vision. Since the male Y chromosome carries no gene for color discrimination, the single gene the female contributes, if it is defective, will cause color blindness. Therefore, half of the female's sons on the average will be color blind. (See Chapter 27, Genetics.)

Incidence. Approximately 7.5 percent of white males, 4 percent of black males, and only 0.5 percent of all females are color blind.

Classifications. There are three inherited types of color blindness:

- Protan—affects red, blue, green color sensitivity
- Deutan—affects green, purple color sensitivity
- Tritan—affects yellow, blue color sensitivity. It is extremely rare.

Screening. This is done by having the child name several colors. If speech development is normal and the child cannot accurately name colors, screening is done with pseudoisochromatic tests which have children trace lines or numbers on colorful backgrounds.

MANAGEMENT

There is no treatment for color blindness. However, it is important to make parents, teachers, relatives, and peers aware that the child's perception of color is not the same as others' with accurate color discrimination. Affected individuals have problems with matching clothing colors, particularly light shades.

Counseling. The nurse practitioner discusses with the family the results of the color vision screening. Individuals who are protan types may not see the red brake lights of cars. They confuse red, brown, and black colors. Deutan types may not be able to distinguish green traffic lights from street lamps. They confuse green, brown, and purple colors.

Conjunctivitis

ASSESSMENT

Definition. Conjunctivitis is an inflammation and infection of the conjunctiva producing erythema, mucoid, or mucopurulent discharge, tearing, itching, and irritation. The discharge occasionally results in caking and sticking together of the lids. Conjunctivitis is classified according to the causative agent or the age at which it occurs.

MANAGEMENT

General. A search for the causative agent is undertaken through smears and conjunctival scrapings for culture. The child is placed on broad-spectrum antibiotics or sulfonamides while awaiting the results of the culture. If the causative agent is not readily identified, the medications are continued until the discharge is gone to decrease the incidence of secondary infection. Topical medications such as drops are given as frequently as every 2 hours. The usual frequency for ointments is every 4 hours. In young children eye ointment is easier to apply, and there is less chance of overdosage. Older children tolerate drops during the day since it does not interfere with vision.

Role of the nurse practitioner. It is of primary importance to assess the degree of infection and to obtain cultures. Health education is provided to the parents as to the etiology, methods of contagion, and the treatment regimen. The correct procedure for instilling topical ophthalmic medications is reviewed.

OPHTHALMIA NEONATORUM

Assessment. This condition is an inflammation of the conjunctiva of the newborn. Accurate diagnosis is essential since the causative agents are numerous. In the newborn, $AgNO_3$ (silver nitrate) conjunctivitis occurs 12 to 24 hours after birth, bacterial conjunctivitis occurs 2 to 5 days after birth, and viral conjunctivitis occurs 5 to 10 days after birth.

Management. Management is according to the causative agent.

NEISSERIA GONORRHOEAE CONJUNCTIVITIS

Assessment. This condition is a rarity in the U.S. due to prophylactic $AgNO_3$ drops or antibiotics placed in the eyes of all newborns. However, if it occurs, it requires prompt diagnosis and treatment since untreated it can cause corneal ulceration, panophthalmitis (inflammation of all eye structures), and occasionally septicemia. Symptoms are copious, purulent discharge, edema of the lids, and intense erythema. Diagnosis is by smear which shows gram-negative intracellular diplococci and a positive culture for *Neisseria*.

Management. Topical antibiotics are given every 1 to 2 hours. Systemic antibiotics are given four times a day for 5 days. The conjunctival sac is irrigated with saline solution and cycloplegics are used in cases where there is corneal involvement.

CHEMICAL CONJUNCTIVITIS

Assessment. This condition is caused by $AgNO_3$ drops, and it is the most common type of ophthalmia neonatorum. Symptoms are erythema, chemosis (edema of the conjunctiva), and a mucoid discharge. It is a sterile inflammation which occurs during the first 24 to 48 hours after birth and clears spontaneously in 3 to 4 days.

Management. There is none except to wipe away discharge from the eye with moist cotton.

ADENOVIRUS CONJUNCTIVITIS

Assessment. This condition is occasionally associated with pharyngitis and preauricular adenopathy. Symptoms are erythema and chemosis of the conjunctiva, mucopurulent discharge, and enlargement of lymphoid follicles on the lower palpebral conjunctiva.

Management. Topical antibiotics or sulfonamides are used to prevent secondary infection but have no other therapeutic value.

INCLUSION CONJUNCTIVITIS (INCLUSION BLENNORRHEA)

Assessment. This condition is caused by the microorganism *Chlamydia oculogenitalis*. Symptoms are acute erythema and edema of the lids with purulent discharge. Conjunctival scrapings are stained with Giemsa solution and show typical cytoplasmic inclusion bodies in epithelial cells. In older children, the conjunctivitis is characterized by early enlargement of the lymphoid follicles of the lower palpebral conjunctiva. The acute phase may last for several weeks and if not treated may progress to a chronic keratoconjunctivitis.

Management. Topical tetracycline ointment and oral sulfonamides are given until 72 hours after the inflammation subsides.

HERPES SIMPLEX CONJUNCTIVITIS

Assessment. This viral conjunctivitis can affect the eye with or without accompanying, generalized herpes infection. Symptoms are discharge, keratitis (inflammation of the cornea), and chorioretinitis (inflammation of the choroid and retina). An ophthalmologist is consulted if there is involvement of the eye structures other than the conjunctiva.

Management. Idoxuridine (IDU) is applied topically when there is corneal involvement. Adenosine arabinoside (Ara-A), an antiviral topical medication is used in cases of IDU-resistant herpes ocular infections.

BACTERIAL CONJUNCTIVITIS

Assessment. The most common causative agents are: *Staphylococcus aureus*, hemolytic *Streptococcus, Neisseria gonorrhoeae, Pneumococcus,* and *Hemophilus influenzae.* Symptoms are copious, purulent discharge which accumulates on lashes causing them to stick together, and erythema of the bulbar and palpebral conjunctiva. Other names used to denote bacterial conjunctivitis are pink eye and acute catarrhal conjunctivitis.

Management. Culture and sensitivity studies are obtained and the appropriate antibiotics are prescribed.

FUNGAL CONJUNCTIVITIS

Assessment. The primary causative agent is *Pseudomonas.* The infection is serious in prematures and can lead to orbital cellulitis, panophthalmitis, and occasionally death from septicemia.

Management. Topical gentamicin, colistin, or polymixin B is given. Occasionally systemic antibiotics are used.

ALLERGIC CONJUNCTIVITIS

See Chapter 28, Allergies.

Dacryocystitis

ASSESSMENT

Dacryocystitis is secondary to dacryostenosis and occurs because of the accumulation of mucus and tears in the lacrimal sac with resulting bacterial infection. Symptoms are excessive tearing without crying, and purulent discharge.

MANAGEMENT

Lacrimal sac massage is instituted and topical antibiotics are applied after cultures are taken. Severe infection of the lacrimal sac is treated with systemic antibiotics. After treatment, probing of the lacrimal duct is occasionally necessary to open it.

Counseling. The technique of massage and the application of topical antibiotics is demonstrated to the parents. See Dacryostenosis.

Dacryostenosis

ASSESSMENT

Dacryostenosis or lacrimal duct obstruction occurs in the newborn period and during infancy. Symptoms are chronic tearing (epiphora) and a mucoid discharge from the lacrimal puncta near the inner canthus.

MANAGEMENT

To remove accumulated tears and mucus from the duct, massage with firm pressure is instituted along the side of the nose toward the eye, four times a day. If tearing or mucoid discharge persists after 6 months of age, the infant is referred to an ophthalmologist for probing to open the lacrimal duct.

Counseling. Parents are shown the technique of massage and are instructed to observe for symptoms of infection. Massage is done three to four times a day.

Emergencies

A pediatrician assesses and manages eye emergencies such as corneal abrasions and nonpenetrating foreign objects. All other emergencies are referred to an ophthalmologist. The role of the nurse practitioner in eye emergencies is to offer accurate information to parents when they call in reference to first aid measures and to make referrals to the appropriate individuals.

COMMON EYE EMERGENCIES

1. Poke in the eye
2. Foreign body
3. Hit in the eye
4. Painful sty (Pascoe 1973, p. 69)

CORNEAL ABRASIONS

Assessment. With any irritation or denudement of the corneal surface an abrasion occurs. Fluorescein strips are used to detect the extent of the abrasion, and they stain epithelial defects light green.

Management. Cycloplegic drops are used to maintain pupillary dilation and to rest the eye. Antibiotic ointment is applied, and the eye is patched for 24 to 48 hours or until the epithelium is healed.

CONJUNCTIVAL FOREIGN BODY

Assessment. The most common site is the furrow immediately behind the margin of the upper lid.

Management. The usual method of removal is to evert the upper lid and with a moist cotton tip applicator lift out the foreign body.

INJURIES

Fracture of the eye orbit. Symptoms are bone tenderness and displacement of the globe. Eye X-rays and ophthalmologist referral are indicated.

Chemical burns of the cornea and conjunctiva. These conditions are irrigated with clear water. Occasionally a topical anesthetic is instilled into the eyes to relieve blepharospasm before the irrigation is started. After irrigation the eye is inspected for obvious injury. Antibiotic ointment is instilled and the eye is re-examined in 24 hours.

Thermal burns of the cornea. This condition is usually caused by a cigarette. The burn becomes a white eschar on the corneal surface. Treatment consists of topical anesthetic application, removal of the eschar with a cotton tip applicator, and the application of antibiotic ointment to the eye.

Hordeolum (Sty)

ASSESSMENT

External hordeolum is an abscess of the sebaceous gland of the eyelash follicle at the lid margin. It is caused by *Staphylococcus aureus*. Symptoms are erythema, edema, and tenderness. Occasionally the abscess ruptures spontaneously.

Internal hordeolum is an abscess of the meibomian glands which are sebaceous glands located in the upper eye lids.

MANAGEMENT

Warm compresses three to four times a day are prescribed for both types of hordeolum. Occasionally antibiotic or sulfonamide ophthalmic medication is used during the acute stage. If spontaneous rupture does not occur, the sty is incised when it is large and edematous.

Counseling. Application of warm compresses is discussed with parents as the most important part of the treatment. Application of eye medication is demonstrated. Washing hands after contamination to prevent recurrence is emphasized.

Nystagmus

ASSESSMENT

Nystagmus is an involuntary movement of the iris and pupil. Intermittent periods of nystagmus in an infant up to 3 months of age are normal. Continuous nystagmus before 3 months of age and nystagmus in older infants and in children is abnormal and is referred for further evaluation.

Types of movements. The following are the most common movements:

- Horizontal, vertical, rotatory, or mixed
- Jerky (rhythmical), slow drifting movement in one direction followed by a quick corrective movement in the opposite direction
- Pendular, to and fro movements equal in each direction with jerking movements when the eyes are moved to the side

Etiologies. Most often the etiologies are associated with defective vision.

- Congenital nystagmus exhibits movements which may be in all directions of gaze. The condition is present at birth, but is not commonly detected before 2 to 3 months of age, and may indicate organic eye disease.

• Neurologic nystagmus exhibits jerky, horizontal, or rotatory movements. They are secondary to lesions in the vestibular apparatus, the cerebellum, or the brainstem.

• Ocular nystagmus exhibits pendular movements which prevent the development of normal fixations. Causes include: albinism, congenital anomalies of the optic nerve, total color blindness, and congenital opacities of the cornea or lens.

Opticokinetic nystagmus. These movements indicate functioning neural receptors in the retina and intact neural pathways and are a normal finding in infants. They are produced by having the infant fixate on a rotating object. The movements are slow in the direction of the moving stimulus and quick in the reverse direction. This procedure is important in assessing the presence of vision in infants.

MANAGEMENT

For intermittent nystagmus occurring past 3 months of age and for continuous nystagmus before 3 months of age, the child is referred for ophthalmologic consultation.

Ptosis

ASSESSMENT

Ptosis is a drooping of the upper eyelid. It may affect one or both eyes. Congenitally the cause is a defective levator palpebral superior muscle. It is often inherited as an autosomal, dominant trait. Acquired causes include birth trauma, encephalitis, pineal tumors, and Horner's syndrome. Occasionally the ptosis can be so severe as to interfere with vision and cause amblyopia.

MANAGEMENT

If the ptosis interferes with vision, surgical correction is advised as soon as possible. If there is no visual compromise, surgical correction is done after 1 year of age.

Counseling. Parents are counseled about the causes and usual treatment regimens. They observe for symptoms of amblyopia: squinting, frequent blinking, and rubbing the eyes.

Refractive Errors

ASSESSMENT

The leading causes of visual impairment in childhood are refractive errors. There are three types:

- Astigmatism, in which light rays diffuse on the retina due to inconsistent curvatures of the cornea; it is associated with hyperopia or myopia
- Hyperopia (farsightedness), in which light rays fall behind the retina due to a short anterior-posterior diameter of the eyeball or due to a lens which is too thin and flat and light rays are not bent adequately
- Myopia (nearsightedness), in which the light rays fall in front of the retina due to a long anterior-posterior diameter of the eyeball or due to a lens which is too thick and the light rays are not bent adequately

At birth most infants are hyperopic and continue to remain so until 5 years of age when the farsightedness gradually decreases. Between 9 and 11 years of age, emmetropia (parallel light rays brought to a pinpoint focus on the retina) is established. At 1 year of age, a child's visual acuity is 20/100, at 2 years of age 20/60, and at 4 years of age 20/20. Pupillary dilation is required for accurate assessment of refractive errors.

Astigmatism. This condition produces headaches, vertigo, frowning when reading, chronically irritated lids, and various degrees of visual defects, according to the amount of hyperopia or myopia present. Significant degrees of astigmatism can be detected through screening for visual acuity with the Snellen chart.

Hyperopia. This condition is more common than myopia and is the natural accommodation of the eyes until approximately 9 years of age. Occasionally one eye may be more hyperopic than the other eye, causing amblyopia. Esotropia is frequently associated with hyperopia in childhood. Efforts to accommodate the visual strain may cause headaches, tired eyes, and blurring vision. Generally, hyperopia is more difficult to diagnose in children because they can accommodate this defect more effectively. Hyperopia is associated with complaints of eye strain and headaches after long periods of reading or writing. It cannot be diagnosed by visual screening with the Snellen charts. It is suspected with the following history: eye strain and pain, headaches, and lines running together when reading. Referral to an ophthalmologist for refraction is indicated.

Myopia. This condition is seen initially between the ages of 9 and 11 years and can be evident by complaints of not seeing the chalkboard at school, holding books close to the face, and not catching a bounced ball at play. It can be diagnosed through visual acuity screening with the Snellen chart.

Other symptoms of refractive errors. These symptoms include: frequent rubbing of the eyes, complaints of double vision, burning and tearing eyes, frowning, words running together while reading, tired eyes (asthenopia), and squinting to create a pinhole effect to help bring the eye into more accurate accommodation.

Screening for refractive errors. This usually cannot be done until the child is 3 to 4 years of age because of the child's inability to understand instructions and general impatience. If visual screening cannot be done adequately at 4 years of age, the parent is instructed to practice the procedure at home, teaching the child to point his/her fingers in the direction of the legs of the "E" on the chart. The visual acuity is then assessed at the next visit.

MANAGEMENT

All children are referred to the ophthalmologist whose visual acuity chart screening shows inability to see half the letters on the 20/40 line after a second screening. Children are also referred whose history indicates hyperopia.

Glasses. The correct treatment for refractive errors is glasses. Their use, however, does not prevent a progression of the visual defect. Visual changes continue to develop because of the ophthalmic changes due to the rapid growth during childhood and adolescence. Therefore, when glasses are worn, yearly ophthalmic examinations are necessary to evaluate the status of the refractive error. After 20 years of age, the same glasses can be worn until middle age.

Counseling. The cause of the visual impairment is discussed with the parents, what objections if any they or the child have in reference to wearing glasses, and the reasons for yearly follow-up eye examinations. The symptoms of poor vision because of refractive errors are reviewed, and the need for repeat visual acuity screening is stressed if the symptoms persist.

Strabismus

ASSESSMENT

Definition. Strabismus is the crossing or squinting of the eyes. It can occur when there is any disorder or disruption of binocular vision.

Pathophysiology. Double vision or diplopia occurs in strabismus because the image viewed does not fall on corresponding parts of the retina in each eye. To avoid diplopia, the child learns to suppress vision in the deviating eye, and ineffectual vision develops. This eye then becomes amblyopic (impaired vision because of disuse). The earlier strabismus is diagnosed, the greater the prevention of amblyopia and the acquisition of normal vision.

Pseudostrabismus. This condition occurs when there are epicanthal folds or a wide bridge across the nose. In these instances, a slight portion of the medial aspect of the eye is covered and the illusion of cross eyes results. Pseudostrabismus is differentiated from true strabismus by the cover-uncover and Hirschberg tests. There is no treatment.

Etiology. The most common cause is imbalance of the muscle alignment of the eyes. Other causes include: brain tumor, infection, retinoblastoma, cataracts, uveitis, ocular injury, and optic nerve atrophy.

Incidence. Strabismus occurs in 5 percent of all children. It can be congenital, and 50 percent of all cases are familial.

Classifications. The following are common types of strabismus:

Nonparalytic (comitant). This is the most common type of strabismus. The deviation is the same in all fields of gaze.

Paralytic (noncomitant). This type of strabismus is due to paralysis of the ocular muscles. The eyes are straight except when moved in the direction of the paralyzed muscles.

Accommodative. There are two types:

1. Convergent. This internal deviation occurs when there is hyperopia and the eyes overaccommodate to remove the error. In doing so, the eyes exert an abnormal degree of overconvergence on the muscles and strabismus develops.

2. Divergent. This external deviation is associated with slight or no refractive error and is often present at birth. The deviation occurs when the child looks at distant objects or daydreams.

Monocular. This type of strabismus is due to paralysis of the ocular muscles. One eye deviates permanently while the other eye fixates normally.

Alternating. In this type of strabismus, either eye is used for fixation while the other eye deviates. Vision develops equally in both eyes since each eye is used for normal vision part of the time.

Terms. The following are used to describe abnormal positions of the eye:

1. Tropias are active frank misalignments of the eyes when the subject is staring straight ahead. Examples are: esotropia, exotropia.

2. Phorias are latent, intermittent misalignments of the eyes which become active (tropias) only when binocular vision is impeded. Examples are: esophoria, exophoria.

History. In the newborn period parents may complain that the infant looks cross eyed. In an older child, in addition to cross eyes, parents may describe frequent blinking, rubbing, squinting, overreaching objects, and tripping. All observations of the parents are investigated. Occasionally parents relate that the preceding symptoms occur only when the child is tired. This situation is due to a latent deviation (phoria) becoming an active deviation (tropia).

Physical examination. Strabismus is evident when there is a positive cover-uncover test. This examination is done by bringing a bright object in front of the child's eyes at a distance of approximately 30 cm. When the child fixes on the object, the nurse practitioner covers one of the eyes with a cover card or the examiner's finger. The second eye is then covered and the uncovered eye is observed for movement. If the uncovered eye moves to fixate while the other eye is covered, there is a strong suspicion that the moving eye has a strabismus. If the child pushes the examiner's hand away while it is covering the good or seeing eye, this can also be a strong suspicion for amblyopia. This examination is most accurate if done after 5 months of age. The Hirschberg test involves shining a penlight into the child's eyes or above the nose. The light reflection should come from corresponding parts of the cornea if strabismus is absent.

MANAGEMENT

The goal of treatment is to determine the etiology and to develop adequate vision in each eye. Conservative management consists of patching the good eye so the deviant eye develops normal vision through continued use. The length of time the eye is patched depends on the age of the child when the diagnosis was made. If before the first year of life, patching may only be used for a few weeks. The successfulness of patching depends on the ability of the child to cooperate with a patch over the eye.

Glasses. Corrective lenses help to focus the object on the retina and relieve accommodative effort. The successful wearing of glasses also depends on the cooperation of the child.

Surgery. Usually surgery is indicated in those children whose strabismus is not corrected by glasses. Occasionally, multiple surgical procedures are necessary to adjust the ocular muscles.

Counseling. Evaluation of pseudo- or true strabismus is made. If pseudostrabismus is present, counseling is directed toward the explanation and the necessity of no treatment. Parents' questions are answered.

After medical consultation and ophthalmologist referral for true strabismus, parents are counseled in reference to their understanding of the etiology and the rationale for management. If the child requires operative treatment, the nurse practitioner remains in contact with the family to reinforce the physician's explanations, to define procedures, to interpret medical and nursing management, and to assist in planning home management.

References

Alexander, M. and M. S. Brown. *Pediatric Physical Diagnosis for Nurses.* New York: McGraw-Hill, 1974.

De Angelis, C. *Basic Pediatrics for the Primary Health Care Provider.* Boston: Little, Brown, 1975.

Goodman, Louis S. and Alfred Gilman. *The Pharmacological Basis of Therapeutics.* New York: Macmillan, 1970.

Graef, J. W. and T. E. Cone, Jr. *Manual of Pediatric Therapeutics.* Boston: Little, Brown, 1974.

Green, M. and R. Haggerty. *Ambulatory Pediatrics II.* Philadelphia: Saunders, 1977.

Kempe, C. H., H. K. Silver, and D. O'Brien, editors. *Current Pediatric Diagnosis and Treatment*, 4th ed. Los Altos, Calif.: Lange Medical Publications, 1976.

Pascoe, D. J., et al. *Quick Reference to Pediatric Emergencies.* Philadelphia: Lippincott, 1973.

Rudolph, A. M., editor. *Pediatrics*, 16th ed. New York: Appleton-Century-Crofts, 1977.

Stern, E. Personal Communication, April 1977.

Vaughan, V. C. and R. J. McKay, editors. *Textbook of Pediatrics*, 10th ed. Philadelphia: Saunders, 1975.

Waechter, E. H. and F. G. Blake. *Nursing Care of Children*, 9th ed. Philadelphia: Lippincott, 1976.

Ziai, M. *Pediatrics*, 2nd ed. Boston: Little, Brown, 1975.

17

The Mouth and Teeth

In the care of the mouth and teeth a wide variety of normal variants and abnormal physical findings present to the examiner. This chapter includes assessment and management of common problems of the mouth and teeth in addition to basic dental information, explanation of normal variants, and preventive measures against dental disease. The nurse practitioner can be responsible for this care and can refer to the physician and the dentist when necessary.

ASSESSMENT

History

PRESENT CONCERNS

Obtain information pertaining to the individual presenting problem following suggestions contained in Chapter 13, Assessment of Presenting Symptom.

517

PAST HISTORY

Obtain information on methods of infant feeding (breast or bottle, length of time), pattern of tooth eruption, history of mouth breathing, thumb sucking (length of time), brushing habits, dental visits, dental problems, mouth diseases, and upper respiratory infections.

BIRTH HISTORY

Obtain information on congenital deformities of the nose and mouth, cleft lip or palate, supernumerary teeth, and maternal medication.

FAMILY HISTORY

Obtain information on congenital deformities, malocclusion, mouth breathing, and periodontal diseases.

NUTRITION HISTORY

Obtain information on carbohydrate and fluoride intake and bottle habits (use at bedtime, what the bottle contains, snacking habits).

Physical Examination

POSITIONING

To obtain an adequate examination of the mouth and throat:

1. Place a cooperative child in a sitting position on the examining table or on the parent's lap.
2. Place an infant or uncooperative child flat on the table. Have the parent hold the child's arms above and beside the head as the examiner immobilizes the child's body with her/his own body and arms.

FACIES

Observe for symmetry, jaw size, swellings, and discolorations.

MOUTH

Observe for ability to open, extent of opening, and odors (see Table 1). To examine the mouth:

1. Use a tongue depressor to inspect under the tongue and between the tongue and the cheeks.
2. Have a young child say "aa" as in "apple" to obtain a clear view of the tonsils, uvula, and epiglottis. Children prefer that a tongue depressor not be used for this purpose.

LIPS

Observe for symmetry, size, color, fissures, bleeding, edema, and hydration.

Common findings. Some common findings are:

1. Cracked, bleeding lips (cheilitis). This is a sign of illness or chapping due to wind and frequent licking of the lips.

Table 1
Mouth Odors and Probable Causes

Odors	Probable Causes
Ammoniacal or stale urine	Uremic conditions
Burnt rope	Marijuana
Camphor	Mothballs
Decaying tissue	Typhoid fever
Fetid	Diphtheria
Garlic	Arsenic poisoning
Offensive breath (halitosis)	Poor oral hygiene and caries; local or systemic infections; mouth breathing or foreign body in nose.
Sweet	Dehydration, malnutrition, or diabetic acidosis

Source: Adapted from B. McVan, "Odors," *Nursing* '77 7:46–49, April 1977.

2. Dry, scaly patches. Observed at lip corners, they may be caused by nutritional deficiencies.
3. Maceration and fissures. Observed at lip corners, they may indicate onset of a fungal infection.

GUMS (GINGIVAE)

Observe for color, texture, bleeding, and lesions.

Normal variants. Some normal variants are:

1. Extension of the septum (alveolar frenulum). Observed on the upper gum, it may cause a separation between the central incisors. It corrects itself with growth.
2. Melanotic (dark pigmentation) line. It is observed along the gums of black children.

Abnormal findings. Some abnormal findings are:

1. Bleeding gums. This may be a sign of poor dental hygiene.
2. Overgrowth of gums (hyperplasia). See this chapter, Gum Hyperplasia.
3. Purple, bleeding gums. This is a sign of scurvy.

BUCCAL MUCOSA

Observe for color, lesions, and hydration.

TONGUE

Observe for movement, papillae changes, dryness, coating, color, and frenulum. See Chapter 4, Frenulum.

Normal variants. Some normal variants are:

1. Fissured tongue. Fissure may run parallel to or at right angles to the central grooves. Ten percent of the population manifests at least two fissures. Fissuring may follow scarlet fever, syphilis, or typhoid fever.

2. Geographic tongue. The dorsum of the tongue shows characteristic smooth, shiny, erythematous areas which are slightly depressed below the surrounding normal papillae. Noticed in 1 to 6 percent of the population, they disappear and reappear in different areas and at different times of a person's life.

Abnormal findings. Some abnormal findings are:

1. Coated tongue. This is caused by the accumulation of food debris and bacteria among hypertrophied filiform papillae. The tongue has a smooth appearance until the age of 5 because the filiform papillae are normally short. In a child under 5 the cause should be sought for any coating of the tongue.

2. Dry coated tongue. This is a result of failure of secretion by the salivary and lingual glands and is one of the best clinical signs of dehydration. The color may vary from white to brown.

3. Furry tongue. This is seen early in states of mild dehydration and low-grade fever.

4. White strawberry tongue. This is a transitional stage from the white coated tongue to the raw red tongue. The appearance is of an unripe strawberry. The engorged and enlarged fungiform papillae appear prominently above the level of the white, desquamating filiform papillae. It is seen early in scarlet fever and other acute states. See Chapter 29, Scarlet Fever.

HARD PALATE

Observe for color, lesions, and high arching.

SOFT PALATE

Observe size and movement of uvula, or if bifid.

TONSILS

Inspect for color, edema, size, symmetry, coating, crypts, and exudate.

Tonsil size. Tonsillar lymphoid tissue is not prominent in the 1 to 2 year old; tonsils appear largest in the 3 to 4 year old; and tissue is again small in the 10 year old. A method for recording tonsillar size is:

1+ edges seen
2+ larger
3+ touching uvula
4+ meeting at midline (kissing tonsils)

POSTERIOR PHARYNX AND EPIGLOTTIS

Inspect for color, swelling, and exudate.

TEETH

Observe number, extra or missing, staining, caries, bite (occlusion), or overbite (malocclusion). See this chapter, Malocclusion and Caries.

Staining. Stains observed on teeth are:

1. *Black stain.* This may occur as a result of iron ingestion. It is a temporary staining which disappears when the diet contains less iron. Iron or acid medications should be taken through a straw. See Chapter 20, Iron Deficiency Anemia.

2. *Green stain.* A greenish color of the enamel may result from intense neonatal jaundice. The deciduous teeth may be completely green except for the portion developed postnatally. Green stains may occur on the labial surfaces of the anterior teeth near the gingivae in children who lack satisfactory care. This can be removed by a dentist.

3. *Yellow-grey, bright yellow, and grey-brown stains.* These discolorations may occur as a result of tetracycline therapy during the period of tooth formation. Tetracyclines have caused tooth defects when administered to the mother in the last trimester of pregnancy while the teeth are forming in utero; through milk from a nursing mother; or directly to the child. Tetracyclines at

levels exceeding 75 mg/kg nearly always cause enamel hyperplasia. Although no treatment is necessary, severe hyperplasia may require dental restoration of teeth.

Dentition

TOOTH DEVELOPMENT

The process of normal tooth development begins in utero and continues into early adulthood. Basic facts of tooth development are as follows:

- Each tooth undergoes four successive periods of development during its life cycle: growth, calcification, eruption, and attrition. Normal eruption and shedding of primary teeth, and eruption of permanent teeth are presented in Table 2.
- Calcification of the central and lateral incisors of the deciduous (primary) teeth begins about the fifth fetal month. These are the first deciduous teeth to erupt at about the infant's fifth or sixth month of age.
- Calcification of the first molars of the permanent (secondary) teeth begins at birth. These are the first permanent teeth to erupt at the child's sixth or seventh year of age.
- Normal variants include premature eruption, delayed eruption, and congenital absence of some teeth.
- The formation of healthy tooth structure is fostered by a diet adequate in protein, calcium, phosphate, and vitamins (especially C and D), and requires strenuous chewing of foods such as hard breads, raw fruit, and vegetables.
- Nutritional disorders and prolonged illness in infancy may interfere with calcification of deciduous and permanent teeth.

IMPORTANCE OF THE PRIMARY TEETH

The primary teeth play an important role for the following reasons:

Table 2
Normal Tooth Eruption and Shedding

Eruption and Shedding of Primary Teeth			Eruption of Permanent Teeth	
Upper	Eruption	Shedding	Upper	
Central incisor	7½ mo	7½ yr	Central incisor	7–8 yr
Lateral incisor	9 mo	8 yr	Lateral incisor	8–9 yr
Cuspid	18 mo	11½ yr	Cuspid	11–12 yr
First molar	14 mo	10½ yr	First bicuspid	10–11 yr
Second molar	24 mo	10½ yr	Second bicuspid	10–12 yr
			First molar	6–7 yr
			Second molar	12–13 yr
			Third molar	17–21 yr
Lower			Lower	
Central incisor	6 mo	6 yr	Central incisor	6–7 yr
Lateral incisor	7 mo	7 yr	Lateral incisor	7–8 yr
Cuspid	16 mo	9½ yr	Cuspid	9–10 yr
First molar	12 mo	10 yr	First bicuspid	10–12 yr
Second molar	20 mo	11 yr	Second bicuspid	11–12 yr
			First molar	6–7 yr
			Second molar	11–13 yr
			Third molar	17–21 yr

Source: Adapted from *Your Child's Teeth.* Chicago: American Dental Association, 1971, p. 11.

- Each primary tooth is needed to occupy a space for a permanent tooth. The most common disturbance in the eruption of teeth is caused by premature loss or extraction of neglected primary or permanent teeth. Early loss of a primary tooth impairs mastication and may result in improper eruption or impaction of the permanent tooth. When teeth are lost prematurely, construction of a space maintainer by the dentist is necessary.
- Speech development depends on primary teeth. Proper pronunciation of at least 18 of the 268 letters requires the proper alignment of the teeth.
- Primary teeth round out the shape of the face by supporting facial muscles and ligaments, contributing to the growth and development of the jaws.

MANAGEMENT

Plaque

Plaque is a colorless, transparent, sticky, organic layer which firmly coats the surface of the teeth. It supports the growth of destructive bacteria that cause decay and periodontal disease. It accumulates along the gums and at the site of cracks and rough spots.

CAUSES OF PLAQUE

High carbohydrate intake, sweet sticky foods taken between meals, and poor dental hygiene contribute to plaque formation. Plaque adheres to enamel in 24 hours.

PLAQUE REMOVAL

Plaque is removed only by brushing and flossing the teeth and should be removed at least once in 24 hours.

Toothbrushing. Toothbrushing will remove plaque from the outer, inner, and biting surfaces of the teeth. Methods of toothbrushing are as follows:

- The parent may first start cleansing the child's teeth by rubbing them gently with gauze wrapped around a finger.
- Children should begin brushing between 18 months to 3 years of age or when they are able to stand at the sink on a stool. An egg timer may be used to help the child to spend enough time at brushing. The child may need help until 4 or 5 years of age.
- The older child may use a "disclosing tablet," a vegetable dye that colors the plaque red and indicates areas where plaque has not been removed.
- Teeth are brushed thoroughly after each meal and after eating sweets. If unable to brush the mouth should be rinsed with water.

- With the bristle tips at a 45° angle against the gum line, the brush cleans the teeth and gums at the same time. Short strokes are used in a gentle back-and-forth scrubbing motion. Chewing surfaces are also brushed with the same scrubbing strokes.

SELECTION OF TOOTHBRUSH.   This includes:

1. Type of brush. A brush with a straight handle, a flat brushing surface, and soft, round-ended bristles is recommended. The head of the brush should be small enough to provide easy access to every tooth. Both hand brushes and powered brushes can be effective for plaque removal; powered cordless brushes may be especially appealing and useful to children.
2. Size of brush. Children need brushes smaller than those designed for adults; however, the handle should be large enough to hold easily.
3. Replacement of brush. Toothbrushes should be replaced when they soften and the bristles are slightly frayed, probably as often as every 2 to 3 months or sooner.

Flossing.   This is the most effective method for removing plaque from between the teeth. Methods used to aid in flossing are as follows:

- The floss is gently guided against the side of the tooth into the space between the teeth until resistance is felt. It is then curved into a C-shape around the side of the tooth and scraped up and down against the surface of each tooth.
- Children may find it easier to hold the floss when the ends have been tied together to form a circle about 10 inches in diameter.
- Care is taken to floss gently but firmly as improper flossing can be injurious to the gums.

Water irrigation.   "Water pik" is recommended for removing food particles which are stuck between the teeth and cannot be removed with brushing or flossing. Water irrigation is especially effective for wearers of braces or permanent bridges. "Water pik" does not remove plaque.

Fluoride

The ingestion of fluoride during the period of tooth development has been shown to reduce significantly the incidence of dental caries, in some cases by as much as 80 percent. To achieve the greatest benefits from fluoride, sources of fluoride must be introduced in infancy and provided systematically until at least 14 years of age.

RECOMMENDED INTAKE

The Committee on Nutrition of the American Academy of Pediatrics (1972) recommends optimal dosage of fluoride supplementation as follows:

Age	Dosage
Birth to 3 years	0.5 mg/day
3 years	1.0 mg/day

METHODS OF FLUORIDE SUPPLEMENTATION

Water fluoridation. The fluoridation of community water supplies is the most efficacious method of assuring consistent intake of fluoride. The optimal level of fluoride concentration in community water supplies is 0.5 to 1.0 parts per million (ppm). The amount of fluoridated water necessary to provide the recommended intake of fluoride is 500 ml (1 pint).

Medicinal fluoride. Fluoride preparations are available either singly or in combination with vitamins. Examples of available preparations are:

- Fluoride alone

Luride drops (Hoyt Laboratories)	0.1 mg/drop
Luride tablets	0.5 mg/tablet
	1.0 mg/tablet

- Fluoride with vitamins.

  Tri-Vi-Flor (Mead Johnson)

  | Drops | 0.5 mg/ml |
  | Chewable tablets | 1.0 mg/tablet |

  Poly-Vi-Flor

  | Chewable tablets | 1.0 mg/tablet |

Topical fluoride applications. This fluoride, which is applied by the dentist, becomes part of the tooth enamel making it more resistant to decay-causing acids. In fluoridated water areas it provides an additional 17 percent protection to the teeth. Parents should know of its importance.

Fluoride toothpastes. The American Dental Association recommends the use of these toothpastes, and reports show that they reduce the incidence of new carious lesions.

DETERMINING THE NEED FOR FLUORIDE SUPPLEMENTATION

The need for and the amount of supplementation depends on the age of the child, the level of fluoride concentration in the local water supply, and the amount of water in the child's diet.

Guidelines for supplementation. Supplementation is necessary and should begin at birth (see below, Breast-Fed Infants) when:

1. Community water contains less than 0.5 ppm
2. The diet does not contain sufficient fluoridated water, as with infants fed cow's milk or ready-to-feed commercially prepared formulas, and the many children who do not drink sufficient water

Breast-fed infants. There is controversy over the issue of when to begin fluoride supplementation in breast-fed infants. Very little fluoride is transmitted in breast milk, yet the reduction in dental caries that has occurred in children in naturally fluoridated communities has occurred without fluoride supplementation during breast feeding (Hess, 1977). Currently, Fomon (1974) and Waitrowski (1975) recommend that fluoride supplementation in the breast-fed infant be delayed until 6 months of age.

Excessive fluoride. Mottling of the teeth occurs when the fluoride content of the water is higher than 2.5 ppm or when a child receives an overdose of medicinal fluoride (over 4 mg/day). See this chapter, Fluorosis. To avoid the possibility of mottling, the prescribed dietary supplement should be adjusted downward in proportion to the concentration of fluoride in the drinking water. The following allowance (adapted from Hess, 1977) is recommended for children 3 years of age or older:

Water Fluoride (ppm)	Adjusted Allowance Fluoride (mg/day)
0.0	1.0
0.2	0.8
0.4	0.6
0.6	0.4

Dental Referral

INITIAL VISIT

It is recommended that the child be seen first at least by age 3. Most children should be seen at an earlier age if possible since 36 percent of children have caries by age 3. Parental attitude creates the mood of the first visit. One should speak of the dentist as a friend who helps to keep the teeth healthy. "Overpreparing," urging, bribing, or forcing the child are not recommended.

LATER VISITS

The child should visit the dentist on a regular basis, at least every 3 or 4 months, during the ages of 4 to 8 because the greatest incidence of caries occurs between these years and because of the speed with which caries develop.

SPECIAL REFERRALS

Referrals are made to the dentist for a child of any age if the following occur:

1. The child falls and injures a tooth or the jaw. The tooth is kept moist and taken to the dentist.
2. The child complains of pain in teeth or gums.
3. The teeth become discolored.
4. Caries is present upon examination.
5. Malocclusion is severe, or the child's tongue thrusts, and the child has not previously had dental care.

COMMON CLINICAL PROBLEMS

Mouth

DROOLING (SALIVATION)

Assessment.   In infancy cells of the salivary glands do not mature until 3 to 6 months of age at which time the flow of saliva is increased. The infant has not learned to swallow efficiently, therefore drooling occurs. Excessive salivation is more evident with teething; as a reflex to anticipated pain; from nausea; or from irritation of lesions in the mouth. It may also follow administration of mercurial compounds and occurs in certain nervous disorders such as encephalitis and chorea.

Management.   The parents are given an explanation of salivation.

GINGIVITIS

Assessment.   Mild inflammation of the gingivae (gums) occurs in two ways:

1. Eruption gingivitis is temporary gingivitis seen during decidu-

ous tooth emergence. See this chapter, Teething in Infancy. Eruption of the permanent teeth is often accompanied by a mild gingivitis possibly because the surrounding gingivae receive little protection from the tooth during early eruption. The gingivae become inflamed by the continued irritative and abrasive action of food.

2. Marginal gingivitis in children is usually associated with poor oral hygiene and, at times, with the presence of abnormal occlusion.

Management. Treatment is aimed at relief of soreness and improvement of oral hygiene.

1. Eruption gingivitis is relieved by mouth rinses using warm normal saline solution.
2. Marginal gingivitis is relieved by improved toothbrushing techniques for removing plaque and by water irrigation for removal of food debris.

THRUSH

Assessment. Oral candidiasis (thrush) is caused by the fungus *Candida albicans*. Infections are transmitted from the vaginal canal of mother; from poorly sterilized bottles or nipples, mother's breast, attendant's hands; or result from long-term suppression of the natural oral flora through infections and use of antibiotics.

SIGNS OF THRUSH. Thrush presents with white, milky, or cheesy patches on the tongue and/or on the buccal mucosa. If scraped, a red, bleeding lesion results. Microscopic examination of cheesy material mixed with 10 percent potassium hydroxide will show hyphae of the organism and will confirm the diagnosis. If diaper rash appears in association with thrush, fungal diaper infection is suspected.

Management. Antifungal agents are used as follows:

1. Installation in the mouth of nystatin (Mycostatin) in suspension in dosage prescribed by the physician.
2. Local applications of 1 percent methylrosaniline chloride (gen-

tian violet) solution, daily, with a soft cotton swab. A fresh swab is used with each application. This treatment is less effective than nystatin and can discolor the skin and clothing. Relapse is not uncommon and calls for further course of medication.

TRAUMA TO THE TONGUE

Assessment. Some causes of trauma to the tongue are accidental biting of the tongue, injuries by sharp objects such as toys, and burns by hot foods. Symptoms may include swelling and redness, blisters, or ulcers which disappear in a few days.

Management. Ice may be used for swelling. A mild antiseptic mouthwash, such as 1 percent tincture of iodine in physiologic saline solution, may be used. Food is kept cool and in liquid form until the trauma is healed.

Dental Problems

BRUXISM (NIGHT GRINDING)

Assessment. Bruxism is involuntary grinding, clenching, or gnashing of the teeth during sleep. It is caused by malocclusion in an effort to find a more comfortable position for the teeth or is triggered by anxiety or emotional disturbance. It can result in especially rapid attrition (the normal wearing of the teeth) and can lead to periodontal disease, facial pain, and, sometimes, loss of teeth.

Management. Treatment consists of:

1. Equilibration. This is done by the dentist who grinds down high chewing surfaces and/or builds up low ones to restore proper alignment. Orthodontia may be required.
2. Exercise. An exercise that helps the problem with psychologic roots is to clench the teeth tightly for 5 seconds, relax for 5 seconds, and repeat six times each day for 2 weeks.
3. Counseling. The cause of the emotional disturbance should be sought.

CARIES (TOOTH DECAY)

Assessment. Dental caries are progressive lesions of the calcified dental tissues characterized by loss of tooth structures.

CAUSATIVE FACTORS. Three definitive factors necessary to produce tooth decay are *bacteria, carbohydrate*, and *plaque*. The bacteria are classified into three groups:

1. Acidogenic organisms that produce the acids upon the tooth surface which decalcify the hard tissues. *Lactobacillus acidophilus* and certain streptococci are the most frequent.
2. Proteolytic organisms that digest the organic matrix after its decalcification and produce the characteristic discoloration and odor of caries.
3. *Leptotrichiae* organisms that form plaque on the smooth surfaces of the teeth where the acidogenic organisms are harbored.

Carbohydrates are the major food factor. These are sticky, refined carbohydrates that are eaten between meals and remain on the tooth surface for long periods of time. Acidogenic bacteria quickly produce acid from these sugars. Mealtime sugars are buffered by saliva and other foods that tend to neutralize the acid.

INCIDENCE. By the age of 6 years from 50 to 97 percent of children have one or more cavities. The average percentage of decayed or filled teeth at this age is 4.5 to 6 percent. The periods of greatest carious activity are 4 to 8 years of age in deciduous dentition and 12 to 18 years of age in the permanent dentition.

SIGNS OF TOOTH DECAY. Caries are seen as discolored areas or actual cavitations in the pits and fissures of the chewing surface of the posterior teeth or between the teeth and, in a badly neglected mouth, at the neck of the tooth at the junction of the gingivae. Many caries are not visible upon inspection of the teeth. Dental equipment and X-rays provide more reliable detection.

Management. Management is directed toward prevention of caries. Preventive measures include:

1. Plaque removal by brushing and flossing after each meal
2. Fluoridation of community water or oral fluoride supplementation by drops or tablets
3. Topical application of fluoride by the dentist
4. Use of toothpastes containing fluoride
5. Early introduction to dental care with frequent supervisory visits
6. Proper, nutritional diet containing limited carbohydrates

FOODS TO RECOMMEND FOR SNACKS. These include food groups as follows:

- Milk group. Milk, cheese, cheese dips, cheese curls
- Meat group. Luncheon meats, salami, smoked sausages, clam dip, nuts of all kinds
- Fruit and vegetable group. Raw fruits and vegetables, unsweetened fruit juices and vegetable juices.
- Bread and cereal group. Crackers, toast, pretzels, corn chips, popcorn, teething biscuits.

FOODS TO AVOID. These include:

- High carbohydrate content foods such as infant formula with added sugar and sweet, sticky snacks taken in between meals ("trigger" foods). These snacks are candy, cake, cookies, pie, pastry, ice cream, sundaes or cones, candied popcorn, candy apples, candy-coated gum, peanut butter and jelly sandwiches, honey graham crackers, dried fruits and raisins.
- Products such as hard candies, lollipops, breath mints, and cough drops that are held in contact with teeth over a period of time.
- Lemons, if they are sucked or eaten, bring teeth into contact with acid.

CONGENITAL ABSENCE OF TEETH (ANODONTIA)

Assessment. Congenital absence of teeth occurs frequently as a genetic anomaly. The permanent absence of the third molars, the upper lateral incisors, and/or the lower and upper bicuspids is attributed to evolutionary causes. Absence of other teeth may be indicative of some hereditary systemic disease such as arachnodactyly, cleido-cranial dyostosis, or congenital ectodermal dysplasia.

Management. Consultation and/or referral are indicated.

DELAYED ERUPTION

Assessment. The first tooth normally erupts between the fifth and twelfth month. A first tooth which does not appear by the twelfth month suggests disturbances of nutrition or endocrine origin. Rickets, Down's syndrome, and congenital syphilis should be ruled out.

Management. Referral to or consultation with the physician is indicated.

FLUOROSIS

Assessment. "Mottling" of the teeth results from excess exposure to fluoride. This occurs when the fluoride content of the community water is over 2.5 ppm or when the diet contains more than optimal levels of fluoride (see this chapter, Fluoride). Fluorosis occurs only in children during the tooth development ages from birth to 14 years. Teeth affected in childhood remain affected throughout life. The types of fluorosis are:

1. Mild fluorosis. "Mottling" of the teeth is a cosmetic defect in which opaque paper-white areas appear on the surface of normally translucent teeth.
2. Moderate fluorosis. This occurs when brown stains begin to appear.
3. Severe fluorosis. This occurs when brown stains appear, the teeth become pitted, and, eventually, the enamel erodes.

Management. There is no actual treatment. Prevention includes a careful assessment of the child's diet, looking for:

1. A diet containing large amounts of fluoridated water, such as

drinking water, foods reprocessed in water, or diets rich in fish, tea, and mineral water

2. An overdosage of supplemental fluorides

GUM HYPERPLASIA

Assessment. This is defined as overgrowth of gums due to prolonged periods of Dilantin therapy, mouth breathing, or vitamin deficiency. The gums may bleed as the child stops brushing thereby aggravating the problem.

Management. Treatment includes meticulous attention to dental hygiene with the use of soft toothbrushes and digital pressure to the gums several times a day.

INJURY TO TEETH

Assessment. Teeth may be broken, cracked, pushed out of alignment, or knocked out of the mouth.

Management. The child is taken to the dentist immediately. The tooth is wrapped in a wet cloth or placed in water and taken with the child. The tooth is replaced in its normal position in hopes that it will reattach itself to the jaw and function normally.

LIP BITING

Assessment. Habitual sucking or nibbling on the lower lip tends to force the lower incisors backwards. This habit may occur as a tensional outlet.

Management. Lip pomade can be applied frequently, to serve as a reminder not to bite lips and to promote healing of chapped mucosa. The abnormal position of the teeth tends to rectify itself spontaneously with growth. It is best not to pay undue attention to this habit. See Chapter 8, Common Clinical Problems.

MALOCCLUSION

Assessment. Malocclusion refers to irregularities of tooth alignment and the improper fitting together of the teeth on chewing. Abnormal jaw relationships, and abnormal and deforming muscle function, both inherited and acquired, may result in malocclusion. Deciduous teeth or first permanent teeth may be widely spaced or may overlap. This is usually temporary as the teeth tend to realign spontaneously with growth. Malocclusion is not common in deciduous teeth.

NORMAL OCCLUSION. This is present when the top posterior teeth (molars) meet and rest snugly on the opposing bottom posterior teeth and when the upper anterior teeth (incisors) barely overlap and touch the bottom anterior teeth. The examiner should observe the jaw structures of the parents as a clue.

CAUSES OF MALOCCLUSION. These include:

1. Incompatibility of tooth size and jaw size that may result in spacing, crowding, or irregularity of teeth
2. Prolonged retention of primary teeth that may result in delayed eruption of permanent teeth
3. Neglected primary or permanent teeth that may be lost prematurely
4. Lip biting, mouth breathing, tongue thrusting, teeth grinding, thumb sucking, or improper sleeping habits over a long period of time. These may exert pressures that interfere with good growth patterns.

Management. Referral is made when malocclusion is present which interferes with the proper chewing of foods, or when there is obvious jaw deformity in the family.

PREVENTION. Preventive measures include:

1. Parental encouragement to meet early sucking needs in the first year and discouragement of weaning to the cup before 1 year to promote better development of mouth and jaw

2. Removal of the thumb or fingers from child's mouth while sleeping
3. Positioning of the child in sleep so his/her cheek does not rest on small, hard, firm objects such as fists or toys

MOUTH BREATHING

Assessment. Mouth breathing may occur as a result of habit or nasal obstruction. The tongue normally lies against the roof of the mouth. When the tongue is suspended between the dental arches or on the floor of the mouth, development of the teeth and jaws are affected. These effects include:

1. Elongation of the face with dropping of the mandible
2. Narrow and pinched nostrils from disuse
3. Dull and drawn expression

Young children normally sleep with their lips open, this is not considered to be mouth breathing. To determine whether a child is mouth breathing, a wisp of cotton is held to the child's nose and mouth.

Management. Referral is made to an otolaryngologist if nasal obstruction is present. Surgical removal of the obstruction (adenoidectomy) and muscular exercises to strengthen the lips and to maintain closure may be necessary. Orthodontia is frequently necessary.

NURSING BOTTLE MOUTH

Assessment. This condition is a form of rampant caries associated with frequent, prolonged use of a nursing bottle containing carbohydrate liquids which are in contact with the teeth. These liquids may be milk, apple juice, or other fruit juices. Nursing bottle mouth may occur in children as early as 18 months of age. The history may reveal that the child has a well-regulated diet and the teeth are brushed, but the child is put to bed with a nursing bottle. The bottle often remains in the mouth most of the night, and/or through naptime.

SIGNS OF NURSING BOTTLE MOUTH. These are:

1. Severe to mild decay of all primary upper anterior teeth
2. Decay of upper and lower first molars and lower primary canine teeth in extensive cases

Management. Prevention includes:

1. Early health education of parents and early dental assessment
2. Elimination of milk or juice in nursing bottle at nap or bedtime. If the child needs additional sucking, water in the bottle is preferable.
3. Guidance. This may be necessary if bedtime sucking continues beyond infancy.

PREMATURE ERUPTION

Assessment. Supernumerary or normal lower deciduous teeth may erupt at birth. Supernumerary teeth are usually loose, lack roots, and may have defective structure.

Management. Teeth that are prematurely erupted are usually removed since they may interfere with nursing or may be aspirated.

TEETHING IN INFANCY

Assessment. Primary or deciduous tooth eruption begins at about 6 months of age with the lower central incisors, closely followed by the lower lateral incisors and the upper central incisors. Teething continues with teeth erupting approximately every 2 months until 2 years of age. See Table 2.

SIGNS OF TEETHING. They are not always clear. Some children teethe without pain and with few physical signs. Other children are uncomfortable, irritable, cry, and rub at the gums. Upon inspection, red and swollen gums are evident.

PHYSIOLOGIC AND DEVELOPMENTAL FACTORS. Occurring coincidentally in the infant are factors which some parents find difficult to disassociate from teething. These factors are:

1. Excessive salivation. This occurs normally at 3 to 4 months of age.
2. Lowering of the level of maternal antibody protection. Fevers do not occur as a result of teething and should be separately assessed.
3. Fussiness, sleep disturbances, and separation anxiety
4. Reaching for and mouthing objects

Management. Chewing on clean, hard objects to relieve tension felt in the gums is recommended. Some favorite objects are:

- Hard, rubber teething rings
- Hard, rubber teething beads
- Ridged rubber or plastic teething toys
- Hard rools or crusts of bread
- Teething pretzels

Rubbing gums with teething lotions which contain benzocaine has been recommended. Rubbing gums with whiskey is a time honored and most frequently recommended treatment. Some teething appliances made of plastic with liquid filling are not recommended since infants may chew through the plastic and may ingest the liquid.

THUMB SUCKING

Assessment. Thumb sucking is suspected if upper incisors markedly protrude over lower teeth. The thumb or other fingers may exhibit calluses. Holding the thumb in the mouth the greater part of the day and/or night can permanently distort the jaws and teeth. The child's age and severity of the habit determine whether or not sucking is harmful to the facial contours and structures. In 75 percent of all cases the dental deformity will be remolded and corrected spontaneously if the thumb sucking ceases before the age of 6.

Sporadic sucking is essentially innocuous, and regular sucking until age 2 or 3 is considered to be normal. Excessive sucking beyond the age of 4 may be caused by an emotional disturbance.

Management. Practical suggestions are:

1. The thumb or fingers may be removed from the mouth after the child is asleep.
2. Parents and well-meaning relatives and friends are cautioned against pulling the thumb from the mouth or against ceaselessly reminding the child to remove it.
3. Unpleasant tasting medications used to coat the thumb or appliances which prevent sucking are ineffective and may cause further emotional damage.

COUNSELING. Factors to consider for counseling about excessive sucking are:

1. The child may need more activity or playtime with other children, or he may need more time alone with parents
2. The child may be jealous of a sibling
3. The child may be left for lengthy periods with a caretaker
4. The child may be bored, tired, thirsty, hungry

TONGUE THRUST

Assessment. Tongue thrust occurs as a result of the habit of bracing the tongue against the upper and lower incisors at each swallow. In time this causes the teeth to protrude. It may be a manifestation of tension. It may interfere with the acquisition of clear speech.

SIGNS OF TONGUE THRUSTING. Suspect tongue thrusting if both upper and lower incisors protrude enough to leave an oval space when the jaw is closed. If this condition is arrested early, the abnormal position of the teeth may rectify itself spontaneously with growth.

Management. Referral to the dentist is made if signs of tongue thrusting are evident. Orthodontia may be necessary.

COUNSELING. The source of tension may need to be discussed with the parents if the habit continues. It is advised not to call the child's attention to the habit.

Resource Information

Resource information can be obtained from these organizations:
1. American Dental Association, 211 E. Chicago Avenue, Chicago, IL 60611.
2. American Society of Dentistry for Children, 211 E. Chicago Avenue, Chicago, IL 60611.
3. College of Physicians and Surgeons, 344 14th Street, San Francisco CA 94118.

References

Alexander, M. M. and M. S. Brown. *Pediatric Physical Diagnosis for Nurses*. New York: McGraw-Hill, 1974.

Bernick, S. M. "What the Pediatrician Should Know About Children's Teeth: Part 4. Baby Bottle Syndrome." *Clin Pediatr* 10:243–244, April 1971.

Committee on Nutrition, American Academy of Pediatrics. "Fluoride as a Nutrient." *Pediatrics* 49:456–459, March 1972.

Council of Dental Therapeutics. *Accepted Dental Therapeutics*. Chicago: American Dental Association, 1976.

Curson, M. E. J. "Dental Implications of Thumbsucking." *Pediatrics* 54:196–200, August 1974.

De Weese, D. D. and W. H. Saunders. *Textbook of Otolaryngology*. St. Louis: Mosby, 1973.

Fomon, S. J. *Infant Nutrition*, 2nd ed. Philadelphia: Saunders, 1974.

Graber, T. W. *Orthodontics, Principles and Practice*. Philadelphia: Saunders, 1966.

Hess, J. "Fluoride Therapy in Children." Unpublished material, Dept. of Pediatrics, Grand Rounds, University of California, San Francisco June 16, 1977.

McVan, B. "Odors." *Nursing '77* 7:46–49, April 1977.

Morris, A. L. and H. M. Bohannon. *The Dental Specialties in General Practice*. Philadelphia: Saunders, 1969.

Prival, M. J. and F. Fisher. "Adding Fluorides to the Diet." *Nursing Digest* 16:53–55, Aug. 1975.

Slattery, J. "Dental Health in Children." *Am J Nurs* 76:1159–1161, July 1976.

van der Horst, R. L. "On Teething in Infancy." *Clin Pediatr* 12:607–610, Oct. 1973.

Vaughan, V. C. and R. J. McKay, editors. *Nelson Textbook of Pediatrics*, 10th ed. Philadelphia: Saunders, 1975.

Waitrowski, E. et al. "Dietary Fluoride Intake of Infants." *Pediatrics* 55:517–522, April 1975.

Your Child's Teeth. Chicago: American Dental Association, 1971.

18

The Respiratory System

The most common cause of illness in infancy and childhood is infection of the respiratory tract. Infections of the upper respiratory tract alone account for more than one half of the acute illnesses treated in pediatric ambulatory health facilities. This chapter provides information to assist the nurse practitioner in the assessment and management of common acute problems of the respiratory tract in collaboration with a physician. Complete discussion of respiratory tract problems is beyond the scope of this chapter and is available in major pediatric textbooks. Related information is found in the corresponding chapters on allergy, the gastrointestinal system, infectious diseases, and the mouth and teeth.

ASSESSMENT

A careful history and physical examination determine whether the child can be managed on an ambulatory basis or whether further investigation is warranted prior to deciding on the plan of management.

History

PRESENT CONCERN

Obtain a precise chronologic history of each presenting symptom. (See Chapter 13, Assessment of the Presenting Symptom).

Cough. Obtain information about onset, duration, type (dry, hacking, moist, barking), progress (better or worse), pattern (day or night), pain (location), postnasal drip, sputum (color, consistency, frequency), associated symptoms (sore throat, respiratory distress, nasal discharge, fever), medications (type, frequency, duration), past history of cough, and exposure (illness in family).

Respiratory difficulty. See this chapter, Respiratory Distress. Obtain information about onset (abrupt, gradual), duration, pattern of respiration (rapid, slow), type of difficulty (inspiratory, expiratory), associated sounds (wheezing, barking cough), nasal flaring, cyanosis, associated symptoms (fever, abdominal pain, rhinorrhea, anorexia, headache, malaise), and past history of respiratory difficulty (diagnosis, treatment).

Rhinorrhea. Obtain information about onset, duration, description of discharge (color, consistency), progress (better, worse), pattern (completely clears and then returns), associated symptoms (sore throat, respiratory distress, fever, cough), medications (type, frequency, duration), previous history of nasal congestion and discharge.

Sore throat. Obtain information about onset, duration, progress (better, worse), treatment (lozenges, salt-water gargles), exposure (illness in other family members), and dysphagia.

PAST HISTORY

Obtain information on immunization status and on previous problems of the respiratory tract (diagnosis, treatment, frequency, hospitalization).

FAMILY HISTORY

Obtain information about familial respiratory tract disorders and illness (allergies, asthma).

HOME ENVIRONMENT

Obtain information on available resources (family, friends, financial), the family's ability to follow a management plan, to make observations of the child's respiratory status, and to return for follow-up care.

Physical Examination

A thorough general physical examination is performed. See Chapter 1, Child Health Assessment. The focus of the examination is to determine the severity of the illness and the location of the abnormality. Table 1 summarizes the signs which are helpful in localizing the respiratory tract abnormality. The key diagnostic technique is observation. Table 2 summarizes the observed physical signs which help to differentiate between an upper and lower airway obstruction.

MEASUREMENTS AND VITAL SIGNS

Obtain weight, temperature, heart rate (see Chapter 19), and respiratory rate.

Respiratory rate. Normal resting respiratory rates are listed in Table 3. Obtain the respiratory rate when the child is quiet and relaxed. Take full 1-minute counts since the rate may normally be uneven. In assessing the rate consider factors such as activity level, anxiety, and fever. The active or febrile infant often has a respiratory rate that is more rapid than the resting rate.

GENERAL APPEARANCE

Assess the overall appearance of the child (prostrate, inactive, apathetic, apprehensive, agitated).

Table 1
Signs Helpful in Localizing Respiratory Tract Abnormality

Site of Abnormality	Signs Evident from Simple Observation of Patient	Signs Evident on Further Exam
Nose	Noisy respirations (nasal congestion) Rhinorrhea Occasional cough (secondary to postnasal drip or associated pharyngitis) No signs of respiratory distress except in young infants who may have obligatory nasal breathing	Nasal mucosa edematous and either red (suggesting infection) or pale (suggesting allergic rhinitis) Nasal discharge (usually thin, clear). Chest clear to auscultation except for transmitted sounds
Paranasal sinuses (ethmoid and maxillary sinuses clinically most significant in children < 6 yrs of age)	Mucopurulent nasal discharge Choking cough (↑ at night, occasionally productive of mucopurulent material) Older children may report postnasal drip and/or pain—frontal, temporal, retro-orbital, or in upper incisors.	Nasal mucosa usually red, edematous Mucopurulent nasal discharge May see mucopurulent discharge in midline of pharynx (postnasal drip)
Pharynx, tonsils	Dysphagia (in severe tonsillopharyngitis) Older children may complain of sore throat; however, sore throat may also result from pain referred from the middle ear, parotid gland	Pharynx red Tonsils enlarged, red, with or without whitish or yellow exudates Petechiae on soft palate (suggesting streptococcal infection) Discrete ulcers on anterior tonsillar pillars or pharynx (suggesting enteroviral infection, herpangina) Anterior cervical lymph node enlargement (with or without tenderness)

Larynx (edema, spasm)	Hoarseness Barking ("croupy") cough Inspiratory stridor Dysphagia, drooling (in epiglottitis) May have signs of respiratory distress (See Croup Syndromes)	Decreased breath sounds Supraclavicular and suprasternal retractions relatively more pronounced (compared to intercostal and subcostal retractions)
Trachea and bronchi (edema, mucus)	Deep ("hacking") cough No signs of respiratory distress unless other areas of respiratory tract are also involved	Rhonchi

Bronchioles (edema, mucus, spasm)	Wheezing (expiratory whistling sound); may be absent in severe airway obstruction
	Hyperexpansion of chest, with increased anterior-posterior diameter and shallow respirations
	May have signs of respiratory distress
		Hyperresonance to percussion
		Decreased breath sounds
		Prolonged expiratory phase
		Musical rales:
		  sonorous
		  sibilant

Alveoli (exudate, edema, collapse)	May have signs of respiratory distress	Over involved lung, *may* have:
		  dullness to percussion
		  decreased breath sounds
		  coarse and fine rales

Pleura	"Splinting" of chest
	May have signs of respiratory distress
		Over involved pleura, *may* have:
		  dullness to percussion
		  decreased breath sounds
		  friction rub

Source: Reprinted with permission from D. S. Rowe, unpublished material, 1973.

Table 2

Differentiation Between Upper and Lower Airway Obstruction by Simple Observation

Physical Sign	Upper Airway Obstruction	Lower Airway Obstruction
Voice	Hoarse[a]	Normal
Cough	Barking (croupy)[a]	Deep (hacking)
Sounds made during breathing	Stridor (high-pitched, crowing sound), more pronounced during inspiration than expiration	Wheezing (whistling sound), more pronounced during expiration than inspiration
Inspiratory/expiratory ratio	Prolonged inspiratory phase	Prolonged expiratory phase
Chest retractions	Supraclavicular, suprasternal, and sternal retractions relatively pronounced (compared with intercostal and subcostal retractions)	Intercostal and subcostal retractions relatively pronounced
Chest configuration	Normal	Increased anterior-posterior diameter
Respiratory rate	Relatively less rapid (rarely over 60/min)	Often very rapid (frequently over 60/min)

Source: Reprinted with permission from E. Waechter and F. Blake, *Nursing Care of Children*, 9th ed. © 1976 by the J. B. Lippincott Company, p. 457.

[a]Hoarseness and a characteristic barking cough are present only when the vocal cords are involved. Children with epiglotitis are usually not hoarse.

Table 3
Normal Resting Respiratory Rate Per Minute

Age (years)	Boys (Mean ± 2 SD)	Girls (Mean ± 2 SD)
0–1	31 ± 16	30 ± 12
1–2	26 ± 8	27 ± 8
2–3	25 ± 8	25 ± 6
3–4	24 ± 6	24 ± 6
4–5	23 ± 4	22 ± 4
5–6	22 ± 4	21 ± 4
6–7	21 ± 6	21 ± 6
7–8	20 ± 6	20 ± 4
8–9	20 ± 4	20 ± 4
9–10	19 ± 4	19 ± 4
10–11	19 ± 4	19 ± 4
11–12	19 ± 6	19 ± 6
12–13	19 ± 6	19 ± 4
13–14	19 ± 4	18 ± 4
14–15	18 ± 4	18 ± 6
15–16	17 ± 6	18 ± 6
16–17	17 ± 4	17 ± 6
17–18	16 ± 6	17 ± 6

Source: From A. Iliff and V. A. Lee, Pulse, respiratory rate, and body temperature of children between 2 months and 18 years, *Child Development,* 1952, 23:238. By permission of The Society for Research in Child Development, Inc.
Data of Iliff and Lee from both fed-sleeping and fasting-awake children.

EAR

Inspect the external canal for discharge (white, cheesy material; thin or thick purulent material) foreign body, lesions. Note pain upon manipulation of the tragus. Examine the tympanic membrane for reddish to greyish-yellow color, absence of the bony landmarks, decreased mobility, and fluid level.

NOSE

Inspect for nasal flaring, discharge, color of the mucous membrane, and foreign body.

PHARYNX AND TONSILS

Inspect for redness, petechiae on the soft palate, discrete ulcers on the anterior tonsillar pillars or pharynx, and exudate on tonsils. Listen for hoarseness. Watch for drooling (epiglottitis).

CHEST

Inspect for pattern of breathing (rate, depth, rhythm, ease), retractions (intercostal, subcostal, supraclavicular, and suprasternal), decreased breath sounds, abnormal auscultatory chest sounds (rales, rhonchi, wheezing), tachypnea, prolonged inspiratory or expiratory phase. See Figure 1 for diagram of retraction scoring.

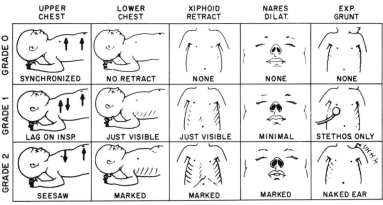

OBSERVATION OF RETRACTIONS

Figure 1. Retraction scoring. An index of respiratory distress is determined by grading each of five arbitrary criteria: grade 0 indicates no difficulty, grade 1 moderate difficulty, and grade 2 maximum respiratory difficulty. The "retraction score" is the sum of these values; a total score of 0 indicates no dyspnea, whereas a total score of 10 denotes maximal respiratory distress. (From W. Silverman, *Dunham's Premature Infants*, 3rd ed., 1961. Courtesy of Paul B. Hoeber Inc.)

Laboratory Procedures

CULTURES

(See Chapter 29, Infectious Diseases.) Nasopharyngeal, sputum, and throat cultures are frequently obtained and often of little help except for identifying beta-hemolytic streptococcus in pharyngitis. For example, a nasal culture will probably show a high bacterial count. This is often mistaken for bacterial disease rather than mere colonization. Interpretation of culture results should consider the origin of the culture (flora of the respiratory tract mucosa normally contain pathogenic organisms) and the possibility of contamination.

CHEST X-RAY

It is usually indicated if the physical examination of the chest reveals any abnormalities or signs of pulmonary dysfunction.

Basic Principles of Infections of the Respiratory Tract

1. Etiologic classification is of limited value due to the large number of different organisms which cause similar clinical symptoms and the few distinctive clinical syndromes.
2. A single organism is capable of producing clinical symptoms of varying severity and extent. The factors that affect the clinical symptoms are: age, sex, previous exposure to the infectious agent, allergy, and nutritional status. For example, illnesses in family members may be simultaneously manifested as the common cold in the parents, bronchiolitis in the infant, and pharyngitis and a subclinical infection in siblings (Vaughan, 1975).
3. Most acute respiratory tract infections are caused by viruses and *Mycoplasma*. The only bacterial agents capable of producing primary nasal or pharyngeal disease are Group A and B

beta-hemolytic streptococci and the diphtheria organism (Vaughan, 1975, p. 937). Lower respiratory illness is also caused mainly by viral agents; however, pneumonia may be caused by the pneumococcus, *Hemophilus influenzae* and, rarely, other bacterial pathogens. Table 4 outlines the ecology of infections, the seasonal pattern, the epidemiology, and the risk of reinfection.

MANAGEMENT

General Measures

FLUIDS

A generous amount of fluids, water in particular, is important. Prevention of dehydration will help prevent thickened mucus. Recommended clear liquids include water, juice, tea, cola, and ginger ale. See Table 2 in Chapter 6 for the amount of fluid required daily.

HUMIDIFICATION

Generally, inspired, humidified air soothes the respiratory mucosa, decreases the viscosity of upper respiratory secretions, and relieves cough and hoarseness of laryngitis. Methods for humidifying air include: steam (boiling water, hot shower) and vaporizer (cool-mist, steam). There is no therapeutic difference between cool-mist and steam vaporizers.

Cool-mist vaporizer. It is preferred for safety reasons, and the mist can be directed toward the child. It is noisier and humidifies the air more slowly than steam vaporizers. Following each use, it is drained and cleaned carefully according to instructions to avoid bacterial overgrowth. As a precaution against excessive moisture, nearby surfaces are protected with towels or absorbent pads.

Table 4

Ecology of Infection with Various Respiratory Tract Pathogens

Group	Serotype	Usual Time of Primary Infection	Person-to-person Spread	Pattern of Infection	Risk of Indicated Illness during Primary Infection	Reinfection
Myxovirus:						
Influenza	A,B	Infancy and childhood; any age for minor antigenic variants	Highly effective	Epidemic—every 2–4 years, usually winter	Influenza—75%	Common with new variants—less common with same variant
Parainfluenza	1,2,3,4	Infancy—type 3 Childhood—types 1,2,4	Highly effective—type 3; less effective—types 1,2,4	Endemic or sporadic—occasionally epidemic (types 1,3)	Febrile respiratory illness—50–75% (types 1,2,3)	Common—can be associated with URI
Resp. syncytial	—	Infancy	Highly effective	Epidemic, every year—fall, winter or spring	Febrile lower respiratory tract illness—45%	Common—often associated with URI
Adenovirus	1,2,3,5,7	Infancy (1,2) Childhood (3,5,7)	Effective (1,2,5) or moderately effective (3,7)	Endemic (occasionally epidemic types 3,7)	Febrile respiratory disease—55–90%	Uncommon
Picornavirus:						
Coxsackie B	—	Infancy and childhood	Moderately effective	Epidemic—summer	Not known	Not known
Rhinovirus	60 or more	All ages	unknown	Endemic sporadic flurries of different types	URI 50%[a]	Occurs
M. pneumoniae	—	2nd and 3rd decades	Ineffective	Endemic or occasionally epidemic	Pneumonia 3—10%[a]	Uncommon

Source: From V. C. Vaughan and R. J. McKay, *Nelson Textbook of Pediatrics*, 10th ed., p. 939, © 1975 by the W. B. Saunders Company, Philadelphia. Table modified from R. M. Chanock and R. H. Parrott: *Pediatrics*, 36:21, 1965.

[a]Data for adult infection.

Steam vaporizer. It emits steam and produces moisture quickly. Additives (designated by manufacturer) are necessary to control the vapor output. The new models are designed to meet safety requirements to prevent tipping over on a 30-degree incline regardless of water level and to prevent water from being scaldingly hot if it should spill. For safety reasons it is still advisable to avoid handling the steam vaporizer unless it is unplugged. It should be placed on the floor to prevent hot steam from reaching the child's face and to avoid accidental tripping. Frequent cleaning is advisable to prevent malfunctioning due to mineral deposits.

COUNSELING. Ideally, vaporizers are purchased before a crisis so a suitable model can be purchased at an economic price. Suggestions for using a vaporizer are:

1. Direct the vapor toward the child
2. Clean unit after each use

MEDICATION

See Chapter 14, Approach to Medications in Childhood.

Cough Suppressants. They are used to depress the cough reflex. They can be useful with a dry, nonproductive, hyperactive, and annoying cough; however, there are very few indications for the use of suppressants. Codeine and dextromethorphan hydrobromide are the common ingredients of suppressant medications.

CODEINE. It is considered to be the most useful narcotic antitussive agent. It has a drying effect on the respiratory mucosa. Side effects include nausea, drowsiness, and constipation. It is contraindicated in children with chronic pulmonary disease.

DEXTROMETHORPHAN HYDROBROMIDE. It is considered to be as effective as codeine but does not depress respiration or predispose to addiction. Side effects are mild and infrequent. The most common complaints are drowsiness and gastrointestinal upset.

Decongestants (sympathomimetics, antihistamines). They are of questionable value, and their use remains controversial (Lampert, 1975; West, 1975). They are either applied topically or administered orally to decrease the edema of the nasal mucosa and to relieve symptoms.

NOSE DROPS. Phenylephrine hydrochloride (e.g., Neo-Synephrine Hydrochloride) is the common ingredient used in topical products. Nose drops must be used with great caution. Overuse may cause rebound edema of the nasal mucosa. They should be avoided during the first 3 months of life.

ORAL PRODUCTS. Pseudoephedrine hydrochloride (e.g., Sudafed) is commonly used in cold products. It should not be used for more than 10 days. Side effects are uncommon, but nervousness, restlessness, or sleeplessness may occur. This medication is not recommended in the presence of high blood pressure, heart disease, diabetes, or thyroid disease without physician consultation. The usual dosage for over-the-counter decongestants is:

- 2 to 5 years: 15 mg, three to four times per day
- 6 to 12 years: 30 mg, three to four times per day
- >12 years: 60 mg, three to four times per day

Expectorants. They are of questionable effectiveness. Glyceryl guaiacolate is the most common ingredient of expectorant medication. It is seldom associated with gastric upset and nausea.

OTHER SYMPTOMATIC MEASURES

1. A bulb syringe is useful for removal of nasal discharge in infants below 3 to 4 months. Drops of physiologic saline prepared by a pharmacist are put into each nostril to liquefy the dried mucus. The bulb is squeezed prior to insertion into the nostril and allowed to suck. The mucus is then squirted onto tissue paper, and the process is repeated as necessary.
2. Hard, sour candies or popsicles relieve cough or sore throat.
3. Warm, saline gargles several times a day relieve sore throat.

4. Fever reduction. See Chapter 13, Approach to Illness in Childhood.

Counseling

The first illness is often a problem of the respiratory system. This is an opportune time to counsel parents about the care of their sick child. Their ideas and practices in the care of their own respiratory illnesses are explored, and good practices are reinforced. Therapeutic measures are practically reviewed. The use of over-the-counter preparations is discussed. See Chapter 14, Approach to Medications in Childhood.

COMMON CLINICAL PROBLEMS

Upper Respiratory Tract

The upper respiratory tract consists of the structures above the larynx: nasal cavity, paranasal sinuses, pharynx, and middle ear.

EPISTAXIS (NOSEBLEEDING)

Assessment. Epistaxis is most often secondary to an upper respiratory infection (URI), dry air, or nose picking. Other causes include:

- Benign or malignant tumor of the nose and paranasal sinuses
- Blood dyscrasias (i.e., leukemia, hemophilia, ITP)
- Dilated vessels in the nasal septum
- Foreign body in the nose
- Nasal polyps
- Severe hypertension
- Trauma

Epistaxis rarely occurs in infancy, but it is common in childhood and decreases after puberty.

Management. Most nosebleeds stop spontaneously. Over 90 percent of them originate in the anterior nasal septum. The following steps are followed to control bleeding:

1. The child is positioned in a sitting posture if possible, and instructed to breathe through the mouth while pressure is applied to the nose.
2. Direct, firm pressure is applied for 2 to 10 minutes from the lateral side of the nose against the septum in the area of Kesselbach's plexus.
3. If bleeding persists, a nose packing by an otolaryngologist may be necessary.
4. Petroleum jelly is applied to the nasal mucosa to alleviate crusting of blood and further excoriation.

Consultation with a physician is indicated if a bleeding site is not identified. If a significant amount of blood was swallowed, the parents are warned that the child might pass a dark, tarry stool or might vomit bloody material.

FOREIGN BODY

Ear

ASSESSMENT. Symptoms may include discharge from the external canal, decreased hearing in the affected ear, and symptoms of inflammation. Failure to remove the foreign body may lead to otitis externa. Examination requires good visualization.

MANAGEMENT. Consultation is obtained. If it is a nonvegetable object, irrigation with water helps to remove the object. If it is a vegetable object, irrigation with water is contraindicated because it may cause the object to swell. A referral to an ENT specialist may be indicated.

Nose

ASSESSMENT. Symptom is unilateral rhinorrhea that is purulent and unresponsive to antimicrobial therapy. Examination requires good visualization. A foreign body that is not removed can induce an acute inflammatory process.

MANAGEMENT. Referral to a physician is indicated if the foreign body cannot be removed easily or if high fever is present. The child may need to be sedated prior to the removal of the object.

Trachea or bronchial tree

ASSESSMENT. Sudden onset of severe coughing without previous history of fever or nasal discharge suggests inhalation of a foreign body. X-rays may be indicated, although a negative X-ray does not rule out the possibility of a foreign body because many substances are not radio-opaque. The cough may become quiescent but may recur later accompanied by fever and possibly dyspnea. Pneumonia may ensue. The problem does not resolve until the foreign body is removed.

MANAGEMENT. ENT and/or surgical consultation is indicated.

IMPACTED CERUMEN

Assessment. The question of how vigorously to pursue visualization of the tympanic membrane is a most common problem. Indication for removal of impacted cerumen include a history of upper respiratory symptoms, fever, or decreased hearing.

Management. To remove cerumen hold the child securely. There are two basic techniques to remove cerumen: dry and wet.

DRY TECHNIQUE. Use a #00 blunt ear curet. Do not use a sharp curet. Gain the cooperation of the child by showing the curet and stroking it lightly over the back of the hand, cheek, and pinna. Clean the canal under direct vision. If the wax is clinging to the walls of the canal, pass the curet beyond it and gently retract the curet with light pressure on the skin of the ear canal. If there is a large mass of wax, pass the curet superior to the mass and position it just behind the mass. Pull the wax mass out of the canal. Parents should be prepared for the possibility of bleeding. The dry technique is successful 95 percent of the time. (Graef, 1974.)

WET TECHNIQUE.   If the wax is pushed firmly against the tympanic membrane, irrigate with water at body temperature. Body temperature is important to avoid vertigo. The wet technique is messier and may frighten children. Do not use this technique if a perforation of the tympanic membrane is suspected because wax may be inadvertently blown into the middle ear.

MEDICATION.   Triethanolamine polypeptide oleate-condensate (Cerumenex) is sometimes prescribed to soften ear wax. Allow the drops to remain in the ear no longer than 15 to 30 minutes because of its potential caustic and allergenic effects. Debrox, hydrogen peroxide, or mineral oil are used to soften hard, dry cerumen. Instill four to five drops two to three times each day for 4 to 5 days. Allow the hydrogen peroxide or mineral oil to remain in the ear for about 15 minutes.

COUNSELING.   Education about ear hygiene is part of routine ambulatory care. Cotton Q-tips are useful for cleaning the external ear, but they should *not* be inserted into the ear canal. If it is necessary to remove cerumen during the clinic visit, the process is explained to the parent and to the child. Prophylactic medication is sometimes prescribed for installation several days prior to the next clinic visit.

INFLUENZA

See Chapter 29.

NASOPHARYNGITIS

Assessment.   In acute nasopharyngitis there is usually a history of recent exposure to a respiratory illness, and the symptoms completely resolve. It is difficult to differentiate allergic rhinitis from recurrent upper respiratory infection. Refer to Chapter 28, Allergic Rhinitis, for more discussion.

INCIDENCE. The number of respiratory infections in children under 6 years ranges from 0 to 15 per year with an average of 7 per year (Dingle, 1964). After the age of 6 the number of colds decreases to 4 to 5 yearly.

ETIOLOGY. Viruses are the primary cause of nasopharyngitis. Refer to Table 4. Of the relatively few bacteria implicated in nasopharyngitis, group A beta-hemolytic streptococcus is the only one that occurs frequently enough to require serious consideration in the general population (Waechter, 1976).

CLINICAL FINDINGS. Nasal congestion, rhinorrhea, and sneezing are the common symptoms. Other symptoms may include fever, sore throat, headaches, muscle aches, intermittent coughing, and decreased appetite. The physical findings include inflammation and edema of nasal mucosal membranes, redness of the pharynx, tonsils, and palpebral conjunctivae, redness and congestion of the tympanic membrane, enlargement of cervical lymph glands.

COURSE OF ILLNESS. The incubation period ranges from 1 to 6 days with an average duration of 2 days. Nasal congestion and cough usually persist for about 1 to 2 weeks. Other symptoms rarely last beyond 2 to 3 days. Persistence of symptoms beyond 2 weeks suggests the possibility of complications.

COMPLICATIONS. The most common complications are secondary bacterial infections of the middle ear and paranasal sinuses. Suppurative cervical adenitis may also occur. A secondary bacterial infection is suspected if fever persists or returns after 3 days.

Management. Management is supportive and symptomatic. See General Measures. Antibiotics are not used except in cases of proven streptococcal infections. Cold preparations and remedies are largely ineffective, and their value remains unproven. Humidification may prevent drying of the nasal mucosa. Nasal mucus can be removed with the bulb syringe in the young infant or with a soft tissue.

COUNSELING. Openly share with parents the current knowledge on nasopharyngitis. Education should include information about the course of illness, signs, and symptoms indicative of bacterial complications and the need for re-evaluation, and the use of medications (see Chapter 14, Approach to Medications in Childhood).

OTITIS EXTERNA (SWIMMER'S EAR)

Assessment. It is a painful infection of the external auditory canal. *Pseudomonas aeruginosa* is the most common causative agent. The common clinical findings are pain upon movement of the tragus, edema, and a whitish cheesy discharge. Otitis externa may follow perforation of tympanic membrane.

Management

MEDICATION. Ear drops containing corticosteroids and antibiotics specific for *P. aeruginosa* and staphylococcus are given as follows: three drops three times per day for 7 to 14 days. Analgesics are given to relieve pain.

COUNSELING. Education is provided about the causes of external otitis, administration of eardrops, and signs and symptoms which indicate the need for further evaluation. Gentle cleansing of the ear canal is done as needed (usually one to two times each week). Cotton is placed in the canal while drainage is present to prevent dermatitis of the pinna. Swimming is not allowed.

PHARYNGOTONSILLITIS

Assessment. It is uncommon in children less than 2 years of age. Thirty to fifty percent of the cases of acute pharyngitis in school age children seen at the health care facility are streptococcal in origin. The incidence of strep pharyngitis increases during the winter and spring months.

ETIOLOGY. Eighty to ninety percent of attacks of acute pharyngotonsillitis are due to viruses (Eichenwald, 1976a). The only common bacterial cause of acute pharyngitis is group A beta hemolytic streptococcus.

CLINICAL PRESENTATION. Distinguishing a viral infection from a bacterial infection requiring antimicrobial therapy is difficult. Table 5 summarizes the major differences. A characteristic scarlatiniform rash sometimes develops within the first 12 hours after the onset of symptoms, and may occur up to 2 days later. (See Chapter 29, Table 1.) The peritonsillar lymph nodes are tender and enlarged. The symptoms usually subside within 24 to 48 hours and rarely continue after 4 to 5 days even without antibiotic therapy.

Table 5
Differentiation of Viral and Streptococcal Pharyngotonsillitis

	Viral Pharyngotonsillitis	*Strep Pharyngotonsillitis*
Age	Any age	Usually over 3 years
Onset	Gradual	Sudden
General appearance	Mild to moderate toxicity and malaise	Moderate to severe toxicity and malaise
Fever	Slight to moderate (38.3°C to 39.4°C)	Moderate to high (38.9°C to 40.6°C)
Symptoms	Cough, conjunctivitis, hoarseness, rhinitis, sore throat	Sore throat, abdominal pain, headache, vomiting
Physical findings	Minimal to moderate tonsillar erythema, none or small exudate (except in infectious mono), minimal to moderate enlargement and tenderness of anterior cervical nodes	Moderate to extensive tonsillar erythema, small to extensive exudate (rule out diphtheria if extensive), petechial mottling of soft palate, moderate to extensive enlargement and tenderness of anterior cervical nodes

Source: Compiled from Eichenwald, 1976a; Green, 1977; and Waechter, 1976.

THROAT CULTURE. A throat culture is the most reliable method of identifying a streptococcal infection. Criteria for when to obtain a throat culture in children below 3 years of age are poorly defined since the incidence is less and complications are uncommon. One guideline is to obtain a throat culture from infants who have a prolonged illness with thin nasal discharge or who have exudative tonsillitis. (Waechter, 1976, p. 450.) Honikman and Massel's (1971) guidelines for obtaining throat cultures in school age children are useful in communities in which streptococcal infection and its complications are common. A throat culture is obtained on any child with:

1. A pure or predominant sore throat and fever of any degree (over 37.3°C orally)
2. Associated oral temperature of 38.3°C or higher

If there is any question about the etiology, a throat culture is taken.

COMPLICATIONS.

Suppurative:

• Cervical adenitis
• Otitis media
• Peritonsillar abscess (uncommon but serious)
• Sinusitis

Nonsuppurative:

• Acute poststreptococcal glomerulonephritis
• Acute rheumatic fever

Management. Medication is best delayed until throat culture results are available, even when strep pharyngitis is strongly suspected. Antimicrobial therapy is still effective in preventing acute rheumatic fever even if treatment is delayed up to 9 days after the onset of symptoms.

ANTIMICROBIAL THERAPY. Penicillin is the drug of choice for 10 days for acute streptococcal pharyngotonsillitis. The choice of route of administration depends on the ability and willingness of the child to take the oral medication and on the parents' ability to comply with the 10-day treatment. See Chapter 14, Compliance.

Erythromycin is given to children with a documented penicillin allergy. Sulfonamides are effective prophylactically but are ineffective in the treatment of streptococcal infections.

SUPPORTIVE THERAPY. See General Measures. For sore throats warm, normal saline gargle several times each day soothes irritated mucosa. Hard, sour candy is useful with a dry, raspy throat since it acts as a demulcent by increasing the flow of saliva. Hot or cold compresses to tender cervical nodes may comfort the child.

EXPOSED CONTACTS. Throat cultures are indicated for symptomatic family members; but if recurrent streptococcal pharyngitis occurs within the family, all family members should be cultured.

COUNSELING. Education should include information about the course of illness, the necessity for a full 10-day course of treatment if strep is the etiologic agent, side effects of the antibiotic, and signs and symptoms indicative of bacterial complications.

SEROUS OTITIS MEDIA

Assessment. It is a noninfectious condition with an accumulation of fluid in the middle ear.

ETIOLOGY. It is caused by allergy, nasopharyngeal inflammation, or barotrauma (such as rapid descent in a nonpressurized aircraft cabin). It is often a sequelae of suppurative otitis media.

CLINICAL FINDINGS. A marked conductive hearing loss that continues for weeks or months is the principal symptom. The fluid produces a sensation of fullness in the ear, decreasing hearing, and a "popping" sound with swallowing. The tympanic membrane is retracted, translucent, and dull. Fluid may or may not be evident behind the drum. Decreased mobility of the drum is evident with pneumatic otoscopy or electronic tympanometry.

Management. Attention is directed toward the identification of the cause of serous otitis media. Oral decongestants are usually prescribed, but their efficacy is unproven. See Decongestants, this chapter. Children with a history of allergies can be treated with a traditional program of environmental control and antihistamines. Insertion of small plastic tubes in the tympanic membrane for chronic conditions does temporarily aerate the middle ear and improve hearing; however, the problem may recur upon removal of the tubes.

SINUSITIS (ACUTE)

Assessment. Acute bacterial sinusitis is seen as a complication of acute viral nasopharyngitis. The signs occur shortly after the acute phase of the illness, just when the child should be improving.

ETIOLOGY. It may be viral or bacterial in origin. In young children *H. influenzae,* pneumococcus, group A streptococcus, staphylococcus are the primary organisms.

CLINICAL FINDINGS. Mucopurulent nasal discharge is the most common finding. Fever, headache, and localized sinus pain are rarely seen in early childhood. A postnasal discharge tends to precipitate coughing attacks. Pain of the upper teeth and cheeks may indicate maxillary sinusitis; increased pain on bending the head forward may indicate frontal sinusitis.

LABORATORY STUDIES. X-ray studies confirm the diagnosis in children after 5 years of age. Prior to this age the X-rays are difficult to interpret.

COMPLICATIONS

- Acute orbital cellulitis
- Meningitis, subdural abscess, epidural abscess
- Cavernous sinus thrombosis

Management. There is no specific therapy for acute viral sinusitis.

MEDICATION

1. A short course of topical decongestant may be helpful in shrinking swollen nasal mucosa and facilitating sinus drainage. See this chapter, Decongestants.

2. Ten to fourteen days of ampicillin therapy is the drug of choice for bacterial sinusitis.

COUNSELING. Parents are educated about the course of the illness, signs and symptoms of secondary bacterial infection (mucopurulent discharge, persistent cough, malaise), and the necessity for the 10 to 14 day course of therapy if antibiotics are prescribed.

SUPPURATIVE OTITIS MEDIA

Assessment. A bacterial infection of the middle ear is the most common infection of infants and children. One factor which is popularly considered to be a cause of the high incidence of middle-ear infection is the anatomic difference in the eustachian tube. In the infant the eustachian tube is shorter and more horizontal compared to the adult.

ETIOLOGY. Causative organisms vary with age. During the first 6 weeks of life, the most common causes are: gram-negative bacilli and staphylococci. In infants and children the most common causes are: *D. pneumoniae* and *H. influenzae. Mycoplasma pneumoniae* and viruses are infrequent isolates.

CLINICAL FINDINGS. Nasal congestion, irritability and cough are often the only presenting symptoms. Fever is absent in 30 to 50 percent of bacterially proven otitis media. Other associated symptoms include vomiting, diarrhea, and difficulty in hearing.

DIAGNOSIS. The diagnosis is based on the abnormal appearance of the tympanic membrane: outward bulging of the tympanic membrane which obscures the normal bony landmarks and light reflex. The redness of the tympanic membrane alone is insufficient evidence to establish the diagnosis of suppurative otitis media.

COMPLICATIONS

- Chronicserous otitis media
- Hearing loss
- Mastoiditis (rare)
- Meningitis (rare)

Management

MEDICATION. Selection of an antibiotic is based on the age of the child.

- Neonatal (birth to 6 weeks). Therapy is aimed at gram-negative bacilli and staphylococci. Ampicillin is combined with kanamycin or gentamicin. Hospitalization is indicated for parenteral therapy and observation for generalized sepsis.
- 6 weeks to 6 years. Therapy is aimed at *D. pneumococci* and *H. influenzae.* Ampicillin is the drug of choice (50 to 100 mg/kg/24 hrs) in four divided doses for 10 days. Alternative choices are Penicillin V combined with sulfisoxazole or erythromycin combined with sulfisoxazole.
- Older children (>6 years). Penicillin or erythromycin alone may be given. To cover the possibility of *H. influenzae,* the antimicrobial therapy recommended for children 6 weeks to 6 years of age may be given.

Decongestants are frequently prescribed as adjuncts to the antibiotic therapy; however, their efficacy has not been proven. See this chapter, Decongestants.

MYRINGOTOMY. It is rarely performed. The major indication for myringotomy is severe ear pain unrelieved by analgesic medication.

FOLLOW-UP. A follow-up visit is scheduled 2 to 3 weeks after the initiation of therapy to re-evaluate the middle ear and check hearing response.

RECURRENT SUPPURATIVE OTITIS MEDIA. Approximately 50 percent of infants and children have at least one other middle-ear infection within 4 months following the diagnosis of the first one, caused by a different organism. This suggests that the second episode is a new infection, not an exacerbation of the previous episode. Referral to an otologist is indicated for frequent recurrent episodes of suppurative otitis media.

COUNSELING. Education should include information about the causes and complications of otitis media, the side effects of the antibiotic, the importance of giving the antibiotic for the entire course of therapy, and the need to return for a follow-up evaluation.

Lower Respiratory Tract

Conditions affecting the larynx, trachea, bronchi, and bronchioles warrant careful evaluation because of the potential interference with ventilation.

RESPIRATORY DISTRESS

Assessment. It indicates lower respiratory tract abnormality and may require emergency measures.

ETIOLOGY

1. Respiratory tract infection (i.e., bronchiolitis, acute epiglottis, spasmodic laryngitis, acute laryngotracheobronchitis, pneumonia).
2. Noninfectious respiratory tract abnormality (i.e., asthma, atelectasis, aspiration, pneumothorax)
3. Cardiac disorders (i.e., congestive heart failure). See Chapter 19.
4. Generalized metabolic disorders (i.e., acidosis, salicylate poisoning)
5. Neurologic disorders (i.e., encephalitis, intracranial hemorrhage, meningitis)
6. Sepsis

CLINICAL EVALUATION. Signs of respiratory distress are: cyanosis, expiratory grunting, inspiratory chest retractions (subcostal, intercostal, suprasternal, supraclavicular), nasal flaring, and tachypnea (the most sensitive indicator). A consistently elevated respiratory rate is more important than the specific rate. Guidelines for determining tachypnea are:

Age	Respiratory Rate
Newborn	> 50
One year	> 36
Five years	> 25
Adolescent	> 22

See Figure 1, Retraction Scoring.

Management. Immediate referral to a physician is indicated. Treatment is directed toward the basic disease as well as the administration of oxygen. (A fire truck may be the quickest source.)

SUPPORTIVE MEASURES. See Chapter 18, General Measures. Oral hydration and humidification are essential. Oxygen therapy is almost always indicated. Specific additional therapy depends on the etiology of the respiratory distress.

COUNSELING. Parents are often frightened when their child is in respiratory distress. Education should include observational guidelines for assessing the condition of the child, including how to count respiratory rates, positions for easier breathing, and possibly pulmonary resuscitation measures.

BRONCHIOLITIS

Assessment. It is a viral infection of the small bronchi and bronchioles characterized by lower airway obstruction. Obstruction is caused by edema, accumulation of mucus, and bronchospasm.

INCIDENCE. It occurs during the first 2 years of life with a peak incidence at 6 weeks of age. The highest incidence occurs during the winter and early spring months.

ETIOLOGY. The causative agent in over 50 percent of the cases is respiratory syncytial virus (RSV). Other viruses include: parainfluenza type 3, adenovirus, and rhinovirus type 2.

CLINICAL PICTURE. The infant suddenly develops respiratory difficulty after 1 to 2 days of coryza and cough. Respiratory difficulty is characterized by prolongation of expiratory phase and wheezing. The acute phase is usually 24 to 48 hours after the onset of wheezing. Usually within a few days the wheezing subsides, but a deep, hacking cough may persist for 2 to 3 weeks. Fever is rarely higher than 38.3°C and may even be absent. The degree of respiratory distress is variable. Physical findings may include tachypnea, cyanosis, flaring of the alae nasi, shallow intercostal and subcostal retractions, and inspiratory rales. See Figure 1 for retraction scoring.

LABORATORY. Chest films are obtained. Blood gas determinations may be necessary to rule out other causes of severe respiratory distress.

DIFFERENTIAL DIAGNOSIS

- Asthma (one injection of epinephrine to test reversible bronchospasm may be helpful)
- Primary pneumonia
- Foreign body aspiration
- Anaphylactic reactions to drugs, food proteins, or other allergic substances
- Poisoning

COMPLICATIONS

- Pneumonia (over 30 percent of hospitalized infants with bronchiolitis have chest X-rays revealing pulmonary infiltrates)
- Atelectasis
- Pneumomediastinum (rare)
- Pneumothorax (rare)
- Subcutaneous emphysema (rare)

Management. If the child is severely ill, hospitalization is indicated for treatment with humidified oxygen and observation of respiratory status. Mild infections can be managed supportively at home.

HYDRATION. See General Measures. Oral fluids are important to prevent dehydration and thickening of mucus in the lower respiratory tract; they are contraindicated in severe respiratory distress because vomiting may be induced and aspiration pneumonia may ensue.

HUMIDIFICATION. See General Measures. Cold steam is traditionally used, although there is good evidence that the water particles do not reach the bronchioles.

MEDICATION. Bronchodilators and corticosteroids have not been proven effective in the management of bronchiolitis. Antimicrobials are not indicated unless a superimposed bacterial pneumonia is present.

COUNSELING. Caring for a child in respiratory distress is a frightening experience for parents. They need clear instructions for managing the child at home. Explanations should be given about the course of the illness and the signs and symptoms which indicate progressive respiratory distress. Often asking parents "What are you most afraid of?" will provide directions for further counseling.

CROUP SYNDROMES

Assessment. The term "croup" refers to syndromes or diseases that present with inspiratory stridor. These conditions are further characterized by a "brassy" or "barking" cough, hoarseness, and respiratory distress. The three forms of the croup syndromes are: acute epiglottitis, spasmodic laryngitis, and acute laryngotracheobronchitis (LTB). Table 6 summarizes the clinical presentation, clinical findings, and treatment for each of these croup syndromes.

ACUTE EPIGLOTTITIS. *This is a medical emergency.* It is a rapidly progressing supraglottic obstruction due most commonly to *H. influenzae.* The child characteristically sits with his chin extended and breathes slowly through the mouth. Swallowing is painful and drooling is common. Examination of the posterior pharynx is deferred until the personnel and equipment are available to perform

Table 6
Croup Syndromes

	Epiglottitis (Acute)	Spasmodic Laryngitis	Acute LTB
Primary age	>3 years	1 to 3 years	6 months to 3 years
Etiology	Usually *H. influenzae*, occasionally pneumococcus or viruses	Uncertain; possibly viral	Virus (RSV, parainfluenzae, influenzae)
Onset	Rapid (4 to 12 hours)	Sudden, usually at night	Gradual (may become progressively severe over 24 hrs)
Presenting complaints	High fever (37.8°C to 40.6°C), acute inspiratory stridor, drooling, dysphagia	No fever, severe inspiratory stridor, "barking" cough, hoarseness	"Barking" cough, hoarseness, grad. increasing inspiratory stridor, low or absent fever
Physical examination	Pharynx inflamed, diminished breath sounds, pallor, inspiratory rhonchi, severe respiratory distress	Diminished breath sounds, labored respirations, respiratory distress, accelerated pulse	Diminished breath sounds, inspiratory rales, respiratory distress, expiratory phase of respiration labored and prolonged
Laryngeal findings	Inflammation of supraglottic structures, grossly edematous, red epiglottis (raspberry)	Spasm of vocal cords (glottic), inflammation minimal	Edema of subglottic area, mildly reddened and mildly edematous epiglottis
Clinical course	Rapidly progressive (within 6 to 12 hours), total airway obstruction	Self-limited, usually within hours but may be recurrent the following night	Moderate airway obstruction may persist, rapid respiratory failure may develop
Bacterial complications	Common when causative agent is *H. influenzae* and pneumococcus	None	Rare
Treatment	Antibiotics and airway maintenance; hospitalization is mandatory; cool-mist; oxygen; tracheotomy or ET tube may be necessary.	Cool or warm humidification; oxygen; relief of laryngospasm may be obtained from racemic epinephrine from IPPB machine.	Cool-mist; oxygen; bed rest; hydration; stridor relieved by racemic epinephrine via IPPB machine; tracheotomy is rarely necessary.

Source: Information gathered from Eichenwald, 1976a; Tooley, 1977; and Vaughan, 1975.

an emergency endotracheal intubation or tracheotomy in the event of complete obstruction.

SPASMODIC LARYNGITIS. This infection causes acute inspiratory obstruction of the vocal cords. The child typically awakens during the night with a barking cough, hoarseness, and marked inspiratory stridor. The attack lasts several hours, subsides, and may recur during the next several nights. The examination of the posterior pharynx reveals minimal inflammation.

ACUTE LARYNGOTRACHEOBRONCHITIS (LTB). This is the most common croup syndrome in young children 6 months to 3 years of age. The child usually has nasal congestion and occasional cough for 1 to 2 days prior to the development of inspiratory stridor. Inspiratory stridor results from edema of the subglottic area. The cautious examination of the posterior pharynx reveals a mildly reddened and mildly edematous epiglottis. The attack reaches maximal severity within 24 hours. Stridor and chest retraction diminish within 3 to 4 days, but the paroxysmal, barking cough may persist for 2 to 3 weeks.

Management

ACUTE EPIGLOTTITIS. See Table 6. Intravenous ampicillin is administered. Improvement occurs within 24 hours after initiating treatment. Within 2 to 5 days the tracheostomy or ET tube can be removed.

SPASMODIC LARYNGITIS. See Table 6. Warm steam from a hot shower can bring immediate relief. If this is unsuccessful, the child is taken to the emergency room. Racemic epinephrine administered by intermittent positive pressure brings relief.

ACUTE LARYNGOTRACHEOBRONCHITIS. See Table 6. Therapy includes cool-mist, hydration, and bed rest. See General Measures. Hospitalization may be necessary. Systemic steroid treatment has been frequently used, but its value has not been proven in controlled trials. Nebulized racemic epinephrine by IPPB causes short-term relief of stridor but may need to be repeated at 4-hour intervals. Emergency tracheotomy or endotracheal intubation may be necessary before the development of severe hypoxia or complete airway obstruction.

COUNSELING. Stridor, coughing, and laryngeal spasms are frightening to the child and to the parents. The child needs the emotional closeness of a protective person. Holding infants and children securely in the arms helps to relax them and to make them feel safe. Education should include information about the course of illness of the specific croup syndrome, observational guidelines for respiratory distress, and supportive measures.

PNEUMONIA

Assessment. It is one of the common serious childhood infections. The presentation of pneumonia is highly variable depending on factors such as the age of the child and the etiologic organism. Any child with suspected pneumonia should be evaluated by a physician. Refer to any standard pediatric textbook for more specific information.

ETIOLOGY. The causative agents are: viruses (cause of the majority of pediatric pneumonias), *Mycoplasma pneumoniae* (common cause in children 5 to 15 years of age), staphylococcus (most common in infants under 2 years), *Diplococcus pneumoniae* (most frequent cause for all ages of the bacterial pathogens). *Mycobacterium tuberculosis* should be considered as the etiologic agent for any age.

CLINICAL PICTURE. The manifestations of pneumonia in infants and children are highly variable. Some children appear very sick while others do not seem ill at all. The most common presenting symptoms are fever and cough. Other symptoms include dyspnea, tachypnea, chills, chest or abdominal pain. Young infants may have just vomiting or diarrhea initially. The physical findings may or may not reveal signs of respiratory distress, rales, or decreased breath sounds over the inflamed area. In spite of the variability of signs and symptoms, pneumonias caused by *D. pneumococcus, Mycoplasma pneumoniae,* and staphylococcus have characteristic clinical pictures.

Mycoplasma pneumonia.   It is more common in older children. The early clinical features include insidious onset, malaise, headache, low-grade fever, sore throat, nonproductive cough, and normal chest findings during the early course of the illness. The chest X-ray findings include interstitial pneumonitis and areas of consolidation.

Pneumococcal pneumonia.   It occurs at all ages. It typically presents after 1 or 2 days of mild nasal discharge and cough with an abrupt high fever and respiratory distress. Inflammatory edema and the exudation of serum and red cells into the alveoli result in early consolidation. The chest X-ray is usually positive for infiltrates. The chest examination may be unremarkable. The white blood cell count is usually elevated.

Staphylococcal pneumonia.   It is a life-threatening illness that is most common in infants under 2 years. The typical history is of an infant who abruptly develops respiratory distress following a variable period of a mild respiratory illness. Within a few hours the infant's condition rapidly deteriorates. The signs include rapidly evolving respiratory distress (see Figure 1, Retraction Scoring), cyanosis, pallor, and abdominal distention. Fever is either low grade or absent. Auscultation of the chest is often not helpful. The chest X-ray may be normal or show only faint focal mottling.

LABORATORY PROCEDURES
- Blood cultures (for etiologic diagnosis)
- Chest X-ray
- Tuberculin skin test (rule out *Mycobacterium tuberculosis*)

UNDERLYING ABNORMALITIES.   The possibility of a foreign body aspiration should be explored with the parents. If pneumonia is recurrent or persistent, consideration is given to the following:

- Asthma
- Bronchiectasis
- Congenital anomalies
- Immune deficiency states

COMPLICATIONS

- Fluid in the pleural space (pleural effusion, empyema)
- Pneumothorax

Management. Consultation and referral to the physician is indicated. The child's age and condition, severity of the symptoms, causative agent, and availability of adequate home care determine the management plan.

INDICATIONS FOR HOSPITALIZATION

- Infants under 6 months of age
- Severe respiratory distress
- Toxic appearance
- Staphylococcal pneumonia
- Inadequate home care

MEDICATION. Antimicrobial therapy depends on the age of the child and on the causative agent. Expectorants and antitussives are of questionable value and may even be unwise. See this chapter, Medication.

SUPPORTIVE CARE. See General Measures. Adequate hydration is necessary to prevent thickening of secretions. A vaporizer may provide some relief but its value is questionable.

Counseling. Education should include information about the course of the illness, side effects of the medication, observational guidelines for respiratory distress, and specific supportive measures.

References

American Pharmaceutical Association. *Handbook of Prescription Drugs,* 5th ed. Washington DC, 1977.

Bass, J. W., et al. "Streptococcal Pharyngitis in Children." *JAMA* 235:1112–1116, March 15, 1976.

Chinn, P. *Child Health Maintenance*. St. Louis: Mosby, 1974.

De Angelis, C. *Basic Pediatrics for the Primary Health Care Provider*. Boston: Little, Brown, 1975.

Dingle, J. F., G. F. Badger, and W. S. Jordan. *Illness in the Home: A Study of 25,000 Illnesses in a Group of Cleveland Families*. Cleveland: Press of Case Western Reserve University, 1964.

Editors of Consumer Reports. *The Consumers Union Guide to Buying for Babies*. New York: Warner Books Edition, 1975.

Editors for Consumer Reports. *The Medicine Show*, rev. ed. New York: Consumers Union, 1976.

Eichenwald, H. P. "Respiratory Infections in Children." *Hospital Practice* 11:81–90. April 1976a.

Eichenwald, H. P. "Pneumonia Syndromes in Children." *Hospital Practice* 11:89–96, May 1976b.

Graef, J. W. and T. E. Cone Jr. *Manual of Pediatric Therapeutics*. Boston: Little, Brown, 1974.

Honikman, L. H. and B. F. Massell. "Guidelines for the Selective Use of Throat Cultures in the Diagnosis of Streptococcal Respiratory Infections." *Pediatrics* 48:573–582, October 1971.

Illiff, A. and V. A. Lee. "Pulse, Respiratory Rate, and Body Temperature of Children Between Two Months and Eighteen Years." *Child Dev* 23:237–245, December 1952.

Lampert, R. P., D. S. Robinson, and L. F. Soyka. "A Critical Look at Decongestants." *Pediatrics* 55:550–552, April 1975.

Levy, J. S. and G. Lovejoy. "Management of Pharyngitis by Pediatric Nurse Practitioners." *Clin Pediatr* 15:415–418, May 1976.

Lipow, H. W. "Respiratory Tract Infections." In M. Green and R. J. Haggerty, editors, *Ambulatory Pediatrics, II*. Philadelphia: Saunders, 1977. Pp. 36–72.

McCracken, G. H., Jr. "Managing Neonatal Infections." *Hospital Practice* 11:49–57, February 1976.

McMillan, J. A., P. I. Nieburg, and F. A. Oski. *The Whole Pediatrician Catalog*. Philadelphia: Saunders, 1977.

Rowe, D. S. "Acute Suppurative Otitis Media." *Pediatrics* 56:285–294, August 1975.

Rowe, D. S. "Signs Helpful in Localizing Respiratory Tract Abnormality," unpublished material. San Francisco: University of California, June 1973.

Rudolph, A., editor. *Pediatrics*, 16th ed. New York: Appleton-Century-Crofts, 1977.

Silverman, W., editor. *Dunham's Premature Infants*, 3rd ed. New York: Hoeber, 1961.

Stool, S. E. and C. S. McConnell Jr. "Foreign Bodies in Pediatric Otolaryngology." *Clin Pediatr* 12:113–116, February 1973.

Tooley, W. H. and H. W. Lipow. "Specific Diseases Causing Obstruction." In A. Rudolph, editor, *Pediatrics*. New York: Appleton-Century-Crofts, 1977. Pp. 1554–1571.

Vaughan, V. C. and R. J. McKay, editors. *Nelson Textbook of Pediatrics*, 10th ed. Philadelphia: Saunders, 1975.

Waechter, E. and F. Blake. *Nursing Care of Children*, 9th ed. Philadelphia: Lippincott, 1976.

West, S., et al. "A Review of Antihistamines and the Common Cold." *Pediatrics* 56:100–107, July 1975.

19

The Heart

Approximately 8 to 10 of every thousand live-born children have a congenital cardiac disorder. Some cardiac defects are detectable at birth or during early infancy, and a few do not become manifest until later in childhood. Many infants with severe defects succumb during the first month of life, but others go undetected until symptoms of cardiac decompensation occur.

The role of the nurse practitioner in relation to the cardiovascular system is to identify those children with signs or symptoms of congenital heart disease and to refer them immediately for medical evaluation. This chapter presents information that will assist the nurse practitioner in screening children for cardiac disease and in providing counsel and support to affected families. A complete discussion of specific congenital cardiac defects is beyond the scope of this book and may be found by consulting the major textbooks listed under References.

ASSESSMENT

Normal Values

Pulse rate, respiratory rate, and blood pressure vary considerably from infancy through childhood. Measurements need to be ob-

581

tained with the child at rest since exercise or crying will affect values. The average pulse rates and blood pressure levels for children are shown in Tables 1 and 2 respectively. Average respiratory rates are found in Chapter 18, The Respiratory System, Table 1. Concern about blood pressure control and the early origins of cardiovascular disease have led to attempts to monitor blood pressure closely from childhood onward. Figures 1 (A and B) are newly developed charts of percentiles of blood pressures for children ages 2 to 18 years. The charts are recommended for use in plotting blood pressures during growth and maturation as a mechanism for determining patterns over time (Blumenthal, 1977). They may be obtained from: National High Blood Pressure Education Program, Landow Building, 13th floor, 7910 Woodmont Avenue, Bethesda, MD 20014.

History

PAST HISTORY

Obtain information on maternal infection during pregnancy (e.g., rubella); fetal distress; Down's syndrome or other genetic syndromes; signs or symptoms of congenital heart disease; heart murmurs, group A beta-hemolytic streptococcal infections, and rheumatic fever.

FAMILY HISTORY

Obtain information on incidence of heart attack (include age of occurrence), high cholesterol levels, type II hyperlipoproteinemia (familial hypercholesterolemia), high blood pressure, stroke, obesity, congenital heart disease in sibling or other family member, and rheumatic fever.

Physical Examination

GENERAL APPEARANCE

Observe activity levels and degree of fatigability. Measure height and weight.

Table 1
Average Pulse Rates at Rest

Age	Lower Limits of Normal		Average		Upper Limits of Normal	
Newborn	70		120		170	
1–11 months	80		120		160	
2 years	80		110		130	
4 years	80		100		120	
6 years	75		100		115	
8 years	70		90		110	
10 years	70		90		110	
	Girls	*Boys*	*Girls*	*Boys*	*Girls*	*Boys*
12 years	70	65	90	85	110	105
14 years	65	60	85	80	105	100
16 years	60	55	80	75	100	95
18 years	55	50	75	70	95	90

Source: From V. C. Vaughan and R. J. McKay, editors, *Nelson Textbook of Pediatrics*, 10th ed., p. 1003. © 1975 by W. B. Saunders Company, Philadelphia.

Table 2
Normal Arterial Blood Pressures at Different Ages

Age	Systolic		Diastolic	
	50th Percentile (mm Hg)	95th Percentile (mm Hg)	50th Percentile (mm Hg)	95th Percentile (mm Hg)
Birth–6 months	80	110	45	60
3 years	95	112	64	80
5 years	97	115	65	84
10 years	110	130	70	92
15 years	116	138	70	95
Adults	120	140	80	90–95

Source: Reprinted with permission from A. M. Rudolph, editor, *Pediatrics*, 16th ed. (New York: Appleton-Century-Crofts, 1977), p. 1485. Adapted from Londe: Clin Pediatr 5:71, 1966; Moss and Adams: Problems of Blood Pressure in Childhood, Springfield, Ill, Thomas, 1962; Zinner et al: *N Engl J Med* 284:401, 1971.

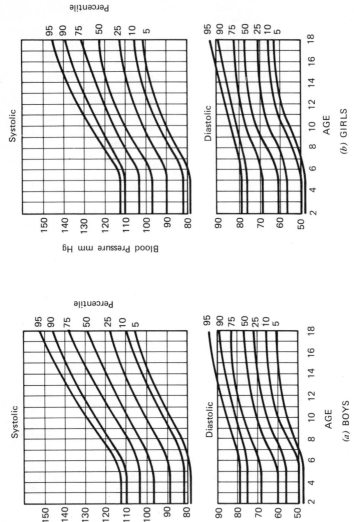

Figure 1. Percentiles of blood pressure measurement (right arm, seated). (*a*) Boys. (*b*) Girls. (Reprinted with permission from S. Blumenthal et al., "Report of the Task Force on Blood Pressure Control in Children," *Pediatrics*, Supplement, Vol. 59, No. 5, Part 2, May 1977, p. 803.)

VITAL SIGNS

Obtain pulse rate, respiratory rate, and blood pressure. If the respiratory rate in a quiet, resting child is above 50, suspicion index should rise.

- Blood pressure. The cuff must cover two thirds of the upper arm or leg and three fourths of the limb's circumference. In children over 1 year of age, systolic pressure in the thighs is usually about 20 mm Hg higher than in the arms.

EYES

Observe for periorbital edema.

SKIN

Observe for pallor, cyanosis, and excessive perspiration.

CHEST

Observe for retractions. Listen for rales. See also Chapter 18, Physical Examination.

HEART

Inspect and palpate for evidence of cardiac enlargement (precordial bulging, distended or pulsating neck veins), location and character of apex beat, and presence of heaves or thrills. Percussion is not generally useful in infants and small children. Auscultate heart sounds for rate and rhythm. Note character and intensity of each heart sound (S_1 and S_2). Listen for extra sounds and note timing, intensity, and pitch. Listen for murmurs and describe timing (systolic or diastolic), location, radiation (use the "inching" technique to follow sound to axillae, back, and neck), quality, and intensity. Note whether the murmur changes with position change from supine to sitting. Grade the murmur according to the following scale:

- Grade 1. Very faint and heard only after the examiner has "tuned in"; may not be heard in all positions
- Grade 2. Quiet but heard immediately upon placing the stethoscope on the chest
- Grade 3. Moderately loud; not associated with a thrill
- Grade 4. Loud and may be associated with a thrill
- Grade 5. Very loud; associated with a thrill
- Grade 6. Heard with the stethoscope off the chest; associated with a thrill (Bates, 1974, p. 114)

ABDOMEN

Palpate for hepatomegaly and splenomegaly.

EXTREMITIES

Observe for clubbing of fingers and toes; edema. Palpate pulses (radial, femoral, carotid, popliteal, and pedal) for regularity and intensity. Absent femoral pulses suggest coarctation of the aorta.

Signs and Symptoms of Congenital Heart Disease

INFANCY

The findings in infancy include anorexia, cyanosis, delayed development, enlarged heart or liver, exertional dyspnea during feeding, failure to gain weight, heart murmurs, persistent tachycardia (over 150 to 200 per minute at rest), rapid respiratory rate (over 50 to 60 per minute at rest), recurrent respiratory infections, and respiratory distress.

CHILDHOOD

In older children additional findings include clubbing of the fingers and toes, decreased exercise tolerance, dyspnea, poor physical development, and squatting.

Signs and Symptoms of Congestive Heart Failure

Any child suspected of congestive failure should be treated as an emergency. Symptoms include dyspnea, fatigue, weakness, irritability, weak cry, poor feeding, and sweating (prominent on exertion). Signs include enlarged heart, hepatomegaly, neck vein distention, tachycardia (pulse over 140 in sleeping infants, over 100 in sleeping older children), tachypnea (50 to 100 or faster), and retractions. Late findings include facial and periorbital edema, pulmonary edema, and pulmonary rales.

Signs and Symptoms of Rheumatic Fever (Acquired Heart Disease)

Rheumatic fever is an inflammatory disease that can cause cardiac damage. It occurs most commonly between 5 and 15 years of age. It is usually a sequel to a preceding group A streptococcal infection.

JONES CRITERIA

The presence of two major or one major and two minor manifestations with evidence of a preceding streptococcal infection indicates a high probability of rheumatic fever (Kempe, 1976, p. 343).

Major manifestations.   These include:

1. Carditis. Significant new murmur, tachycardia, evidence of congestive heart failure, and enlarging heart
2. Polyarthritis. Two or more joints affected by heat, redness, swelling, severe pain, and tenderness
3. Chorea. Emotional lability and involuntary movements appearing most often in prepubertal girls usually several months after streptococcal infection
4. Erythema marginatum. Macular erythematous rash with a serpiginous pattern primarily on the trunk and extremities
5. Subcutaneous nodules. Joints, scalp, and spine are affected

Minor manifestations. These include:

1. Clinical findings of:
   - Previous rheumatic fever or streptococcal infection
   - Fever
   - Arthralgia

2. Laboratory findings of:
   - Increased erythrocyte sedimentation rate (ESR) or C-reactive protein (CRP)
   - Increased white blood count (WBC) and anemia
   - Prolonged PR and QT intervals on electrocardiogram (ECG)
   - Increased antistreptolysin titer (ASLO)

MANAGEMENT

An infant or child who manifests any of the preceding signs or symptoms is referred for medical evaluation. The diagnosis of congenital or acquired heart disease requires specialized medical management and supervision. Once the referral is made, the role of the nurse practitioner remains active. The objectives of care are:

1. To provide on-going preventive and health maintenance services in collaboration with the physician
2. To provide support for the family during diagnosis and treatment
3. To assist the family to understand the diagnosis and treatment plan
4. To provide opportunity for family members to express their feelings and concerns
5. To provide the teaching necessary for parents to care for the child at home including:
   - Reduction of the work load of the heart
   - Reduction of respiratory distress

- Recognition of symptoms of congestive heart failure
- Prevention of respiratory infections
- Maintenance of nutrition

6. To initiate public health nursing referral where indicated

COMMON CLINICAL PROBLEMS

The Innocent Murmur

ASSESSMENT

By far the most common clinical situation encountered in pediatric primary care settings is the identification of innocent heart murmurs in infants and young children. An innocent heart murmur is a cardiac murmur occurring in the absence of significant heart disease or structural abnormality of the heart. At least 30 percent of children may have innocent murmurs detected at a single, random examination (Vaughan, 1975, p. 1002).

General characteristics of innocent murmurs. The characteristics of innocent murmurs which help to distinguish them from significant murmurs include the following:

- Usually systolic in timing except for the venous hum
- Duration usually short
- Loudest usually at the lower left sternal border or at the second or third left intercostal space
- Variation in loudness and presence from visit to visit
- Usually soft (no more than grade 2/6) and localized
- Rarely transmitted
- Changes in loudness with position change
- Heard best in the recumbent position, during expiration and after exercise, except the venous hum
- Heart sounds normal

- Normal pulses, respiratory rate, and blood pressure (Caceres, 1967, pp. 99–100).

Additional features. With increased body temperature there is increased heart rate, increased cardiac output, and increased velocity of flow. Consequently, the intensity of innocent murmurs may increase during acute infections associated with fever. Soft murmurs also may develop during acute illness or severe anemia and disappear during convalescence.

Types of innocent murmurs. Common innocent murmurs are described.

1. Still's murmur is a soft, low-pitched, mid-systolic, musical murmur heard best at the apex and lower left sternal border with the child lying down.
2. Basal ejection systolic murmur is a blowing systolic murmur heard best at the pulmonic area (upper left and upper right sternal borders) with the child lying down. It will get softer when the child sits up.
3. Carotid bruit is a very common, soft, early systolic murmur heard above the clavicles along the carotid arteries with the child lying down.
4. Physiologic peripheral pulmonic stenosis is a systolic murmur heard best in the axillae and back. It disappears by 3 to 4 months of age as the pulmonary arteries enlarge.
5. Venous hum is a humming, continuous, systolic/diastolic murmur heard best just below the clavicles with the child sitting up. It can be abolished by having the child lie down.

MANAGEMENT

Since innocent murmurs do not indicate heart disease and require no treatment, the clinical issue that arises is *whether* and/or *what* to tell the parents. Many parents have difficulty in understanding the meaning of an innocent murmur and the information that their new baby or young child has a heart murmur, however innocent, generates fear and anxiety. One study (Bergman, 1967) revealed that in a group of children with innocent murmurs, 40 percent had been restricted in normal activities by their parents. The parents had misinterpreted the diagnosis and believed their children had "something wrong" with the heart or heart disease. The philosophy basic to this book is that parents should be fully informed about their children's health status and be participants in decisions about care. Yet, the decision to inform parents of the presence of an innocent murmur needs to be made on an individual basis.

Informing parents. In deciding when and how to inform parents about an innocent murmur the following factors should be considered:

1. Knowledge of the family

   - Is there a family history of heart disease? If so, who has or had it and what was the outcome?
   - How much anxiety can be expected?
   - Is this the first visit of the child and family? It can be argued that the first well-baby visit is not the time to discuss an innocent murmur due to the many normal anxieties faced by new parents during this period of adjustment.
   - If the family is known, how have illness situations been handled in the past?
   - Are the parents calm, overreactive, faced with other stresses?
   - What is the level of understanding of the parents?
   - Are there language or other communication barriers? The dangers of misinterpretation of information are present even without language barriers.

2. Source of health care and follow-up

   - Does the family plan to receive further health care at the specific agency or office?
   - Will the child be followed by one primary person or team?
   - What other health care facilities are used by the family? If the parents use another agency (e.g., the local emergency room) when the child is ill, it is likely that they will be questioned about the murmur. If they have not been informed previously, this may result in increased anxiety over the

child's condition, anger at not having been told before, and suspicion that previous caretakers "missed" the murmur.

Parent counseling. When the decision is made to inform the parents it must be stressed that the innocent murmur is a normal phenomenon that may be exaggerated at times; that the child does *not* have heart disease; and that no restrictions are necessary. The murmur can be described as the sound that blood makes while moving through the heart. A helpful analogy is to compare the sound with that made by water flowing through a garden hose; usually it is not heard unless a person's ear is very close to the hose or unless there is a kink in the hose obstructing the flow of water. Ample opportunity for questions and discussion must be provided at the time and at subsequent visits to ensure correct interpretation of this common clinical finding.

Patent Ductus Arteriosus (PDA)

ASSESSMENT

Patent ductus arteriosus is a common congenital cardiac anomaly which occurs as an isolated defect or is frequently associated with maternal rubella during early pregnancy and with small preterm infants. Because the ductus fails to close soon after birth, aortic blood is shunted (left-to-right) into the pulmonary artery and is recirculated through the pulmonary circulation. Consequently the left ventricle must work harder to meet the needs of the peripheral tissues.

Clinical signs and symptoms. Findings vary with the size of the defect.

1. Small defects. A small opening will usually not affect physical growth and development. The only finding may be a murmur that is similar to a venous hum.

2. Larger defects. With larger defects and shunts, symptoms may be progressive exertional dyspnea, left ventricular failure, or congestive heart failure. Physical signs include a wide pulse

pressure, prominent radial pulses, and limited growth and activity. The classic murmur is a machinery, humming, harsh sound beginning in systole, reaching maximum intensity at the end of systole, and waning in diastole, heard best under the left clavicle and in the pulmonic area.

MANAGEMENT

Spontaneous closure of the ductus after infancy is extremely rare and even asymptomatic PDAs are not benign. Life expectancy is reduced and subacute bacterial endocarditis is a frequent complication. Therefore, surgical closure of the defect is usually indicated.

Resource Information

Information on educational materials and services available for children with cardiac conditions can be obtained from:
1. American Heart Association, 44 E. 23rd Street, New York, NY 10010.
2. Crippled Children's Services, State Health Departments.

References

Bates, B. *A Guide to Physical Examination*. Philadelphia: Lippincott, 1974.

Bergman, A. B. and S. J. Stamm. "The Morbidity of Cardiac Nondisease in Schoolchildren." *N Engl J Med* 276:1008–1013, May 4, 1967.

Blumenthal, S., et al. "Report of the Task Force on Blood Pressure Control in Children." *Pediatrics*, Supplement 59(5), Part 2, May 1977.

Caceres, C. H. and L. W. Perry. *The Innocent Murmur*. Boston: Little, Brown, 1967.

Friedberg, D. Z. and S. B. Litwin. "The Medical and Surgical Management of Patients with Congenital Heart Disease." *Clin Pediatr* 15:324–333, April 1976.

Friedman, S. "Some Thoughts about Functional or Innocent Murmurs." *Clin Pediatr* 12:678, December 1973.

Kempe, C. H., H. K. Silver, and D. O'Brien. *Current Pediatric Diagnosis and Treatment*, 4th ed. Los Altos, California: Lange Medical Publications, 1976.

Nadas, A. S. and D. C. Fyler. *Pediatric Cardiology*, 3rd ed. Philadelphia: Saunders, 1972.

Rudolph, A. M., editor. *Pediatrics*, 16th ed. New York: Appleton-Century-Crofts, 1977.

Vaughan, V. C. and R. J. McKay, editors. *Nelson Textbook of Pediatrics*, 10th ed. Philadelphia: Saunders, 1975.

20

The Hematopoietic System

The hematopoietic system is complex and disorders can involve many organs and organ systems. The disorders most commonly encountered in primary pediatric settings are neonatal jaundice and the anemias of childhood including hemolytic disease of the newborn, nutritional anemias, and the hemoglobinopathies. This chapter presents information basic to understanding jaundice and anemia, normal blood values related to these conditions, and data necessary for assessment and management. With such information the nurse practitioner can provide appropriate health education to individuals, families, and groups regarding prevention of anemia and explanation of common blood disorders.

ASSESSMENT

Normal Blood Values

Red blood cell values at different ages are presented in Table 1. Different agencies and laboratories may have established slightly

Table 1
Red Blood Cell Values at Various Ages: Mean and Lower Limit of Normal (-2 SD)

Age	Hemoglobin (g/dl)		Hematocrit (%)		Red Cell Count (10¹²/liter)		MCV (fl)		MCH (pg)		MCHC (g/dl)	
	Mean	-2 SD	Mean	-2 SD	Mean	-2 SD	Mean	-2 SD	Mean	-2 SD	Mean	-2 SD
Birth (cord blood)	16.5	13.5	51	42	4.7	3.9	108	98	34	31	33	30
1–3 days (capillary)	18.5	14.5	56	45	5.3	4.0	108	95	34	31	33	29
1 week	17.5	13.5	54	42	5.1	3.9	107	88	34	28	33	28
2 weeks	16.5	12.5	51	39	4.9	3.6	105	86	34	28	33	28
1 month	14.0	10.0	43	31	4.2	3.0	104	85	34	28	33	29
2 months	11.5	9.0	35	28	3.8	2.7	96	77	30	26	33	29
3–6 months	11.5	9.5	35	29	3.8	3.1	91	74	30	25	33	30
0.5–2 years	12.0	10.5	36	33	4.5	3.7	78	70	27	23	33	30
2–6 years	12.5	11.5	37	34	4.6	3.9	81	75	27	24	34	31
6–12 years	13.5	11.5	40	35	4.6	4.0	86	77	29	25	34	31
12–18 years: female	14.0	12.0	41	36	4.6	4.1	90	78	30	25	34	31
male	14.5	13.0	43	37	4.9	4.5	88	78	30	25	34	31
18–49 years: female	14.0	12.0	41	36	4.6	4.0	90	80	30	26	34	31
male	15.5	13.5	47	41	5.2	4.5	90	80	30	26	34	31

Source: Reprinted with permission from A. M. Rudolph, editor, *Pediatrics*, 16th ed. (New York: Appleton-Century-Crofts, 1977), p. 1111. Compiled from the following sources: Dutcher: *Lab Med 2:32, 1971*; Koerper et al: *J Pediatr 89:580 1976*; Marner: *Acta Paediatr Scand 58:363, 1969*; Matoth, et al: *Acta Paediatr Scand 60:317, 1971*; Moe: *Acta Paediatr Scand 54:69, 1965*; Okuno: *J Clin Pathol 25:599, 1972*; Oski and Naiman: *Hematological Problems in the Newborn*. Saunders, 1972, p 11; Penttilä et al: *Suomen Lääkärilehti 26:2173, 1973*; and Vieri et al: *Br J Haematol 23:189, 1972*. Emphasis is given to recent studies employing electronic counters and to the selection of populations that are likely to exclude individuals with iron deficiency. The mean ± 2 SD can be expected to include 95 percent of the observations in a normal population.

different standards depending on the population sampled and the methods of sampling and analysis used. These standards are those used at the University of California Medical Center, San Francisco, California.

History

PRESENT CONCERNS

Presenting symptoms are evaluated according to the guidelines outlined in Chapter 13, Assessment of Presenting Symptom.

PAST HISTORY

Factors to be elicited in the past history include any blood loss, jaundice, bruising, or petechiae at birth or later; anemia, pallor, irritability, malaise, weight loss, chemical ingestions, drugs, recurrent infections, and parasitic infections. A nutrition history is obtained. See Chapter 6, Nutrition History.

FAMILY HISTORY

Important factors in the family history include race; geographic country of origin; any previous infants with jaundice, anemia, or exchange transfusions; familial diseases (e.g., sickle cell anemia); maternal blood type, Rh factor, and maternal nutritional status during pregnancy.

Physical Examination

GENERAL APPEARANCE

Observe physical development and nutritional status. Obtain height, weight, and vital signs.

SKIN

Observe for pallor, jaundice, bruises, petechiae, and hematomas.

EYES, MOUTH, NOSE, THROAT

Observe sclera, conjunctiva, and mucous membranes for color and evidence of bleeding.

HEART

Palpate and auscultate for murmurs, tachycardia, and signs of congestive failure.

ABDOMEN

Palpate for hepatomegaly and splenomegaly.

Metabolism of Bilirubin

When red blood cells break down, hemoglobin is released and further broken down into iron, protein, and bilirubin. Iron and protein are stored and re-used by the body. The bilirubin resulting from this breakdown of hemoglobin is unconjugated, indirect bilirubin. Unconjugated bilirubin is fat soluble, not water soluble, so it cannot be excreted by the kidneys. Being fat soluble it can permeate the membranes and enter tissues (i.e., subcutaneous and brain tissue) where it can become neurotoxic at certain concentrations. This is especially dangerous in premature infants who lack subcutaneous fatty tissue.

The normal mechanism for converting unconjugated to conjugated bilirubin begins with the binding of unconjugated bilirubin to serum albumin. It is then transported to the liver, and there is acted upon by enzymes (e.g., glucuronyl transferase) and converted to direct, conjugated bilirubin. Direct bilirubin, which is water soluble, is soluble in body fluids and is easily excreted through bile ducts to the gut. It does not enter the cells so is not toxic.

Jaundice

Jaundice results from the accumulation in the skin of bilirubin pigment. Jaundice can be detected clinically when bilirubin levels exceed 4 to 5 mg/dl.* It is best assessed in daylight. In infants with dark pigmented skin, it can be detected in the sclera and posterior palate and by blanching the palms and soles. The causes of jaundice are:

1. Any factor that increases the load of bilirubin to be metabolized by the liver (e.g., erythroblastosis fetalis, hemolytic anemias, infection)
2. Any factor that may damage or may reduce the activity of the enzyme, bilirubin glucuronyl transferase (e.g., anoxia, infection)
3. Any factor that may compete for or block the enzyme (e.g., drugs such as nitrofurantoin or other substances requiring glucuronic acid conjugation for excretion)
4. Any factor leading to absence or decreased amounts of the enzyme (e.g., genetic defect, prematurity) (Vaughan, 1975, pp. 375–376).

Common Laboratory Procedures for Jaundice

Data useful in the assessment of jaundice include the following:

1. Total serum bilirubin. This is the sum of unconjugated and conjugated bilirubin. Normal values of total bilirubin are:

---

*dl = deciliter. It is a new unit of measurement and one deciliter equals 100 ml. See Appendix for table of new measurements in current use.

Age	Term Infant	Premature Infant
Birth	<2 mg/dl	<2 mg/dl
0–1 day	<6 mg/dl	<8 mg/dl
1–2 days	<8 mg/dl	<12 mg/dl
3–5 days	<12 mg/dl	<16 mg/dl
Thereafter	<1 mg/dl	<2 mg/dl

After the newborn period total bilirubin is normally less than 1 mg/dl.

2. Direct bilirubin. This measures the amount of conjugated bilirubin. After 1 month of age values are 0 to 0.3 mg/dl.
3. Indirect bilirubin. This measures the amount of unconjugated bilirubin. Normally, 90 percent of total bilirubin is in unconjugated form. After 1 month of age values are 0.1 to 0.7 mg/dl.
4. Direct Coombs test. This detects the presence of antibody attached to red blood cells. A positive result in the newborn indicates that the newborn's red blood cells are coated with maternal antibodies and is diagnostic of isoimmunization (e.g., Rh incompatibility, ABO incompatibility).
5. Indirect Coombs test. This is used to detect antibodies in serum by mixing serum with cells of known antigenic type. A positive result indicates maternal antibody in the infant's blood but does not confirm incompatibility with the infant's red blood cells. It is not used often in infants.

Anemia

Anemia is defined as "a lower than normal value for hemoglobin or hematocrit or number of red blood cells per cubic millimeter. The lower limits of the normal range is set two standard deviations below the mean at any given age" (Rudolph, 1977, p. 1114). See Table 1. Since anemia is a manifestation of an underlying process it is important that the cause be determined.

Etiologic classification of anemias (from Rudolph, 1977, p. 1115):
I. Impaired Production of Red Cells and Hemoglobin
 A. Nutritional anemias

    1. *iron deficiency*
    2. *megaloblastic anemia*
  B. *Anemia of infection and chronic disease*
  C. *Aplastic and hypoplastic anemia*
II. *Accelerated Destruction of Red Cells*
  A. *Extracorpuscular* [sic] *defects* •
    1. *erythroblastosis fetalis*
    2. *autoimmune and drug-induced hemolytic anemia*
    3. *abnormalities of the vasculature or plasma*
    4. *splenic enlargement*
  B. *Intracorpuscular defects*
    1. *abnormalities of hemoglobin structure and synthesis*
    2. *abnormalities of the red cell membrane*
    3. *abnormalities of red cell metabolism*
III. *Blood Loss*

Common Laboratory Procedures for Anemia

Information in this section comes primarily from the data of Dallman and Koerper. (See this chapter, References.) Laboratory data useful in assessment of anemia include the following:

1. Hematocrit. This is a measurement of the percentage of red blood cells in the total blood volume.

2. Hemoglobin. This is a measurement of the concentration by weight of hemoglobin in each deciliter of whole blood. With the use of electronic counters, the hemoglobin is a more accurate measurement than the hematocrit.

3. Red blood cell count (RBC). This is the measurement of the number of red blood cells found in each cubic millimeter of blood.

4. RBC indices. Indices provide an estimate of the size (volume), amount of hemoglobin, and hemoglobin concentration of the average red blood cell:

    • Mean corpuscular volume (MCV) is the volume of the average RBC expressed in femtoliters (fl).

    • Mean corpuscular hemoglobin (MCH) is the absolute

amount of hemoglobin by weight in the average RBC expressed in picograms (pg).

- Mean corpuscular hemoglobin concentration (MCHC) is the concentration of hemoglobin in the average RBC expressed in grams per deciliter. See Table 1 for normal values of the above.

5. Peripheral blood smear. A stained smear of blood gives information about the morphology (size, shape) and hemoglobin content (color) of the red blood cell, the level of platelets, indices, and types of leukocytes present. Terms used to describe red blood cells are:

- Anisocytosis: cells of unequal size.
- Poikilocytosis: cells of abnormal shapes.
- Microcytic: cells that are smaller than usual.
- Hypochromic: cells that are paler than normal.

6. Reticulocyte count. Reticulocytes are young, newly formed RBCs that normally comprise about 1 percent of total RBCs. An increase may indicate that the bone marrow is compensating for some problem by producing more RBCs.

7. Free erythrocyte protoporphyrin (FEP). The FEP rises in conditions that interfere with the final step in the synthesis of heme, the combination of iron and protoporphyrin. When the RBC does not have enough iron to make heme, the FEP becomes elevated and rises markedly as the concentration of hemoglobin falls. It rises before anemia becomes severe enough to be detected by traditional means (e.g., hemoglobin and blood smear). Values above 3 μg/gm of Hgb are abnormal and occur in iron deficiency, chronic inflammatory disease, and lead intoxication.

8. Serum iron (SI). This measurement indicates iron concentration in serum or plasma. It is not the most helpful test because values fluctuate during the day, being higher in the morning. Mean values for children are 30 to 70 μg/dl; and for adults are 65 to 110 μg/dl (Koerper, 1977a).

9. Total iron binding capacity (TIBC). This indicates how many binding sites are available for iron. Normal values for children and adults are 200 to 400 μg/dl.

10. Ratio of serum iron to total iron binding capacity (SI/TIBC). This ratio is expressed as percent saturation and is more helpful than either measure taken separately. In iron deficiency the SI decreases, and the TIBC increases, resulting in a lower percent saturation. In young children levels below 10 to 12 percent indicate restriction in the rate of hemoglobin production, and in adults levels below 16 percent are abnormal.

11. Serum ferritin concentration (SF). This indicates the level of iron stores in the liver, spleen, and bone marrow. Ferritin is a large molecule that carries iron to storage sites. When iron is deficient none will go for storage since it is being used to synthesize hemoglobin. In children beyond 6 months of age the normal range is 7 to 140 ng/ml. Values below 7 ng/ml are present only in iron deficiency.

12. Stool examination for occult blood. Guaiac testing is only sensitive enough to pick up more than 5 ml of occult blood. The benzidine test is very sensitive. A 1+ reaction (4+ is maximum) is considered normal and not indicative of occult blood (Levin, 1971).

COMMON CLINICAL PROBLEMS

Jaundice in the Newborn (Hyperbilirubinemia)

The nurse practitioner provides well-baby and/or follow-up care for infants who have had some form of hyperbilirubinemia and often is the first to identify breast-feeding jaundice in normal newborns. See Chapter 4, Dermal Icterus Index. The information presented here will assist the nurse practitioner in monitoring the progress of such infants and in explaining the infant's condition to parents. Before beginning such explanations it is essential to ask the parents to describe their understanding of what happened while the infant was in the nursery and what they were told about the infant's condition.

PHYSIOLOGIC JAUNDICE

Assessment. Jaundice is the result of the breakdown of fetal red cells plus the immaturity of liver enzymes to conjugate and to excrete bilirubin (see this chapter, Metabolism of Bilirubin, and Jaundice). Jaundice appears in the full-term infant on the second to fourth day, may reach levels of 6 to 10 mg/dl, and resolves by the seventh day. In the premature infant jaundice appears on the third or fourth day, may reach levels of 10 to 12 mg/dl by the fifth to seventh day, and resolves by the ninth day or longer. The infant is otherwise healthy. Levels of bilirubin exceeding 10 mg/dl in the term infant and 14 mg/dl in the premature infant suggest that other factors are superimposed on the normally occurring physiologic jaundice (Rudolph, 1977, p. 1077). See below, Hyperbilirubinemia of the newborn.

Management. The infant needs adequate hydration. Phototherapy is usually not required in physiologic jaundice.

HYPERBILIRUBINEMIA OF THE NEWBORN

Assessment. This is a more severe form of physiologic jaundice and suggests additional contributing factors such as blood group incompatibility, cephalohematoma, or infection. The primary problem usually is deficiency or inactivity of bilirubin glucuronyl transferase causing abnormal elevation of unconjugated bilirubin. Jaundice appears during the first week and may persist. Bilirubin levels may exceed 15 mg/dl and present the dangers of kernicterus. The incidence of bilirubin levels higher than 15 mg/dl is greater in low-birth-weight infants.

LABORATORY. Laboratory assessment of newborns with hyperbilirubinemia includes:

1. Maternal blood group and Rh type
2. Infant blood group and Rh type, and direct Coombs test
3. Total and direct-reacting serum bilirubin
4. Hemoglobin or hematocrit

5. Reticulocyte count and white blood count
6. Red cell morphology
7. Urinalysis and culture (Rudolph, 1977, p. 1078)

Management. Photography and/or exchange transfusion may be indicated.

PHOTOTHERAPY. Blue light waves appear to assist the breakdown of unconjugated bilirubin in the skin into nontoxic, excretable by-products. The infant is undressed and placed under a bank of fluorescent lights. The eyes are carefully patched to protect them from the intense light. Position is changed systematically so all body surfaces are exposed. Loose stools, lethargy, skin rashes, and temperature changes are side effects of phototherapy. The therapy is usually discontinued in 1 to 3 days when unconjugated bilirubin has been reduced to levels considered safe in terms of the infant's age and condition.

Parents need ample explanations of what is happening to their infant, and opportunities to care for and feed the infant during hospitalization.

EXCHANGE TRANSFUSION. Infants who have had exchange transfusions for blood group incompatibilities need to be observed closely for 6 to 8 weeks to monitor the degree of anemia. Serial hematocrit or hemoglobin determinations are performed until a sustained rise is demonstrated. Supplemental iron and/or blood transfusion may be necessary.

BREAST-FEEDING JAUNDICE

Assessment. One of every 200 breast-fed infants develops severe and prolonged hyperbilirubinemia which is thought to be caused by the secretion of a substance in the mother's milk which inhibits the activity of bilirubin glucuronyl transferase. Increased bilirubin levels develop by the seventh day and may peak at 2 to 3 weeks of age. Levels may reach 15 to 20 mg/dl. The infant is otherwise well and kernicterus has not been reported with breast-feeding jaundice.

Management. If bilirubin exceeds 20 mg/dl during the first 3 weeks it is recommended that breast-feeding be discontinued for 2 to 4 days to allow the enzyme to become active. Resumption of nursing may produce only a small increase and then a slow decline in bilirubin. If the child is well and the bilirubin is less than 20 mg/dl and falling, there is no need to interrupt breast-feeding (Rudolph, 1977, p. 1081).

COUNSELING. The breast-feeding mother will worry that her milk is not good for the infant or is harming the infant and may be anxious about resuming breast-feeding. Clear explanations, and ample encouragement and support are required. The mother will need instruction on manual expression of milk during the period of formula feeding.

HEMOLYTIC DISEASE OF THE NEWBORN (ERYTHROBLASTOSIS FETALIS)

Assessment. This condition results from exaggerated erythrocyte destruction.

Rh INCOMPATIBILITY. The hemolytic process occurs as the result of:

1. Immunization of an Rh-negative woman caused either by the inherited Rh factor in the red blood cells of her fetus or by transfusion of Rh-positive blood resulting in the production of anti-Rh antibodies by her immune system
2. Transplacental transfer of the woman's anti-Rh antibodies to the fetus causing hemolysis of the red blood cells and other pathologic processes both in utero and in the neonatal period (Lin-Fu, 1975, p. 6).

The hemolysis causes an increased load of unconjugated bilirubin to be metabolized by the liver, and hyperbilirubinemia may develop rapidly. Jaundice at birth or appearing during the first 24 hours should be considered to be due to erythroblastosis fetalis until proven otherwise. Firstborn babies are usually not affected since the degree of maternal sensitization is slight unless the mother has previously been transfused with Rh-positive blood or has had an abortion. Subsequent infants are at greater risk, often are severely affected, and may require multiple exchange transfusions.

ABO INCOMPATIBILITY. Usually the mother is type O and the infant is type A or B. These incompatibilities result in milder disease and often require no treatment other than phototherapy. Occasionally exchange transfusion may be required. Jaundice may be the only clinical manifestation and appears during the first 24 hours.

Management. The goals of management are:

1. To prevent death of the affected infant from the complications of severe anemia and to avoid the toxic effects of hyperbilirubinemia, namely, kernicterus. Exchange transfusions and phototherapy are the major therapeutic modes.

2. To prevent immunization of Rh-negative women by the injection of Rh immunoglobulin (RhoGAM), an IgG containing high titers of anti-Rh antibodies. This is possible only in nonsensitized women. The recommendation of both the U.S. Public Health Service and the American College of Obstetricians and Gynecologists is that any Rh-negative woman whose serum does not contain anti-Rh antibodies be given an intramuscular injection of Rh-immunoglobulin within 72 hours after delivery or abortion. The dangers of immunization following abortion often have been overlooked, but studies indicate that transplacental hemorrhages do occur during both spontaneous and induced abortions (Lin-Fu, 1975, p. 13).

KERNICTERUS

Assessment. Kernicterus refers to the neurologic damage that occurs when unconjugated bilirubin is deposited in certain brain tissues. Symptoms usually develop during the first week of life and include lethargy, poor feeding, weak Moro reflex, high-pitched cry, and opisthotonos. Advanced and terminal symptoms are apnea, convulsions, and respiratory arrest. Mortality is high, and survivors show various signs of central nervous system damage. The risk of kernicterus exists with serum bilirubin levels above 18 to 20 mg/dl. Low-birth-weight and premature infants may be susceptible at lower levels.

Management. Prevention of kernicterus is the best management. Exchange transfusions and phototherapy are indicated to keep unconjugated bilirubin levels below neurotoxic levels.

Anemia

PHYSIOLOGIC ANEMIA OF INFANCY

Assessment. At birth the normal newborn has high hematocrit and hemoglobin levels which gradually decline to a low point (Hgb 9 to 11 gm/dl) between 2 and 3 months of age. See Table 1. At about 3 to 4 months of age the bone marrow begins active erythropoiesis, and levels begin to increase. The same phenomenon operates in premature infants, but the drop in hemoglobin levels is more severe and may go to 7 to 8 gm/dl.

Management. No medical intervention is indicated unless the anemia is severe. The premature infant may require a blood transfusion if hemoglobin falls to 6 to 7 mg/dl and/or if the infant shows signs of early heart failure. On general principle it is important that all premature infants receive dietary sources of iron, folic acid, and Vitamin E so normal hematopoiesis can occur. See Chapter 6, Nutritional Needs of the Low-Birth-Weight Infant, and Iron Nutrition in Infancy.

IRON DEFICIENCY ANEMIA

Assessment. This condition results when the body lacks sufficient iron for hemoglobin synthesis.

ETIOLOGY. Lack of sufficient iron can be the result of:

1. Insufficient iron stores at birth due to prematurity, twinning, blood loss from perinatal hemorrhage, or a severely iron-deficient mother

2. Insufficient iron in the diet to meet demands for expanding body mass and blood volume
3. Blood loss after birth due to hemorrhage or to chronic cow milk-induced enteric blood loss. The latter is considered to be the possible etiology in 25 to 50 percent of the cases and is caused by the combination of ingestion of large quantities of whole nonheat-treated cow milk plus intestinal sensitivity to a protein component in the milk.
4. Parasitic infestation

INCIDENCE. It is most prevalent between 6 months and 3 years of life and during the adolescent growth spurt but is increasingly being found in school age children. Although it is found in children from all socioeconomic groups, the highest incidence of anemia is found in lower socioeconomic populations.

PHYSIOLOGY. Iron deficiency develops in predictable stages over a period of time. "Depletion of iron stores is followed by a fall in *serum transferrin saturation*, which ultimately results in the decreased production of hemoglobin that is clinically recognized as *anemia*" (Rudolph, 1977, p. 1122). As hemoglobin production decreases the newly formed cells become smaller (low MCV) and less well filled with hemoglobin (low MCH). The anemia that develops is a delayed manifestation of iron deficiency and becomes clinically evident only after months of suboptimal hemoglobin production, since red cells that were produced under conditions of iron adequacy live out their normal 120-day life span (Rudolph, 1977, p. 1122).

CLINICAL SIGNS AND SYMPTOMS. Infants with slowly developing anemia usually do not show any clinical symptoms and appear well. They are frequently identified by routine screening tests during health supervision visits. Children with moderate to severe anemia (Hgb below 6 to 7 gm/dl) may exhibit pallor, fatigue, listlessness, constipation, or anorexia. They are sometimes described by their parents as "obnoxious." They may be poor feeders and refuse to take solids. They may be fat and have poor muscle tone, or may be underweight. Pica may be present. Children with severe untreated anemia (Hgb 2 to 3 mg/dl) may be very irritable and develop tachycardia, cardiac murmurs, cardiorespiratory distress, and cardiac failure. Preliminary reports suggest that iron deficiency can affect attention span, alertness, and learning in young children (Smith, 1974).

NUTRITION HISTORY. Essential to the diagnosis is a thorough diet and nutrition history. Use of a 24-hour diet recall is helpful (see Chapter 6, Nutrition History). The history will probably reveal a diet high in milk intake (over 1 quart per day) and low in iron-containing solid foods.

LABORATORY. Laboratory investigation includes the detection of mild iron deficiency, documentation of anemia, and differentiation between iron deficiency and thalassemia minor.

Detection of mild iron deficiency. Mild iron deficiency is not reliably detected by traditional laboratory procedures (e.g., hemoglobin, peripheral blood smear). The tests that are most helpful in identifying mild deficiency are the MCV (using an electronic counter), FEP, and serum ferritin (see this chapter, Common Laboratory Procedures for Anemia).

Detection of iron deficiency anemia. The recommended approach includes:

1. Complete blood count. It will reveal low values for hemoglobin, hematocrit, RBC, MCV, and MCH. The MCHC goes down only when the hemoglobin is 8 gm/dl or lower.
2. Peripheral blood smear. It will show hypochromic, microcytic cells with marked variation in size and shape, but only when the anemia has become moderate to severe.
3. Reticulocyte count. This may be normal in mild anemia and low in moderate to severe anemia.
4. Stool guaiac or benzidine tests. At 2 months of age up to 80 percent of infants being fed fresh cow milk will have stools positive for occult blood. By 6 months of age, 60 percent will have positive findings, and by 1 year of age, 20 percent will have positive findings (Koerper, 1977).

Differentiation between iron deficiency and thalassemia minor. The determination of MCV values by electronic particle counter is becoming more widespread in screening programs for childhood anemias. When the MCV is low, the differential diagnosis is chiefly between iron deficiency and thalassemia minor (see this chapter, Beta Thalassemia). Figure 1 illustrates the diagnostic process that will differentiate between the two. Another differentiating factor is the red blood cell count. If the MCV is low and the RBC is low, iron deficiency can be assumed. If the RBC is over 5.5 million/cu mm, thalassemia minor needs to be investigated (Koerper, 1977).

Management. The management of iron deficiency includes prevention of the condition, screening for early identification of iron deficiency states, and treatment of actual cases.

PREVENTION. Prevention of iron deficiency is the best management and involves provision of adequate exogenous sources of iron. See Chapter 6, Iron Nutrition in Infancy.

SCREENING. The process outlined in Figure 1 represents a new approach to identifying iron deficiency with a high degree of accu-

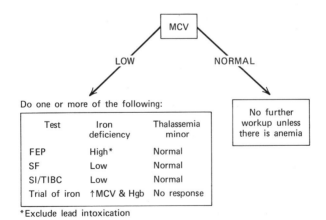

Figure 1. Screening for childhood anemia based on the MCV. (Reprinted with permission from P. R. Dallman, "New Approaches to Screening for Iron Deficiency," *J Pediatr* 90:678–681, April 1977.)

racy. A hemoglobin is also obtained, and the likelihood of iron deficiency is greater if both the Hgb and MCV are low. In settings where the electronic counter is not available, screening is done by obtaining hemoglobin and hematocrit levels. Screening is performed between 6 and 18 months of age and yearly thereafter through adolescence, especially in females with heavy menstrual losses.

TREATMENT. When clinical and laboratory assessment reveals iron deficiency anemia the plan of management includes specific medication therapy and parent counseling as follows:

Medication. The procedures for therapy and follow-up are described.

1. Iron in the ferrous form is the drug of choice. Recommended doses of oral iron are presented in Table 2. Available liquid oral iron preparations are listed in Table 3. In mild anemia medication is given for 3 to 4 months or for 2 months after Hgb reaches normal levels so that iron stores can be replenished. The more severe the anemia, the longer the treatment.

2. The child should be seen 7 to 10 days after institution of iron therapy and at 1-month intervals until the anemia has been corrected. In moderate to severe anemia, the reticulocyte count will show a response within 3 to 10 days if the anemia is truly

Table 2
Recommended Doses of Oral Iron in Infants

Hgb (gm/dl)	Dose (elemental iron/kg/day)	Comments
9–10	2–3 mg	Can be given in a single dose
8	3–4 mg	Can be given in a single dose
< 8	6 mg	Given in divided doses to decrease side effects
< 5	6 mg	Consider admission to hospital for transfusion; danger of cardiac problems, congestive failure

Source: M. Koerper, Personal communication, April 1977.

Table 3
Common Oral Iron Liquids

Proprietary Name	Active Ingredient	Elemental Iron (mg/cc)
Mol-Iron Liquid	Ferrous sulfate	10
Mol-Iron Drops	Ferrous sulfate	25
Feosol Elixir	Ferrous sulfate	8
Fer-In-Sol Syrup	Ferrous sulfate	6
Fer-In-Sol Drops	Ferrous sulfate	25
Fergon Elixir	Ferrous gluconate	7
Chel-Iron Liquid	Ferro cholinate	10
Chel-Iron Drops	Ferro cholinate	25
Ferrolip Pediatric Syrup	Ferro cholinate	4
Ferrolip Pediatric Drops	Ferro cholinate	25
Ferro Drops	Ferrous lactate	25

Source: Reproduced with permission from R. H. Levin, "Iron Deficiency Anemia in the Pediatric Patient," *J Am Pharm Assoc* N.S.11(12): 675, December 1971.

based on iron deficiency, and if the medication is being given and absorbed. Hemoglobin should be checked once a month and should rise 0.5 to 1 gm/dl per month. If no therapeutic response is present after 1 to 2 monhts of reliably administered iron, therapy should be stopped, and other causes of anemia should be investigated.

3. Once blood levels have returned to normal, medication should be continued an additional 6 to 8 weeks to replenish iron stores. The child should be seen again at the end of treatment and hematocrit, hemoglobin, and indices checked.

Parent counseling. Parents need instructions on medication therapy and diet modification.

Medication. Instructions may be written and given to parents. Points to include are:

1. The exact dose and how to measure it should be written out.

2. Medication should be given between meals for better absorption. Giving it shortly after meals is helpful in reducing gastric irritation.

3. Large amounts of milk should be avoided since milk can interfere with absorption.

4. If the taste is unpalatable, the medication can be given with juice. Older children may prefer chewable tablets.

5. The teeth may be temporarily stained, but this can be reduced by placing the medicine with a dropper on the back of the tongue, by using a straw, and by rinsing the mouth or brushing the teeth after taking the medication.

6. The stools may turn black.

7. The full course of medication must be taken, even though the child is well.

8. The medicine must be kept out of reach since accidental ingestions can result in serious side effects including hemorrhage and death. See Chapter 14, Parent Teaching Related to Medications.

Diet. Education of parents regarding feeding practices is essential and should be on-going.

1. Breast feeding or the use of infant formula should be encouraged during the first year. Fresh cow milk should be avoided.

2. Daily milk intake should be restricted to one third of the total calories. This would limit milk intake of young children to little more than 1 pint per day.

3. Iron supplementation. See Chapter 6, Iron Nutrition in Infancy.

4. A list of iron-containing solid foods should be provided and their use encouraged. See Chapter 6, Iron Nutrition in Infancy.

5. Parents must be supported in their efforts to change or to modify feeding patterns.

SICKLE CELL ANEMIA AND TRAIT

Assessment. Each person inherits one gene from each parent that governs the synthesis of hemoglobin. The protein (globin) portion of the normal adult hemoglobin A molecule contains two pairs of polypeptide chains (two alpha chains and two beta chains). The sickle cell hemoglobin molecule (Hgb S) is abnormal and results from a single amino acid substitution on the beta chain caused by inheriting a defective co-dominant gene.

SICKLE CELL TRAIT.   If only one co-dominant gene is inherited, Hgb S will be formed in small proportion to Hgb A (35 percent S to 60 percent A). This person is said to be heterozygous and has sickle cell trait, a benign condition which does *not* cause anemia and disease. Trait is present in 8 to 10 percent of American blacks, and a decreased incidence is found in some Mediterranean and Latin populations. Hemoglobin and hematocrit values are normal. Sickling does not occur except in rare instances when hypoxia may occur from shock or flying at very high altitudes in unpressurized aircraft.

SICKLE CELL ANEMIA.   If two co-dominant genes are inherited, Hgb S will account for up to 70 to 90 percent of the hemoglobin. This person is homozygous and will have sickle cell anemia which is a severe, chronic, hemolytic anemia.

Incidence.   At birth, one in 625 American blacks has sickle cell anemia. In adult blacks the incidence is one in 1875 due to the mortality of the disease (Bailey, 1974, p. 139).

Clinical picture.   The presence of Hgb S with decreased oxygen concentration deforms the normal red blood cell into an abnormal crescent-shaped cell. These cells lead to increased blood viscosity, retarded capillary flow, damage to the fragile cells, and increased red cell destruction. The degree of anemia remains fairly constant unless red blood cell production decreases (aplastic crisis) or blood viscosity increases (vaso-occlusive crisis). Symptoms usually do not appear until the latter part of the first year of life since the presence of large amounts of fetal hemoglobin (Hgb F) in the early months tends to obscure the presence of Hgb S. The child is asymptomatic for periods of time until a crisis occurs. Crises are precipitated by infection, dehydration, trauma, hypoxia, exposure, and strenuous exertion. Vaso-occlusive crises are the most common and symptoms include anorexia, pallor, weakness, jaundice; severe pain and swelling in the hands, feet, abdomen, joints, and extremities; fever; and anemia. Chronic anemia and repeated vaso-occlusive episodes lead to varied and severe problems as children grow older; they are extremely susceptible to infection, and many die in early adulthood.

Laboratory.   Hemoglobin ranges from 6 to 9 gm/dl. Reticulocyte count is elevated to 5 to 25 percent. Indirect bilirubin is elevated.

GENETIC IMPLICATIONS.   The mode of transmission of sickle cell trait and anemia is autosomal co-dominant (see Table 4). It is *co-dominant* because there *are* effects of the trait as well as of the disease. Definite probabilities exist with each pregnancy that the offspring will inherit the disease, the trait, or neither.

Management.   Management includes treatment of the child with sickle cell anemia and screening for detection of sickle cell trait.

SICKLE CELL ANEMIA.   Management of crises and prevention of further crises are the important components of care.

Vaso-occlusive crisis.   The child requires pain medication and increased fluid intake.

General management.   In addition to regular health maintenance care, prevention of vaso-occlusive and anemic crises is the goal. Measures include:

1.   Avoiding dehydration.

Table 4
Transmission of Sickle Cell Disease

Genotype of Parents	Probability of Abnormal Hemoglobin in Offspring		
	Normal	Trait	Disease
1 parent with trait	50%	50%	0
Both parents with trait	25%	50%	25%
1 parent with trait, 1 parent with disease	0	50%	50%
Both parents with disease	0	0	100%

Source: Reproduced with permission from L. S. Brunner and D. S. Suddarth, *The Lippincott Manual of Nursing Practice* (Philadelphia: J. B. Lippincott Co., 1974), p. 1164.

2. Treating fevers as emergencies. If an unexplained fever over 38°C occurs, blood cultures should be obtained and antibiotics should be begun immediately. Parents may keep penicillin at home and treat the first sign of fever or infection. This is because of the high incidence of sudden onset of pneumococcal septicemia which can be overwhelming and cause death in a matter of hours.

3. Avoiding low-oxygen environments. Flights on regular pressurized aircraft are permitted, but unpressurized aircraft are not advised. Prolonged underwater swimming or breath holding can also precipitate problems.

SCREENING. Screening for sickle cell is a complicated issue and many differences of opinion exist. The most reasonable approaches to prevention of transmission and prevention of morbidity are presented.

Sickle cell anemia. Neonatal screening for detection of infants with sickle cell anemia is suggested to counsel parents regarding optimal infant care and early detection of crises. This may reduce the high risk of morbidity and mortality in children between 6 months and 3 years of age. There is a special procedure available that can differentiate trait from disease at birth (Bailey, 1974; Smith, 1973).

Sickle cell trait. The purpose of screening for trait is to identify those parents or prospective parents who are carriers and may produce offspring with sickle cell disease and to provide the information and counseling necessary for these persons to make informed decisions about childbearing.

When to screen. The question about when to perform screening is currently at issue. Many agencies perform screening for sickle cell on all Afro-American children during the latter part of the first year of life. Since screening before 1 year of age may be inaccurate if levels of fetal hemoglobin persist, some authorities recommend that screening be performed after 1 year of age (Koerper, 1977).

Implications of early screening. Identification of infants and young children with sickle cell trait means that parents must be educated about the consequences of childbearing. Parents then have the responsibility of informing their children when they reach childbearing age. Unless continuity of health supervision is maintained, the risks of parental misinterpretation of such information, of placing unnecessary restrictions on themselves and on their children, and the anxiety and worry produced are real dangers.

Screening in adolescence. Recommendations by some authorities suggest that screening programs be directed toward adolescents who have been exposed to an educational program which accurately describes the consequences of sickle cell trait and disease and the reproductive alternatives available to persons with the genetic trait (birth control, abortion, artificial insemination, or assumption of a 25 percent risk with each pregnancy of producing a child with sickle cell disease). This approach runs the risk of being too late in populations where sexual activity results in early adolescent pregnancies. Additional recommendations for screening are at the time of entry into the armed forces, during routine antepartum care, as a part of premarital examinations, and when persons are admitted to the hospital (Smith, 1973). Screening must be voluntary and performed only with informed consent.

Positive results. Every person with a positive screening test should have a hemoglobin electrophoresis test to provide definitive information on the types of hemoglobin present. Sickle cell prep and Sickledex do not differentiate between trait and disease.

Counseling. Points to include in counseling persons with sickle cell trait are:

1. Individuals with the trait must be counseled that they do *not* have the disease, that they do *not* have to alter their normal life activities, and that their life span is normal.

2. There is reason to mention risks associated with unusual hypoxia. It has been reported that unaccustomed, vigorous exercise at high altitudes (over 4000 feet) resulted in the deaths of four black males (Smith, 1973). Increased risk of vaso-occlusive episodes also exists when flying in unpressurized aircraft or when snorkeling or diving if hypoxia occurs.

3. Persons with trait may be blood donors but should acknowledge the presence of trait so the blood will not be used for newborn exchange transfusions.

4. Before undergoing anesthesia, persons with trait should inform health personnel.

5. Screening information is kept confidential.

RESOURCES. Information on sickle cell disease and trait is available from the following resources:

1. Chief, Health Staff, Job Corps, Manpower Administration, U.S. Department Labor, Washington, DC
2. Foundation for Research and Education in Sickle Cell Disease, 423-431 West 120th Street, New York NY 10027.
3. The National Foundation—March of Dimes, P. O. Box 2000, White Plains NY 10602.

BETA THALASSEMIA

Assessment. Beta thalassemia is a hereditary defect in the rate of production of the beta globin portion of the hemoglobin molecule. It is inherited as an autosomal co-dominant trait in a manner similar to sickle cell disease (see Table 4). The defect results in decreased production of normal beta chains of hemoglobin. The defect is found in persons of Mediterranean and Oriental origin with a 1 percent incidence in American blacks.

BETA THALASSEMIA MAJOR (COOLEY'S ANEMIA). This is the homozygous condition in which there is severely deficient production of the beta chain of hemoglobin and overproduction of the delta chain. Red blood cells have a shortened life span and reduced hemoglobin levels.

Clinical signs and symptoms. These result from severe, progressive hemolytic anemia and chronic hypoxia and develop during the second 6 months of life. They include pallor, irritability, poor growth, greenish brown complexion, and enlarged liver and spleen. Hypertrophy of the blood-forming tissues results in widening of the flat bones of the face and skull which gives a characteristic facies and causes bone pain. Puberty rarely occurs. Prognosis is poor due to side effects of frequent transfusions. Cardiac failure develops in late childhood and adolescence.

Laboratory. These children have low hemoglobin levels (about 6 gm/dl), low MCVs and low red blood cell counts.

BETA THALASSEMIA MINOR (THALASSEMIA TRAIT). This is the heterozygous condition in which there is a mild deficiency in the production of the beta chain of hemoglobin. Mild hypochromic anemia occurs which may be confused with iron deficiency. See this chapter, Iron deficiency anemia. Most children are asymptomatic.

Laboratory. Smaller red blood cells are produced resulting in a low MCV. To compensate for the small cells the body produces more red cells and the RBC is high (over 5.5 million/cu mm). Hemoglobin and hematocrit levels are normal or slightly below normal.

Management. Management depends on whether the condition is homozygous or heterozygous.

BETA THALASSEMIA MAJOR. The management of beta thalassemia major includes:

1. Transfusions of packed red blood cells are given often enough to keep the hemoglobin above 10 to 11 gm/dl. This level should permit a reasonable level of activity, school attendance, alleviation of the severe symptoms of anemia, and fairly normal growth and development in early childhood.

2. Iron-chelating agents to relieve the effects of iron overload (hemosiderosis) are being evaluated and are only being used under research protocol.

3. Splenectomy is often necessary because of massive splenomegaly, but this procedure predisposes the young child to severe septicemia.

4. Counseling. The child must receive on-going support from parents and care providers. Any chronically ill child worries about self-image, repeated medical procedures, being different from peers, and ultimate survival. Parents also need support to cope with the changes in family life occasioned by the care of a chronically ill child, to help the child lead as normal a life as possible, and to deal with their fears about the child's anticipated death.

BETA THALASSEMIA MINOR. The management of beta thalassemia minor involves identifying carriers, providing genetic counseling, and avoiding inappropriate iron therapy.

Screening. Screening for thalassemia trait is indicated in high-risk populations to facilitate genetic counseling (see Chapter 27, Genetics). The process for distinguishing beta thalassemia minor from iron deficiency is presented in Figure 1. If the MCV is low and the RBC is over 5.5 million/cu mm, a hemoglobin electrophoresis is done to determine the presence of increased levels of Hgb A_2 and/or Hgb F, which occur in the beta thalassemias.

ALPHA THALASSEMIA TRAIT

Assessment. This condition is common in southeast Asia, and from 2 to 7 percent of American blacks are heterozygotes for alpha thalassemia. The condition is due to deletion of one or more of the four alpha globin genes normally present and results in decreased synthesis of alpha chains. Thus, there are four possibilities of clinical expression as indicated in Table 5.

CLINICAL IMPLICATIONS. Alpha thalassemia trait is most often confused with beta thalassemia and/or iron deficiency anemia.

Table 5
Alpha Thalassemia

Condition	No. of Genes Deleted	Hgb	MCV	RBC	Clinical Findings
Silent carrier of thalassemia	1	nl	nl	nl	None
Alpha thalassemia trait	2	nl–sl ↓	↓	↑	Microcytosis, occasional mild anemia
Hgb H disease	3	mod ↓ (8–10) gm/dl	↓	nl	Chronic hemolytic anemia
Homozygous alpha thalassemia	4				Anemic and hydropic in utero and are stillborn or die at birth

Source: M. Koerper, Personal Communication, April 1977.

Hemoglobin electrophoresis which is normal in alpha thalassemia will distinguish between alpha and beta thalassemia. Neither alpha nor beta thalassemia will respond to iron therapy.

Management. It is suggested that black newborns be screened for alpha thalassemia. If the MCV at birth is less than 94 fl/dl, a hemoglobin electrophoresis should be performed. Approximately 67 percent of these infants will be heterozygotes for the trait (McMillan,

Table 6
Drugs Provoking Hemolysis in G-6-PD Deficient Red Cells

Acetanilid
Acetophenetidin (phenacetin)
Acetylsalicylic acid (aspirin)
N_2 acetylsulfanilamide
Antipyrine
Colamine
Fava bean
Furazolidone
Isoniazid
Naphthalene (moth balls)
Naphthoate
Nitrofurantoin (Furadantin)
Pamaquine
Para-aminosalicylic acid
Phenacetin
Phenylhydrazine
Primaquine
Probenecid
Pyramidone
Quinine
Quinidine
Salicylazosulfapyridine
Sulfamethoxypyridazine (Kynex)
Sulfacetamide
Sulfisoxazole (Gantrisin)
Sulfoxone
Synthetic vitamin K compounds
Thiazolsulfone

Source: Adapted with permission from J. W. Graef and T. E. Cone, Manual of Pediatric Therapeutics (Boston: Little, Brown, 1974), p. 325.

1977, p. 132). If a child is found to possess alpha thalassemia trait, the parents should be screened to determine the chances of producing a child with all four alpha globin genes missing.

GLUCOSE 6-PHOSPHATE DEHYDROGENASE DEFICIENCY (G-6-PD)

Assessment. This genetically inherited condition is a deficiency of the enzyme G-6-PD in red blood cells which results in hemolysis of red cells after exposure to certain substances having oxidant properties. Although it is a sex-linked trait, female carriers may also be symptomatic (see Chapter 27, X-Linked Inheritance). About 10 percent of American black males and 2 percent of American black females have the defect. It occurs also in Mediterranean, Middle Eastern, and Oriental populations. Symptoms of hemolytic anemia usually occur only during severe infection or following exposure to the offending substances listed in Table 6. They resolve following discontinuation of exposure. Occasionally the anemia may be severe enough to require transfusion.

Management. Prevention of hemolysis by avoiding offending substances is the best treatment. This requires identification of persons with the enzyme deficiency and education of such persons regarding drugs to be avoided. A list of substances should be given to every affected family. A screening blood test is available and should be performed on all black children and those of Mediterranean, Middle Eastern, and Oriental extraction.

References

Bailey, E. N., et al. "Screening in Pediatric Practice." *Pediatr Clin North Am* 21: 123–165, February 1974.

Brunner, L. S. and D. S. Suddarth. *The Lippincott Manual of Nursing Practice.* Philadelphia: Lippincott, 1974.

Committee on Nutrition, American Academy of Pediatrics. "Iron Supplementation for Infants." *Pediatrics* 58:765–767, November 1976.

Dallman, P. R. "New Approaches to Screening for Iron Deficiency." *J Pediatr* 90:678–681, April 1977.

Fost, N. and M. M. Kaback. "Why Do Sickle Cell Screening in Children?" *Pediatrics* 51:742–744, April 1973.

Frankenberg, W. K. and A. F. North. *A Guide to Screening for the EPSDT Program under Medicaid.* Washington, D.C.: Social and Rehabilitation Service, Dept. of HEW, 1974.

Frankenberg, W. K. and B. W. Camp. *Pediatric Screening Tests.* Springfield, Ill.: Thomas, 1975.

Graef, J. W. and T. E. Cone. *Manual of Pediatric Therapeutics.* Boston: Little, Brown, 1974.

Haddy, T. B., et al. "Iron Deficiency with and without Anemia in Infants and Children." *Am J Dis Child* 128:787–793, December 1974.

Koerper, M. Personal communication, April 1977.

Koerper, M. A. and P. R. Dallman. "Serum Iron Concentration and Transferrin Saturation in the Diagnosis of Iron Deficiency in Children: Normal Developmental Changes." *J Pediatr* 91:870–874, December 1977.

Koerper, M. A., M. C. Mentzer, G. Brecher, and P. R. Dallman. "Developmental Changes in Red Blood Cell Volume: Implications in Screening Infants and Children for Iron Deficiency and Thalassemia Trait." *J Pediatr* 89:580, October 1976.

Levin, R. H. "Iron Deficiency Anemia in the Pediatric Patient." *J Am Pharm Assoc* N.S.11(12):670–676, December 1971.

Lin-Fu, J. S. *Prevention of Hemolytic Disease of the Fetus and Newborn Due to Rh Isoimmunization.* Rockville, Md.: DHEW Publication No. (HSA) 75-5125, 1975.

McFarlane, J. M. "Everyday Care of the Child with Sickle Cell Anemia." *Pediatric Nursing* 2:9–11, January/February 1976.

McMillan, J. A., P. I. Nieburg, and F. A. Oski. *The Whole Pediatrician Catalog.* Philadelphia: Saunders, 1977.

Rudolph, A. M., editor. *Pediatrics,* 16th ed. New York: Appleton-Century-Crofts, 1977.

Smith, N. J. *Iron Nutrition in Infancy: Report of the Sixty-Second Ross Conference on Pediatric Research.* Columbus, Ohio: Ross Laboratories, 1970.

Smith, N. J. and E. Rios. "Iron Metabolism and Iron Deficiency in Infancy and Childhood." *Adv Pediatr* 21:239–280, 1974.

Smith, W. B., W. C. Mentzer, and P. R. Dallman. "Identifying and Counseling Patients with Sickle Trait." *Calif Med* 119:1–7, July 1973.

Vaughan, V. C. and R. J. McKay, editors. *Nelson Textbook of Pediatrics,* 10th ed. Philadelphia: Saunders, 1975.

21

The Gastrointestinal System

Parents are frequently concerned during infancy and childhood about commonly occurring maladjustments of the gastrointestinal (GI) system such as regurgitation, constipation, diarrhea, and abdominal pain. While these conditions occasionally cause only minor problems, they can also herald the beginning of more serious pathologic conditions. The nurse practitioner is continuously alert to the presence of symptoms that indicate more serious progression of disease processes, obtains medical consultation when indicated, and discusses with parents the management.

ASSESSMENT

Normal Values

BOWEL MOVEMENTS

There is a wide variation in stool patterns from individual to individual. Frequency and consistency are determined to a large extent on the type and amount of oral intake and on the variability in the GI pattern of absorption and motility. There is no correct number of bowel movements an individual should have over a period of days. Color of stools also varies according to oral intake and physiology of the GI tract. Normally stools are brown. Black stools may indicate the presence of blood, iron, or bismuth preparations. Red stools may indicate frank bleeding of the large intestine or anal fissures or may be due to certain foods such as undigested beets. Clay-colored stools may indicate biliary obstruction. For normal patterns of stools in infancy, see Chapter 8, Constipation in Infancy.

History

PAST

Obtain information on past illnesses: colic, infant feeding problems, constipation, melena, surgical procedures, failure to thrive, chronic diarrhea, indigestion, vomiting, family allergies, and foreign travel.

PRESENT

Obtain information regarding the age of the child; initial symptoms: progression, severity, and duration; the quality of pain: radiating, dull, or sharp; symptoms associated with eating, drinking and if relieved by such; number and consistency of bowel movements; family's feelings in reference to normalcy of elimination; presence of blood, mucus, or pus in the stools; medications taken; previous treatments; current oral intake; presence of vomiting and description: color, projectile or nonprojectile.

BIRTH

Discuss: complications of pregnancy, labor, and delivery, gestational age, birth weight, early elimination patterns, description of bowel movements, and feeding problems in the hospital: poor sucking, copious regurgitation, vomiting.

FAMILY

Discuss familial diseases (cystic fibrosis, celiac disease); family members with similar symptoms of the presenting complaint.

Physical Examination

The nurse practitioner performs a complete physical examination. See Chapter 1, Child Health Assessment.

Laboratory

STOOL ANALYSIS

Examination of the stool is helpful evaluating disease entities such as bacterial and parasitic infections, malabsorption, and ulcerative colitis. Frank examination of the stool includes inspection for:

- Mucus, blood, or pus; this could suggest a bacterial infection.
- White flecks and beanlike curds; this could indicate a protein allergy.
- Oil in stool; this could indicate steatorrhea indicative of cystic fibrosis and celiac disease.

Other examinations of the stool include:

- pH and reducing substances (sugar); pH below 6.0 and sugar in the stool could indicate disaccharide intolerance.
- Stool smear for leukocytes; their presence could indicate bacterial infection or ulcerative colitis.
- Stool for ova and parasites; a positive result indicates infection.
- Stool for bacterial culture
- Seventy-two hour stool collection for quantitative fat determination; a fat content of more than 10 percent of fat ingested in the previous 24 hours could indicate the presence of malabsorption.

OTHER LABORATORY EXAMINATIONS

- Complete blood count to rule out infection, anemia
- Sweat test to rule out cystic fibrosis
- Disaccharide tolerance test to rule out disaccharide intolerance
- Xylose tolerance test to rule out small bowel malabsorption
- Barium enema to rule out Hirschprung's disease, malrotation, and colitis

MANAGEMENT

Diet

Diet therapy is an important aspect of any management plan in the GI system. Depending on the specific disease entity, the dietary management may include nothing by mouth, clear liquids, a modified or routine diet.

Counseling

Disease of the GI tract, while extremely common, can occasionally become life threatening. Examples include intractable diarrhea, undetected malabsorption syndromes, appendicitis, Hirschprung's disease, and intestinal obstruction. The nurse practitioner educates parents about the symptoms of severe illness: dehydration, extreme lethargy, severe abdominal pain, copious blood in the stools, severe vomiting, and abdominal distension. Parents are counseled to seek medical consultation if these conditions occur.

Hospitalization

In situations when hospitalization occurs, the nurse practitioner continues to offer psychologic support, explanations of the medical regimen, and plans with the parents and hospital staff for discharge and follow-up care.

Ambulatory Care

If ambulatory management is indicated, the nurse practitioner follows closely with the parents the progression of symptoms, is alert to increased symptoms of illness, and reinforces explanations of management.

Medications

LAXATIVES

Laxatives are rarely used for simple constipation. Instead families are counseled in establishing proper bowel habits, increasing high residue foods in the diet, and increasing the oral fluid intake. Laxatives are never used in infants. In school age children they are used when constipation is a symptom of conditions like encopresis and anal fissures.

Stimulant. These laxatives increase the peristaltic activity of the intestine by irritation of the mucosa. Examples are cascara and senna compounds.

Emollient. These laxatives permit the mixture of fat and water in the intestines which helps soften the stool. An example is dioctyl sodium sulfosuccinate (Colace).

Lubricant. These laxatives soften the stools by preventing colonic reabsorption of water. Examples of lubricants are mineral oil and olive oil. With prolonged use mineral oil is absorbed through the GI tract and can penetrate the mesenteric lymph nodes, liver, and spleen causing chronic inflammation (American Pharmaceutical Association, 1977, p. 43). If given with meals, mineral oil may interfere with the absorption of calcium and vitamins A and D.

ANTIEMETICS

Medications to control vomiting are rarely used in infants and children because they can mask symptoms diagnostic of potentially serious diseases such as intestinal obstruction. Judicious use of antiemetics is at the discretion of the physician.

ANTIDIARRHEALS

Occasionally medications are used in the management of diarrhea in older children, but never in infants and toddlers. Medications do not lessen the amount of fluid loss and mask the severity of the diarrhea by making the stools appear more firm. Some medications decrease abdominal cramps and bowel motility. The following are some commonly used drugs:

- Opiates (paregoric and tincture of opium) increase smooth muscle tone and decrease bowel motility.
- Absorbents (Kaopectate) absorb excess water in the stools.
- Antispasmodics (Lomotil) decrease bowel motility.
- Lactobacillus preparations (yogurt) are thought to help restore normal flora in the colon after acute infections.

COMMON CLINICAL PROBLEMS

Anal Fissures

ASSESSMENT

Definition. Anal fissures are small tears in the anal mucosa and occur as a result of the passage of hard stools. Occasionally, children will try to hold back stools because of painful defecation with resulting increased constipation. Occasionally, small streaks of bright red blood are seen in the bowel movement.

Physical examination. With a good light and a magnifying lens, fissures can usually be seen with the child in knee-chest position and with the buttocks spread apart. A digital examination is done to rule out anal sphincter stenosis.

Differential diagnosis. Anal fissures account for over 50 percent of all causes of rectal bleeding. Other causes include intussusception, volvulus, diarrhea, and ulcerative colitis. Rarely is malignancy a cause of rectal bleeding in childhood. Gross red blood in stools is usually associated with lower intestinal bleeding, while tarry stools are usually associated with gastric or small intestinal bleeding.

MANAGEMENT

Diet. The diet is increased in roughage-containing foods such as fibrous vegetables, fruits, and bran flakes.

Medication. The consistency of the stool is altered to permit passage through the rectum without difficulty. Stool softeners, such as mineral oil, between meals so as not to interfere with Vitamin A and D absorption, and dioctyl sodium sulfosuccinate (Colace), are prescribed.

Sitz baths. These warm tub baths reduce anal discomfort and are prescribed three times a day.

Counseling. Parents are counseled to continue the medication regimen until stools are soft. Dietary management is reviewed. In cases where the anal sphincter is tight manual dilation by the child or parent while the child is taking a sitz bath is recommended.

Appendicitis

ASSESSMENT

Definition. Appendicitis is an inflammation of the small appendage of the cecum.

Symptoms. Frequently, the symptoms are varied, vague, and atypical. However, the child usually complains of persistent, localized lower-right-quadrant pain. There may or may not be vomiting, slight fever, anorexia, diarrhea, or constipation. Physical examination reveals signs of peritoneal irritation such as rebound tenderness on palpation of the abdomen.

Differential diagnosis. Other causes of abdominal pain include viral and bacterial gastroenteritis, urinary and pelvic infections, food poisoning, and respiratory disease.

Laboratory. Blood leukocytes seldom reveal values greater than 15,000/cu mm. Chest X-ray and urinalysis are obtained to rule out respiratory and urinary tract infection which can cause abdominal pain.

Physical examination. A complete physical is done including a rectal examination.

MANAGEMENT

Appendectomy is performed and the prognosis is excellent. If the appendix ruptures, either localized or generalized peritonitis results, and the treatment is intensive antibiotic therapy.

Constipation

ASSESSMENT

Definition. Constipation is frequently interpreted by parents as straining, grunting, or any difficulty with stool passage especially during infancy. While these symptoms are frequent, true constipation is defined as hard, rocklike bowel movements regardless of difficulty of passage.

Etiology. The most common cause during infancy is dietary mismanagement. Other causes in childhood include faulty habits (retaining stool), pain on defecation, cultural beliefs, frequent use of laxatives and enemas, and psychogenic problems related to elimination. Medical causes include Hirschsprung's disease, hypothyroidism, renal-tubular acidosis, anal fissures, and strictures.

Physical examination. Occasionally on examination a distended abdomen and a rectum full of feces is present.

MANAGEMENT

Diet. During infancy and childhood the amount of water and high residue foods such as fruits, fibrous vegetables, and bran flakes is increased.

Medication. For chronic constipation the lower bowel is cleansed with enemas and stool softeners are prescribed. See this chapter, Medications.

Encopresis

ASSESSMENT

Definition. Encopresis is fecal incontinence without any organic cause. The bowel movements are usually constipated and some children have fecal impactions. Children with primary encopresis have never been toilet trained, while children with secondary encopresis had at one time established complete control of bowel patterns.

Etiology. Chronic constipation or psychogenic problems such as an attention-gaining behavior or regression are frequent causes of encopresis. Rarer causes include spinal cord lesions and anorectal stenosis (Green, 1977).

Epidemiology. Generally the condition appears in children over 5 years of age, and males are more commonly affected. Children state that they are unaware that they are having a bowel movement.

Some children are compulsive about neatness, have a large amount of stress in their lives, have dysfunctional parental relationships, and are loners.

Physical examination. A complete physical is done including rectal examination for anal strictures.

MANAGEMENT

Bowel routine. The establishment of a regular bowel routine is mandatory. Fecal impactions are removed through enemas, and a high residue diet is prescribed.

Medication. Stool softeners are given daily to ensure easy passage of stool and to help retrain bowel habits.

Family therapy. If the condition continues the family is referred for therapeutic counseling and investigation of psychogenic causes.

Role of the nurse practitioner. In management the nurse practitioner provides education in reference to adequate nutrition, monitors compliance to the medication regimen, and allows the family to discuss feelings of frustration and anger.

Diarrhea

ASSESSMENT

Definition. Diarrhea is defined as watery, copious bowel movements which are usually green in color and have a foul odor. Occasionally the diarrhea contains blood, pus, or mucus, and this can indicate bacterial infection. Diarrhea is prevalent during infancy and childhood and is of particular concern during the first 12 months of life because of the infant's inability to tolerate fluid losses which result in dehydration and electrolyte imbalance.

Etiology. There are multiple causes of diarrhea:

- Nonbacterial, nonspecific, or viral
- Dietary mismanagement

- As a symptom of other illnesses: otitis media, urinary tract infection, meningitis (in infants)
- Complication of antibiotic therapy: ampicillin, neomycin, tetracycline
- Bacterial: *Salmonella, Shigella,* enteropathic *Escherichia coli*
- Malabsorption: mono- and disaccharide deficiencies; cystic fibrosis, celiac disease
- Milk allergy
- Food poisoning
- Chronic ulcerative colitis
- Chronic giardiasis
- Intestinal obstruction

History. In assessing diarrhea the following are included:

- Caretakers definition of diarrhea
- Onset of symptoms
- Number and size of bowel movements in 24 hours
- Consistency and color including presence or absence of blood, pus, mucus, or water ring
- History of exposure in family, community
- Current oral intake
- Presence or absence of other symptoms: fever, irritability, cold, cough, lethargy, anorexia, vomiting, pain, or frequency in voiding
- Symptoms of dehydration
- Treatment regimens at home
- Parental degree of concern

Physical examination. A complete physical examination is done to rule out the presence of contributing disease conditions. The degree of hydration is evaluated. Special attention is given to the following areas:

- Skin: dry, hot
- Head: anterior and posterior fontanelle: bulging, full, flat, or sunken
- Mouth: mucous membranes, moist or dry

- Eyes: orbits sunken, presence or absence of tearing
- Neck: supple or rigid
- Ears: presence of middle-ear infection
- Abdomen: presence or absence of organomegaly, tenderness, bowel sounds
- Neurologic: tone, normal, hypo- or hyperactive; symmetry of movement, general state of awareness

Complications. The following can be severe complications of diarrhea.

DEHYDRATION. This condition is defined as the percentage of body weight lost as water. For example, a child who is 10 percent dehydrated has lost 100 cc of water for every kilogram of body weight. The majority of children with diarrhea are less than 5 percent dehydrated. Clinical signs of dehydration are:

Body weight lost as water	Symptoms
5 percent	Dry mucous membranes, lack of tear formation
7–10 percent	Decreased skin turgor, sunken eyes, sunken fontanelle, increased pulse rate
10–15 percent	Low blood pressure

METABOLIC ACIDOSIS. This condition occurs because of excessive fluid and electrolyte losses. The bicarbonate concentration and the pH of the blood decreases causing hyperventilation, tachypnea, tachycardia, and extreme irritability. Blood electrolyte studies show a low bicarbonate level and a relatively normal chloride level.

Indications for referral. It is difficult to assess the problem of diarrhea over the phone if parents or the caretakers are unfamiliar to the nurse practitioner. Newborns with diarrhea and children with increased symptoms of illness are seen in the primary health care facility.

MANAGEMENT

Goals. The goals of management are to provide decreased irritation to the GI tract, to prevent dehydration, and to correct electrolyte imbalances.

Diet. Diet modification is a major management component of diarrhea.

LIQUIDS. Clear liquids are prescribed for 24 hours and include water with nonlactose sugar, apple juice, flat, diluted ginger ale, and flavored gelatin. Commercial preparations such as Lytren or Pedialyte contain carbohydrates and electrolytes in correct amounts and are also prescribed.

AMOUNTS. Amounts of clear liquids given are approximately 150 cc per kilogram of body weight up to 1 year of age. For fluid requirements over 1 year of age see Chapter 6, Table 2, Daily Fluid Requirements. If vomiting is present, small amounts of fluids are given frequently, 15 to 30 cc every 30 to 60 minutes. With diarrhea large amounts of fluids are given infrequently.

FOOD PROGRESSION. If diarrhea continues after 24 hours without clinical evidence of dehydration, solids such as rice cereal, applesauce, and bananas are added to the diet to promote bulk in the stools. If the diarrhea is decreasing, the diet is slowly advanced on the second or third day to include half-strength formula. If the diarrhea has been prolonged some authorities recommend a soy formula for several months because of secondary lactose intolerance.

Medication. See this chapter, Medications.

Stool culture. Cultures are obtained on all children whose symptoms last longer than 5 days, whose history is positive for exposure to bacterial gastroenteritis, and whose stools contain blood, mucus, or pus.

Secondary lactose intolerance. Because of gastrointestinal inflammation, lactase, the enzyme which changes lactose into the simple sugars fructose and galactose, cannot function properly. This leads to transient intolerance of lactose with secondary diarrhea. Since human and cow milk contain lactose as the carbohydrate, a nonlactose soy formula is substituted until the diarrhea is abated. See this chapter, Malabsorption: Disaccharide Deficiencies.

Counseling. Monitoring the temperature is discussed with the parents. The amount and frequency of oral fluids are reviewed. Parents are counseled to observe for increased symptoms of illness: reduced fluid intake, increased water in bowel movements, fever, lethargy, symptoms of dehydration and electrolyte imbalance, irritability, and anorexia.

Indications for hospitalization. Medical consultation is necessary and possible hospitalization is indicated if the client is an infant and exhibits symptoms of dehydration, electrolyte imbalance, or sepsis.

Enteropathic *Escherichia coli* Gastroenteritis

ASSESSMENT

Etiology. *E. coli* are gram-negative bacteria which normally inhabit the GI tract. Only some serologic types are pathogenic. *E. coli* gastroenteritis is more common with poor sanitary conditions and with a contaminated water supply.

Symptoms. Variable symptoms are present ranging from mild diarrhea to fever, vomiting, and copious stools which are green, watery, and foul smelling. Occasionally stools contain mucus, but blood and pus are usually absent.

MANAGEMENT

Diet. Clear liquids or intravenous fluids are prescribed if the child is hospitalized until fluid and electrolyte imbalances are corrected. A diet then may be eaten as tolerated.

Medication. The management of choice is antibiotic therapy by mouth, or systemically, depending on the age of the child and the severity of the disease. Since some types of pathogenic *E. coli* are resistant to antibiotics sensitivity studies are necessary.

Counseling. Parents are counseled to observe for symptoms of increased illness and secondary infection. Sanitary measures are discussed which include hand washing after toilet use and after contact with infected materials.

Salmonella Gastroenteritis

ASSESSMENT

Etiology. *Salmonella* are gram-negative bacteria which commonly infect mammals, birds, and reptiles. They are transmitted between animals and man through contaminated food and water and through infected pet turtles.

Symptoms. Diarrhea is the primary symptom and occasionally it contains blood or pus. The *Salmonella* bacillus is destroyed by the inflammatory cells of the GI tract, hence the disease is self-limited and usually lasts 5 to 7 days.

Diagnosis. A stool culture is obtained.

MANAGEMENT

Diet. Clear liquids or intravenous fluids are prescribed if the child is hospitalized until fluid and electrolyte imbalances are corrected. A diet then may be eaten as tolerated.

Medication. There is no evidence that antibiotics shorten or reduce the severity of the illness, and there is some evidence that antibiotics may even prolong the carrier state. They are used when there is evidence of secondary infection and in children with chronic bowel or sickle cell disease.

Counseling. Parents are counseled that the bacillus is shed in the stools of asymptomatic children for weeks to months. Some children become chronic carriers and periodic stool cultures are necessary. If children return to school while carriers, they are counseled about handwashing after toilet use.

Shigella Dysentery

ASSESSMENT

Etiology. The etiologic agents of the genus *Shigella* are divided into types: *S. dysenteriae, S. flexneri, S. boydie*, and *S. sonnei*. All may cause dysentery in humans. Some types of *Shigella* produce extraintestinal infections such as those in the urinary tract.

Symptoms. Variable symptoms range from mild (loose stools, slight or absent fever), to severe (watery green stools with blood or mucus, abdominal pain, vomiting, headache, rigid neck, and delirium).

Diagnosis. A stool culture is obtained.

MANAGEMENT

Diet. Clear liquids or intravenous fluids are prescribed if the child is hospitalized until the fluid and electrolyte imbalances are corrected. A diet then may be eaten as tolerated.

Medication. Antibiotics by mouth or systemically are the treatment of choice. Sensitivity studies are necessary to ascertain resistant strains.

Counseling. Parents are counseled to observe for symptoms of increased illness and/or secondary infection. Follow-up appointment includes repeat stool cultures.

Malabsorption: Disaccharidase Deficiencies

ASSESSMENT

Definition. The disaccharides lactose and sucrose are broken down by specific enzymes called disaccharidases, which are located in the brush border of the epithelial cells of the small intestine. The enzymes change lactose, sucrose, and maltose to glucose, galactose, and fructose for absorption from the GI tract. In disaccharidase deficiency, the disaccharidases are impaired, and the disaccharides cannot be absorbed. It is speculated that the unabsorbed disaccharide causes an increased osmotic load in the colon, leading to increased intestinal fluid secretion and diarrhea (Lebenthal, 1975).

Classification and etiologies. Disaccharide deficiencies are classified into primary and secondary etiologies.

PRIMARY. The primary deficiencies are congenital and are characterized by the absence of the enzyme in the small intestine. Primary sucrase deficiency is the result of an autosomal recessive disorder. The genetic inheritance of primary lactase deficiency is not yet known.

SECONDARY. The secondary deficiencies occur in any disease involving damage to the mucosa of the small bowel which results in impaired action of the enzymes. Examples are gastroenteritis, ulcerative colitis, irritable colon, cystic fibrosis, celiac disease, malnutrition, and impaired GI tract functioning after gastric surgery. Drugs such as neomycin, kanamycin, and colchicine also affect the mucosa of the small bowel. While all the disaccharidases are affected, lactase is the most severely damaged and is the slowest to recover.

Incidence. Primary sucrase and lactase deficiency is extremely rare. Secondary lactase deficiency occurs in approximately 10 percent of American whites and in 60 to 80 percent of American blacks. Secondary sucrase deficiency symptoms are usually masked by those of lactase.

Symptoms. In infants, watery diarrhea is the most striking symptom. It is usually frothy and copious. Other symptoms are vomiting, abdominal distension, and dehydration. In more severe cases, failure to thrive, electrolyte imbalance, metabolic acidosis, lethargy, and irritability are evident. In older children symptoms include intermittent diarrhea and abdominal pain. Steatorrhea, excessive fat in the stool, occurs in some children, and it is usually an indication that the intestinal mucosa has suffered extensive damage.

Laboratory. The following tests are done:

REDUCING SUBSTANCES. The stool is examined for the presence of undigested sugar (reducing substance). In testing the stool for the presence of lactose 10 drops of water and 5 drops of watery stool are mixed. One Clinitest tablet is added, and the test is read the same as when testing urine for sugar.

In testing the stool for the presence of sucrose 10 drops of 1 normal hydrochloric acid and 5 drops of stool are mixed. The mixture is allowed to react for a few minutes before the Clinitest tablet is added. The test is read the same as when testing urine for sugar.

pH. The stool is also tested for pH since in disaccharide intolerance the pH is less than 6.0. These tests if positive, however, are not considered diagnostic of disaccharide malabsorption.

DISACCHARIDE TOLERANCE TEST. A more specific test of disaccharidase function is the oral disaccharide tolerance test. Two grams of lactose or sucrose per kilogram of body weight are given orally. A rise in blood glucose of 20 to 25 mg/100 ml or greater indicates normal hydrolysis of disaccharides. A blood glucose rise of less than 20 mg/100 ml indicates that the disaccharide has not been hydrolyzed and remains unabsorbed from the GI tract. A complication of this test can be severe diarrhea.

Physical examination. A complete physical is done.

MANAGEMENT

Diet. For lactase deficiency a lactose-free diet is prescribed. Since lactose is the sugar in human and cow milk the child is placed on a soy formula. Foods are also excluded which contain lactose such as whey, dry milk solids, and dairy products. Parents are instructed to read labels on all products including baby food preparations to make sure that they do not contain lactose.

In sucrase deficiency the diet is more complicated since sucrose is present in many foods including various fruits, vegetables, cooked and dry cereals, and canned foods. Oral antibiotic preparations and aspirin contain sucrose.

Counseling. The nurse practitioner counsels parents about dietary management. After gastrointestinal infections the nurse is aware that several months are needed for the small intestine to regenerate sufficiently for the disaccharidase to return to normal function. Therefore dietary management is continued for 3 to 4 months. Table 1 shows the composition of various carbohydrates in liquid preparations.

Table 1
Composition of Various Carbohydrates in Liquid Preparations

Lactose	Sucrose	Glucose	Corn Syrup (contains glucose, maltose, dextrin)
Breast milk	Nutramigen	Pregestimil	Lofenalac
Cow milk	Meat Base	Lytren	Nursoy
Goat milk	Neomullsoy	Oral electrolyte solution	Prosobee
Similac	Nursoy		Soyalac
Similac PM	Prosobee		Isomil
Enfamil	Soyalac		Portagen
SMA	Isomil		Bakers
Lonalac	Portagen		
Bakers			

Pyloric Stenosis

ASSESSMENT

Etiology. The circular muscle of the pylorus valve of the stomach is thickened and elongated, causing disruption in passage of stomach contents into the small intestine. Spasm of the valve occurs causing projectile vomiting.

Epidemiology. This condition occurs in approximately 1 in 500 births. Males are four times more affected, and firstborns are more susceptible than later children.

Symptoms. The most common are:

- Projectile vomiting after feeding. Vomiting most commonly begins after the third to fourth week of life, and it might not occur after every feeding.
- Slow weight gain or weight loss
- Avidly hungry infant
- Dehydration
- Constipation

Physical examination. Occasionally the hypertrophied pyloric valve can be palpated in the upper right quadrant of the abdomen and is felt as an olive-sized tumor. The abdomen is observed for distension in the upper right quadrant. Gastric peristaltic waves due to gastric contractions are occasionally observed after feeding. They are seen as rhythmical waves moving across the abdomen.

Diagnostic studies. An abdominal X-ray shows a large gas-filled stomach. Fluoroscopy with barium shows an elongated and narrowed pylorus valve with a delayed opening. However, many authorities rely on the history of sudden occurrence of projectile vomiting, the presence of visible peristaltic waves, and a palpable pyloric mass as symptoms diagnostic of the condition.

MANAGEMENT

Surgery. Dehydration and electrolyte imbalance is corrected before surgery. The operation consists of an incision into the hypertrophied pyloric valve (pyloromyotomy). Depending on the extent of the surgery, the infant may be fed intravenously for several hours or for 1 to 2 days. When oral feedings are begun they are instituted slowly and in small amounts.

Counseling. The nurse practitioner is alert to the symptoms of pyloric stenosis. Since this condition occurs frequently with firstborn children, emotional support to anxious parents is offered. The nurse encourages the parents to hold and to care for the infant and offers explanations about management procedures during hospitalization. Support and routine health education continue after hospital discharge.

Regurgitation

ASSESSMENT

Definition. Regurgitation is a common occurrence in the first year of life. It is the nonforceful, nonprojectile, effortless expulsion from the stomach of a small quantity of liquid or food after feeding. Refer to Chapter 8, Spitting-Up, for more information.

Etiology. Regurgitation is caused by air swallowed with food, overfeeding, allergy to cow milk or a relaxed stomach cardiac sphincter muscle. Because of the lax muscle, milk is expulsed with bubbling. Occasionally significant regurgitation continues past 6 months of age, and close observation of weight gain is necessary.

Diagnostic studies. An upper gastrointestinal series is helpful in determining the severity of the regurgitation if the condition continues past 12 months of age and in assessing the presence of anatomic anomalies. Hemoglobin determination is sometimes necessary because of occasional iron deficiency anemia from coexistent esophagitis secondary to hydrochloric acid bathing the lower esophagus.

Physical examination. A complete physical is done.

MANAGEMENT

Counseling. Parents are counseled to thicken oral liquids with cereal and to bubble the child frequently during feeding. The child remains upright after feeding for 30 minutes.

Stomach ache

ASSESSMENT

Etiology. Organic causes of stomach ache are found in less than 10 percent of all cases. They include:

- Cholelithiasis
- Constipation
- Malrotation of the bowel
- Meckel's diverticulum
- Parasitic infection
- Peptic ulcer
- Regional enteritis
- Ulcerative colitis
- Urinary tract infection or anomaly

Other causes include:

- Idiopathic
- Psychogenic

  1. Attention mechanism
  2. Phobias
  3. Stress
  4. Unconscious diversion to keep family from solving other problems

Epidemiology. Complaints of stomach ache occur in 1 of 10 children. The most common ages are 5 to 10 years.

Symptoms. The most common symptom is pain usually around the umbilicus or in the lower abdomen. Pain in this area is less likely to have an organic cause than pain that is lateral. The pain is not usually related to stressful situations, does not awaken the child from sleep, and is rarely related to meals. Frequency varies from several times a day to weekly or monthly. Occasionally there is pain in other areas of the body. This usually indicates a psychogenic rather than an organic cause.

Physical examination. A complete physical is done. Occasionally this procedure has reassuring qualities for the parents in knowing that a thorough examination was completed even though no organic cause is found.

Laboratory. Diagnostic studies are considered after evaluating the results of the physical examination, the chronicity of the symptoms, and the psychosocial milieu.

MANAGEMENT

Organic. If organic lesions are found, appropriate management is initiated. If no evidence of organic or familial dysfunction is found, the child is periodically seen for re-evaluations, since an organic pathologic condition may be more easily diagnosed at a later date.

Psychogenic. If physical and laboratory values are normal, the presence of family dysfunction is further investigated. Common factors to consider are recent death or separation of family members, amount and frequency of illness in the family, marital disharmony, too strict or too inconsistent discipline, lack of attention toward the child, alcoholism or drug abuse, and financial problems. If serious family dysfunction is evident, the family is referred to a behavioral pediatrician for further counseling.

Vomiting

ASSESSMENT

Definition. Vomiting is the forceful retching of gastric contents. It may be projectile or nonprojectile. Projectile vomiting may indicate serious organicity such as pyloric stenosis or increased intracranial pressure. Vomiting is occasionally confused with regurgitation. See this chapter, Regurgitation.

Etiology. In association with the GI tract, the following etiologies are considered:

- Chalasia
- Intestinal obstruction
- Overfeeding
- Pyloric stenosis

In association with infection, the following etiologies are considered:

- Gastroenteritis
- Meningitis
- Parasitic
- Respiratory
- Septicemia
- Urinary tract

Other causes of vomiting include:

- Congenital adrenal hyperplasia
- Diabetic acidosis
- Drugs: digitalis, aspirin, some antibiotics, sulfonamides
- Increased intracranial pressure

History. Include the following information:

- Age of the child
- Frequency, amount, and time of occurrence

- Length of time symptom is evident
- Nature of vomitus: color, presence of blood, mucus, pus
- Projectile or nonprojectile
- Forceful or effortless
- Other associated symptoms: diarrhea, respiratory infection, dehydration, fever, constipation
- Feeding techniques: frequency of burping, sitting up after feeding.
- Home treatment: use of medications, types of food given

Physical examination. A complete physical is done.

MANAGEMENT

Diet. After a serious organic pathologic cause is ruled out, management begins with dietary modifications. Infants and children are given clear liquids for 6 hours initially. See this chapter, Diarrhea, Dietary Management. Liquids are given in small amounts 15 to 30 cc, frequently every 30 to 60 minutes. If the child retains fluids over a period of time larger amounts of clear liquids are added. After 12 to 24 hours bland foods may be added such as cooked cereal, applesauce, crackers, and bananas. If vomiting continues after 6 hours the child is seen in the health care agency.

Medication. Rarely are antiemetics or sedatives used to control vomiting in infants and children. These medications cause drowsiness and therefore decrease the fluid intake. They also can mask possible serious progression of the vomiting. See this chapter, Medications.

Counseling. The nurse practitioner monitors the frequency of vomiting along with the parent, educates the parent in reference to increased symptoms of illness, and assesses parents' understanding of dietary management. Parents are counseled to bring infants below 6 months of age who exhibit true vomiting to the acute care facility to investigate etiologies and to assess hydration.

References

American Pharmaceutical Association. *Handbook of Nonprescription Drugs,* 5th ed. Washington D.C.: American Pharmaceutical Association, 1977.

Fitzgerald, J. F. "Encopresis, Soiling, Constipation: What's to be Done?" *Pediatrics* 56:348–349, September 1975.

Graef, J. W. and T. E. Cone, Jr. *Manual of Pediatric Therapeutics.* Boston: Little, Brown, 1974.

Grant, M. and W. M. Kubo. "Assessing a Patient's Hydration Status." *Am J Nurs* 75:1306–1311, August 1975.

Green, M. and R. J. Haggerty. *Ambulatory Pediatrics II.* Philadelphia: Saunders, 1977.

Hamilton, J. R., et al. "Recent Developments in Viral Gastroenteritis." *Pediatr Clin North Am* 22:747–755, November 1975.

Kempe, C. H., et al. *Current Pediatric Diagnosis and Treatment.* Los Altos, Calif.: Lange Medical Publications, 1976.

"Lactose Intolerance in Infancy: A Review of the Problem and Its Dietary Management." Evansville, Ind.: Mead Johnson Laboratories, 1975.

Lebenthal, E. "Small Intestinal Disaccharidase Deficiencies." *Pediatr Clin North Am* 22:757–766, November 1975.

Levine, M. D. "Children with Encopresis: A Descriptive Analysis." *Pediatrics* 56:412–416, September 1975.

McMillan, J. A., et al. *The Whole Pediatrician Catalogue.* Philadelphia: Saunders, 1977.

Problems Relating to Feeding in the First Two Years. Columbus, Ohio: Ross Laboratories, 1977.

Rudolph, A. M. editor, *Pediatrics,* 16th ed. New York: Appleton-Century-Crofts, 1977.

Smith, D. W. and R. E. Marshall. *Introduction to Clinical Pediatrics.* Philadelphia: Saunders, 1972.

Waechter, E. H. and F. Blake. *Nursing Care of Children,* 9th ed. Philadelphia: Lippincott, 1976.

Wallach, J. *Interpretation of Diagnostic Tests,* 2nd ed. Boston: Little, Brown, 1974.

22

The Urinary System

The two major functions of the kidneys are to excrete most of the end-products of body metabolism and to control the concentrations of most of the components of body fluids. Urinary disorders (including congenital malformations, structural anomalies, and infections of the urinary tract) are significant in relation to their potential for interrupting these functions and contributing to renal disease. For this reason, any deviations from normal urinary function should be evaluated in collaboration with the physician. This chapter presents information on assessment of the urinary tract with special emphasis on two common problems in primary care pediatrics—enuresis, and urinary tract infection.

ASSESSMENT

Normal Values

BLADDER CONTROL

Ninety-nine percent of infants urinate within the first 48 hours of life. Voiding is completely involuntary until sometime during the

651

second year of life when bladder sensation develops. Complete neuromuscular control of urination is achieved in most children by 4 to 5 years of age.

BLADDER CAPACITY

Approximate bladder capacity in infants and children is as follows (Schauffler, 1958):

At birth	60 cc
3 months	115 cc
1 year	285 cc
12 years	840 cc

ROUTINE URINALYSIS

The specimen should be the first morning specimen (because it is concentrated) and should be examined within a few hours of collection.

General appearance. The urine should be clear. If it is cloudy, it may be abnormal sediment or may be an "old" specimen.

Color. Normal urine is pale yellow or amber. Pink or reddish color may indicate red blood cells, ingestion of beets, blackberries, certain vegetable dyes and drugs. Orange-red or reddish-brown color may indicate bilirubin, blood. Red or red-brown is the most common abnormal color.

Odor. Acetone odor indicates ketonuria. Ammonia or fecal odor indicates bacterial infection.

Specific gravity. Normal values are 1.010 to 1.030. Abnormally low values indicate lack of ability to concentrate urine. Abnormally high values indicate dehydration.

pH. Urine is usually acidic (5-6) in the fasting state. Normal range is 4.6 to 8.

Glucose, protein, ketones, blood. Screening tests for these substances should be negative. However, approximately 5 percent of children will have a trace or 1+ protein which can be caused by exercise, fever, dehydration, infection, cold temperatures. It is usually transient. A second specimen (first morning specimen) should be examined and if proteinuria is persistent or above 2+, the child needs further evaluation.

Sediment. The specimen is centrifuged and examined microscopically for sediment.

- Red blood cells. More than 2 to 3 cells per high power field is abnormal. A repeat specimen is obtained.
- White blood cells. More than 5 cells per high power field is abnormal and indicates a suppurative process. A repeat specimen is obtained with special care in cleansing the perineal area. *Pyuria* is defined as 10 or more leukocytes per cubic millimeter in an uncentrifuged sample of a clean catch, midstream urine specimen, *or* 5 to 10 leukocytes per high power field on a centrifuged specimen (Bailey, 1974, p. 147).
- Epithelial cells. These are seen commonly but probably are urethral or vaginal cells.
- Casts. These are clumps of cells formed in the nephron, and their presence indicates some pathologic state in the kidney. Physician consultation is indicated. Red cell casts suggest glomerular injury and renal bleeding; white cell casts suggest pyelonephritis; hyaline casts suggest proteinuria of glomerular origin; granular casts suggest a degenerative process.
- Crystals. These are normally not present. Most are of no significance although some acid urine crystals may be suggestive of kidney stones.
- Bacteria. Bacteriuria is evaluated by direct microscopic examination of the urinary sediment. Any bacteria present in an unspun specimen is indication for obtaining a urine culture and consideration of urinary tract infection.

History

FAMILY HISTORY

Obtain information on incidence of renal disease, deafness, hypertension, structural abnormalities of the urinary tract, and syndromes having associated urinary tract abnormalities.

PAST HISTORY

Obtain information on congenital anomalies; infections, especially streptococcal infections; abdominal pain or mass; vomiting; diarrhea; fever of undetermined origin; failure to thrive; changes or abnormalities in micturition including frequency, dribbling, dysuria, urgency, enuresis, daytime incontinence, increased or decreased urine volume; change in color or odor or urine; edema; toilet training.

Physical Examination

GENERAL

Obtain vital signs, blood pressure. Evaluate growth patterns.

SKIN

Observe for pallor, sallow complexion, dehydration, and edema.

EARS

Inspect for low-set or deformed ears.

CARDIOVASCULAR

Check for tachypnea, hypertension, and circulatory congestion.

ABDOMEN

Palpate for enlargement of kidneys, costal-vertebral angle (CVA) tenderness, flank or suprapubic tenderness, abdominal masses, and ascites.

GENITALIA

Observe for abnormalities of the external genitalia.

NEUROLOGIC

Examine for innervation abnormalities in the lower extremities.

MANAGEMENT

Every child with symptoms or findings suggestive of urinary tract anomaly or kidney disease must be referred for thorough evaluation. Parents and child need interpretation of diagnostic procedures and treatment plans. They also need education aimed at preventing urinary infections. See this chapter, Urinary Tract Infection.

COMMON CLINICAL PROBLEMS

Enuresis

ASSESSMENT

Enuresis is involuntary urination in a child whose age and development are such that control would be expected. *Primary* enuresis occurs in children who have never achieved bladder control. *Secondary* enuresis occurs in children who previously have achieved bladder control for at least 3 months to 6 months and then lose it. *Enuresis* usually refers to involuntary wetting during sleep; *diurnal enuresis* refers to wetting during the day and when it occurs in children over 5 years of age, a significant pathologic state must be suspected. Since the complete neuromuscular control of urination is attained by most children by 4 to 5 years of age, the diagnosis of enuresis should be made for involuntary urination beyond the age of 5 years in girls and 6 years in boys.

Incidence. Twenty-five percent of children will have some relapse bedwetting that usually occurs at times of illness or stress and is self-limiting. Beyond this, surveys indicate that up to 15 percent of 6 to 7 year olds and 3 percent of 13 to 14 year olds may still wet the bed more than once a month (Starfield, 1972). Males are affected more than females in all age groups.

Etiology. Etiology is complex and not completely understood, but several factors are thought to contribute.

1. Developmental delay. An inherited tendency toward delayed development of adequate neuromuscular control is thought to be a major factor in primary enuresis. Strong familial tendencies exist; these children have small functional bladder capacity sometimes called "irritable bladder," and most are cured spontaneously as maturation occurs (Cohen, 1975). Twenty-five percent of children having one enuretic parent will themselves be enuretic and 50 percent if both parents were enuretics.

2. Organic factors. Most cases of enuresis involve no organic basis, but organic etiology must be ruled out. Disorders that may cause enuresis include obstructive lesions of the genitourinary tract, urinary tract infections, lumbosacral disorders which affect bladder innervation, conditions in which the ability to concentrate urine is impaired (e.g., diabetes mellitus, diabetes insipidus, sickle cell anemia, and allergic disorders).

3. Deep sleep. One hypothesis suggests that some enuretic children have a high threshold for nocturnal arousal (Waechter, 1976).

4. Psychologic-emotional factors. Situational crises (e.g., death of a parent, birth of a sibling, move to a new surrounding) may cause temporary regression in bladder control. Too early, too vigorous or other inappropriate approaches to toilet training may result in enuresis. Enuresis may also be symptomatic of more serious behavioral disorders, significant family stress, or psychopathology. Parental attitudes commonly associated with an enuretic child are punitiveness, neglect, oversubmissiveness, and perfectionism.

History. A detailed account of the enuresis includes information regarding:

1. Number of nights per week or month that bedwetting occurs
2. Fluid intake

3. Sleep patterns
4. Voiding patterns
5. Any related events or stress
6. Occurrence at home and/or away from home
7. Management techniques used by family
8. Child's response to enuresis—ask the *child*
9. Family attitudes and response to enuresis
10. Emotional climate in the home
11. Details of toilet training
12. Presence or absence of family history of enuresis

Past medical history, review of systems, and physical examination should include areas mentioned previously in this chapter.

Laboratory. Routine urinalysis and measurement of specific gravity after an overnight fast are performed. Functional bladder capacity should be measured as a baseline. Functional bladder capacity is determined by having the child refrain from voiding as long as possible and then measuring the amount voided. Adequate nighttime bladder control cannot be attained if bladder capacity is significantly less than 10 ounces. Urine culture is obtained if suspicion of infection exists. If an underlying organic disorder is suspected, appropriate blood and urine studies should be carried out with referral to the appropriate specialists.

MANAGEMENT

Most children will be best managed by the primary care provider who has rapport with the family since a positive relationship may be the most important therapeutic tool. The approach must be geared to the individual situation considering the child's age, severity of symptoms, and severity of family disruption. Since the cause of the enuresis is often obscure or difficult to assign with certainty, the most frequent approach to therapy is to attempt to alleviate the symptom. The method chosen must be planned with the child's and family's active participation and consent. If the child is not interested in nor motivated to achieve control, all attempts will fail. Regardless of the method chosen, it must be presented and undertaken with optimism for success.

Counseling and support. These are imperative for every child and family dealing with enuresis. Expression of the feelings of both child and parents should be encouraged and acknowledged. Parents need to be reassured that the child cannot help the enuresis, and that it isn't their fault. If punitive or shaming techniques have been used in the past, parents should not be made to feel more guilty but need explanations that this approach just does not work. The objectives of counseling should include:

1. Parental understanding of the multifactorial nature of enuresis
2. Parental acceptance of the child and the symptoms to provide maximum emotional support
3. Conveyance to the child and family of a sense of optimism
4. Acceptance by the child of the symptom accompanied by identification of the child's strengths in other areas of functioning
5. Development of an appreciation in the child that control of the enuresis can be achieved (Cohen, 1975)

Psychotherapy is indicated when there is evidence of significantly disturbed parent-child relationships.

Simple measures. Activities such as restricting fluids after supper, voiding before bedtime, and rousing to void before the parents' bedtime and at other intervals during the night are frequently suggested, but there is no evidence that they hasten the onset of a spontaneous cure. They may even result in additional conflict between parent and child.

Conditioning. Devices such as the Enuretone apparatus are being used more frequently in children over 8 years of age. A bed mattress device sensitive to moisture is connected to an alarm bell which goes off and wakes the child upon initiation of wetting. Over time this can condition the child to awaken before voiding. Relapses occur frequently, but dryness is attained more quickly and even permanently with a second course. The child may develop a rash on the buttocks or perineum. Use of this technique may be impractical in homes where the sleep of other family members becomes a problem. Studies have shown that this procedure is not psychologically harmful to children (Cohen, 1975).

Medications. Imipramine (Tofranil) has been successful in the control of enuresis in a significant number of cases. The mode of action is unclear but is thought to be either an anticholinergic effect on bladder muscle or an antidepressant effect on the central nervous system. Side effects are nervousness, sleep disorders, and mild GI disturbances. More alarming are the toxic effects, sometimes fatal, which have been associated with accidental ingestion of an overdose by a younger sibling of the enuretic child. Many physicians are wary of prescribing this drug also because of the increasing abuse of mood-altering drugs.

Bladder training. School age children with decreased functional bladder capacity have responded well to a regimen of bladder training. Starfield (1972) has developed a procedure which involves the child in a 6-month program. Once a day the child holds urine for as long as possible. The child drinks a lot of fluid during this period. When the child must void, the urine is measured and the amount recorded in a daily log. Dry nights are also recorded. The recording serves as reinforcement for the child. Wall charts can be kept and the child encouraged to break previous records. In Starfield's study one third of children were cured, and all children had increased functional bladder capacity after 6 months.

Urinary Tract Infection (UTI)

ASSESSMENT

Bacterial infections occur both in the presence of structural abnormalities in the urinary tract and in normal urinary tracts.

Incidence. During infancy about 1 percent of children will develop bacteriuria, and about two thirds of these are boys. After infancy the incidence is much more common in girls. It has been conservatively estimated that from 5 to 10 percent of girls and less than 1 percent of boys will have at least one UTI before 18 years of age (Kunin, 1977). Recurrent infections, abnormalities of the urinary tract, and infections of the upper urinary tract (pyelonephritis) carry guarded prognoses as far as renal damage is concerned.

Etiology. Bacteria enter the urinary tract either through the blood stream (more common in young infants who cannot localize infections well) or through the urethra. Infection may develop in the urethra (urethritis), bladder (cystitis), or kidney (pyelonephritis).

PREDISPOSING FACTORS. Predisposing factors to invasion of bacteria through the urethra are:

1. Shortness of female urethra
2. Obstructive uropathy
3. Foreign bodies
4. Fecal contamination, poor perineal hygiene
5. Stasis or urine, incomplete emptying of the bladder
6. Chemical irritants, bubble bath, detergent
7. Pinworms
8. Indwelling catheters, catheterization
9. Sexual intercourse
10. Pregnancy

COMMON ORGANISMS. The most common organisms which infect the urinary tract are:

1. *Escherichia coli* which accounts for 80 to 85 percent of acute uncomplicated infections and 50 to 70 percent of recurrences.
2. Gram-positive organisms (e.g., *Staphylococcus aureus*) which account for 5 to 10 percent of uncomplicated infections.
3. *Klebsiella, Enterobacter, Pseudomonas,* and *Proteus* which occur less commonly and are associated with more complicated infections (i.e., with presence of structural abnormalities).

Clinical signs and symptoms. Presenting signs and symptoms vary considerably and onset may be gradual or abrupt. A large number of children are asymptomatic, and infection is detected on routine urine screening. Infants may have nonspecific symptoms and may appear lethargic, irritable, and septic with vomiting, diarrhea, fever, and failure to thrive. Young children may have GI symptoms of anorexia, vomiting, diarrhea, abdominal pain; fever, irritability, loss of previously attained bladder control, urgency, frequency, burning on urination, dribbling, foul-smelling urine. Fever, chills, and flank pain may occur when the infection is in the kidney.

Laboratory.   The diagnosis is confirmed primarily by the presence of bacteria on urine culture. The presence of more than 100,000 (10^5) colonies of a single bacteria per ml of urine in a correctly collected and plated specimen indicates infection. One such culture in a child with symptoms is the minimal criterion for confirmation of infection. If the colony count is between 10,000 and 100,000 per ml, a repeat specimen is obtained. In an asymptomatic child at least three consecutive cultures with greater than 100,000 colonies of the same bacteria per ml should be obtained to confirm the diagnosis. If a suprapubic tap (direct aspiration of the bladder) has been performed, the presence of *any* bacteria indicates infection. Positive urine cultures are also tested for sensitivity of the organisms to drugs.

Specimen collection.   The importance of correct technique in obtaining urine for culture cannot be overemphasized. In infants it is difficult to obtain adequate samples due to the obvious possibilities for contamination. In children who are toilet trained, a midstream urine after cleansing of the external genitalia is usually sufficient. If the specimen cannot be cultured within 30 minutes, it is refrigerated and plated within 24 hours. If the specimen is brought from home it should be kept on ice en route.

MANAGEMENT

After diagnosis of a urinary tract infection, nurse practitioners are involved in coordinating treatment and follow-up with the child and family. The goals of management are:

1.   Eradication of the infection
2.   Prevention and/or treatment of recurrences
3.   Identification and correction of structural anomalies (Margileth, 1976)

Medication.   Choice of medication, dosage, and length of course will be decided by the physician based on the offending organism, age and weight of the child, whether the infection is the first or a recurrent one, and sensitivity of the organism to the drug. Usually the drug is prescribed for 2 weeks in a first infection. Longer courses may be necessary in recurrent or complicated infections.

The school nurse should be informed when children are on long-term drug therapy.

Medications commonly used are:

1. Sulfisoxazole (Gantrisin)

   • Organisms. Effective against *E. coli, Klebsiella, Proteus,* and *Staphylococcus*

   • Contraindications. Not to be used in infants less than 2 months of age, in pregnancy or lactation, or in persons with G-6-PD deficiency (see Chapter 20, G-6-PD)

   • Side effects. Blood dyscrasias, allergic reactions, GI symptoms, and occasionally CNS reactions

   • Practical points. It is low in cost. It must be stored in the refrigerator. Increased fluid intake is necessary during the course of medication to prevent crystalluria and stone formation.

2. Ampicillin

   • Organisms. Effective against *E. coli, Proteus*

   • Contraindications. Not to be used in persons with previous hypersensitivity to penicillin or during pregnancy

   • Side effects. GI symptoms, particularly diarrhea, and hypersensitivity with skin rash

   • Practical points. It is low in cost. Reconstituted suspensions are stable for 7 days at room temperature and for 14 days with refrigeration.

3. Nitrofurantoin (Furadantin)

   • Organisms. Effective against *E. coli, Staphylococcus aureus, Klebsiella, Proteus, Pseudomonas* and enterococci

   • Contraindications. Not to be used in infants under 1 month of age, during pregnancy or lactation, or in persons with G-6-PD deficiency.

   • Side effects. GI distress, hypersensitivity reactions (pulmonary), skin rashes, hemolytic anemia; 10 to 15 percent of children develop nausea and vomiting

   • Practical points. It is moderate in cost. The suspension can be given with water, milk, juices, or food to decrease GI irritation.

4. Cephalexin (Keflex)

- **Organisms.** Effective against *E. coli, Proteus, Klebsiella*
- **Contraindications.** Not to be used in pregnancy or in persons with hypersensitivity
- **Side effects.** Diarrhea and other GI symptoms, hypersensitivity reactions
- **Practical points.** It is more expensive than other medications. It can be given without regard to meals.

Supportive care. During the symptomatic period children need increased fluids and increased rest.

Follow-up care. Once drug therapy has been initiated the child is seen in 48 to 72 hours to determine if the symptoms have subsided and to reculture the urine. Urine should be sterile at this time. If not, a new medication may need to be selected. The child should then be seen shortly after completing the course of medication (within 1 to 2 weeks) and another urine culture obtained. If this culture is negative, the infection is considered cured. Since the recurrence rate of UTIs is high, long-term follow-up is indicated. A suggested protocol is as follows (Rowe, 1975):

After resolution of infection, follow-up visits are scheduled at:

1 month	Culture, urinalysis
3 months	Culture, urinalysis
6 months	Culture, urinalysis
12 months	Culture, urinalysis, and physical exam
18 months	Culture, urinalysis
24 months	Culture, urinalysis, and physical exam
Annually	Culture, urinalysis, and physical exam

Indications for further diagnostic studies. Significant urinary tract abnormalities have been discovered via radiologic examinations in approximately 15 percent of children at the time of their first diagnosed UTI. Yet, there is considerable debate over the indications for such studies and other urologic procedures. Existing guidelines suggest that when there is no evidence of urinary tract dysfunction except infection (Rowe, 1975):

1. All males have an intravenous pyelogram (IVP) and voiding cystourethrogram (VCUG) after resolution of the first infection.
2. Females less than 1 year of age have an IVP and VCUG after resolution of the first infection.
3. Females from 1 year to menarche have an IVP after resolution of the first infection.
4. Postmenarchal females have an IVP after the second documented infection.
5. Postmenarchal females with clinical signs of pyelonephritis or a history suggesting previous undocumented UTIs have an IVP after resolution of the first documented UTI.

PREPARATION FOR DIAGNOSTIC PROCEDURES. Should any child be required to undergo IVP or VCUG, the nurse practitioner must tackle the significant task of preparing both the child and the family for these intrusive procedures. In addition to teaching and support geared to the child's developmental level some additional suggestions are:

1. The child must be assured, especially if loss of bladder control is one of the symptoms, that the tests are not punishment.
2. The nurse practitioner needs to investigate and to be familiar with the way children are handled in the radiology unit. Efforts to assure humane treatment of children may need to be a larger project for the nurse practitioner.
3. Where possible the parent and child should be accompanied through the procedures. Often student nurses are available and can learn as well as act as advocate for the family.
4. The child and parent must be given the opportunity to express their feelings, perceptions, and fears before and after the procedures.

Prevention

SCREENING. The objective of screening is to identify those children with asymptomatic bacteriuria. Routine screening is recommended primarily for girls as early in life as 1 to 2 years of age, and retesting between the ages of 5 to 7 years. Several direct culture techniques which are simple, inexpensive, and can be performed at home are currently on the market (Kunin, 1977, p. 168). In addition a nitrite dip-strip test is available for use at home (Kunin, 1976).

PARENT TEACHING. Perineal hygiene in girls should be taught from infancy. The technique of wiping from front to back should be stressed. Abundant fluid intake and regular voiding practices are important as is complete emptying of the bladder with each voiding. Harsh detergents and bubble baths may irritate perineal and urethral tissue and lead to inflammation and infection. In children who have had one UTI, parents need to know that subsequent symptoms should be promptly investigated and regular follow-up carefully obtained. Because the severity of symptoms in childhood is poorly correlated with the ultimate course, follow-up into adulthood is advised. Parents may ask about giving the child cranberry juice since it has some ability to suppress bacteria in the urine. It takes 2 gallons of cranberry juice per day to suppress bacteria in an adult which makes it an unrealistic and unnecessary therapy (Bergman, 1969).

References

Bailey, E. N., et al. "Screening in Pediatric Practice." *Pediatr Clin North Am* 21:123–165, February 1974.

Bergman, A. B., editor. *Urinary Tract Infections in Childhood: Report of the First Ross Roundtable on Critical Approaches to Common Pediatric Problems.* Columbus, Ohio: Ross Laboratories, 1969.

Cohen, M. W. "Enuresis." *Pediatr Clin North Am* 22:545–560, August 1975.

"Feelings and Their Medical Significance: Enuresis." *Ross Timesaver* 18(5), September–October 1976. Columbus, Ohio: Ross Laboratories.

Kunin, C. M. *Detection, Prevention and Management of Urinary Tract Infections*, 2nd ed. Philadelphia: Lea and Febiger, 1974.

Kunin, C. M. "The Natural History of Recurrent Bacteriuria in Schoolgirls." *N Engl J Med* 282:1443–1448, June 25, 1970.

Kunin, C. M. "Urinary Tract Infections." In M. Green and R. J. Haggerty, editors, *Ambulatory Pediatrics II*. Philadelphia: Saunders, 1977. Pp. 165–171.

Kunin, C. M., et al. "Detection of Urinary Tract Infections in 3- to 5-Year Old Girls by Mothers Using a Nitrite Indicator Strip." *Pediatrics* 57:829–835, June 1976.

Margileth, A. M., et al. "Urinary Tract Bacterial Infections: Office Diagnosis and Management." *Pediatr Clin North Am* 23:721–734, November 1976.

Rowe, D. S. "Urinary Tract Infections in Children," unpublished material. San Francisco: University of California, November 1975.

Schauffler, G. C. *Pediatric Gynecology*, 4th ed. Chicago: Yearbook publishers, 1958.

Starfield, B. "Enuresis: Its Pathogenesis and Management." *Clin Pediatr* 11:343–350, June 1972.

Vaughan, V. C. and R. J. McKay, editors. *Nelson Textbook of Pediatrics*, 10th ed. Philadelphia: Saunders, 1975.

Waechter, E. H. and F. G. Blake. *Nursing Care of Children*, 9th ed. Philadelphia: Lippincott, 1976.

23

The
Genitalia

Genital problems are not uncommon in childhood and, regardless of severity, must be assessed and managed with gentleness and sensitivity because of the degree of concern likely to be felt both by parents and children. Examination of the genital organs in the neonatal period must be done with care and with attention to the parent's spoken or unspoken concerns. Many new parents will have questions and/or fears about the appearance of their infant's genitals and may be hesitant to touch or to manipulate the genital area for proper hygiene. The first examination with the parents present is an excellent opportunity for demonstrating techniques of care and for eliciting concerns. Obviously, such an approach is used for any child regardless of age.

ASSESSMENT

History

MALE

Factors to ascertain in the male are any history of pain in the penis, testicles, or rectum; disturbances in micturition; hematuria; urethral discharge or bleeding; swelling; and inflammation.

FEMALE

Factors to ascertain in the female are any history of itching, burning, irritation, discharge, or pain in the perineal area; menstrual history. See Chapter 10, Health Care of the Adolescent.

Physical Examination

EXTERNAL GENITAL ORGANS, MALE

Inspect for size, configuration, symmetry, cleanliness. Note presence or absence of circumcision. If uncircumcised, gently check retractibility of the foreskin to observe position of the urethral meatus. Note size of the meatus and any discharge from it. Palpate genital area for masses. Note presence of phimosis, hypospadias, hydrocele, hernia, and cryptorchidism (see this chapter, Common Clinical Problems).

Testes. Palpate testes for location and size. The testes may have to be "milked down" from the inguinal canal. The environment and the examiner's hands should be warm as an active cremaster reflex may simulate cryptorchidism. To abolish this reflex have the child sit crosslegged on the examining table. Parents may have more success in palpating the testes at home with the child in a warm bath.

Scrotum. Note the size of the scrotum and any swelling or fullness. Any swelling of the scrotum other than the testicle should be checked by transillumination. The room is darkened and a beam of light from a flashlight is directed from behind the scrotum through the mass. Transmission of light will appear as a red glow. Swellings caused by serous fluid will transilluminate; those caused by blood or tissue will not.

Older males. Note pubertal changes. Check pubic hair for pediculosis.

EXTERNAL GENITAL ORGANS, FEMALE

Inspect for size, configuration, symmetry, and cleanliness. Separate the labia fully to inspect clitoris, urethral meatus, vaginal orifice, and hymen. Note mucous or skin tags. Note presence of vaginal discharge, vulvar or labial adhesions, imperforate hymen, clitoral hypertrophy, presence of hair and distribution, pubertal changes. Palpate area for any masses. Check pubic hair for pediculosis.

COMMON CLINICAL PROBLEMS

Adhesions, Labial and Vulvar

ASSESSMENT

Adhesions are usually associated with the hypoestrogenic state of childhood or with vulvovaginitis.

MANAGEMENT

They are readily lysed mechanically and prevented from recurring by using dienestrol cream (Rudolph, 1977, p. 1340).

Circumcision

ASSESSMENT

Circumcision is the surgical removal of the prepuce (foreskin) from the penis. Although the most common surgical procedure in male infants in the United States, the medical indications for circumcision have not been established. Parents elect the procedure because of religious or cultural beliefs, social pressure, custom, cosmetic purposes, or because it has "always been done."

Arguments in favor of circumcision. Rationale put forth by those who favor circumcision states that circumcision:

1. Promotes cleanliness of the glans penis and will result in decreased incidence of cervical carcinoma in sexual partners
2. Prevents penile cancer
3. Prevents balanitis (infection of the foreskin), adhesions, phimosis, and occlusion of the urethral meatus

Arguments against circumcision. Those who do not favor routine circumcision state that:

1. The level of hygiene in both male and female does seem to be a factor in the etiology of cancer of the cervix, but "noncircumcision is not, of itself, of primary etiologic significance" (AAP, 1975, p. 611).
2. Cancer of the penis can be prevented by circumcision but also by good penile hygiene.
3. There is no convincing evidence that circumcision reduces the incidence of cancer of the prostate.
4. The only medical indications for circumcision are extreme phimosis that could lead to obstructive uremia or intractable paraphimosis.
5. Two to ten percent of males with true phimosis may need circumcision before starting school.
6. Significant complications occur in 1 of 500 newborns circumcised (Gee, 1976, p. 826).

Contraindications. Contraindications to circumcision are:

1. Exstrophy of the bladder
2. Epispadias or hypospadias. The foreskin may be needed if plastic surgery is necessary.
3. Ambiguous genitalia
4. Neonatal illness
5. Premature birth
6. Familial bleeding disorders

Complications. Complications of circumcision include:

1. Hemorrhage
2. Meatal ulceration leading to meatal stenosis
3. Local infection that can lead to septicemia, significant hemorrhage, or mutilation
4. Cautery burns
5. Urethral fistula, as a result of too deeply placed sutures
6. Trauma to penis, amputation of the glans, excessive removal of penile skin.

MANAGEMENT

Care of the circumcision. When performed in the immediate neonatal period (after 24 hours of age), the incision is covered with sterile dressing and petrolatum, or Vaseline gauze, to prevent infection and to prevent irritation from the penis sticking to the diapers. Parents should observe for: adequacy of urinary stream, hematuria, bleeding, signs of infection. The incision usually heals quickly within 3 to 4 days.

Counseling. It is the responsibility of the nurse practitioner to provide parents, before delivery, with factual options regarding circumcision. The known long-term medical effects of circumcision and noncircumcision should be presented. Ultimately it is the parents who make the final decision. Education for penile hygiene is necessary if noncircumcision is elected (see this chapter, Phimosis). Some parents may have concerns or emotional fears about manipulating the child's penis during cleansing. Assistance with verbalizing such discomfort and demonstration of cleansing techniques will reassure these parents.

Cryptorchidism

ASSESSMENT

Cryptorchidism is the absence of one or both testes from the scrotal sac. It is important to differentiate undescended from retractile testes. Retractile testes can be manipulated into the bottom of the scrotum. Undescended testes may represent delayed descent, prevention of descent by mechanical lesions (e.g., adhesions, narrow inguinal canal, fibrous bands, or diversion of descent into the perineum or femoral area). They are usually unilateral. Twenty percent are bilateral and are frequently associated with hernias. Endocrine causes are rare. Secondary sex characteristics develop normally as androgen production usually is normal.

Incidence. Approximately 4 percent of term male newborns and 30 percent of premature males have undescended testes at birth, but during the first weeks and months of life about 80 percent of all undescended testes will be in the scrotum. Spontaneous descent after infancy is uncommon and even if it does occur, damage to the testes may have occurred. Late descent is neither to be expected nor desired.

MANAGEMENT

Any child with undescended testes is referred to à physician for evaluation and treatment. Differences of opinion exist as to the best age for medical and surgical treatment.

Medical treatment. In the case of *bilateral* undescended testes, medical treatment consists of a series of injections of human chorionic gonadotropin to precipitate descent of the testes when the child is about 5 years of age. One third of the children so treated will respond. If the testes do not descend, surgery is performed. Medical treatment is not recommended in unilateral cryptorchidism.

Surgical treatment. Orchidopexy is the surgical procedure for bringing the testis down into the scrotum. Since some cellular changes and degeneration are found to occur in the undescended testis after 5 to 6 years of age, it is recommended by many authorities (Vaughan, 1975, and Rudolph, 1977, p. 1339) that surgery be performed by 5 years of age. It cannot be said with certainty that correction of the condition will absolutely prevent infertility or sterility as some testes may have been defective to begin with.

Counseling. Whatever the course of management selected, the nurse practitioner is a key figure in interpreting the plan to both child and parents and in preparing them for eventual surgery. See this chapter, Hypospadias. The child and parents should be helped to verbalize their concerns about possible defective sexual ability.

Hydrocele

ASSESSMENT

A hydrocele results from the accumulation of peritoneal fluid in the scrotal sac. Normally, in utero, as the male testis descends toward the scrotum, it is preceded by a sac of peritoneal tissue called the processus vaginalis. Once the testis reaches the scrotum the processus vaginalis atrophies and is usually obliterated at the time of birth.

Noncommunicating hydrocele. Frequently at birth some residual peritoneal fluid remains after closure of the processus vaginalis. This is called a *noncommunicating hydrocele*. The scrotal sac appears full, fluctuant, tense, and clear on transillumination. The fluid gradually absorbs during the first year of life and no treatment is necessary. Since the processus vaginalis is closed off, there is no danger of hernia.

Communicating hydrocele. A *communicating hydrocele* exists when the processus vaginalis remains open. Fluid may not be noticed in the scrotum until some time after birth. The patent passageway to the abdomen is often associated with an inguinal hernia and surgical repair is more frequently required.

MANAGEMENT

Parents need simple, clear explanations of the enlarged scrotum. Parents are frequently frightened by the size of the scrotum, fearing that it means their sons will have abnormally large genitals in adulthood. Assurance that the fluid will resorb during the first year brings great relief. With a communicating hydrocele, parents must be instructed to observe for signs of potential inguinal hernia.

Hypospadias

ASSESSMENT

In hypospadias the urethral opening is on the ventral (lower) surface of the penis. In mild cases the opening is on the glans or corona. In severe cases the urethra opens on the shaft of the penis, at its base, or on the perineum. It is frequently associated with chordee, a ventral bowing of the penis. Incidence is about 1 in 500 male infants. Most cases are mild.

Clinical signs. The child is unable to urinate with the penis in the normal elevated position and usually must sit to void.

MANAGEMENT

Surgery is indicated to correct the chordee and to reposition the urethral opening. Since the foreskin is used in this repair, infants with this condition must not be circumcised. It is essential that the repair be performed prior to school entry so the boy will be able to void standing up like his peers.

Preparation for surgery. Preparation of the young child for genital surgery must consider the age of the child, stage of development, level of understanding, fears and fantasies, correction of misconceptions, assurance that he is not to blame for his condition nor being punished for anything—especially masturbation—opportunities for expression of feelings verbally or through play, and assistance to parents so they can fully prepare and support their child.

Paraphimosis

ASSESSMENT

Paraphimosis occurs when the prepuce has been retracted, usually by the parent, child, or vigorous examiner, and cannot readily be replaced over the glans. Blood supply to the glans is constricted; edema, bluish discoloration, pain, and dysuria result. Gangrene can occur.

MANAGEMENT

Application of cold compresses to reduce swelling is indicated. Physician consultation is obtained. If manual attempts to replace the foreskin are unsuccessful, surgical release may be required.

Phimosis

ASSESSMENT

Phimosis occurs when the preputial opening of the foreskin is narrowed so that the foreskin cannot be retracted over the glans of the penis. Straining at urination may result. In most normal uncircumcised males there is some degree of adherence of the foreskin during the first year which will disconnect by 1 year of age. In fact, at birth only 4 percent of males have a fully retractable foreskin; at 6 months of age 15 percent; at 1 year of age 50 percent; and it is not until 3 years of age that most males have a completely retractable foreskin (Preston, 1970).

MANAGEMENT

If this adherence does not interfere with urination, no manipulations are necessary. If mild phimosis exists the parent may be instructed to clean the penis carefully and to use gentle retraction during the bath to widen the opening or release the adhesions. If the phimosis is severe, the preputial opening may be widened by incision, or circumcision may be performed.

Vulvovaginitis, Nonspecific

ASSESSMENT

Vulvovaginitis refers to infections of the vulva, vagina, and occasionally the urethra. Such infections are most frequent after the second year of life and are the result of poor hygiene, pinworms, local varicella lesions, local trauma from insertion of foreign bodies, or masturbation. *Streptococci, Staphylococcus aureus,* or *Trichomonas* organisms are frequently found. Symptoms may include urinary frequency, enuresis, inflammation with discharge, excoriation, swollen mucous membranes.

MANAGEMENT

Local cleansing measures (baths, saline irrigations) are effective in treating many infections. Specific local therapy may be indicated to acidify vaginal secretions (e.g., instillation of dilute acetic acid solutions, vaginal suppositories). Systemic antibiotic therapy is occasionally warranted.

References

American Academy of Pediatrics, Committee on Fetus and Newborn. "Report of the Ad Hoc Task Force on Circumcision." *Pediatrics* 56:610–611, October 1975.

Bates, Barbara. *A Guide to Physical Examination.* Philadelphia: Lippincott, 1974.

Gee, W. F. and J. S. Ansell. "Neonatal Circumcision: A Ten-Year Overview." *Pediatrics* 58:824–827, December 1976.

Preston, E. N. "Whither the Foreskin?" *JAMA* 213:1853–1858, September 14, 1970.

Redman, J. F. and N. K. Bissada. "How to Make a Good Examination of the Genitalia of Young Girls." *Clin Pediatr* 15:907–908, October 1976.

Rudolph, A. M., editor. *Pediatrics*, 16th ed. New York: Appleton-Century-Crofts, 1977.

Sorrells, M. L. "Letter to the Editor." *Pediatrics* 56:339, August 1975.

Terris, M., F. Wilson, and J. H. Nelson. "Relation of Circumcision to Cancer of the Cervix." *Am J Obstet Gynecol* 117:1056–1066, December 1973.

Vaughan, V. C. and R. J. McKay, editors. *Nelson Textbook of Pediatrics*, 10th ed. Philadelphia: Saunders, 1975.

24

The Skeletal System

Minor orthopedic abnormalities and developmental variants are common problems for management in pediatric ambulatory care. Although definitive diagnosis and treatment of orthopedic problems fall within the realm of the orthopedist, early detection of these conditions is the responsibility of the nurse practitioner. This chapter describes the most common orthopedic problems with emphasis on methods of assessment.

ASSESSMENT

History

PRESENT CONCERN

See Chapter 13, Assessment of Presenting Symptom.

PAST HISTORY

Obtain information about injuries or deformities, webbing of the neck, fractures, nerve injuries, shoulder or arm paralysis, hip or

679

feet deformities or problems, and nutrition pertinent to vitamin D and calcium intake.

BIRTH HISTORY

Obtain information about congenital abnormalities, birth injuries, abnormal presentation (breech), prematurity, or anoxia in the neonatal period.

FAMILY HISTORY

Obtain information about congenital abnormalities of the hip, feet or back problems, limps, painful joints, or "twisted spine."

Physical Examination

The general screening examination in infancy and childhood includes components of the skeletal examination. This can be found in Chapter 1, Child Health Assessment. Specific screening examinations for hip, leg, and spinal disorders can be found in this chapter under the specific problem. Included here are examination techniques for assessing range of motion of limbs, flexibility of foot and ankle joints, posture, and gait.

EXAMINATION FOR RANGE OF MOTION

Full range of motion (extension, flexion, and rotation) of limbs and joints, both active and passive, is performed. Range of motion is described by degrees of a circle with neutral position at 0° (see Figure 1). Note deviations, rigidity, stiffness, or pain.

Normal limits. Normal limits of range of motion are:

Shoulder abduction	0°–90°
Shoulder backward extension	0°–60°
Shoulder forward flexion	0°–180°
Shoulder rotation	0°–90°

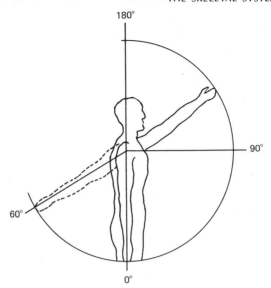

Figure 1. Range of motion of limbs described by degrees of a circle. (Reproduced with permission from "Joint Motion: Method of Measuring and Recording," Chicago: American Academy of Orthopaedic Surgeons, 1965, p. 33.)

Hip flexion and extension (knee flexed over chest)	0°–120°
Hip extension (leg extended and back)	0°–30°
Ankle dorsiflexion, newborn	0°–30°
Ankle dorsiflexion, adolescent	0°–10°
Ankle plantar flexion	0°–30°–45°
Foot inversion	0°–35°
Foot eversion	0°–15°

EXAMINATION FOR FLEXIBILITY OF FOOT AND ANKLE

Flexibility of the foot and ankle is examined both actively and passively (Figure 2) and by eliciting the tonic foot reflexes. Tonic foot reflexes are elicited by using an ordinary applicator and lightly

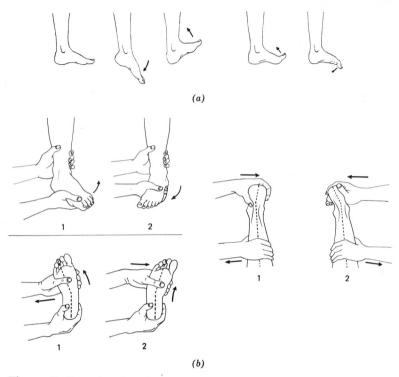

Figure 2. Examination for flexibility of the foot. (*a*) Active flexion of foot and toes. (*b*) Passive flexion of foot; (1) eversion, (2) inversion. (Reproduced with permission from R. J. Ducroquet, et al, La marche et les boîteries, Paris: Masson, 1965; English translation: Lippincott, 1968.)

stroking areas of foot indicated in Figure 3. Observe foot or ankle joints for rigidity, stiffness, or pain. Rigidity is indicated by eversion or inversion when the foot does not move beyond the neutral position (Figure 3) and does not respond to toe-grasping or by dorsiflexing.

EXAMINATION FOR POSTURE

To examine for posture (see Figure 4):

1. Have the child undress to panties

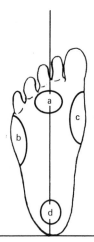

Figure 3. Tonic foot reflexes. Areas of foot stroked to elicit tonic foot reflexes: (a) plantar or toe-grasping, (b) eversion, (c) inversion, (d) dorsiflexion. Midline bisects the second and third toes indicating the neutral position of the foot. (Adapted from G. P. Furlong and G. W. Lawn, "Evaluation of Foot Deformities in the Newborn," *GP* 31:89–97, November 1965, p. 89.)

2. Observe from the front, back, and sides
3. Note the following:
    - From the front, whether the pelvis and hips are level, shape of the legs, amount of space between the knees and ankles, and whether the feet turn in, out, or pronate
    - From the back, curvature, masses of the spinal column, level of the hips and shoulders, whether the hips and shoulders are level, and whether the legs are straight over the heels
    - From the side, whether the head is held straight over the shoulders with the chin in, chest up and over the hips, abdomen taut, buttocks tucked in, and feet straight forward

EXAMINATION FOR GAIT

To examine a child for gait:

1. Observe the child walking backward and forward

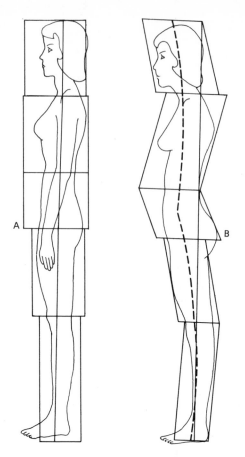

Figure 4. Good and poor standing posture. (A) In good standing posture, the weight-bearing line (line of gravity) passes just anterior to the ear, through the shoulder joint, just posterior to the hip joint, and slightly behind the patella; it strikes the floor just anterior to the external malleolus. (B) Poor standing posture illustrating malalignment of the body segments and a distorted weight-bearing line. Note forward position of the head, round shoulders, increased lordosis, and protruding abdomen. (From C. B. Larson and M. Gould. *Orthopedic Nursing*, 8th ed., St. Louis: C. V. Mosby, 1974. Credit: M. Joan Popp, University Microfilms, 300 N. Zeeb Road, P. O. Box 1346, Ann Arbor, Michigan 48106. Copyright registration No. A912364S.)

2. Note deviations of gait, knock-knees, bowlegs, or pronation of feet. For a description of abnormal gaits see this chapter, Limps.

Normal gait of a child beginning to walk. Characteristics of early gait are as follows:

1. Normal base width heel to heel is 15 to 20 cm
2. Feet turn out and the femurs are in eversion. As the child ages and step becomes steadier the femurs turn in to their normal base width.
3. Steps off with knee bent, leg held high, and arms held up for balance. Sometimes a child pushes off with one foot, slightly dragging the other, and this is considered to be a normal deviation.

Normal gait of an older child. Characteristics of mature gait are as follows:

1. Normal base width is 5 to 10 cm heel to heel
2. Pelvis rotates 40° forward in the swing phase of gait
3. Knee remains flexed during all components of gait
4. Pelvis and trunk shift laterally approximately 1 inch

Potential Orthopedic Risks

DISLOCATIONS AND FRACTURES

Parents and health personnel need reminding that some common habits can lead to these problems:

1. Radial head dislocations. These can be caused by pulling, jerking, or swinging infants and toddlers by their arms, or by taking them down from one's shoulders after a "piggy back" ride.
2. Fractures and injuries. Playground equipment can be hazardous to children. Parents must locate a safe place where children can play. Centrifugal swings, teeter-totters, swings with wooden seats, black-top playground surfaces, trampolines, and skateboards are particularly hazardous.

DEVELOPMENTAL PROBLEMS

Positioning and "poor" posture contribute to these potential risks:

1. Femoral anteversion. In infancy this may be caused by the child's sleeping on haunches with buttocks in the air and feet turned in. In an older child it is caused by sitting in "TV squat," or "tailor fashion" on haunches with legs tucked under and feet turned in. Infants should sleep in different positions, on back and both sides. Older children should be taught to sit "yoga" style.

2. Muscular "hip pockets." These are common upper thigh bulges often seen in adolescent girls and adult women. These are caused by standing or walking with the knees rigid and hyperextended (locked) as a result of poor posture. Good posture can be maintained with emphasis on taut abdominal and gluteal muscles and flexed knees.

3. Pronated feet, lordosis, and knock knees. These defects may develop in young children and adolescents due to obesity. Obesity can also cause fatigue, backache, or limps.

Commonly Used Terms

ABDUCTION. Drawing away from the midline.

ADDUCTION. Drawing together, or toward the midline.

ANTEVERSION. Displacement so the whole axis is directed farther forward than normal.

DORSIFLEXION. Movement of toes/foot or fingers/hand toward the dorsal surface (up).

DYSPLASIA. Abnormality of development.

EPIPHYSIS. A part or process of a bone that ossifies separately and later becomes ankylosed to the main part of the bone.

EVERSION. A turning out or inside out.

EXTERNAL ROTATION. Turning anterior surface of limb out or laterally.

INTERNAL ROTATION. Turning anterior surface of limb in or medially.

INVERSION. A turning up, supination.

LUXATION.   Complete displacement of a part, dislocation.

MALLEOLUS.   Either of the two rounded prominences on either side of the ankle joint, lateral (external or outer) and medial (internal or inner).

PLANTAR FLEXION.   Movement of the toes/foot or fingers/hand toward the plantar surface (down).

PRONATION.   Palmar surface of hand turned downward or toward posterior surface of the body; plantar surface of foot turned outward.

SUPINATION.   Palmar surface of hand turned upward or toward anterior surface of the body; plantar surface of foot turned inward.

TORSION.   The act or state of twisting.

VALGUS.   Deviation away from the midline.

VARUS.   Turned inward to an abnormal degree.

MANAGEMENT

Counseling

Early identification of skeletal abnormalities is important to prevent future problems, for example, dislocation of the hip. When abnormalities are detected at birth, parents will need information and counseling beginning in the early postpartum period. This is a very sensitive time, especially for parents of a first child, and the nurse practitioner needs to be aware of factors which may be involved:

1. Parents, particularly mothers, normally experience feelings of inadequacy as they adjust to their infants. If abnormalities, even minor, are discovered, strong feelings of guilt and frustration may develop as the parents react to the suggestion that their child is not perfect. These feelings must be appreciated and dealt with in a delicate manner.

2. The nurse practitioner may be taken unaware by the discovery of an abnormal finding and feel overanxious. It may be expe-

dient to take a few minutes to collect one's thoughts by continuing with the examination, then returning to the area in question before giving an explanation.

3. The findings may not be definitive until there is further evaluation. While this may make the parents more anxious, their anxiety can be greatly eased if the nurse practitioner intervenes to smooth the way to the appropriate consultant. For example, if an additional appointment has to be made with an orthopedist, the nurse can make the call to the clinic or physician to facilitate the process.

Besides providing support and understanding the nurse practitioner may choose to be available at all times for parental questions or problems.

Exercise

Daily exercise is essential to good growth and development by providing muscular activity to stimulate the flow of blood to carry oxygen throughout the body. Exercise for fun and competition can be superior to forced exercise.

INFANCY

The infant exercises by kicking, stretching, crying, and squirming. This activity should occur several times a day on a firm surface, without the restriction of clothes and with the child in the supine position. Limits must be set for safety when the child begins to crawl and to walk, but the baby needs more space than is provided by a "play-pen" which is mainly a convenience for the parent.

TODDLERS AND PRESCHOOLERS

These children need safe areas indoors and outdoors in which to run, to climb, and to explore. Neighborhood parks can provide this space if the child is confined to apartment living. A method designed to exercise and straighten the spine consists of a removable bar placed in a doorway from which a child can hang freely by the hands.

SCHOOLS

Most schools provide opportunities for organized exercise and for group and competitive sports. Ice-skating classes and dancing classes are excellent choices for obtaining exercise. Afterschool exercise is important if the child has been sitting for most of the day.

PARENTS

Parents can encourage active forms of play, participation in school sports, and act as examples to their children. Activities and sports children can continue for the rest of their lives such as swimming, bicycling, hiking, dancing, tennis, skiing, soccer, and kickball are good forms of exercise for the entire family.

Posture

GOOD POSTURE

Good posture exists when body alignment is such that the musculoskeletal system of the body can function with efficiency and with a minimum of effort. See Figure 4. It is nonfatiguing, painless, and can be maintained for periods of time. It creates a more pleasing appearance and also provides for correct functioning of the weightbearing joints. It lessens the possibility of strain to joints and ligaments by preventing uneven distribution of body weight.

FACTORS INFLUENCING POSTURE

Of factors which influence posture there are three that supersede all others in their prevalence and frequency:

1. Familial-hereditary. These include postures, variations in ligamentous laxity, and muscle tone.
2. Structural abnormalities. These may be congenital or acquired; skeletal, muscular, or neurologic; static or progressive.

3. The posture of habit and postural training by parental control or educators. These lay the groundwork of ultimate adult posture.

POOR POSTURE

Some factors which influence poor posture are:

1. Obesity. This may produce sway-back (lordosis), knock-knees, or pronated feet.
2. Chronic illness or chronic fatigue. These may lead to slumping or sagging.
3. Unusual tallness. This may make some adolescents insecure and cause slouching or ducking of the head.
4. Insecurity or lack of self-esteem. These may be due to criticism at home, difficulties in school, or an unsatisfactory social life.
5. Diseases. Among these are rickets, poliomyelitis, tuberculosis of the bone, or developmental problems such as scoliosis or slipped epiphysis.

MAINTAINING GOOD POSTURE

Parents should be encouraged to help the child to maintain good posture from birth. Some areas for education include:

1. Bedding. Use of firm mattresses beginning with the crib, the bassinet, or the carriage is recommended. No pillow is necessary for babies.
2. Lying position. Lying in the prone position is not recommended. When the child sleeps in the prone position the feet are often adducted, the buttocks are elevated, the hips and knees are in complete flexion, and the child is at risk for tibial torsion. Later these children tend to sit on the adducted feet and may prolong the presence of metatarsus adductus or femoral anteversion (Ponseti, 1966, p. 709).
3. Sitting position. Back and feet should be supported while the child is sitting at the table, in a high chair, on a toilet seat, or in a car seat. Poor sitting positions help to develop lordosis, protruding abdomens, and rounded backs. Infants should not be

propped or left sitting in canvas swings for long periods of time.

4. Infant and baby equipment. Infant carriers, slings, infant seats, swings, and strollers are not considered to be potentially risky for posture if they are used as directed and for short periods of time.

5. Child's self-esteem. Parents need to understand its importance for the child's well-being.

6. Proper diet and exercise. Proper nutrition is important for the normal growth and development of bones and muscles. See this chapter, Exercise.

7. Parental example. This should include posture, diet, and exercise.

8. TV watching. Activity level of children and adolescents has dropped severely in recent years and is attributed to long hours of television watching.

9. Regular health visits and physical examinations. These should be conducted on a regular basis.

Shoes

FIRST SHOES

Neither high top nor low quarter shoes are necessary until the foot needs warmth or protection. Booties, slippers, fabric shoes, or moccasins can be used to keep the feet warm. They do not give support, but permit full motion of the foot if they are not so small or tight as to turn under the toes. Care should be taken that the soles are not too slippery for a child attempting to walk.

LATER SHOES

After the child walks and needs protection for the feet, shoes should have a thin leather sole sufficient to protect the foot, and uppers and soles flexible enough to permit normal motion and use of muscles. High-top shoes help to keep the shoe on the foot and are used if the child tends to pronate or walks on toes beyond an initial period.

Low quarter shoes. These shoes should be narrow enough in the heel to fit snugly, and long and broad enough so the ball of the foot is accommodated at the widest part of the shoe. They should be flexible enough to bend at this point and give good support. The big toe should be a thumb's width from the end of the shoe in the weightbearing position. The width is determined in the weightbearing position by the pinch test. The leather over the widest part should be supple enough and wide enough to allow a small amount to be pinched.

Sneakers and sandals. These shoes are adequate if they do not interfere with the movement of the foot or if the child does not have foot problems. There is no evidence that they cause "fallen arches."

High-heeled shoes. These shoes may cause in-toeing if worn for long periods of time by throwing the body forward and resulting in poor posture, calluses, and strained metatarsal arches.

EVALUATION OF SHOES

When the child is being examined the shoes should be carefully observed for worn areas on the soles and heels. These areas should be evenly centered. If corrective shoes are used, the length of time since they were prescribed should be ascertained and their need reassessed if 2 or more years have elapsed. Ill-fitting shoes can cause corns (due to pressure on the little toe), calluses, and over-riding toes. Painful feet and limps in children are most commonly caused by ill-fitting shoes.

Cast Care

Parents need help with caring for a child in a cast. Some suggestions for improved care include not only care of the cast but also care of the child's skin and the child's well-being.

CARE OF THE CAST

Casts must be kept clean, dry, and free from odors and sharp edges. Suggestions for care are:

1. Loose cotton can be placed under the cast edges. This can be removed and replaced as necessary to keep the cast dry or clean.
2. Plastic material may be used on the cast edges to maintain dryness.
3. Hair-dryer may be used for drying small areas.
4. Edges of the cast may be overlapped with small strips of adhesive tape to keep edges clean and free from sharp areas. They are replaced as necessary.
5. Dirty areas can be washed with Zephiran Chloride 1:1000 to clean and to eliminate some of the odor-causing bacteria.

CARE OF THE SKIN

Daily bathing keeps the child clean and comfortable. Special care of the skin includes:

1. More frequent cleaning of the anal area of an infant or young child who wears diapers
2. Massaging areas of redness with rubbing alcohol. Alcohol is not used if the skin is broken.
3. Avoiding oils and lotions since they cause maceration
4. Avoiding powders since they cake and crumble causing irritation
5. Positioning the crib at a tilt to prevent the infant or child from lying in accumulated urine
6. Keeping the skin exposed to the air

CARE OF THE CHILD

Special measures are as follows:

1. The child who wears a cast should be kept cool, preferably indoors. Insects and heat are a problem outdoors.

2. The physician or medical clinic should be called if the child develops pressure sores, a fever, or a foul odor from the cast.
3. The child's position should be changed frequently if immobilized. The body should be kept in good alignment.
4. Small babies need to be played with, held, and cuddled.
5. The child should be given an opportunity to talk about the experience of being immobilized.

COMMON CLINICAL PROBLEMS

Most of the common problems, except for the very minor ones, are treated by the orthopedist. Quick detection and rapid referral are in the province of the nurse practitioner. Assessment of specific symptoms and signs is included with many of these common problems.

Birth Injuries

BRACHIAL PALSY

Assessment. Brachial palsy occurs when traction for vertex delivery is exerted on the head during delivery of the shoulder; for breech delivery when the head is extracted by strong lateral flexion of the trunk and neck. Injury to the brachial plexus may cause paralysis of the upper arm with or without paralysis of the forearm and hand. Most commonly the injury is limited to the fifth or sixth cervical nerves. The infant loses the power to abduct the arm from the shoulder, to rotate the arm externally, and to supinate the forearm. The usual position is adduction and internal rotation of the arm with pronation of the forearm. Recovery can be expected by 18 months in mild cases. Poorer prognosis exists when the entire plexus is involved or when the lower plexus is involved.

SIGNS OF BRACHIAL PALSY. Extension of the forearm is retained, the biceps reflex is absent, and the Moro reflex is absent on the affected side. On examination the arm which lies limply close to the body and does not come around when stimulated for Moro reflex is a key sign.

DIFFERENTIAL DIAGNOSIS. Cerebral injury, dislocation, epiphyseal separation of the humerus, fracture of the arm or clavicle, and septic arthritis of the shoulder must be ruled out.

Management. The arm and joints are put through full range of motion several times daily. Referral may be made to a physiotherapist or the parent is taught to mimic the actions of the other arm as a model.

COUNSELING. The nurse practitioner supports the parents by providing explanations sufficient to their understanding of the problem, by assisting them to reach the orthopedist as needed, by making sure that the exercises are done, and by requesting the aid of the public health nurse when necessary. Parents need to understand that this child is to be played with, held, and cuddled. Parents also need to be reassured that it is not their fault or the result of "poor performance" during labor and delivery.

FRACTURE OF THE CLAVICLE

Assessment. Fracture of the clavicle occurs during a difficult delivery of the shoulders. The clavicle is fractured more frequently than any other bone.

CLINICAL SIGNS. Signs of a fractured clavicle are:

1. Infant fails to move the affected side
2. Crepitus may be elicited
3. The Moro reflex is absent
4. Spasm of the sternocleidomastoid muscle is present
5. Callus forms within a week and may be the first observed clinical sign presenting as a mass on the affected side
6. Diagnosis is confirmed by X-ray

Management. Treatment, if any, may be immobilization of the arm and shoulder of the affected side. Parental support is given with explanation of the cause, callus formation, treatment, and prognosis. Parents need to understand that this child is to be played with, held, and cuddled. See this chapter, Brachial Palsy.

FRACTURES OF OTHER LONG BONES

Assessment. These bones include the humerus, femur, forearm, or leg.

CLINICAL SIGNS. Signs of fractures are:

1. Spontaneous movements of the affected limb ("pseudo-paralysis") are usually absent
2. The Moro reflex is absent in the involved extremity
3. Callus may be felt as a mass
4. Associated nerve damage may be present
5. Diagnosis is confirmed by X-ray

Management. Treatment may vary. Some methods are:

1. Humerus. Strapping arm to side or chest, or application of a spica cast
2. Femur. Application of Bryant's traction or Buck's extension
3. Forearm or leg. Application of splints

COUNSELING. Parents need support with explanations of cause, callus formation, treatment, and prognosis. They need to understand that this child is to be played with, held, and cuddled. See this chapter, Brachial Palsy.

FOLLOW-UP. At subsequent health visits the nurse practitioner can inspect the child for cleanliness, abrasions of the skin due to appliances, and inspect the splints or straps for tightness or sharp edges. Reassurance and added support are given the parents at each visit.

TORTICOLLIS

Assessment. Congenital muscular torticollis is unilateral contracture of the sternocleidomastoid muscle. It is an asymmetrical deformity of the head and neck, in which the head is tilted toward the side with the shortened muscle and the chin rotated toward the opposite side. Torticollis means "twisted neck." "Wryneck," a lay term, is used to describe torticollis arising from any cause. The condition is more common in girls than in boys. The majority resolve spontaneously within the first year of life.

ETIOLOGY. The immediate cause of the deformity is fibrosis within the sternocleidomastoid muscle in which there is subsequent contracture and shortening. The question is now being raised whether breech presentation is a predisposing factor.

CLINICAL SIGNS. Signs of torticollis are:

1. Firm swelling (mass) 1 to 2 cm in diameter is present in the midportion of the sternocleidomastoid muscle.
2. The child tilts head toward the affected side and rotates it toward the opposite shoulder.
3. Possible facial deformity is present with the affected side smaller.

Management. Correction can be obtained by persistent stretching in the opposite direction. Parents are advised to position the baby in the crib with the head turned away from light (window). The infant will attempt to turn toward the light thereby stretching and exercising the neck muscles.

COUNSELING. See this chapter, Brachial Palsy.

Congenital Orthopedic Deformities

CONGENITAL HIP DISLOCATION (CHD)

Assessment. Congenital hip dislocation or subluxation is complete or partial displacement of the femoral head out of the acetabulum. The basic abnormality is hip dislocation. Secondary to the dislocation, representing a recovery stage, is hip dysplasia or acetabulum dysplasia.

ETIOLOGY. CHD is not related to trauma or to other musculoskeletal disease. The potential for dislocation exists at birth. It is a multifactorially determined trait which becomes manifest under the influence of certain environmental factors. Among the genes involved are those which tend to produce ligamentous laxity. Levels of female hormones may be elevated in affected infants.

Incidence. The incidence varies greatly with genetic background. Reports of instability of one or both hips range from 1:60 to 1:1000 live births. There is a strong familial tendency with greater risk in a sibling. There is a higher incidence in firstborns, breech deliveries, and in girls.

SIGNS OF CHD IN INFANCY. Primary signs include dislocation of the femoral head by the examiner (Barlow's maneuver) and reduction of the femur by the examiner (Ortolani's maneuver). See this section, Screening for CHD. These maneuvers are performed to demonstrate the instability of the joint and are best performed in the nursery or in the first week when the infant is more "floppy." After this period contracture of the muscle begins to take place.

Secondary signs are better noted after the first week, and are:

1. Limitation of full abduction of the hip. See this section, Screening for CHD.
2. Apparent shortening of the femur. See this section, Screening for CHD.
3. Asymmetry of thigh, labial, and inguinal creases. These signs are insignificant if occurring alone. Occasional inguinal or labial creases and 33 percent of thigh creases are normal.
4. Prominent trochanter on the affected side
5. Hollow over the acetabulum. This may be felt with the thumb in the groin of the affected side.
6. Diagnosis by X-ray in the neonatal period may or may not be reliable as the femur may slip in or out with maneuvering.

SIGNS OF CHD IN THE OLDER CHILD. These signs include:

1. Limitation of abduction with obvious adductor contracture
2. Apparent short leg
3. Delayed walking

4. Limp with waddling gait. Gait is flat-footed with the knee on the normal side slightly bent.
5. Positive Trendelenburg sign. See this section, Screening for CHD.
6. Diagnosis is confirmed by X-ray.

SIGNS OF BILATERAL CHD IN THE OLDER CHILD. These include:

1. Marked lordosis
2. Prominent abdomen
3. Very prominent buttocks, "cute little wiggle or bottom"
4. Bilateral prominent trochanters
5. Very wide perineum and stance
6. Limited abduction bilaterally
7. Diagnosis is confirmed by X-ray

SCREENING FOR CHD. There are several signs that need careful screening. Such screening is accomplished by the various maneuvers described below.

Dislocation of the femoral head (Barlow's maneuver). With one hand grasping the symphysis in front and the sacrum in back, lateral pressure is applied to the medial thigh with the thumb of the other hand while longitudinal pressure is applied with the palm to the knee on the side being examined. The hip, which has been flexed 90° is then abducted. A positive sign is a sensation of abnormal movement, indicating dislocation of the femoral head from the acetabulum. The hands are reversed for examining the other hip.

Reduction of the femur (Ortolani's maneuver). After provocation of a dislocation by Barlow's maneuver, the hip should be abducted to about 80° while the proximal femur is lifted anteriorly with the fingers placed along the lateral thigh. A positive sign is a sensation of a jerk or snap with reduction into the socket. A click is not necessarily heard and a click heard without a sensation of abnormal motion is probably not significant.

Limitation of full abduction of the hip. With the child flat on the back, the hips are abducted one at a time, then together. A phase of limited abduction is normal for 20 percent of children (Sharrard, 1971, p. 163). Many black children have tight adductor tendons, but the incidence of CHD in black children is low (Williams, 1975) to virtually nonexistent (Specht, 1974). Assessment is as follows:

1. Normal limits of hip abduction are:

Some children with comfort	70–80°
Most children	60°
Some children	<60°

2. "Grey" area of limits of hip abduction is 40–60°. Assessment should include whether or not it is bilateral, the state of relaxation of the child, and whether or not it is consistently present on repeated examinations.
3. Suspicious (abnormal) limits are in the range of 20–40°.
4. Positive sign for CHD is limitation of abduction in the range of 0–20°. See Figure 5.

   Apparent shortening of the femur.   This is assessed using the following maneuvers:

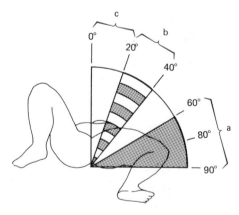

Figure 5. Degrees of abduction of the hip: (a) normal limits, (b) abnormal (suspicious) limits, (c) positive sign for CHD. (Adapted from M. O. Tachdjian, *Pediatric Orthopedics*, Vol. 1, Philadelphia: Saunders, 1972, p. 136.)

1. Allis' sign. With the child lying on the back with pelvis flat and both knees flexed and feet planted firmly, the knees are observed. If a knee projects further anteriorly, the femur is longer; if a knee is higher than the other, the tibia is longer.

2. With the child lying on the back both legs are extended out straight with pressure on the knees. The heels are matched together and observed for equal or unequal length.

3. Trendelenburg sign. With the child standing on one leg, the pelvis is observed. When the child stands on the abnormal leg, the pelvis drops on the normal side (the gluteal fold lowers). Observe dimples overlying the posterior superior iliac spine for rise or fall. See Figure 6.

PROGNOSIS OF CHD. This is dependent on the age of the child when diagnosed and treated as follows:

1. If treated in first 6 months, there is a good chance of complete recovery.

2. If treated at 6 months to 1 year, there is variation in the prognosis. The child may or may not have a normal hip.

3. If treated after walking age, the child will continue to have problems.

Management. In infancy early identification and referral are the most important aspects of management.

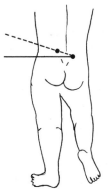

Figure 6. Positive Trendelenburg sign. (Adapted from J. D. Lowell, et al., "Congenital Hip Dysplasia," *Clin Pediatr* 3:279–287, May 1964, p. 282.)

REFERRAL. Immediate referral is made upon finding positive signs. Intervention may be necessary to assure that child is seen by the orthopedist within 24 hours. Positive findings which require referral are:

1. Positive primary signs (dislocation and reduction of femur, Barlow's and Ortolani's maneuvers).
2. Several secondary signs. These include limitation of abduction, apparent shortening of the femur, unequal gluteal and labial folds, and higher trochanter.
3. Apparent shortening of the femur. This is referrable with or without other findings.
4. Limited abduction of the hip, 20° or less.

TREATMENT. Initial treatment consists of reducing the hip(s), proving it is reduced by X-ray, and maintaining reduction through some means of abduction as follows:

1. Double or triple diapering may be advised if borderline subluxation is suspected. To keep down the cost factor the parent is taught to put one diaper on with plastic material or pants between it and the extra diapers. The diapers are folded into rectangles and doubled over in the front.
2. A Frejka splint is used for the infant under 3 months. This is a square pillow filled with kapok and held in place by a "romper-like" garment. It maintains the thighs in flexion, abduction, and external rotation but allows for some movement. The splint must be removed and reapplied after each diaper change. Plastic pants may be worn to protect the splint. A second cover is needed for laundering purposes. The splint may be worn 3 to 10 months until a normally developed hip joint is shown on X-ray.
3. Abduction braces may be used if the hip is not stable after treatment with a splint.
4. Traction is usually necessary to stretch the leg muscles and tendons and place the femoral head in a better position for reduction before application of a cast. This is usually necessary in the treatment of a child over 3 months of age.
.5. A spica cast is used following traction. The legs are put in flexion and abduction.

6. Surgery may be necessary in those hips that do not reduce through gentle manipulation and traction or in those that do not stay reduced.

ROLE OF THE NURSE PRACTITIONER. Early detection and fast referral are of the utmost importance. From discovery of the first positive sign, support and reassurance are given to the parents. This should be accomplished by explaining the cause, treatment, and prognosis of CHD, and by keeping in close contact with the family through the period of further diagnostic measures and treatment. If possible the nurse practitioner should be present when the child visits the orthopedist or is hospitalized. The parents are given an opportunity to express their feelings. Close relationship with the orthopedist is maintained regarding treatment and progress.

FOLLOW-UP. At subsequent health visits the nurse practitioner can:

1. Remove the splint or harness to examine the skin for cleanliness, excoriation, abrasion, or pressure sores
2. Examine the cast for cleanliness, wetness, tightness, or sharp edges. See this chapter, Care of the Cast.
3. Explain the need for the child to be played with, held, and cuddled. Suggest different methods for sitting in the cast to eat and to play.
4. Request earlier follow-up appointment with the orthopedist at own discretion
5. Request visits to family from the public health nurse as necessary

METATARSUS ADDUCTUS (VARUS)

Assessment. In metatarsus adductus the forefoot is turned in or adducted, the longitudinal arch may be exceptionally high, and the space between the first and second toes may be wider than normal. The origin is usually congenital. This toeing-in (pigeon-toe) occurs as a result of rigidity and tightness of the muscles and ligaments of the forefoot. It is commonly associated with tibial torsion. It is most common in a mild form, and many straighten spontaneously with growth.

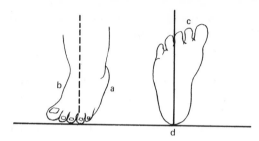

Figure 7. Signs of metatarsus adductus: (a) convex lateral border of foot, (b) concave medial border of foot with possible wrinkling, (c) space may exist between the large toe and second toe, (d) midline bisects third and fourth toes.

CLINICAL SIGNS. Signs of metatarsus adductus are described in Figure 7. In addition the forefoot does not move past neutral position. See Figure 3.

SCREENING FOR METATARSUS ADDUCTUS. The examination consists of testing the foot for flexibility and eliciting tonic foot reflexes, especially eversion reflex. See this chapter, Examination for Flexibility of Foot and Ankle.

Management. Detection and referral before 3 months may improve the results of treatment.

REFERRAL. Referral is made when rigidity and tightness prevent the foot from moving past the neutral position.

TREATMENT. Reversing shoes is not recommended since it merely pushes the toes over and may start a new foot problem. In the interim before the child reaches the orthopedist the parent can be instructed to elicit the eversion reflex as a passive stretching exercise at each diaper change. Other treatment consists of:

1. Casts. These may be applied in rigid and not "relaxed" metatarsus adductus. Casts are changed periodically, the average number is four.
2. Dennis-Brown splint. These splints are sometimes used following casting and remain on for several months or longer.
3. Passive stretching.

COUNSELING. Much of the outcome of treatment depends on the parents' understanding. The nurse practitioner can keep close contact with the orthopedist to better understand and to explain the dynamics of the splinting or casting. It is important to know:

1. Angles of the splint
2. Amount of time to be spent in splint daily
3. Activities which are permitted child

FOLLOW-UP. On subsequent health visits:

1. Review the procedures, teach care of the skin and diapering, and explain the need for child to be played with, held, and cuddled.
2. Inspect a cast for sharp edges, cleanliness, and dryness. See this chapter, Care of the Cast.
3. Inspect the skin for cleanliness or for the presence of pressure sores.
4. Remove the splint to examine the child. Observe for cleanliness, for abrasions on the feet, and evidence of tight straps or shoes. If the feet show evidence of abrasions or pressure, consult with the orthopedist about altering the angle of the splint.

PES PLANUS (FLAT FEET)

Assessment. In pes planus the longitudinal arch of the foot appears flat on the floor when the child is weight bearing. Nearly all infants and the majority of young children exhibit pseudo flat feet. Flat feet are described as:

1. Pseudo flat feet. The plantar fat pad is normal until ages 2 to 3 years. The feet are flexible and exhibit hypermobility of the joint and an anatomical low arch. Pseudo flat feet are strongly familial.
2. Rigid flat feet. Extremely uncommon, this foot presents with tightness of the heel cord or *tarsal coalition* (a cartilaginous fibrous or bony connection between various bones). It is congenital but not visualized at birth.

SCREENING FOR PES PLANUS. The procedure is as follows:

1. Observe the feet in weighted and unweighted positions.

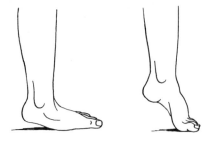

Figure 8. Pseudo flat feet. The flat arch disappears with child on toes. (Reprinted with permission from R. J. Ducroquet, et al., La marche et les boîteries, Paris: Masson 1965; English translation: Lippincott, 1968.)

2. Stand the child on his toes. In flexible flat foot the arch disappears with weight bearing. It reappears when the child stands on his toes. See Figure 8.
3. Elicit dorsal and plantar flexion to rule out tight heel cord.
4. Elicit eversion and inversion flexion to rule out tarsal coalition. For range of motion of ankles see this chapter, Examination for Flexibility of Foot and Ankle.

Management. Referral is indicated for rigid flat feet. Shoe wedges, special heels, and shoe inserts are not recommended for hypermobile flat feet. Exercises are not necessary as this is not a muscular problem.

Developmental Variants

Children can be afflicted with a variety of different congenital and developmental abnormalities of the legs, feet, and toes. Unborn babies lie cramped in utero. As a result, for the first week or two, a leg or foot may present in a distorted asymmetric position. A minimal degree of inversion or eversion is not significant. Joint laxity or hypermobility and torsional (twisting) forces on the limb are responsible for a number of variants seen in young children.

GENU VALGUM (KNOCK-KNEES)

Assessment. Knock-knees are described as a more than 10 to 15° deviant axis of the thighs and calves. "Physiologic" knock-knees are considered to be familial, developmental, and are associated with pronated feet, ligamentous relaxation, and overweight. Severe genu valgum (12 inches or more between the malleoli with femoral condyles touching) may be attributed to rickets or epiphyseal injury. Knock-knees are considered normal from ages 2 to 6 while physiologic genu varum is correcting itself and overcompensation is occurring.

SCREENING FOR GENU VALGUM. The procedure is as follows:

1. Elicit range of motion of legs and flexibility of ankles. See this chapter, Physical Examination.
2. With the child standing observe axis of thighs and calves. Normally they are parallel with a 10° to 15° deviance. See Figure 9.
3. From the front and back observe the space between the knees. Normally this is approximately 1½ inches.
4. From the front and back observe the space between the ankles. Normally the space between the medial malleoli at the heels is approximately 2 inches.

Management. Referral is made if the knees are touching and the ankles are widespread with a corresponding axis deviation of thigh and calf of more than 10° to 15°.

TREATMENT. This is directed at the pronation with inner heel wedges and arch supports and at weight reduction.

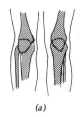 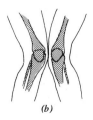 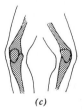

(a)   *(b)*   *(c)*

Figure 9. Axis of thigh and calf: (a) normal axis, (b) deviant axis exhibiting knock-knees (genu valgum), (c) deviant axis exhibiting bowlegs (genu varum). (Adapted from R. J. Ducroquet, et al., La marche et les boîteries, Paris: Masson, 1965; English translation: Lippincott, 1968.)

FOLLOW-UP. On subsequent health visits the nurse practitioner should re-examine for genu valgum and should assess the continued need for corrective shoes with the appropriate referral.

GENU VARUM (BOWLEGS)

Assessment. Genu varum is due to a deviant axis of the thighs and calves. See Figure 9. Bowlegs are defined as:

1. "Physiologic" bowlegs. This condition often occurs with internal tibial torsion and normal genu valgum. It is congenital, familial, or postural in origin. It is common and considered normal until the ages of 2 or 3 with spontaneous correction occurring with growth.
2. "Pathologic" bowlegs. This condition is rare and may be due to rickets, epiphyseal injury, achondroplasia, Morquio's disease, or Blount's disease.

SCREENING FOR BOWLEGS. The same procedure is followed as for knock-knees. See this chapter, Screening for Knock-knees.

Management. Referral is made if the knees are widely spaced and the axis deviation of thigh and calf is more than 10° to 15°. See this chapter, Internal Tibial Torsion. The risks of not treating are degenerative arthritis and bunions in later life.

TREATMENT. This varies with the consulting physician. Children with a strong familial pattern are generally treated with a Dennis-Brown splint.

FOLLOW-UP. See this chapter, Internal Tibial Torsion.

INTERNAL TIBIAL TORSION

Assessment. Internal tibial torsion is usually accompanied by metatarsus adductus and may occur as a result of:

1. Twisting or torsion of the tibia due to lying in "position of comfort" in utero with relaxed tendons. It may continue as a distorted asymmetric position for a few weeks after delivery.

2. External forces applied to the tibia such as sleeping or sitting in position with haunches up, feet turned in. If these forces are removed, there is a natural tendency for the condition to improve. If the child continues these postural habits, then the deformity may persist.

SCREENING FOR INTERNAL TIBIAL TORSION. The procedure is as follows:

1. Examine the legs for range of motion and flexibility of the ankle. Elicit the tonic foot reflexes. See this chapter, Physical Examination.
2. Hold the knee firmly with the foot in the neutral position. Observe the medial and lateral malleoli. See Figure 10. The normal angle between them is approximately 15 to 20°.

Management. Referral is made if the angle between the malleoli is much less than 15 to 20°, and if there are positive findings for metatarsus adductus. See this chapter, Metatarsus Adductus.

TREATMENT. This varies with the consulting physician. The nurse practitioner may recommend:

1. Changing sleeping position of the infant from supine to prone or onto side
2. Changing position of the young child who sits on feet to a "yoga" position
3. Cutting holes in the heels of infant's shoes and tying them together. This will change the tortional force

FOLLOW-UP. If a Dennis-Brown splint is used in treatment, it may be removed to examine for cleanliness, abrasions, or evidence

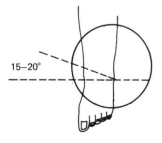

15–20°

Figure 10. Normal angle between medial and lateral malleolus.

of tight straps or shoes. If evidence is present, consult with the orthopedist for changing the angle of the splint.

OVERRIDING TOES

Assessment. In infancy this is usually a hereditary problem. In the older child it may occur as the result of ill-fitted shoes. See this chapter, Shoes.

Management. It may be corrected by splinting the overriding toe to an adjoining toe.

PRONATION

Assessment. Pronation is a common postural disturbance evidenced by flattened or depressed position of the longitudinal arch. It presents as "walking on the inside of the foot" and is usually familial. Pronation may be seen in the normal child under age 3, and with overweight children.

SCREENING FOR PRONATION. This is determined by eliciting range of motion of feet and ankles and observing for tight heel cords. From the back observe child walking. Normally ankles are directly over heels. Shoes may be observed for wear on the inner aspects.

Management. Referral is made if the child is over age 3, is overweight, or if pronation is associated with other foot problems such as genu valgum.

TREATMENT. This includes high-top shoes, with a hard sole and an inner heel wedge with a longitudinal arch. If associated with tight heel cord, exercise may be necessary.

TOEING-IN

Assessment. Toeing-in may be due to:

1. Metatarsus adductus. If not found at an earlier age, it presents

when child first starts to walk. This common problem is discussed fully in this chapter, Metatarsus Adductus.

2. Internal tibial torsion. See this chapter, Internal Tibial Torsion.

3. Increased femoral anteversion. This condition presents as toeing-in and appearance of bowlegs at the age of 3 to 4 years, and is due to rotational deformities of the hip. These children may have as much as 90° internal rotation of the hips in extension and sharply restricted external rotation. Normal internal rotation at birth is 38° to 60°; for adults it is 19° to 20°.

SCREENING FOR TOEING-IN. See this chapter, Metatarsus Adductus, and Internal Tibial Torsion.

Management. See this chapter, Metatarsus Adductus, and Internal Tibial Torsion. In addition attention is given to sitting and sleeping positions. The child needs to be taught the "yoga" position for sitting on the floor. An infant should sleep on back or sides.

Spinal Problems of Children

KYPHOSIS

Assessment. Kyphosis is an exaggerated convex curve in the thoracic region of the spine. It represents a developmental lesion and may cause backache and pain. It may be secondary to congenital deformity such as scoliosis, tumor, trauma, infection, decompressive laminectomy, the chondrodystrophies, or cretinism and achondroplasia.

Management. Referral is made immediately on detection of kyphosis. Deformities that are minimal and mobile can be treated with Milwaukee braces. Congenital kyphosis needs early surgical intervention. Parents need help with understanding the cause and treatment.

LORDOSIS

Assessment. Lordosis is an exaggerated concave curve in the lumbar region of the spine. It represents a developmental lesion. Severe lordosis may cause a limp and pain. The lumbar lordosis is caused largely by the failure of hip flexors to stretch and elongate. Normally children with protuberant abdomens have a slight degree of lumbar lordosis, and it is normally observed more in black children.

Management. Referral is made if the lordosis causes a limp and/or pain.

SCOLIOSIS

Assessment. Scoliosis is described as an S-shaped lateral curvature of the spine with rotation of the vertebral bodies. There are two basic classifications:

1. Structural scoliosis. This means a curve that is less flexible and not usually completely or nearly completely corrected by postural changes (such as with bending X-rays). Structural scoliosis includes:

   - Congenital scoliosis. These curves include hemivertebral, vertebral failure of formation, failure of segmentation, and extra ribs. These curves often have a poorer prognosis.
   - Paralytic scoliosis. Mainly associated with polio, it is now seen with other neuromuscular disorders. These children usually have secondary lung dysfunction problems. This type tends to become worse after bony maturity.
   - Idiopathic scoliosis. This is the most common variety. It has a high familial history. Once thought to be a disease of adolescence, it is now also found at the 4 to 9-year-old level.

2. Functional or nonstructural scoliosis involves no specific structural change. It may be due to shortening of one leg as a result of an old fracture; asymmetrical growth of the legs; flexion fractures about the hip, knee, ankle, or foot; poor posture; or pain.

INCIDENCE. Scoliosis occurs in 5 to 10 percent of the general population; of this 15 percent occurs in the 10-year-old to adult group. It is more frequent in girls than in boys with a large percentage of occurrence in siblings.

SCREENING FOR SCOLIOSIS. Early detection and early treatment are necessary to prevent secondary lung pathology and future back ailments. Pain is not a presenting symptom. The procedure for examination is as follows:

1. Dressed in underwear have the child bend in a 50 percent forward flexing position, with shoulders drooping forward, and arms and head dangling. Observe the child from above the head. Inspect for any lateral curvature of the spine and for any prominence of projection of the rib cage which appears only on one side. This examination should start at the earliest age possible as projection of the rib cage is detectable before the spine curvature is visible. See Figure 11.

2. With the child standing erect and with weight equal on both feet observe for:
   - Difference in levels of shoulders, scapulas, and hips
   - Prominence of either scapula or hip
   - Differences in the size of the spaces between the arms and the trunk
   - A curve in the vertebral spinous process alignment. If given permission, the examiner may mark each process with a pen to aid in detection.

Common factors that may delay detection are failure of healthy-looking youngsters of preadolescent age to have yearly physical examinations; the process of curvature is slow and may not be noticed by child or family; or children have fears of being different from their peers and do not report a change. A common observation by parents is the need to alter hems in dresses or to alter sleeve length.

Management. Referral is made immediately on detection of a curve or an increased muscle mass in the posterior thoracic region.

TREATMENT. The aim of treatment is to prevent increasing deformity. Treatment includes the following:

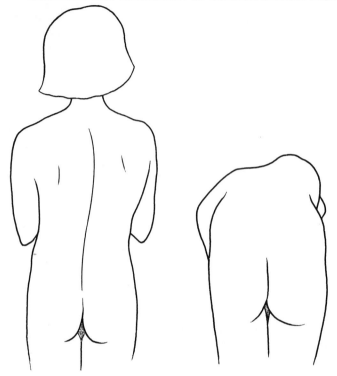

Figure 11. Examination for scoliosis. Structural scoliosis is best demonstrated observing the child bending over. (Reprinted with permission from Report of the Third Ross Roundtable on Critical Approaches to Common Pediatric Problems. In collaboration with the Ambulatory Pediatric Association, 1972.)

1. The Milwaukee brace, in general, is prescribed for structural curves that show some mobility or correction with bending in a child who hasn't reached maturity and whose curve is severe.
2. Traction and casting before surgery may be helpful.
3. Surgery may be indicated if the curve continues to progress.

ROLE OF THE NURSE PRACTITIONER.   This includes:

1. Explaining the problem and the need for immediate referral and treatment. The speed of the child's growth and development causes the problem to worsen rapidly.

2. Attending the child's first referral visit for one's own understanding of the process of treatment and for support to the child and family

3. Preparing the child and parents for hospitalization by arranging a visit to the hospital so procedures of treatment can be explained and the child can be shown some of the equipment to be used

4. Visiting the child in the hospital and maintaining a close relationship with ward personnel and physician

5. Contacting the public health nurse as necessary for home care

6. Being available at all times to the family for support and information

7. Being aware of the psychologic aspects of scoliosis treatment and providing guidance to the family in this area

8. Offering an opportunity to teenagers to discuss their feelings

FOLLOW-UP.   At follow-up visits the following are included:

1. The braces and harness are observed for sharp edges or tightness; the skin is examined for pressure sores.

2. For more comfort in braces the child is advised to wear a T-shirt or undershirt under the brace to keep leather from chafing the skin. Bras may be worn under the T-shirt. Underpants may be worn over the brace since elastic and wrinkles cause pressure sores.

PSYCHOLOGICAL ASPECTS OF SCOLIOSIS.   Because of the disabling effects of scoliosis and the need for long-term treatment these youngsters and their families face multiple problems of adjustment.

Problems for the children.   These include:

1. Lowering of self-esteem as they see themselves as "different"

2. Handling feelings of hostility and anger over the need for treatment, curiosity of strangers, and invasion of privacy

3. Trying to understand fully the problem and treatment

4. Worrying about acceptance by peers and friends, and concern about attractiveness to the opposite sex

5. Wondering about their physical, occupational, and sexual future
6. Worrying about clothes, and participation in sports and schoolwork

Problems for the parents. These include:

1. Guilt for not detecting the problem sooner
2. Concern about inflicting unnecessary pain and treatment on the child
3. Necessity to face the child's hostility and anger
4. Concern about siblings and their need for attention and consideration
5. Concern about expenses
6. Need to express their own feelings

Some helpful suggestions. Independence for the child should be fostered by the parents and by medical personnel. Hospital, clinic, and medical office personnel should show friendly support and interest in child's progress. Improvement of self-image may occur if the child is given an opportunity to master a new hobby or sport or to go to camp for the summer.

LIMPS

Assessment. The cause of a limp may be an organic problem or a simple problem such as a shoe which is ill-fitting, abnormally worn, or has a wrinkled lining. Socks, also, should be investigated for wrinkles or holes. A limp is usually associated with accompanying pain which may be referred to the knee or leg.

CAUSES OF LIMPS IN CHILDREN. These are as follows:

1. 1 to 2 years: Congenital dislocation of hip, cerebral palsy
2. 2 to 5 years: Monarticular synovitis, muscular dystrophy
3. 5 to 12 years: Legg-Perthe's disease
4. 12 to 15 years: Slipped femoral epiphysis
5. All age groups: Osteomyelitis, trauma, neurologic disorders

(polio and peroneal muscular atrophy) spinal deformity, rheumatoid arthritis, tumors, and functional disorders.

SCREENING FOR LIMPS. This includes:

1. Examination of posture and gait. See this chapter, Physical Examination.
2. Observation of general coordination both walking and running
3. Observation of method of arising from the supine to the erect position
4. Thorough neurologic assessment. See Chapter 25, Physical Examination.
5. Inspection of the spine, pelvis, and joints of the lower extremities
6. Measurement of leg length and inspection of shoes for wear
7. Test for Trendelenburg sign for hip flexion deformity. See this chapter, Screening for CHD.

COMMON ABNORMAL GAITS. Among the common abnormal gaits are:

1. Spastic gait. This gait is associated with hemiplegia or diplegia of cerebral palsy. The spastic hemiplegic tends to walk on the toe of the affected leg and the spastic diplegic tends to scissor. See Chapter 25, Cerebral Palsy.
2. Trendelenburg or "waddle" gait. This is a short leg limp associated with a pelvic tilt in standing and bending of the normal knee in walking.
3. Drop-foot gait. This gait is high-stepping with the toes clearing the floor (seldom seen today with the disappearance of poliomyelitis).
4. Antalgic gait. This gait may represent an attempt to avoid a painful lesion in the lower extremity, so the child tends to get off that leg as quickly as possible in what is virtually a hop.
5. Bizarre gaits. These may occur in a normal child who is unconsciously mimicking an abnormal gait in a member of the family or friend.

Management. Except for a minor limp due to a shoe problem the diagnosis and treatment of a limp is managed collaboratively with a physician.

Resource Information

Some helpful publications and their sources are as follows:
1. Cast Care Booklet, Children's Rehabilitation Center, University of Virginia Hospital, Route 250 West, Charlottesville, VA, 22903.
2. "Straight from the Start"—booklet on posture for infants and children   Bureau of Maternal and Child Health, 760 Market St., Room 739, San Francisco, CA, 94102.

References

Aegarter, E. and J. A. Kirkpatrick. *Orthopedic Diseases.* Philadelphia: Saunders, 1975.

Ahstrom, J., editor. *Current Practice in Orthopaedic Surgery*, Vol. 6. St. Louis: Mosby, 1975.

Alexander, M. M. and M. S. Brown. *Pediatric Physical Diagnosis for Nurses.* New York: McGraw-Hill, 1974.

Blount, W. P. *Fractures in Children.* Baltimore: Williams & Wilkins, 1954.

"Common Orthopedic Conditions in Childhood," Report of the Ross Roundtable on Critical Approaches to Common Pediatric Problems. In collaboration with the Ambulatory Pediatric Association, Seattle, Washington, August 20, 1972.

Ducroquet, R., J. Ducroquet, and P. Ducroquet. *Walking and Limping.* Philadelphia: Lippincott, 1968.

Dunn, B. H. "Common Orthopedic Problems of Children." *Pediatric Nursing* 1:7–10, November–December 1975.

Furlong, G. P. and G. W. Lawn. "Evaluation of Foot Deformities in the Newborn." *GP* 31:89–97, November 1965.

Gustafson, S. R. and D. B. Coursin, editors. *The Pediatric Patient.* Philadelphia: Lippincott, 1968.

Hill, R. M. and L. S. Romm. "Screening for Scoliosis in Adolescents." *American Journal of Maternal Child Nursing* 2:156–159, May–June 1977.

Hoppenfield, S. *Physical Examination of the Spine and Extremities.* New York: Appleton-Century-Crofts, 1976.

"Joint Motion: Method of Measuring and Recording." Chicago: American Academy of Orthopaedic Surgeons, 1965.

Lane, P. "A Mother's Confession—Home Care of a Toddler in a Spica Cast: What It's Really Like." *Am J Nurs* 71:2141–2143, November 1971.

Larson, C. B. and M. Gould. *Orthopedic Nursing*, 8th ed. St. Louis: Mosby, 1974.

Lowell, J. D., et al. "Congenital Hip Dysplasia." *Clin Pediatr* 3:279–287, May 1964.

Mignogna-Love, S. "Scoliosis." *Nursing '77* 7:50–55, May 1977.

Ponseti, J. V. and J. R. Becker. "Congenital Metatarsus Adductus: The Results of Treatment." *J Bone Joint Surg* 48A:702–711, June 1966.

Salter, R. B. *Textbook of Disorders of the Musculoskeletal System.* Baltimore: Williams & Wilkins, 1970.

Sharrard, W. J. *Paediatric Orthopaedics and Fractures.* Oxford: Blackwell Scientific Publications, 1971.

Specht, E. "Congenital Dislocation of the Hip." *American Family Physician* 9:88–96, February 1974.

Tachdjian, M. O. *Pediatric Orthopedics*, Vols. 1 and 2. Philadelphia: Saunders, 1972.

Vaughan, V. C. and R. J. McKay, editors. *Nelson Textbook of Pediatrics*, 10th ed. Philadelphia: Saunders, 1975.

Williams, R. A. *Textbook of Black-Related Diseases.* New York: McGraw-Hill, 1975.

25

The Neuromuscular System

Neuromuscular problems are not uncommon in childhood and encompass a broad range of symptoms and defects. The consequences of central nervous system pathology are also variable; they may be minimal (the child who experiences one simple febrile seizure) or they may involve major and life-long sequelae (the child with cerebral palsy or mental retardation). Early identification of such problems is critical for optimum management.

The nurse practitioner is involved in identifying children with neuromuscular problems and, in the role of primary care provider, is in a position to offer long-term support, education, and guidance to affected families. Because of a strong background in growth and development, the nurse practitioner can work with the child, family, school personnel, and other involved professionals to maintain a focus on those aspects of the child that are normal in order to promote optimum development.

This chapter presents information on the systematic assessment of the neuromuscular system and the management of some common neuromuscular problems. Refer to Chapter 24, The Skeletal System, and Chapter 26, Language and Learning Disabilities for related information.

ASSESSMENT

History

PRESENT CONCERNS

Presenting symptoms include delayed development, feeding problems, head enlargement, muscle weakness, vomiting, abdominal pain, seizures, visual or auditory changes, vertigo, changes in personality or behavior, changes in activity, changes in achievement, pain or paresthesias (numbness, tingling), ataxia, changes in gait, abnormal sphincter function, and abnormal involuntary movements.

Obtain information in accurate chronologic detail beginning at the earliest onset of symptoms and including descriptions of symptoms and associated events as follows:

1. Has the symptom been present since birth?
2. If not, when did it first appear?
3. Did the symptom develop suddenly or slowly?
4. How has the symptom progressed?
5. Are there periods when the child is entirely well?
6. Has development arrested?
7. Has previous attainment of function been lost?
8. In older children, has there been a deterioration in school performance, irritability, or emotional lability?

BIRTH HISTORY

Obtain information on complications of pregnancy (illness, infections, drugs, irradiation, injuries, bleeding), previous abortions, labor and delivery (duration, presentation, anesthesia, forceps), gestational age, birth weight, Apgar scores, resuscitation, trauma, jaundice, infections, convulsions, muscle tone (stiffness, limpness), and congenital anomalies.

PAST HISTORY

Obtain information on previous illnesses, injuries (especially head trauma), fevers, headache, convulsions, vision and hearing development, motor development, behavior or personality changes, and school performance.

GROWTH AND DEVELOPMENT HISTORY

Obtain information on serial weight, height, and head circumference; developmental milestones, personality development, and behavior.

FAMILY HISTORY

Obtain information on family members with similar symptoms, neurologic diseases, abnormal gaits, causes of death, "spells," motor or sensory disturbances, mental retardation, inherited disorders, patterns of growth and development, congenital anomalies, and institutionalizations.

Physical Examination

The complete neurologic examination in infancy and childhood includes components of the entire general physical examination as well as the specific elements of the neurologic examination. All the observations made during an encounter with a child contribute to determining the integrity of the nervous system.

SCREENING NEUROLOGIC EXAMINATION

The complete neurologic examination is complex, time consuming, and unnecessary in most instances. The data collected by history and general physical examination indicate whether or not a complete neurologic evaluation is warranted. A reasonable screening neurologic examination is presented in Chapter 1, Child Health Assessment.

COMPONENTS OF THE NEUROLOGIC EXAMINATION

Behavior and mental status. Assessment begins with a general description of the child's abilities and responsiveness as follows:

1. State of consciousness. Assess alertness by response to commands, name, speech, and pinprick. Note irritability, drowsiness, or lethargy.
2. Orientation. Ask the child to identify self by name, place, and approximate time of day. Check short-term memory; for example, "What did you have for lunch today?"
3. Affect. Note appropriateness of mood, ability to relate to others, depression, remoteness, flat affect, euphoria, or lability.
4. Intellectual abilities. Depending on age and developmental level assess:

   • Expressive speech. Assess the child's spontaneous verbalizations for fluency, vocabulary, and grammar; ability to name objects and colors and to repeat phrases verbatim.
   • Receptive speech. Have the child carry out verbal commands.
   • Memory. Ask the child to repeat digits or phrases. Ask what was eaten for dinner the preceding night.
   • Ability to read. Ask the child to read from graded reading paragraphs. See Chapter 26, Educational Testing.
   • Ability to write, to draw, and to copy shapes. Geometric shapes can be copied as follows:

   > Circle or cross at 3–4 years
   > Square   at 4–5 years
   > Triangle   at 5–6 years
   > Diamond   at 6–7 years

   • Ability to add and subtract
   • In the child under 6 years of age many of these areas can be assessed using the Denver Developmental Screening Test. See Figure 1.

Cranial nerve function. The twelve pairs of cranial nerves innervate muscles of the eyes, face, and swallowing, and carry somatic sensory fibers from the face and from the special sensory organs. They are described as follows:

1. Cranial nerve I (Olfactory nerve)
   Function: Determines the sense of smell
   Assessment: Be sure both nasal passages are patent. Have the child close eyes. Occlude each nostril in turn and test the open nostril by presenting a variety of familiar odors (e.g., peppermint, peanut butter, coffee, onions, or oranges). Colds and allergies with nasal congestion can interfere.

2. Cranial nerve II (Optic nerve)
   Function: Transmits visual signals; necessary for vision
   Assessment: Test for visual acuity and visual fields and perform funduscopic examination. See Chapter 16, The Eye.

3. Cranial nerves III, IV, and VI (Oculomotor, Trochlear, and Abducens nerves)
   Function: Innervate all eye muscles; control constriction and dilation of the puils and elevation of the eyelids.
   Assessment: Test for extraocular movements (EOMs) by having the child follow a finger with the eyes while it is moved to all quadrants of vision. Eye movements should be conjugate with both eyes fixed on the finger. Note any nystagmus. Check pupillary reaction to light by shining a light at one pupil. Observe constriction of the pupil receiving the light and consensual constriction of the other pupil. Note unequal pupil size. Note ptosis.

4. Cranial nerve V (Trigeminal nerve)
   Function: Conveys sensation, including touch and pain, to the face; innervates the muscles of mastication; contains the sensory component of the corneal reflex.
   Assessment: Test sensory function by applying light touch (cotton wisp), pressure, temperature (test tubes filled with hot and cold water), and pain (pinprick) to the forehead, cheeks, and jaws. Test motor function by having the child bite hard on a tongue blade as an attempt is made to withdraw it. Test the corneal reflex by touching the cornea with a wisp of cotton. Both eyes should close.

5. Cranial nerve VII (Facial nerve)
   Function: Innervates most of the facial muscles, lacrimal gland, and stapedius muscle of the ear; provides the sense of taste to

1. Try to get child to smile by smiling, talking or waving to him. Do not touch him.
2. When child is playing with toy, pull it away from him. Pass if he resists.
3. Child does not have to be able to tie shoes or button in the back.
4. Move yarn slowly in an arc from one side to the other, about 6" above child's face. Pass if eyes follow 90° to midline. (Past midline; 180°)
5. Pass if child grasps rattle when it is touched to the backs or tips of fingers.
6. Pass if child continues to look where yarn disappeared or tries to see where it went. Yarn should be dropped quickly from sight from tester's hand without arm movement.
7. Pass if child picks up raisin with any part of thumb and a finger.
8. Pass if child picks up raisin with the ends of thumb and index finger using an over hand approach.

9. Pass any enclosed form. Fail continuous round motions.
10. Which line is longer? (Not bigger.) Turn paper upside down and repeat. (3/3 or 5/6)
11. Pass any crossing lines.
12. Have child copy first. If failed, demonstrate

When giving items 9, 11 and 12, do not name the forms. Do not demonstrate 9 and 11.

13. When scoring, each pair (2 arms, 2 legs, etc.) counts as one part.
14. Point to picture and have child name it. (No credit is given for sounds only.)

   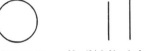

15. Tell child to: Give block to Mommie; put block on table; put block on floor. Pass 2 of 3. (Do not help child by pointing, moving head or eyes.)
16. Ask child: What do you do when you are cold? ..hungry? ..tired? Pass 2 of 3.
17. Tell child to: Put block on table; under table; in front of chair, behind chair. Pass 3 of 4. (Do not help child by pointing, moving head or eyes.)
18. Ask child: If fire is hot, ice is ?; Mother is a woman, Dad is a ?; a horse is big, a mouse is ?. Pass 2 of 3.
19. Ask child: What is a ball? ..lake? ..desk? ..house? ..banana? ..curtain? ..ceiling? ..hedge? ..pavement? Pass if defined in terms of use, shape, what it is made of or general category (such as banana is fruit, not just yellow). Pass 6 of 9.
20. Ask child: What is a spoon made of? ..a shoe made of? ..a door made of? (No other objects may be substituted.) Pass 3 of 3.
21. When placed on stomach, child lifts chest off table with support of forearms and/or hands.
22. When child is on back, grasp his hands and pull him to sitting. Pass if head does not hang back.
23. Child may use wall or rail only, not person. May not crawl.
24. Child must throw ball overhand 3 feet to within arm's reach of tester.
25. Child must perform standing broad jump over width of test sheet. (8-1/2 inches)
26. Tell child to walk forward, ⌒⌒⌒⌒→ heel within 1 inch of toe. Tester may demonstrate. Child must walk 4 consecutive steps, 2 out of 3 trials.
27. Bounce ball to child who should stand 3 feet away from tester. Child must catch ball with hands, not arms, 2 out of 3 trials.
28. Tell child to walk backward, ←⌒⌒⌒⌒ toe within 1 inch of heel. Tester may demonstrate. Child must walk 4 consecutive steps, 2 out of 3 trials.

DATE AND BEHAVIORAL OBSERVATIONS (how child feels at time of test, relation to tester, attention span, verbal behavior, self-confidence, etc,):

Figure 1. Directions for Administering the Denver Developmental Screening Test. (Reprinted with permission from W. K. Frankenburg and J. B. Dodds, *Journal of Pediatrics* (St. Louis) 71(2):185, 1967. © 1969, William K. Frankenberg, M.D., and Josiah B. Dodds, Ph.D., University of Colorado Medical Center.)

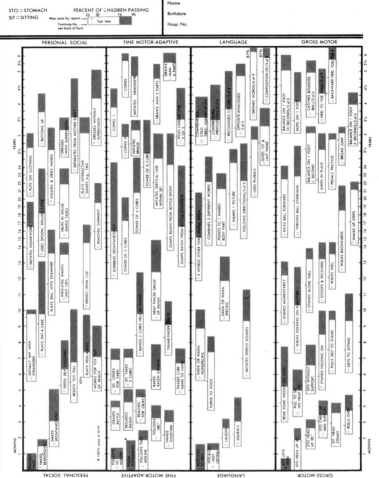

Figure 1. (continued) Denver Developmental Screening Test.

the anterior two thirds of the tongue, and sensation to the external auditory canal

Assessment: Ask the child to smile, to look at the ceiling, to raise the eyebrows, to show teeth, to squint, to wrinkle the forehead, and to puff out the cheeks. Note strength and symmetry. Note faulty tearing or ringing in the ears. Test taste by using sugar and salt.

6. Cranial nerve VIII (Auditory-vestibular nerve)
   Function: Controls hearing and balance
   Assessment: Test for hearing acuity, bone conduction, and air conduction. See Chapter 26, Language and Learning Disabilities. Testing for vestibular function is not routinely done. It involves instilling cold water into the external ear canal to elicit vertigo or nystagmus.

7. Cranial nerves IX and X (Glossopharyngeal and Vagus nerves)
   Function: Innervate muscles in the mouth and throat and control swallowing and phonation
   Assessment: Have the child elevate the palate voluntarily (say "ah"), swallow, and speak. Elicit the gag reflex. Note hoarseness, pooling of secretions in oropharynx, or excessive drooling. Note position of uvula.

8. Cranial nerve XI (Spinal accessory nerve)
   Function: Provides motor supply to sternocleidomastoid and trapezius muscles
   Assessment: Have the child elevate the shoulders against pressure of the examiner's hands. Have the child turn the head to one side and resist the examiner's attempts to turn it in the opposite direction.

9. Cranial nerve XII (Hypoglossal nerve)
   Function: Innervates muscles of the tongue
   Assessment: Have the child stick out the tongue and observe it for symmetry. Note any tremors or fasciculations (involuntary contractions or twitchings). Have the child press the tongue against each cheek as the examiner pushes in on the cheek.

Motor function. The motor system is assessed for size (bulk), tone, strength, and abnormal movements as follows:

1. Size. Inspect and palpate for distribution of muscle mass and symmetry in muscle mass. Note any reduction in muscle mass, hypertrophy, or atrophy of muscles.

2. Tone. Observe posture and adequacy of movement during normal activities. Do both active and passive range of motion and note *tone* (the resistance offered to the examiner's movements). Note involuntary resistance, spasticity, flaccidity, rigidity, or limitations of range of motion.

   • Spasticity: increased resistance to passive movement which gives way suddenly (clasp-knife response)
   • Rigidity: an increase in resistance throughout passive movements of a joint

3. Strength. Have the child stand up from a lying position and walk on tiptoes and heels. This tests strength in the lower extremities, back, and hips. To test shoulder muscles, lift the child with hands in the child's axillae. Test upper extremity muscle groups by having the child move fingers, hands, arms, and shoulders against resistance. Have the child reach up to comb hair.

4. Abnormal movements. Observe for *tremors* (rapid, regular, repetitive involuntary movements, usually of the distal extremities). Some tremors occur with the child at rest; some occur only when voluntary motion is attempted (intention tremor). Most commonly, tremors may occur in infants, in bursts and without obvious cause. Observe for *chorea* (quick, irregular, jerking and writhing movements; often in trunk, major joints, and face; with irregular gait and associated with decreased muscle tone), *tic* (a stereotyped sudden movement always involving the same muscle group), *athetosis* (a slow writhing movement, more marked in the distal extremities; consisting of alternating supination-pronation and flexion-extension of limbs; and associated with increased muscle tone), *dystonia* (involuntary, sustained spasms; slow twisting movements of the neck, limbs, and trunk; a tendency toward hyperextension of the joints especially when trying to walk; abnormal posture). These involuntary movements are accentuated during emotional stress and disappear during sleep. Other abnormal movements are constant overshooting of movements and clonic or tonic convulsive movements.

Cerebellar function. The cerebellum controls balance and coordination. Assessment includes tests of fine motor coordination, gait, and posture control as follows:

1. Fine motor coordination. Young children can be observed while playing, stacking blocks, picking up raisins, dressing, undressing, buttoning, manipulating toys, and drawing. After 4 to 6 years of age tests of rapid alternating movements are used including: rapid supination and pronation of hands; touching finger to nose to examiner's finger (note tremor, past-pointing); touching finger to nose with eyes closed; touching each finger to thumb of same hand; and touching index finger to adjacent thumb crease. Have the child run the heel of one foot down the shin of the opposite leg. These movements should be done smoothly.

2. Gait. Observe gait and standing position. Normal gait is narrow-based with smooth movements; balance is easy and arms swing at sides. Have the child walk a line in toe-to-heel fashion. If there is difficulty with this, have the child stand with feet together, eyes closed, and arms folded across chest. Note ability to maintain upright posture with minimal swaying. This is the Romberg test, and the child should be able to maintain balance without the aid of vision. Have the child walk normally and turn around rapidly. Note ataxia.

3. Posture control. By the age of 4 to 5 years the child should be able to stand on one foot for 5 seconds; by 6 years stand on one foot for 5 seconds with arms folded across chest; and by 7 years stand on one foot with eyes closed.

Sensory function. Sensory assessment is limited in the infant and young child but in older children (4 to 5 years and above) includes the *primary sensory modalities*: superficial tactile sensation (touch), pain, temperature, vibration, pressure, and response to motion and position; and *secondary (cortical) sensation*: two-point discrimination, point localization, stereognosis, and graphesthesia. The child's eyes are closed during assessment which is conducted as follows:

1. Primary sensations:

   • Superficial tactile sensation. Stroke various parts of the body with a piece of cotton and compare responses. Check symmetrical areas.
   • Pain. Observe reaction to light pin prick.

- Temperature. Touch various parts of the body with a cold tuning fork and observe responses.
- Vibration. Touch vibrating tuning fork to various body parts and have the child note when vibration ceases.
- Pressure. Apply pressure to calves, arms, and Achilles' tendon and observe the child's response.
- Motion and position. Grasp the child's toe or finger and move upward and backward. Have the child identify the direction of movement.

2. Secondary cortical sensation:

- Two-point discrimination. Check the child's ability to tell whether two parts of the body are being touched simultaneously.
- Point localization. Have the child identify what spot on the body is being touched.
- Stereognosis. Place a familiar object (key, paper clip, coin, comb) in the child's hand and have the child identify by feel.
- Graphesthesia. Have the child identify numbers or letters written on the palm of the hand with the examiner's finger.

Reflex function. Superficial, deep tendon, and pathologic reflexes are evaluated for presence, symmetry, and strength. Primitive reflexes are discussed in Infant Neurologic Examination which follows. Reflex changes or abnormalities can indicate spinal cord lesions and disorders of peripheral nerves or muscles. Assessment is as follows:

1. Superficial and deep tendon reflexes. Table 1 lists superficial and deep tendon reflexes, where to apply the stimulus, and expected reactions. Superficial reflexes are elicited by stroking the skin. Deep tendon reflexes are elicited by stretching the tendon by a quick tap with a reflex hammer. Reflexes are graded on a scale of 0 to 4 plus, with 1, 2, and 3 being normal. Absence of reflexes or exaggerated reflex response indicates dysfunction (Waechter, 1976, pp. 632–633).
2. Pathologic reflexes. The Babinski reflex and ankle clonus reflex are described in Table 2.

Table 1
Deep and Superficial Reflexes

Reflexes		Stimulus	Normal Results	Involved Segment
Deep	*Superficial*			
Biceps muscle	—	Tap biceps tendon.	Forearm flexes at elbow.	C5-C6
Forearm pronator muscles	—	Tap palmar side of forearm medial to styloid process of radius.	Forearm pronates.	C6
Triceps muscle	—	Tap triceps tendon.	Forearm extends at elbow.	C6-C7
Brachioradial muscle	—	While holding forearm in semipronated position, tap styloid process.	Forearm flexes at elbow.	C7-C8
Finger (flexion)	—	Tap palm at tip of fingers.	Fingers flex.	C7-T1
Abdominal muscles	—	Tap inferior thorax, abdominal wall, and symphysis pubis.	Abdominal wall contracts; leg adducts when symphysis pubis is tapped.	T8-T12
	Abdominal muscles	Stroke upper, middle, and lower skin on abdomen.	Abdominal muscles contract with retraction of umbilicus toward stimulated side.	T8-T12
	Cremasteric muscle	Stroke medial upper leg in adductor region.	Testicles move up.	L1-L2
Adductor muscle	—	Tap medial condyle of tibia.	Leg adducts.	L2-L4
Quadriceps muscle (knee jerk)	—	Tap tendon of quadriceps femoris muscle.	Lower leg extends.	L2-L4
Triceps sural muscle (ankle jerk)	—	Tap Achilles tendon.	Plantar flexion of foot occurs.	L5-S2
	Plantar area	Stroke lateral side on sole of foot.	Plantar flexion of toes occurs.	S1-S2

Source: From B. L. Conway, *Pediatric Neurological Nursing* (St. Louis: C. V. Mosby, 1977), p. 139.

INFANT NEUROLOGIC EXAMINATION

At birth and during the infancy period the neurologic examination is modified since the central nervous system is immature and functions largely at subcortical levels (brainstem and spinal cord). Neurologic development is characterized mainly in terms of motor development and performance. The most significant elements of the infant neurologic examination are described.

Head circumference. This is checked routinely during the first 3 years of life for abnormal head size. See Chapter 1, Child Health Assessment.

Transillumination of the skull. In a darkened room a flashlight beam is applied to the skull at various points. Local or generalized areas of transillumination beyond the periphery of the flashlight indicate the need for referral.

Anterior fontanelle. It is usually soft and slightly depressed with the infant in a sitting position. A tense and bulging fontanelle indicates increased intracranial pressure. The anterior fontanelle is usually closed by 18 months to 2 years of age. See Chapter 1, Child Health Assessment.

General appearance. Positioning, activity, quality of cry, alertness, and response to environmental stimuli are noted and described. Spontaneous activity should be symmetrical. Orientation may be assessed by recognition of the mother's face and later of familiar objects and people.

Head, eyes, ears. Auscultate for bruits. Palpate fontanelles and sutures. Observe for dimples, clefts, and asymmetry. Note close-spacing or wide-spacing of eyes, epicanthal folds. Note a small or recessive chin, low set ears. Head control is poor in the neonate although when lying on the abdomen the newborn can turn the head and lift the face. Head control is stable by 4 months.

Neck and back. Palpate for masses, asymmetry, or injury (fractured clavicle, brachial plexus injury). Note dimpling at the base of spinal cord.

Table 2
Infant Reflexes

Reflex	How to Elicit	Response of Infant	Clinical Implications
Acoustic blink	Produce a sharp loud noise (a clap of the hands) about 30 cm from the head.	By second or third day of life infant will blink both eyes. Disappearance of reflex is variable.	Absence may indicated decreased hearing.
Ankle clonus	Flex the leg at the hip and knee, sharply dorsiflex the foot, and maintain pressure.	Rhythmic flexions and extensions of the foot at the ankle	Abnormal if more than 10 beats during the first 3 months; or more than 3 beats after 3 months. Sustained clonus indicates upper motor neuron disease.
Babinski	Stroke lateral aspect of the plantar surface of foot from heel to toes. Use a blunt object.	Hyperextension or fanning of toes occurs. As myelinization is completed, the normal response becomes flexion (downward curling) of all toes; the positive (pathologic) sign is hyperextension (dorsiflexion) of the great toe with or without fanning of the remaining toes.	After 2 years of age a positive sign is the most significant clinical sign of the presence of an upper motor neuron (pyramidal tract) lesion.
Blinking	Shine a light suddenly at the infant's open eyes	Eyelids close in response to light. Disappears after first year.	Absence may indicate poor light perception or blindness.
Landau	Suspend infant carefully in prone position by supporting infant's abdomen with examiner's hand.	By 3 months of age the expected response consists of extension of head, trunk, and hips. Head is slightly above horizontal plane. Disappears by 2 years of age.	If newborn collapses into a limp concave position, it is abnormal.

Moro	1. With infant in supine position, gently support head and lift it a few cm off the surface. As soon as neck relaxes, suddenly release the head and let it drop back to the surface, *or* 2. Produce sudden loud noise, or jar the table or crib suddenly.	Normal response is present at birth and is one in which the arms extend outward, the hands open, and then are brought together in midline. The legs flex slightly. Usually disappears by 3 to 4 months. Infant may cry.	Asymmetry indicates possible paralysis. Absence suggests severe neurologic problem. Persistence beyond 4 months may indicate neurologic disease. If it lasts longer than 6 months, it is definitely abnormal.
Neck righting	With infant in supine position turn head to one side.	Infant's trunk rotates in direction in which head is turned. Appears at 4 to 6 months. Disappears at 24 months.	Absent or decreased reflex may indicate spasticity.
Palmar grasp	With infant's head positioned in midline, place examiner's index fingers from ulnar side into infant's palm and press against palm.	Normal response is flexion of all fingers around examiner's fingers. Present at birth and disappears by 4 months when infant is ready to reach.	Note symmetry and strength. Persistence of grasp beyond 4 months suggests cerebral dysfunction.
Parachute	Infant is held in a prone position and is quickly lowered toward the surface of the examining table or floor.	Normal response is extension of arms, hands, and fingers, as if to break a fall. Appears by 9 months and persists.	Asymmetry or absence of response is abnormal.
Perez	Infant is held in a suspended prone position in one of the examiner's hands. The thumb of the other hand is moved firmly from sacrum along entire spine.	Normal response is extension of head and spine, flexion of knees on the chest, a cry, and emptying of the bladder. Present at birth and disappears by 3 months.	Absence indicates severe neurologic disease.
Placing	Infant is held erect and the dorsum of one foot touches the undersurface of the examining table top.	Infant flexes hip and knee and places stimulated foot on top of the table. Present at birth and disappears by 6 weeks or variable.	Absent in paralysis or in infants born by breech delivery.

Continued on next page

Table 2 *(Continued)*

Reflex	How to Elicit	Response Of Infant	Clinical Implications
Plantar grasp	Examiner's finger is placed firmly across base of infant's toes.	Toes curl downward. Present at birth and disappears by 10 to 12 months	Absent in defects of lower spinal column. Infant cannot walk until this reflex disappears.
Rooting	Infant is held in supine position with head in midline and hands against chest. Examiner strokes perioral skin at corner of mouth or cheek.	Infant opens mouth and turns head toward stimulated side. Present at birth and disappears by 3 to 4 months (awake); by 7 months (asleep).	Absence indicates severe CNS disease or depressed infant.
Rotation test	Infant is held upright facing examiner and rotated in one direction and then the other.	Infant's head turns in the direction in which the body is being turned. If head is restrained the eyes will turn in the direction in which the infant is turned.	If head and eyes do not move, it indicates a vestibular problem.
Spontaneous crawling (Bauer's response)	Infant is lying prone and examiner presses soles of feet.	Infant makes crawling movements. Present at birth.	Crawling is absent in weak or depressed infants.
Stepping	Infant is held upright and soles of feet are put in touch with solid surface.	Infant "walks" along surface. Present at birth and disappears at 6 weeks.	Absence indicates depressed infant, breech delivery, or paralysis.

Sucking	With infant in supine position place nipple or finger 3 to 4 cm into mouth.	Vigorous sucking of finger or nipple. Present at birth and disappears by 3 to 4 months (awake) and 7 months (asleep). Tongue action should push finger up and back. Note rate of suck, amount of suction, and patterns or groupings of sucks.	Absence in term infants indicates CNS depression. Weak reflex may lead to feeding problems.
Tonic neck	With infant in supine position passively rotate head to one side.	Arm and leg on side to which head is turned extend, and opposite arm and leg flex (fencer's position). Present sometimes at birth but usually by 2 to 3 months. Disappears by 6 months.	Obligatory response is always abnormal. Persistence beyond 6 months is abnormal and indicates central motor lesions, e.g., cerebral palsy.
Trunk incurvation (Galant's)	Infant is held prone in examiner's hand. With the other hand the examiner moves a finger down the paravertebral portion of the spine, first on one side, then on the other.	Infant's trunk should curve to the side being stimulated. Present at birth and disappears by 2 months.	Presence of spinal cord lesions will interrupt this reflex.
Vertical suspension positioning	Infant is held upright, head is maintained in midline.	Legs are flexed at the hips and knees. Present at birth and disappears after 4 months.	Scissoring or fixed extension indicate spasticity.

Source: Adapted from M. L. Erickson, *Assessment and Management of Developmental Changes in Children* (St. Louis: C. V. Mosby, 1976), pp. 62–66; and B. L. Conway, *Pediatric Neurological Nursing* (Philadelphia: J. B. Lippincott, 1977).

Extremities. The normal newborn has increased flexor tone and holds hands in a clenched fist position with extremities drawn up on the trunk. Note palmar creases. Move each body joint through range of motion noting symmetry, tone, and dislocations.

Neuromotor function. This develops in cephalocaudal progression. A simple schema for assessment, keeping individual variation in mind, is as follows:

Age (± 2 weeks)	Activity	Progression
1 month	Eyes focus and follow	Eyes
2 months	Social smile	Face
3 months	Early head control	Neck
4 months	Reaches	Arms, hands
5 months	Trunk control	Trunk
6 months	Sits when placed	Trunk, legs
7 months	Uses thumb to grasp	Fingers
10 months	Stands with support	Legs
12 months	Walks with support	Legs, feet

More complete information on growth and development of infants and young children is found in the section, Developmental Assessment, which follows.

Sensory function. The newborn perceives tactile stimuli both soothing and painful. Visual acuity is poor, but the newborn follows large moving objects and will blink in response to a bright light. Pupils are equal and react to bright light. The normal newborn startles to a sudden, loud noise, and other auditory stimuli evoke changes in spontaneous motor activity.

Reflex function. A large number of primitive reflex patterns are found in the normal newborn or appear shortly after birth. Absence of these reflexes may indicate general depression of central or peripheral motor functions. Asymmetrical reflexes may indicate focal lesions. Abnormal persistence of these reflexes beyond the point when voluntary motor functions should be present indicates general developmental lag or central motor lesions. Table 2 describes certain of these reflexes and how to assess them.

Developmental Assessment

NORMAL GROWTH AND DEVELOPMENT

The term, development, incorporates two concepts: (1) observable increases in size and structure of an organism over time and (2) progressive changes in an individual's adaptation to the environment (Waechter, 1976, p. 50). Children universally follow the same pattern of development and over the years developmental standards have been established based on studies of the age levels at which normal children achieve various motor, language, adaptive, and social behaviors. Excellent and comprehensive summaries of growth and development during the infancy and preschool periods, the Waechter Developmental Guides, are presented in Tables 3 and 4. The information contained in these tables should be an integral part of the repertoire of all pediatric care providers.

DEVELOPMENTAL SCREENING

A critical part of the neurologic examination is assessment of developmental functioning. Several screening tests are available which can be used to determine which children need more comprehensive developmental evaluation. Interpretation of the results of screening tests requires recognition of the range of normality, individual variations, and the variables present in the test situation.

Denver Developmental Screening Test. This test (see Figure 1) has gained wide acceptance as an economical, simple, and accurate tool for developmental screening of children from birth to 6 years. It gives a quick visual picture of the child's strengths and weaknesses in four areas of behavior: gross motor, fine motor, language, and personal-social. All test materials, including the instruction manual, can be obtained from: LADOCA Project and Publishing Foundation Inc., East 51st Street and Lincoln Street, Denver, CO 80216.

The developmental profile. This tool can be used from birth through 12 years of age to determine objectively a child's level of functioning. It consists of 217 items that, to large extent, can be

Table 3

Waechter Developmental Guide: Summary of Average Development during the First Year

Age	Physical and Motor Development	Intellectual Development	Socialization and Vocalization	Emotional Development
1 month	Physiologically more stable than in newborn period Waves hands as clenched fists Objects placed in hands are dropped immediately Momentary visual fixation on objects and human face TNR position frequent and Moro reflex brisk Able to turn head when prone, but unable to support head Responds to sounds of bell, rattle, etc. Makes crawling motions when prone Sucking and rooting reflex present Coordinates sucking, swallowing, and breathing	Reflexive No attempt to interact with environment External stimuli do not have meaning	Cries, mews, and makes throaty noises Responds in terms of internal need states Interested in the human face	Response limited generally to tension states Panic reactions, with arching of back and extension and flexion of extremities Derives satisfaction from the feeding situation when held and pleasure from rocking, cuddling, and tactile stimulation Maximal need for sucking pleasures Quiets when picked up
2 months	Moro reflex still brisk Posture still toward TNR position Has visual response to patterns	Recognition of familiar face Indicates inspection of the environment Beginning to show anticipation before feeding	Beginnings of vocalization: coos Beginning of social smile Actively follows movement of familiar person or object with eyes	Maximal need for sucking pleasures Indicates more active satisfaction when fed, held, rocked

		Crying becomes differentiated Vocalizes to mother's voice Visually searches to locate sounds of mother's voice	Maximal need for sucking pleasure Wish to avoid unpleasant situations Not yet able to act independently to evoke response in others
Eye coordination to light and objects Follows objects vertically and horizontally Responds to objects placed on face Listens actively to sounds Able to lift head momentarily from prone position Turns from side to back Able to swallow pureed foods	Shows active interest in environment Can recognize familiar faces and objects such as bottle; objects, however, do not have permanence Recognition is indicative of recording of memory traces Beginning of play with parts of body Follows objects visually Beginning ability to coordinate stimuli from various sense organs Shows awareness of a strange situation	More ready and responsive smile Facial and generalized body response to faces Preferential response to adult voices Has longer periods of wakefulness without crying Beginnings of prelanguage vocalizations: babbling and cooing Laughs aloud and shows pleasure in vocalization Shows anticipatory preparation to being lifted Turns head to follow familiar person Ceases crying when mother enters the room	
3 months Frequency of TNR position and vigor of Moro response rapidly diminishing Uses arms and legs simultaneously, but not separately Able to raise head from prone position; may get chest off bed Holds head in fairly good control Beginning differentiation of motor responses Hands are beginning to open and objects placed in hands are retained for brief inspection; able to carry objects to mouth Indicates preference for prone or supine position "Stepping" reflex disappears Landau reflex appears			

Continued on next page

Table 3 (Continued)

Age	Physical and Motor Development	Intellectual Development	Socialization and Vocalization	Emotional Development
	Eyes converge as objects approach face Has necessary muscular control to accept cereal and fruit			
4 months	Ability to carry objects to mouth Inspects and plays with hands Grasps objects with both hands Turns head to sound of bell or bottle Reaches for offered objects Eyes focus on small objects Beginning eye-hand coordination Ability to pick up objects Rooting reflex disappears; TNR disappearing Sits with minimal support with stable head and back Turns from back to side Breathing and mouth activity coordinated in relation to vocal cords Holds head up when pulled to sitting position Begins to drool	Recognizes bottle on sight Becomes bored when left alone for long periods of time Actively interested in environment Indicates beginnings of intentionality and interest in affecting the environment Indicates beginning anticipation of consequences of action	Vocalizes frequently and vocalizations change according to mood Begins to respond to "no, no" Enjoys being propped in sitting position Turns head to familiar noise Chuckles socially Demands attention by fussing; enjoys attention	Interest in mother heightens Baby is affable and lovable Shows signs of increasing trust and security

5 months	Ability to recover near objects	Able to discriminate strangers from family	Enjoys play with people and objects	Other members of the family become important as the baby's emotional world expands
	Reaches persistently	Turns head after fallen object	Smiles at mirror image	Beginning ability to postpone gratification
	Grasps with whole hand	Shows active interest in novelty	More exuberantly playful, but also more touchy and discriminating	Awaits anticipated routines with happy expectation
	Ability to lift objects	Attempts to regain interesting action in environment		Beginning exploration of mother's body
	Beginning use of thumb and finger in "pincer" movement	Ability to coordinate visual impressions of an object		
	Able to sustain visual inspection	Beginning differentiation of self from environment		
	Able to sit for longer periods of time when well supported			
	Beginning signs of tooth eruption			
	Ability to sleep through night without feeding			
	Moro reflex and TNR finally disappear			
6 months	Ability to pick up small objects directly and deftly	Increasing awareness of self	Very interested in sound production	Beginning sense of "self"
	Ability to lift cup by handle	Responds with attentiveness to novel stimuli	Playful response to mirror	Increased growth of ego
	Grasps, holds, and manipulates objects	Beginning ability to recognize mother when she is dressed differently	Laughs aloud when stimulated	
	Ability to pull self to sitting position	Objects begin to acquire permanence; will search for lost object for brief period	Great interest in babbling which is self reinforcing	
	Beginning to "hitch" in locomotion		Beginning recognition of strangers	
	Momentary sitting and hand support			
	When lying in prone position, supports weight with hands			
	Weight gain begins to decline			
	Ability to turn completely over			

Continued on next page

Table 3 (Continued)

Age	Physical and Motor Development	Intellectual Development	Socialization and Vocalization	Emotional Development
7 months	Ability to transfer objects from one hand to another Holds object in one hand Gums or mouths solid foods; exploratory behavior with food Ability to bang objects together Palmar grasp disappears Bears weight when held in standing position Sits alone for brief periods Rolls over adeptly	Ability to secure objects by pulling on string Repeats activities that are enjoyed Discovers and plays with own feet Drops and picks up objects in exploration Searches for lost objects outside perceptual field Has consciousness of desires Growing differentiation of self from environment Rudimentary sense of depth and space	Vocalizes four different syllables Produces vowel sounds and chained syllables Makes "talking sounds" in response to the talking of others Crows and squeals	Beginning to show signs of fretfulness when mother leaves or in presence of strangers Shows beginning fear of strangers Orally aggressive in biting and mouthing
8 months	Ability to ring bell purposively Ability to feed self with finger foods Beginning tooth eruption Sits well alone Ability to release objects at will	Uncovers hidden toy Increased interest in feeding self Differentiation of means from end in intentionality Has lively curiosity about the world	Listens selectively to familiar words Says "da da" or equivalent Babbles to produce consonant sounds Vocalizes to toys Stretches out arms to be picked up	Plays for sheer pleasure of the activity Anxiety when confronted by strangers indicates recognition and need of mother; attachment behavior begins to be obvious and strong
9 months	Rises to sitting position Creeps and/or crawls, maybe backward at first Tries out newly developing motor capacities	Ability to put objects in container Examines object held in hand; explores objects by sucking, chewing, and biting	Responds to simple verbal requests Plays interactive games, such as peek-a-boo and patty cake	Mother is increasingly important for her own sake; reacts violently to threat of her loss

744

Age	Physical/Motor	Cognitive	Language/Social	Emotional
10 months	Ability to hold own bottle Drinks from cup or glass with assistance Beginning to show regular patterns in bladder and bowel elimination Good ability to use thumb and finger in pincer grasp Pulls self to feet with help Ability to unwrap objects Pulls to standing position Uses index finger to poke and finger and thumb to hold objects Finger feeds self; controls lips around cup Plantar reflex disappears Neck-righting reflex disappears Sits without support; recovers balance easily Pulls self upright with furniture	Beginnings of imitation Looks at and follows pictures in book	Extends toy to another person without releasing Responds to own name Inhibits behavior to "no, no" or own name Beginning to test reactions to parental responses during feeding and at bedtime Imitates facial expressions and sounds	Begins to show fears of going to bed and being left alone Increasing interest in pleasing mother Active search in play for solutions to separation anxiety
11 months	Ability to hold crayon adaptively Ability to push toys Ability to put several objects in container; releases objects at will Stands with assistance; may be beginning attempts to walk with assistance Beginning ability to hold spoon "Cruises" around furniture	Works to get toy out of reach Growing interest in novelty Heightened curiosity and drive to explore environment	Repeats performance laughed at by others Imitates definite speech sounds Uses jargon Communicates by pointing to objects wanted	Has powerful urge toward independence in locomotion, feeding; beginning to help in dressing Experiences joy when achieving a goal and mastering fear Reacts to restrictions with frustration, but has ability to master new situations with mother's help (weaning)

Continued on next page

Table 3 (Continued)

Age	Physical and Motor Development	Intellectual Development	Socialization and Vocalization	Emotional Development
12 months	Turns pages in book; can make marks on paper Babinski sign disappears Beginning standing alone and toddling "Cruises" around furniture Lumbar curve develops Hand dominance becomes evident Ability to use spoon in feeding	Dogged determination to re-move barriers to action Further separation of means from ends Experiments to reach goals not attained previously Concepts of space, time, and causality begin to have more objectivity	Jabbers expressively Has words that are specific to parents Few, simple words Experimentation with "pseudo-words" of great interest and pleasure	Ability to show emotions of fear, anger, affection, jealousy, anxiety Baby is in love with the world

Source: Reprinted with permission from E. H. Waechter and F. G. Blake, *Nursing Care of Children*, 9th ed. (Philadelphia: J. B. Lippincott, 1976), pp. 276–279.

746

Table 4

Waechter Developmental Guide: Summary of Toddler Development

Age	Physical Development	Intellectual and Verbal Development	Emotional and Social Development
18 months	Anterior fontanel closed	Imitates words	Imitates behavior of parents
	Trunk long, legs short and bowed	Uses some words to indicate needs, mainly gestures	Beginning to test limits
	Protruding abdomen	Ability to point to objects named by adult	Extremely dependent on parents, yet beginning to strive for autonomy
	Walks upstairs with help, creeps downstairs	Follows directions, understands requests	Plays "pretending" games, such as peek-a-boo, sleeping
	Turns pages of a book	Imitates adult behavior	Play and imitation fused
	Holds cup with digital grasp, lifts cup	Ability to retrieve toy out of reach through experimentation	Explores house area—into "everything"
	Beginning to use spoon, but may turn bowl downward	Follows a toy through several hiding places	Plays alone, but near others
	Walks without support and with balance	Beginning of symbolic thought	Will have bowel movement when placed on potty at appropriate time
	Can build a tower of 3 cubes	Egocentrism in thought and behavior	Indicates wet pants
	Picks up small beads and places in receptacle	"Magical thinking" present	
	Scribbles spontaneously, uses whole hand	Global organization of mental processes	
	Closes small box	Short attention span	
		Imitates nonliving objects, absent objects, and humans	
		Invention of new "means"; symbols increasingly covert	
		Beginning sense of time in anticipation and memory	
		Infers causes from observing effects	

Continued on next page

Table 4 (Continued)

Age	Physical Development	Intellectual and Verbal Development	Emotional and Social Development
2 years	Holds glass in one hand Steady gait, runs Weight is about 28 pounds Protruding abdomen less noticeable Has about 16 teeth Can build a tower of 6 cubes Inserts spoon in mouth correctly	Arranges several words together in sentences "Telegraphic" speech Refers to self by pronoun Beginning to learn about time sequences Searches for new ways to solve problems, "invents means" Global organization of thought processes Increasing attention span Obeys simple commands Beginnings of symbolic thought	"Rituals" and stability of routine important Extremely vulnerable to changes in physical environment Extreme use of "no" as assertion of self Negativism Extremely resistant to restrictions on freedom "Loves" and "hates" intensely Beginning cooperation in toileting—anticipates need to eliminate Extremely possessive with toys Consumed by own wishes Extreme reaction to separation from parents Striving for autonomy prominent Temper tantrums decreasing Dawdling Resistant to bed time; use of transitional object Interested in other children, but has no social skills—parallel play
2½	Walks up and downstairs, one step at a time Throws a ball overhand Can jump in place Beginning to ride a kiddie car	"Telegraphic" speech continues Speech resembles monologue Increase in vocabulary Beginning knowledge of past, present, and future	Solitary and parallel play Dawdling continues Temper tantrums continuing, but lessening in quantity and quality Ritualistic behavior at peak

3	Pours from pitcher, may spill Teething almost complete Can build a tower of 8 cubes	Egocentrism in thought and behavior Beginning ability to reflect on own behavior	Use of "transitional object" to reduce anxiety—e.g., security blanket Fears prominent Extreme reaction to separation from parents; beginning to work on fear of separation Prominent striving for autonomy Continuing negativism Daytime bladder control with accidents when absorbed in play Beginning to acquire nighttime bladder control
	Walks downstairs, alternating feet Hops on one foot Swings and climbs Balances on one foot Rarely needs assistance in eating Rides a tricycle Fine motor control increasing, enjoys painting, coloring, etc. Eruption of deciduous teeth completed	Increased attention span Uses regular plurals Can give first and last name Begins to ask "why" Exploration of the environment outside the home Vocabulary: 1,000 words; speech fluid; sentences of 4 words Centers attention on one aspect of a situation Transductive reasoning	Nighttime bladder control is fairly reliable, but not complete; takes responsibility for toileting, occasional accidents Reduction of ritualistic behavior Beginning interaction with others in play, sharing toys Dramatizes, expresses imagination in play Interest in conforming to parental expectations Greater independence in activities Beginning awareness of sex role Sense of self as an individual Consolidation of autonomy Increased ability to separate from parents for short periods

Source: Reprinted with permission from E. H. Waechter, and F. G. Blake, *Nursing Care of Children,* 9th ed. (Philadelphia: J. B. Lippincott, 1976), pp. 386–387.

obtained by report from any individual familiar with the child. The items are grouped into five scales: physical, self-help, social, academic, and communication. The results provide an individual profile that can be used to stimulate development in weak areas. The tool is available from: Psychological Development Publications, 7150 Lakeside Drive, Indianapolis, IN 46278.

The Neonatal Behavioral Assessment Scale. Developed by T. Berry Brazelton, M.D., this tool is discussed in Chapter 5, Assessment of Parent-Child Interaction.

Normal Laboratory Values

CEREBROSPINAL FLUID

Lumbar puncture and examination of cerebrospinal fluid (CSF) is probably the most important laboratory procedure in the evaluation of neurologic disorders. Normal values include:

- Appearance: Colorless, odorless
- Specific gravity: 1.007 to 1.009
- Pressure: 50 to 180 mm of water (with child relaxed and in lateral recumbent position)
- Cell count: WBC 0 to 5/cu mm
- Protein: 15 to 45 mg/dl
- Sugar: Varies with level of serum glucose. CSF value is about 50 to 75% of the serum glucose level
- Culture: negative

Meningeal Signs

Inflammation of the meninges is a serious condition in infants and young children and must be identified as early as possible. Two specific maneuvers are used to detect meningeal inflammation:

1. Kernig's sign. With the child in the supine position, flex one leg at the hip and knee, then straighten the knee. Note resistance

or pain. If either is present, it suggests meningeal inflammation. This is a difficult sign to evaluate in infants under 6 months.

2. Brudzinski's sign. With the child in the supine position, flex the neck. Note pain or resistance in the neck and flexion of the hips and knees. This sign indicates meningeal irritation.

Other meningeal signs include stiffness of the neck (nuchal rigidity), inability to touch chin to chest, and inability to sit up normally (stiffness of the back).

Neurologic "Soft" Signs

These are discussed in Chapter 26, Language and Learning Disabilities.

COMMON CLINICAL PROBLEMS

Breath Holding

ASSESSMENT

Breath-holding attacks are periods of apnea followed by brief unconsciousness which usually occur in response to emotional insult or unexpected painful stimuli. There are two types:

1. Cyanotic breath-holding attack. A situation that precipitates fear, anger, or frustration leads to violent crying. The crying is interrupted by a sudden gasp, apnea, cyanosis, rigidity, and frequently brief unconsciousness with loss of body tone. Opisthotonos and convulsive movements may occur if unconsciousness is prolonged. Prompt restoration to full awareness follows. Complete episodes last less than 1 minute. Episodes lasting longer than 1 minute may indicate epilepsy.

2. Pallid breath-holding attack. In this type a sudden painful ex-

perience precipitates apnea, pallor, and loss of consciousness. Opisthotonos and seizure activity with incontinence may or may not occur. Spontaneous recovery occurs promptly. Neurologic findings are normal in most children.

The parent-child relationship should be evaluated to determine the presence or absence of disturbances which may be contributing to the incidence of attacks.

Incidence. Up to 5 percent of children experience breath-holding attacks. Age range is from 6 months to 6 years with peak incidence from 1 to 3 years of age. A history of breath holding in a near relative is present in approximately 25 percent of the cases.

Differential diagnosis. Features that distinguish breath-holding spells from idiopathic epilepsy are described in Table 5.

MANAGEMENT

Medication. Treatment with anticonvulsants is not indicated unless there is evidence of epilepsy.

Counseling. Breath-holding attacks are terrifying to most parents and frequently lead to oversolicitation and overprotectiveness by parents. This can lead to manipulative behavior by the child. It is important to reassure parents that the attack will spontaneously cease and that the child will resume breathing. They do not have to slap the child on the back, do mouth-to-mouth resuscitation, or call an ambulance. The child should not be punished for having an attack. The most effective approach includes an attitude of calmness during the attack and a subsequent ignoring of the attack. Parents initially need tremendous reassurance and support to develop this approach.

Referral. Unprovoked apneic attacks and children whose breath-holding results in frequent loss of consciousness or convulsions need to be referred for further evaluation.

Table 5

Differentiation between Epilepsy and Breath-holding Attacks

	Grand Mal (Idiopathic Epilepsy)	Anoxic Convulsion (Breath-holding Spell)
Age of onset	Rarely in infancy	Often begins in infancy
Family history	None or positive for epilepsy	Often positive for breath-holding spell or fainting
Precipitating factors	Usually absent (or specific sensory stimuli or nonspecific stresses)	Usually present (specific emotional or painful stimuli)
Occurrence during sleep	Common	Never
Posture	Variable	Usually erect
Sequence and patterns	Single cry (may be absent) with loss of consciousness→tonic→clonic phases, cyanosis may occur later in attack; flushed at first, pale after attack	Long crying or single gasp, cyanosis or pallor→loss of consciousness→limpness→clonic jerks→opisthotonos→clonic jerks
Perspiration	Warm sweat	Cold sweat
Heart rate	Markedly increased	Decreased, asystole, or slightly increased
Duration	Usually >1 minute	Usually 1 minute or less
Incontinence and tongue biting	Common	Uncommon (but may occur)
Postictal state	Confusion and sleep common	No confusion. Fatigue common
Interictal EEG	Usually bilateral discharges	Usually normal
Ictal EEG	Generalized, high-voltage polyspike discharges, gradually subsiding into slow waves and depression for several minutes	Isoelectric pattern preceded and followed by diffuse high-voltage delta waves, promptly reverting to normal pattern upon recovery of consciousness

Source: Adapted with permission from C. T. Lombroso and P. Lerman, "Breathholding Spells (Cyanotic and Pallid Infantile Syncope)," *Pediatrics* 39:579, April 1967. Copyright 1967, American Academy of Pediatrics.

Cerebral Palsy

ASSESSMENT

Cerebral palsy is the comprehensive term used to designate a group of nonprogressive neuromotor disorders which are the result of antecedent insults to the central nervous system. In addition to motor deficits, cerebral palsy may include mental retardation (50 to 75 percent), seizures (60 percent), speech disorders, visual disorders (more than two thirds), and auditory disorders.

Etiology. In many cases the exact etiology is never determined, but causative and risk factors include:

1. Prenatal factors. Maternal anoxia, maternal bleeding, Rh or ABO incompatibility, irradiation during pregnancy, maternal infection (rubella, toxoplasmosis, cytomegalic inclusion disease), and injuries
2. Perinatal factors. Prematurity, asphyxia, cerebral trauma, hemorrhage, low birth weight, and kernicterus
3. Postnatal factors. Trauma, hemorrhage, anoxia, meningitis, and encephalitis

Incidence. Approximately 25,000 children each year are affected, or 1 to 2 of every 1000 births.

Clinical manifestations. The clinical findings are related to the area of the brain that has been damaged and are described according to the nature of the observed motor deficit as follows:

1. Spastic cerebral palsy. This is the most common type (70 to 75 percent of affected children); it is due to involvement of upper motor neurons and is characterized by increased muscle tone, exaggeration of deep tendon reflexes, clonus, abnormal persistence of neonatal reflexes, and a tendency toward contractures.

    • Spastic quadriplegia. All four extremities are affected. Mental retardation, convulsions, speech defects, and swallowing disorders are commonly associated.

- Spastic hemiplegia. Both extremities on one side are involved with the upper extremity more severely affected.
- Spastic diplegia. Scissoring of the legs, tightening of the Achilles' tendon, flexion contractures of the knees, and toe gait are characteristics. All four extremities are involved but the lower extremities are more severely affected. It is frequently associated with low birth weight.
- Atonic diplegia. It is characterized by hypotonia, normal or increased deep tendon reflexes, marked delay in developmental milestones, and mental retardation. Muscle tone changes with age and by late childhood may be normal or hypertonic.
- Spastic paraplegia. Both legs are involved and the upper extremities are normal.
- Monoplegia (one extremity involved) and triplegia (three extremities involved) are rare.

2. Dyskinetic cerebral palsy. This type is the result of basal ganglia or extrapyramidal tract lesions and occurs in 15 to 20 percent of affected children. It causes impairment of volitional activity by uncontrolled, uncoordinated, and purposeless movements that disappear during sleep. Athetoid movements are the most common. Speech and swallowing are impaired, and walking exaggerates the involuntary movements. The combination of motor handicap and disturbed speech may lead to the faulty impression of mental retardation. Intellectual ability must be carefully evaluated before assuming mental defect.

3. Ataxic cerebral palsy. Two to five percent of affected children have this type which is the result of a cerebellar lesion and is characterized by ataxic signs from early childhood. Hypotonia and decreased tendon reflexes are present in infancy. Later the child develops a wide-based gait, has difficulty turning rapidly, and performs coordinated rapid movements (e.g., finger-to-nose test) poorly. Prognosis for improvement is better than for other types.

4. Mixed cerebral palsy. More than one form of cerebral palsy may be present in the same child. The combination of spasticity and athetosis is most common.

Presenting symptoms. In infancy the common presenting symptoms are feeding problems, sucking and swallowing difficulties, prolonged drooling, early handedness, irritability, motor delay, decreased spontaneous movements, hypertonicity, asymmetry, and persistent toe-walking (Taft, 1977). The presence of any of these symptoms plus the presence of any of the risk factors listed earlier indicate the need for a careful and thorough neurologic evaluation.

MANAGEMENT

The management of cerebral palsy depends on the child's age, the type of cerebral palsy, the extent of involvement, the presence or absence of related abnormalities (e.g., seizures), and the degree of mental functioning. Problem areas can be categorized generally in the areas of: feeding, safety, physical care, promotion of optimum development, and adjustment of the child and family to lifelong disability. An extensive guide to management is Finnie's book, *Handling the Young Cerebral Palsied Child at Home*. See Resource Information.

Feeding. Difficulties in sucking and swallowing are often present in the infant and may be combined with hyperextension of the neck and spasticity in the extremities. This makes the feeding situation frustrating and challenging. The nurse practitioner must acknowledge the difficulties the parents are having and plan a joint effort with them to improve the feeding experience. Suggestions for improving the feeding situation include the following:

- Maintain the infant in a flexed position, sitting cross-legged in the mother's lap to minimize the pathologic extensor reflexes
- Provide a feeding environment that is quiet, calm, and non-stimulating
- Develop patience and a slow pace
- Place food on the back of the tongue for easier swallowing
- Cut food into small pieces
- Serve foods that stick to the spoon; e.g., mashed potatoes, apple sauce
- Slowly guide the spoon to the child's mouth

- Obtain necessary special equipment; e.g., special handles, non-skid plate and glass holders
- Use a straw for liquids
- Try to disregard the mess

Safety. Routine safety measures are discussed in Chapter 9, Accident Prevention and Safety. The child with ataxic cerebral palsy or associated seizures may need special head gear to protect against head injury due to falls. Seizure precautions are discussed in this chapter under Epilepsy.

Physical care. Frequent change of position lessens irritability and increases comfort. Prevention of contractures is accomplished by appropriate exercises, passive range of motion, encouragement of active motion via play, and the use of splints, braces, and back supports. Medications to reduce spasticity and abnormal movements and to relax skeletal muscle are occasionally used but are frequently unsuccessful.

Promotion of optimum development. Provision of routine health maintenance care is important and assists the family to focus on the child's assets. Suggestions for age-appropriate activities and interactions contribute to promotion of developmental potential.

Adjustment of the family to lifelong disability. The nurse practitioner provides primary care to many children with severe and chronic handicapping conditions and can help parents, over time, to understand their feelings and to adjust to the situation. Questions that help to elicit parental feelings are*:

What is your understanding of the cause?

Do you think you are/were at fault?

Was this child a planned baby?

When did you first find out that there was something wrong?

What did the doctor say at first? Did you understand what the doctor said at the beginning?

---

*From C. U. Battle, "Chronic Physical Disease: Behavioral Aspects," *Pediatr Clin North Am* 22:525–531, August 1975, © 1975 by the W. B. Saunders Company, Philadelphia.

How long after the birth of the baby did you see your child? (if there is a birth defect)

What do you think about your child's problem?

How does your husband/wife feel about it?

What did your mother say?

Did anyone suggest institutionalizing your child?

Did you ever think it would have been better if the baby had died?

Did you feel uneasy about showing your baby to relatives and friends?

Were your friends helpful? Do they stay away?

Was the baby difficult to care for in early infancy?

Do you and your husband/wife feel the same way about your child's condition?

What do you disagree about?

Do you feel comfortable now about taking your child out in public?

Do you and your husband/wife share in the care of the child?

Do you ever get an opportunity to be away from home to do something you would like for yourself?

Does anyone ever babysit for your child?

How often do you and your husband/wife go out together?

Do you feel that this child takes up most of your time?

Do you think that your normal children resent the time you spend with your child?

What worries you about the future of your child? What are your plans for the future of your child?

Coordination of care. The total management of the child with cerebral palsy or any chronic handicapping condition involves several disciplines and separate specialists. Integration and coordination of care by the nurse practitioner who is the continuity figure for the family are important role functions. Additional information on assisting families with chronically ill children is found later in this chapter under Epilepsy.

Dermal Sinus

ASSESSMENT

Interference with the development of the spinal cord during the first three weeks of gestation results in defects of closure of the neural tube. Spina bifida and meningomyelocele are examples of severe defects. Dermal sinus tracts are small closure defects. They are epithelial-lined sinus tracts which may be located at any point along the spine but are most common in the lumbosacral area or the occipital region of the head. They are significant if they penetrate into the subarachnoid space as this can be a route of entry for bacteria and recurrent meningitis. Most dermal sinuses, including the low sacral pilonidal cysts, end blindly and do not communicate with the nervous system. They are, however, prone to periodic local infection.

Clinical signs. Skin markings along the spinal column include dimpling, tufts of hair, or small hemangiomas.

MANAGEMENT

Sinus tracts above the sacral level should be surgically explored and excised. Noncommunicating pilonidal cysts require careful hygiene to prevent infection.

Developmental Delay

ASSESSMENT

Developmental delay is a term frequently used to describe a wide spectrum of clinical findings that may (or may not) indicate abnormalities in the functional status of infants and young children. It is a symptom of subnormal function of the central nervous system whether due to damage, altered physiology, environmental deprivation, or abnormally slow maturation. When developmental delay is suspected thorough developmental history and neuro/developmental assessment are indicated. See this chapter, Physical Examination, and Developmental Assessment. It is of critical importance, however, to recognize that individual variations exist within established norms, and that development is influenced by both heredity and environment. Consequently, it is often difficult to assess with certainty the significance of developmental variations.

Types of developmental delay. Some guidelines for considering various forms of developmental delay are as follows:

1. Multiple, global, or major delay in all areas usually signifies an underlying central nervous system disorder, e.g., mental retardation, cerebral palsy. It may also indicate severe systemic illness causing weakness, malnutrition, emotional disturbance, deprivation or other difficult environmental factors, or benign congenital hypotonia (see this chapter, Hypotonia). And finally, it may indicate prematurity and failure of the examiner to correct for gestational age. The weeks a child is born prematurely are subtracted from the chronologic age to determine age norms.

2. Specific delays in any one of the areas of development indicate specific disorders or may, in fact, be normal variations in which case the child eventually catches up.

3. Delayed gross motor function occurs in cerebral dysfunction; muscle, spinal cord, or peripheral nerve disorders; or other physical disorders, e.g., a dislocated hip.

4. Delayed fine motor function may indicate sensory loss, blindness, or peripheral nerve disorders.

5. Delayed speech occurs with brain disorders, hearing loss, bilingualism, and lack of stimulation.

6. Poor social and adaptive behavior implies diffuse brain disturbance or psychosocial disturbance.

MANAGEMENT

Obvious delays. Obvious delays in development are readily identified and with careful history and physical examination can often be specifically diagnosed and appropriately managed. Children who are mentally retarded present complex management challenges to family, health professionals, and community. Major areas of management are similar to those discussed elsewhere (see this chapter, Cerebral Palsy, Epilepsy). Detailed discussions of comprehensive management can be found in Barnard and Erickson, 1976 (see this chapter, References).

INFANT STIMULATION AND PRESCHOOL EXPERIENCE. Up to 80 percent of developmental retardation occurs in children from environmentally deprived backgrounds. Since the majority of intellectual development occurs before school age, the importance of infant stimulation programs and preschool learning and socialization experiences is great. All children with developmental delays should be referred to such programs.

Subtle delays. The subtle delays are more difficult to assess and to manage. Many times nurse practitioners are faced with children who present marginal or subtle findings of developmental delay, who, based on the nurse's experience and intuition, just do not seem "quite right," or about whom an experienced parent is concerned. When thorough examination fails to reveal any significant findings, the concern does not go away. These are uneasy situations to manage. There are no definite rules to follow, but experienced nurse practitioners should pay attention to their hunches and provide close follow-up until subsequent development either confirms or negates the concern. A suggested protocol for following such children is as follows:

1. Consult with the physician and consider referral to the neurologist when abnormal developmental screening (DDST) persists for more than two visits scheduled at least 1 month apart.

2. Evaluate the parent-child relationship. See Chapter 5, Assessment of Parent-Child Interaction.

3. Make a home visit to evaluate the child in the normal environment.

4. Consider referral to community resources providing play and stimulation experiences.

Epilepsy

ASSESSMENT

Epilepsy refers to a symptom complex characterized by recurrent, paroxysmal attacks of unconsciousness or impaired consciousness, usually with a succession of tonic or clonic muscular spasms or other abnormal behavior, produced by abnormal and excessive neuronal discharge occurring in the brain. If the cause is known the disorder is termed *organic* epilepsy; if the cause is unknown (the majority of cases), it is termed *idiopathic* epilepsy. Approximately 7 percent of children will have had one or more seizures by the age of 5 years (Green, 1977).

Classification of seizures. An extensive discussion of the various forms of seizures is beyond the scope of this book, but since the nurse practitioner may be providing primary care services to children being treated for epilepsy, and since long-term medications are prescribed according to the type of seizure, the classification of seizures based on cerebral localization is presented (Waechter, 1976, p. 651):

International Classification of Epileptic Seizures
  I. *Partial seizures that begin locally (focal)*
    A. *Simple: motor, sensory, or autonomic*
    B. *Complex: temporal lobe*
    C. *Partial seizures that rapidly become generalized*
 II. *Generalized seizures without local onset*
    A. *Absences, petit mal*
    B. *Myoclonic jerks*
    C. *Infantile spasms*
    D. *Clonic*
    E. *Tonic*
    F. *Tonic-clonic*
    G. *Atonic drop attacks (brief), atonic absence (longer)*
    H. *Akinetic (loss of movement), no loss of tone*
III. *Unilateral (or mainly unilateral), usually in children*
IV. *Undefined*

Causes of seizures. The etiologic factors associated with epilepsy are multiple and are presented in Table 6.

History. The history is obtained bearing in mind the etiologic factors listed in Table 6. Additionally, the history of the paroxysmal episode is especially important for accurate diagnosis. Information to be obtained includes:

1. Events preceding the attack. What was the child doing prior to the attack? Was the child anxious, excited, or crying? Was there an aura, warning sensation, or change in mood? Did the child become dizzy, drowsy, or uncoordinated? What was happening in the environment? What was the time of day?

2. Events during the attack. How long did the attack last? What was the position of the head, trunk, and extremities? Where did the movements begin and what kind of movements were involved? What were the eye movements like? Were there pupillary changes? Was there cyanosis, perspiration, or drooling? Did the jaw clamp shut? Was there any respiratory problem, loss of consciousness, or incontinence?

3. Events after the attack (postictal state). Was there drowsiness, sleep, or rapid recovery? Was there any impairment in speech or motor function? Could the child recall any events during the seizure?

4. Related information. If not the first attack, how often do attacks occur? Is the child receiving medication? If so, what type and dose?

5. Consider other causes of paroxysmal behavior (e.g., breath-holding attacks, syncope, migraine headaches, or sleep disturbances).

Physical examination. A thorough general physical examination and complete neurologic examination are performed.

Laboratory. The data obtained from the history and physical examination will determine which laboratory procedures are indicated. Electroencephalogram (EEG) is routinely performed. Additional procedures include skull X-rays, lumbar puncture, blood and urine chemistries, brain scan, arteriography, and pneumoencephalography.

Table 6
Etiologic Factors Associated with Epilepsy

Prenatal Factors
  Genetic
    Genetic epilepsy
    Inborn errors of metabolism
      Carbohydrate: glycogen
        storage disease,
        hypoglycemia
      Protein: phenylketonuria,
        maple syrup urine disease
      Fat: cerebral lipidoses,
        leukodystrophies
    Heredofamilial diseases:
      myoclonus epilepsy
  Congenital structural anomalies
    Porencephaly
    Vascular malformations
    Neurocutaneous syndrome
    Developmental defects of brain
  Fetal infections
    Viral encephalopathy: rubella,
      cytomegalic inclusion disease
    Protozoan
      meningoencephalitis:
      toxoplasmosis
  Maternal diseases
    Toxemia of pregnancy
    Chronic renal disease
    Diabetes mellitus
    Radiation during pregnancy
    Drug usage and drug
      intoxication
    Trauma

Perinatal Factors
  Trauma
  Hypoxia
  Jaundice
  Infection
  Prematurity
  Drug withdrawal

Postnatal Factors
  Primary infection of central
    nervous system
  Infectious diseases of childhood
    with encephalopathy (eg,
    measles, mumps)
  Head trauma
  Circulatory diseases
    Vascular anomalies
    Occlusive diseases: arterial,
      venous
    Hemorrhage
    Hypertensive encephalopathy
  Toxic encephalopathy
    Thallium
    Lead
    Convulsogenic drugs: INH,
      steroids
  Allergic encephalopathy
    Immunization reactions
    Drug reactions
  Physical and metabolic
    encephalopathies
    Fever and febrile convulsions
    Anoxia and hypoxia
    Prolonged convulsions with
      cyanosis
    Electrolyte disturbance
    Acute porphyria
    Hypoglycemia
    Hypocalcemia
    Hypomagnesemia
    Hyponatremia and
      hypernatremia and others
    Pyridoxine deficiency or
      dependency
  Degenerative diseases of the
    brain
  Tumors

Source: Reprinted with permission from A. M. Rudolph, editor, *Pediatrics*, 16th ed. (New York: Appleton-Century-Crofts, 1977), p. 1842.

MANAGEMENT

The acute convulsive episode. Major objectives of care are protection of the child from injuries and observation of the event. Protective measures during a seizure are as follows:

1. Maintain an airway
2. Loosen restrictive clothing around the neck
3. Position the child on the side to prevent aspiration of secretions
4. Do not restrain body movements
5. Protect the mouth, tongue, and teeth if possible. Padded tongue depressors are used to prevent injury to the tongue and other oral tissues but are useful only during the initial moments of a seizure before the teeth clamp down. If the teeth have already shut, do not force the jaw open as it can cause further damage to mouth and teeth.
6. Provide oxygen and suction as necessary in a prolonged seizure
7. Comfort and reassure the child and parents as the child rouses from the episode

Long-term management. This is directed at prevention of seizures and promotion of normal psychosocial development in the child and family. It is a collaborative effort involving the family, nurse practitioner, physician, school personnel, and other appropriate professionals.

MEDICATION. With the correct choice of medication and sufficient dosage, approximately 60 percent of epileptic attacks can be completely controlled. The duration of drug therapy depends on the nature and severity of the underlying disease but generally is long term (i.e., several years). Management of drug therapy is the role of the physician, but the nurse practitioner needs to be aware of the drugs used to identify drug-related problems and to teach the child and family effectively. Only the most commonly used medications are discussed here.

1. Phenobarbital
   Use: Most commonly used anticonvulsant in children because

of its broad spectrum (focal, generalized, and psychomotor seizures), low toxicity, and low cost

Side effects: Drowsiness, skin rash, fever, and ataxia; paradoxical hyperactivity and irritability occur in some infants and young children

2. Diphenylhydantoin (Dilantin)

Use: Effective in treatment of generalized tonic-clonic (grand mal), focal, and psychomotor seizures

Side effects: Gum hypertrophy occurs in about 50 percent of children. Good dental hygiene and firm massage of the gums help to alleviate the symptom. Nausea and vomiting can be minimized by giving the drug after meals. Ataxia, incoordination, diplopia, and tremor are other side effects. Hypersensitivity reactions (rash, fever, and glandular involvement) may occur.

3. Ethosuximide (Zarontin)

Use: Drug of choice in the treatment of petit mal epilepsy

Side effects: Anorexia, abdominal pain, hiccoughs, drowsiness, and skin rash, and irritability. Aplastic anemia is a rare side effect.

Comment: The drug comes only in 250 mg capsules. In young children the drug may be dissolved in 1 to 2 ounces of fluid, but this mandates that the child drink all the fluid and demands careful calculation of the small pediatric dose. Another suggestion for improved accuracy is to freeze and then to cut the capsule into desired amounts (Conway, 1977, p. 243).

Teaching related to medication.   When teaching the child and family about the medication therapy:

1. Stress the importance of taking the medication as prescribed and the necessity for long-term therapy, even after seizures are controlled

2. Include the fact that it may take several months of regulation before control is achieved

3. Elicit feelings and attitudes about drug therapy

4. Stress safety precautions relative to storage of drugs at home

5. Discuss side effects and when to call for assistance

6. If the child is school age, plan for administration of the drug at school and involve the teacher and school nurse

7. See Chapter 14, Approach to Medications in Childhood

COUNSELING. General guidelines and considerations in the supportive counseling of families include:

1. Presentation and interpretation of the diagnosis. Both parents should be present.

2. Explanation of treatment and follow-up plans. Repeated opportunities must be provided for parents and child to ask questions.

3. Consideration of the impact of the diagnosis. The care provider should try to comprehend the illness as a human experience from the family's point of view.

4. Consideration of the prior life-style of the family and the effect of adaptations to long-term illness

5. Exploration of attitudes about epilepsy. Reactions of guilt, denial, shame, hostility, and fear can be expected. Most fears will be unspoken so parents and child need assistance to verbalize them.

6. Provision of support during an initial period of dependency as the family begins to face the problem and adapt

7. Planning of normal activities consistent with safety

8. Review of medications, what to do during an acute seizure, and seizure precautions

9. Anticipation of crisis periods requiring extra support for the family (e.g., school entry, adolescence)

10. Planning with parents and child for informing school personnel

11. Provision of information on specific resources (e.g., epilepsy organizations). See this chapter, Resource Information. Assistance in overcoming social, educational, legal, and economic obstacles will be necessary.

More detailed information on counseling is available in major references (Vaughan, 1975; Conway, 1977).

Febrile Seizures

ASSESSMENT

Up to 5 percent of children will develop a febrile seizure during childhood. It is important to distinguish whether the seizure is a simple benign febrile seizure or a nonbenign seizure. The characteristics of each type are listed in Table 7.

Prognosis. About 30 to 50 percent of untreated children who have had a first febrile seizure have another febrile seizure (Green, 1977). The second and third seizures can be very severe. The occurrence of more than one febrile seizure increases the probability of subsequent nonfebrile seizures but that risk is quite low (about 3 percent).

Table 7
Characteristics of Benign and Nonbenign Seizures

	Simple, Benign	Nonbenign
Character	General, major motor, symmetrical, clonic; duration less than 5 minutes; single occurrence	Similar to simple seizure but duration more than 5 minutes; repeated seizures during one febrile illness; may be asymmetrical or focal
Family history	History of simple febrile seizure in one third of cases	History of nonfebrile seizures
Age	6 months to 3 years; may be up to 5 years	Wider age range. Onset may be before 6 months or after 5 years
Past history	Birth, developmental, injury, illness history usually not significant	May be positive or negative
Physical examination	Negative; EEG normal; skull films normal	Physical exam, EEG, and skull films may be positive.
Precipitating illness	Extracranial; abrupt rise in temperature with fever over 39.5°C	May have intracranial infection. May have lower seizure threshold.

MANAGEMENT

The goals of management are to prevent recurrence of seizures, to lower fevers during acute illness (see Chapter 13, Approach to Illness in Childhood), and to treat the underlying infection.

Prevention of recurrent seizures. Current recommendations are for daily phenobarbital in all children after their first febrile seizure until the age of 5 to 6 years (Rudolph, 1977, p. 1854; Wolf, 1977, p. 384). This effectively prevents recurrence.

Immunizations. In children with a history of febrile seizures immunizations may be postponed and/or given in fractional doses.

Counseling. See this chapter, Epilepsy.

Handedness

ASSESSMENT

Handedness is never established before 1 year of age and usually by 18 months to 2 years. If a young infant demonstrates handedness before this age, concern and attention must be directed toward the opposite hand to determine paralysis, palsy, or other neuromuscular problem preventing use of the extremity.

The more frequent problem related to handedness is the desire and/or concern of parents that the child learn to use a preferred extremity, usually the right hand. The reasons for this social-cultural preference for the right hand remain mysterious.

MANAGEMENT

Parents need to be reassured that natural dominance is most appropriate, will be fairly consistent by 6 years of age and fully stable by 10 years. Mixed dominance or the use of one hand for one task and the other hand for another task are of no significance.

Headache

ASSESSMENT

Headache in children requires careful assessment of both organic and psychosocial factors since the cause may be benign or very serious. A useful classification of the types of headache (adapted from Vaughan, 1975, p. 1425) is as follows:

1. Vascular headache
   - Migraine
   - Headache secondary to fever
   - Hypertensive headache
2. Headache related to epilepsy
3. Headache related to changes in intracranial pressure
   - Brain tumor headache
   - Low CSF pressure headache
4. Headache due to inflammatory disease of the central nervous system, e.g., meningitis
5. Tension headache
6. Headache related to psychiatric disease
7. Headache due to eye strain
8. Headache due to sinusitis, ear infection, allergies, impacted teeth, or severe dental caries
9. Headache due to drugs, e.g., glue sniffers, "uppers"

History. Data obtained by history should reflect the causes of headache outlined above. Morning headache in children and localization of pain (e.g., occipital pain) are suspicious of brain tumor. Most children do not accurately detail their symptoms of headache. Functional headache should be considered in a child who offers great detail about the headache. Organic headache is usually intermittent; functional headache is more apt to be continuous and generalized. Low CSF pressure headaches are usually due to persistent leak of CSF after a spinal tap and appear as the child sits or stands up. The pain is relieved when the child lies down.

Physical examination. General physical examination and neurologic examination are performed. Facial expression (e.g., depression) should be noted. Blood pressure, careful funduscopic, visual-field, and visual-acuity examinations are important. The young child who cannot describe symptoms may demonstrate behaviors such as irritability, troubled facial expression, ear pulling, headbanging, or rolling.

Migraine headache. Approximately 3 percent of children have recurrent paroxysmal migraine headaches. Initial symptoms usually appear between 6 to 12 years of age. A positive family history is present in 60 to 90 percent of children.

- Common migraine is the most frequent type. There is no aura, the pain is steady, severe, throbbing, usually unilateral, and may last several hours.

- Classic migraine includes a prodome or aura, frequently visual (e.g., "sparkling lines"). The aura is followed by throbbing, unilateral pain which can become generalized and by nausea or vomiting. The pain may last for several hours; the child may withdraw into a quiet, darkened room and go to sleep.

MANAGEMENT

The management of headache varies with the cause. For detailed information see *Postgraduate Medicine,* September 1974. The entire issue is devoted to headache.

Counseling. Most cases of recurrent headaches occur in school age and adolescent children, are tension related, and include a psychosocial component. Thus the counseling role of the primary care provider is the most important aspect of management. Such counseling requires a family approach with investigation and understanding of the past and current family situation, identification of current stresses, and empathetic discussion of the relationship between feelings and symptoms.

Migraine headache. Migraine headaches are managed with a combination of medication and support.

MEDICATION. Aspirin or acetaminophen should be tried first. Phenobarbital in maintenance doses is used in some young children if they consistently are missing out on normal activities. A combination of ergotamine and caffeine (Cafergot) is widely used in older children and adolescents and is administered early in the attack.

COUNSELING. Most children do reasonably well on medication. The benign nature of the condition should be stressed. The environment may need modification if there are precipitating events or if the secondary gain that accrues to the child in terms of sympathy and attention results in more frequent headaches.

Hypothyroidism, Congenital

ASSESSMENT

Congenital hypothyroidism results from deficient production of thyroid hormones. Since thyroid hormones are critical for normal physical and mental development, the consequences of thyroid deficiency are severe physical and mental retardation. Although the severity of symptoms and their reversibility depend on the degree and length of thyroid deprivation, thyroid replacement therapy, if begun in the early newborn period, can have positive effects on growth and development. Thus early identification is extremely important.

Early signs. Warning signs in the immediate newborn period include:

1. Gestation over 42 weeks and/or birth weight greater than 4.0 kg
2. Large posterior fontanelle
3. Respiratory distress
4. Hypothermia, 35°C or less
5. Peripheral cyanosis
6. Hypoactivity, lethargy, poor feeding

7. Lag in stooling beyond 20 hours of age
8. Abdominal distention and/or vomiting
9. Jaundice beyond 3 days of age
10. Edema

The presence of three or more of these signs is highly suspicious of congenital hypothyroidism and a T4 (thyroxine) blood test should be performed.

Signs during the first 3 months of life. If the diagnosis is not made in the nursery, the following signs may develop in the first 3 months (adapted from Smith, 1975):

1. A feeling of coldness to the touch
2. Mottling of the skin*
3. Decreased activity
4. Feeding problems
5. Enlarged tongue
6. Hoarse cry
7. Constipation*
8. Dry skin
9. Umbilical hernia*
10. Unusually large anterior fontanelle for age*
11. Poor growth

MANAGEMENT

Dessicated thyroid medication is given as replacement therapy on a continuous basis.

Hypotonia (The Floppy Infant)

ASSESSMENT

Hypotonia, or decreased muscle tone, is a frequent presenting symptom in a variety of neuromuscular disorders. The clinical

---

*Present in at least 50 percent of patients.

picture of limpness in the neonatal and early infancy period and subsequent delay in achieving motor milestones is produced by problems at the cerebral, spinal, peripheral, or muscular levels. The most common causes are probably nonspecific mental retardation, perinatal hypoxia, and chromosomal disorders (e.g., Down's syndrome, hypothyroidism). There is a form called *benign congenital hypotonia* in which the infant is hypotonic at birth but appears normally alert, has depressed deep tendon reflexes, and has delayed sitting and walking, but has normal muscle fibers, no muscle atrophy, and eventually develops normally. Also, infants of mothers who have received depressant medications may appear hypotonic. Infants with congenital laxity of the ligaments (double-jointed) may appear hypotonic at birth. Recently, attention has been directed toward botulism as a cause of infant hypotonia and weakness (Pickett, 1976; Arnon, 1977). *Clostridium botulinum* toxin was recovered from the feces of six infants under 4 months of age whose clinical findings included constipation followed by neurologic signs of weakened sucking, swallowing, and crying; diminished gag reflex, and generalized weakness.

Evaluation of muscle tone. The hypotonic infant shows the following characteristics:

1. May exhibit poor sucking
2. When supine, lies in a frog-leg position with hips abducted and knees flexed. This position is normal following breech delivery.
3. When eliciting the Landau reflex, droops or collapses over the examiner's hand and looks like an inverted "U"
4. May have absent or depressed deep tendon reflexes
5. Exhibits increased range of joint movement
6. Has muscles that feel flabby to palpation

Laboratory techniques. These include muscle biopsy, EEG, electromyography, serum enzymes, nerve conduction velocity studies, spinal tap, and T4 (thyroxine) test.

MANAGEMENT

The underlying cause determines total management. If the cause is benign, the parents may be completely reassured. The majority of nonbenign causes of hypotonia involve long-term neuromuscular problems, and management includes those principles already discussed elsewhere in this chapter.

Lead Poisoning (Plumbism)

ASSESSMENT

Lead poisoning occurs when abnormal amounts of lead are absorbed in the body. Normal blood lead levels are 50 to 40 μg/dl and result from normal exposure to lead in food, water, and air. Levels above 40 μg/dl represent "undue" exposure and absorption, and may lead to symptoms of lead poisoning. Clinical lead poisoning exists with levels above 80 μg/dl. The amount of lead ingested, the degree of exposure, and repeated ingestions over time are factors that affect the manifestation of clinical symptoms.

Symptoms. In young children the symptoms usually develop insidiously and progressively. Hyperirritability, anorexia, decreased activity, ataxia, vomiting, weight loss, anemia, constipation, personality changes, and developmental delay or reversal make up the constellation of early signs. Late manifestations are acute encephalopathy (cerebral edema, convulsions, coma) which is most common in children 1 to 3 years of age and occurs with lead levels over 100 μg/dl; and chronic encephalopathy in older children including seizure disorders, hyperkinetic behavior disorders, and developmental regression.

Sources of lead. Ingestion and/or inhalation of lead occurs most commonly from flaking lead-based paint and from plaster or putty in dilapidated housing. Other sources include:

1. Artists' oil paints
2. Face powders
3. Fruit tree spray insecticides
4. Fumes and dust from leaded gasoline and from burning casings of storage batteries
5. Lead nipple shields
6. Lead-soldered cooking utensils

7. Lead shots, fishing weights, leaded jewelry
8. Leaded paint used in newspapers, magazines, books
9. Pottery glazed with lead
10. Water stored in lead-lined containers

These sources alone rarely cause symptomatic lead poisoning but do contribute to increased lead absorption.

MANAGEMENT

Increased lead absorption and lead poisoning. Children with elevated blood lead levels (over 40 to 50 μg/dl) are referred for further medical evaluation. Treatment is described by Haggerty (1977).

Screening. Screening for increased lead absorption can prevent death and disability from lead poisoning by:

1. Identifying children who have absorbed undue amounts of lead from their environment
2. Reducing their exposure to lead by removing hazards from the environment or removing susceptible children from the hazardous environment
3. Medically treating those children who have ill effects or are in danger of developing ill effects of absorbed lead (Frankenburg, 1974)

WHO TO SCREEN. Children to be screened include all children between 1 and 6 who live in poorly maintained buildings built before 1950; who visit relatives, friends, or babysitters; or who obtain day care in such buildings. Other children who should be screened are those who:

1. Are known to be exposed to other sources of lead
2. Exhibit pica
3. Exhibit unexplained, aberrant behavior, central nervous system symptoms, gastrointestinal symptoms, or anemia
4. Are members of a household in which another member has developed lead poisoning
5. Are residents of inner cities

WHEN TO SCREEN. Children at risk should be screened yearly after their first birthday. In very high-risk environments children from 1 to 3 years of age ideally should be screened two or three times a year (Frankenburg, 1974, p. 189). Children with lead levels near or slightly above normal, who continue to be exposed to lead hazards, need to be retested and examined frequently until lead hazards are removed or until they mature sufficiently to avoid such hazards.

POSITIVE RESULTS. Children with positive screening tests (blood lead levels over 40 to 50 μg/dl) should be evaluated by a physician skilled in the diagnosis and treatment of lead poisoning.

Environmental control. Local governmental agencies, community and professional groups must act together to identify hazards and to work for housing rehabilitation and environmental control. When a child at risk cannot be separated from the sources of lead (usually the home), the family can take measures to reduce the hazards by:

1. Frequent cleaning of floors, window sills, and bannisters
2. Damp mopping and dusting
3. Covering hazardous surfaces (repainted cribs, window sills) with wall board or heavy contact paper.

Resource Information

Books for Parents

Brown, D. L. *Developmental Handicaps in Babies and Young Children: A Guide for Parents.* Springfield, Ill.: Thomas, 1972.

Finnie, N. R. *Handling the Young Cerebral Palsied Child at Home,* 2nd ed. New York: Dutton, 1975.

Lagos. J. C. *Seizures, Epilepsy and Your Child.* New York: Harper & Row, 1974.

Stewart, M. A. and S. W. Olds. *Raising a Hyperactive Child.* New York: Harper & Row, 1973.

Strauss, S. *Is It Well With the Child? A Parents Guide to Raising a Mentally Handicapped Child.* Garden City, NY: Doubleday, 1975.

Organizations

Literature and information on available resources can be obtained from a variety of national organizations:

1. American Epilepsy Foundation, 77 Reservoir Road, Quincy, MA 02169.
2. Epilepsy Foundation of America, 1828 L Street N.W., Washington DC 20036.
3. Muscular Dystrophy Associations, Inc., 1790 Broadway, New York, NY 10019.
4. National Association for Retarded Children, 420 Lexington Avenue, New York, NY 10017.
5. National Epilepsy League, 203 N. Wabash Avenue, Chicago, IL.
6. National Multiple Sclerosis, Inc., 257 Park Avenue South, New York, NY 10010.
7. National Society for Crippled Children and Adults, Inc. (Easter Seals), 2023 W. Ogden, Chicago, IL 60612.
8. United Cerebral Palsy Association, 66 E. 34th Street, New York, NY 10016.
9. United Epilepsy Association, 113 W. 57th Street, New York, NY 10019.

References

Alexander, M. M. and M. S. Brown. "Physical Examination: Part 17, Performing the Neurologic Examination." *Nursing 76* 6:38–43, June 1976.

Arnon, S. S., et al. "Infant Botulism: Epidemiological, Clinical and Laboratory Aspects." *JAMA* 237:1946–1951, May 2, 1977.

Barnard, K. E. and H. B. Douglas. *Child Health Assessment Part 1: A Literature Review.* DHEW Pub. No. (HRA) 75–30. Bethesda, Md.: U.S. Dept. HEW, Public Health Service, HRA, Bureau of Health Resources Development, Division of Nursing, December 1974.

Barnard, K. E. and M. L. Erickson. *Teaching the Child with Developmental Problems: A Family Care Approach,* 2nd ed. St. Louis: Mosby, 1976.

Bates, B. *A Guide to Physical Examination.* Philadelphia: Lippincott, 1974.

Battle, C. U. "Chronic Physical Disease: Behavioral Aspects." *Pediatr Clin North Am* 22:525–531, August 1975.

Berman, P. H. "Management of Seizure Disorders with Anticonvulsant Drugs: Current Concepts." *Pediatr Clin North Am* 23:443–459, August 1976.

Chisholm, J. J. "Management of Increased Lead Absorption and Lead Poisoning in Children." *N Engl J Med* 289:1016–1018, November 8, 1973.

Conway, B. L. *Pediatric Neurological Nursing.* St. Louis: Mosby, 1977.

Diamond, S., et al. "Symposium Issue: Current Concepts of Headache." *Postgraduate Medicine* 56(3), September 1974.

Erickson, M. L. *Assessment and Management of Developmental Changes in Children.* St. Louis: Mosby, 1976.

Frankenburg, W. K., A. D. Goldstein, and B. W. Camp. "The Revised Denver Developmental Screening Test: Its Accuracy as a Screening Instrument." *J Pediatr* 79:988–995, December 1971.

Frankenburg, W. K. and A. F. North. *A Guide to Screening for the EPSDT Program under Medicaid.* Washington DC: Social and Rehabilitation Service, Dept. HEW, 1974.

Green, J. B. "Seizures." In M. Green and R. J. Haggerty, editors, *Ambulatory Pediatrics II.* Philadelphia: Saunders, 1977. Pp. 306–320.

Green, M. "Headaches." In M. Green and R. J. Haggerty, editors, *Ambulatory Pediatrics II.* Philadelphia: Saunders, 1977. Pp. 153–158.

Haggerty, R. J. "Accidental Poisoning." In M. Green and R. J. Haggerty, editors, *Ambulatory Pediatrics II.* Philadelphia: Saunders, 1977. Pp. 260–270.

Haynes, U. *A Developmental Approach to Casefinding.* Public Health Service Publication No. 2017. Washington DC: U.S. Dept HEW, Public Health Service, Maternal and Child Health Service, 1969.

Kempe, C. H., H. K. Silver, and D. O'Brien. *Current Pediatric Diagnosis and Treatment.* Los Altos Calif.: Lange Medical Publications, 1976.

Lombroso, C. T. and P. Lerman. "Breathholding Spells (Cyanotic and Pallid Infantile Syncope)." *Pediatrics* 39:563–581, April 1967.

Peterson, H. de C. "Diagnosis of Hypotonia in Children: Types, Differential, Diagnosis and Management." *Pediatric Annals* 5:30–38, May 1976.

Pickett, J., et al. "Syndrome of Botulism in Infancy: Clinical and Electrophysiologic Study." *N Engl J Med* 295:770–772, September 30, 1976.

Rudolph, A. M., editor. *Pediatrics,* 16th ed. New York: Appleton-Century-Crofts, 1977.

Smith, D. W., et al. "Congenital Hypothyroidism—Signs and Symptoms in the Newborn Period." *J Pediatr* 87:958–962, December 1975.

Taft, L. T. "Cerebral Palsy." In M. Green and R. J. Haggerty, editors, *Ambulatory Pediatrics II.* Philadelphia: Saunders, 1977. Pp. 294–305.

Vaughan, V. C. and R. J. McKay, editors. *Nelson Textbook of Pediatrics,* 10th ed. Philadelphia: Saunders, 1975.

Waechter, E. H. and F. G. Blake. *Nursing Care of Children,* 9th ed. Philadelphia: Lippincott, 1976.

Wolf, S. M., et al. "The Value of Phenobarbital in the Child Who Has Had a Single Febrile Seizure: A Controlled Prospective Study." *Pediatrics* 59:378–385, March 1977.

26

Language And Learning Disabilities

Approximately 10 to 30 percent of all school aged children experience learning difficulties in school. The causes are complex, multifactorial, and often intangible. Language and learning disabilities are discussed together here because of the interrelationship of language and learning processes.

The 1969 Children with Specific Learning Disabilities Act defines learning disabilities:

> Children with special learning disabilities exhibit a disorder in one or more of the basic psychological processes involved in understanding or in using spoken or written language. These may be manifested in disorders of listening, thinking, reading, writing, spelling, or arithmetic. They include conditions which have been referred to as perceptual handicaps, brain injury, minimal brain dysfunction, dyslexia, developmental aphasia, etc. They do not include learning problems which are due primarily to visual, hearing, or motor handicaps, to mental retardation, emotional disturbance, or to environmental disadvantage.

This chapter will highlight information for the nurse practitioner on the early identification, referral, and management of children with language and learning disabilities. For a comprehensive review of language and learning disabilities the reader is referred to the reference list at the end of this chapter.

ASSESSMENT

The comprehensive evaluation of a child with a language and learning disability involves specialists in language, education, psychology, and family dynamics. The nurse practitioner in collaboration with the pediatrician often functions as the primary coordinator of the evaluation and provides follow-up with the school and the family.

Initially the nurse practitioner gathers observational reports from the school, performs a thorough history and physical examination, and uses selected neurodevelopmental screening tools. If further evaluation is indicated, the nurse practitioner may choose to refer the child.

History

A complete history is done with careful attention to the areas listed below (see Chapter 1, Child Health Assessment).

PARENTAL CONCERN

Allow the parents to describe their concerns in their own words. Elicit a description and onset of the child's behavior which presents problems for them. Look for a pattern of difficulty and stress. Be alert to concerns of difficulty sleeping or feeding, poor health, delayed speech acquisition, poor coordination or concentration, short attention span, restlessness, and behavioral problems.

SCHOOL

Inquire about the child's successes and difficulties in school, most difficult subject, easiest subject, dislike for or reluctance to attend school, poor grades, complaints about performance or academic skills from the teacher, problems in peer relationship, and poor self-concept.

FAMILY HISTORY

Obtain history of familial reading, spelling, speech or behavior disorders, child-rearing practices within the family, parental ideas about discipline, conflicts in the management of the child, life-style, and psychologic disorders.

PREGNANCY AND BIRTH HISTORY

Obtain information about complications during pregnancy, prenatal ingestion of medication, labor or delivery (hypoxia, prematurity), nature of the labor, and condition of the baby at delivery.

INFANCY

Obtain information on temperament characteristics, attachment behaviors, colic, feeding problems, abnormal crying, excessive sleeping, and increased irritability.

DEVELOPMENTAL HISTORY

Obtain information about specific growth landmarks (sit, walk, tie shoes, ride a tricycle, ride a bicycle), language development (onset, quality and quantity of babbling and consonant sounds, use of isolated words, phrases, sentences, ability to use meaningful words in speech, ability to let parents know what is wanted, ability to follow directions, different native tongue or dialect), toilet training, temper tantrums, approach to new tasks, and motor coordination (small and large muscle). Look for signs of maturational delay.

PAST MEDICAL HISTORY

Inquire about history of frequent colds, chronic ear infections, hoarseness, serious illness or hospitalizations, seizures, medications used, lead poisoning, chronic illness, physical handicaps, enuresis, encopresis, and accidents.

Physical Examination

A complete physical examination is performed (refer to Chapter 1, Child Health Assessment). Vision (see Chapter 16) and hearing are tested. Significant physical findings for language difficulties are: cleft palate, submucous cleft (a large notch in the upper hard palate), a bifid uvula, tongue thrust, malocclusion, or tongue paralysis. Significant physical findings for learning difficulties are discussed below.

Supplementary Neurologic Evaluation

Refer to Chapter 25, The Neuromuscular System, for the neurologic examination. A supplementary neurologic evaluation is done to measure higher cortical function and elicit "soft" neurologic signs. The term "soft" neurologic signs has been used to describe perceptual or cognitive behaviors that are present beyond the usual chronologic age in development, such as the persistence of left-right confusion beyond 9 years of age. It has also been used in the description of nonspecific entities such as clumsiness (Conway, 1977). "Soft" neurologic signs reflect developmental and maturational differences in the central nervous system and may indicate abnormalities in the maturational development of the central nervous system of the child. While they do not necessarily indicate a pathologic condition or injury, the presence of these signs may indicate maturational delay. The evaluations of fine-motor coordination, special sensory skills, and laterality and orientation in space are excerpts from the amplified neurologic examination used at the Child Study Unit, University of California, San Francisco.*

---

*Adapted from H. F. Gofman and B. W. Allmond: Learning and Language Disorders in Children. Part II: The School-Aged Child, in Gluck, L. (ed.): *Current Problems in Pediatrics*, September 1971. Copyright © 1971 by Year Book Medical Publishers, Inc., Chicago. Used by permission.

EVALUATION OF FINE-MOTOR COORDINATION

Observe the child during:

A. Undressing, unbuttoning.

B. Tying shoes.

C. Rapid alternating touch of fingertips by thumb.

D. Rattle of an imaginary doorknob.

E. Unscrewing of an imaginary light bulb.

F. Pencil grasp and use; penmanship.

G. Rapid tongue movements.

H. Hand grip.

I. Inversion of both feet. (Look for similar movements of the hands. See below.)

J. Repeating several times rapidly: kitty, kitty, kitty; pa, ta, ka. (Accurate reproduction of these sounds generally indicates adequate articulatory coordination.)

Note:

a. The child's general facility and coordination with these small muscle tasks.

b. On items C, D, E, H, and I, any marked movement of other parts of the body that mirror or duplicate movements of the test side. Such movements are called associated motor movements, mirror movements, adventitious overflow movements, or synkinesia. When marked they are felt to represent, particularly after 8 to 10 years, a lack of normal cortical inhibition.

c. Excessive pressure on the pencil point or a pencil held too lightly. Fingers placed directly over the point, or fingers placed too far (greater than 1 inch) from the point may all indicate difficulty with the coordination of fine musculature within the hands.

d. Presence of dysdiadochokinesia, noting speed, accuracy, and sequencing of maneuvers.

EVALUATION OF SPECIAL SENSORY SKILLS

A. Dual Simultaneous Sensory Tests (face-hand testing). With the child's eyes closed (but first demonstrating items 1 and 2 below with child's eyes open), simultaneously:

   1. Touch both cheeks.
   2. Touch both hands.
   3. Touch right cheek and contralateral hand.
   4. Touch right cheek and homolateral hand.
   5. Touch left cheek and contralateral hand.
   6. Touch left cheek and homolateral hand.

Note:

a. Rostral dominance: failure to perceive hand stimulus when the face is simultaneously touched. Approximately 80 percent of normal children are able to perform this test without rostral dominance by age 8 years.

B. Finger localization test (finger agnosia test). Touch two fingers or two spots on one finger simultaneously with the child's eyes closed, after demonstrating first with eyes open. Ask the child: "How many fingers am I touching—one or two?"

Note:

a. The number of correct responses in four trials for each hand: six correct answers out of eight are accepted as a "pass." Half of all children pass this test by age 6 years, 90 percent by age 7½ years. This test reflects a child's orientation in space, concept of body image, praxic ability, and sensation to touch and position sense.

EVALUATION OF CHILD'S LATERALITY AND ORIENTATION IN SPACE

A. Imitation of Gestures. Have the child imitate the following gestures performed by the examiner, emphasizing first that the child must use the same hand as the examiner:

   1. Extend index finger.

2. Extend little and index finger.

3. Extend index and middle finger.

4. Touch two thumbs and two index fingers together simultaneously.

5. Form two interlocking rings, thumb and index finger of one hand with thumb and index finger of other hand.

6. Point index finger of one hand down toward the cupped fingers of the opposite hand held below.

Note:

a. Difficulty with fine finger movements, manipulation, and/or reproduction of correct gesture.

b. After approximately age 8 years, marked right-left confusion with regard to examiner's right and left. This test reflects a child's ability with finger discrimination, postural praxis, awareness of self-image, and right-left, front-back, up-down orientation.

B. Following directions. Ask the child to:

1. Show me your left hand.

2. Show me your right ear.

3. Show me your right eye.

4. Show me your left elbow.

5. Touch your left knee with your left hand.

6. Touch your right ear with your left hand.

7. Touch your left elbow with your right hand.

8. Touch your right cheek with your right hand.

9. Point to my left ear.

10. Point to my right eye.

11. Point to my right hand.

12. Point to my left knee.

Note:

a. Items 1 through 8 are mastered by approximately age 6 years; items 9 through 12 are mastered by approximately age 8 years.

b. Aside from correct versus incorrect responses, any difficulty with following the sequence of directions.

EVALUATION OF PERCEPTUAL-MOTOR FUNCTION

Visual-motor. Ask the child to copy a circle, square, triangle, and diamond. Observe the child's ability to draw the shapes in a smooth motion, turn corners, especially at right angles, change directions, and accurately reproduce the figure. Also observe eye-hand coordination, spatial and directional organization, and visual-motor coordination. See Chapter 25, Behavior and Mental Status for the average skill response by age.

Auditory-motor. Ask the child to reproduce in writing the verbal phrases and sentences heard; for example: "My name is _____." "Write the numbers from 1 to 10." "Write the letters of the alphabet." "A cat saw a bird." Observe the child's ability to complete the task, to produce and to organize the symbols, and to space the letters. Note any letter or word reversals. A child of 6 years is able to print the first and last names, write the numbers from 1 to 10, and the letters of the alphabet. By 7 years of age the figures are in a horizontal line and become more evenly spaced. By 8 years of age reversals are infrequent.

Gross motor. Ask the child to lie down in a supine position, stand, walk about 30 steps forward and backward, walk about 25 steps on alternating heels, stand on one foot and hop, skip, and gallop. Observe posture, head tilting, position of hands, legs, toes, straightness of spinal column, exaggerated or asymmetric arm swinging, clumsiness, or problems in balance. By 6 years the child is able to walk on alternating heels. By 8 years the child is able to stand on one foot, hop, skip, and gallop.

ELECTROENCEPHALOGRAM (EEG)

An EEG is sometimes indicated to provide for a more complete evaluation of the nervous system, to confirm the "organic" nature of the learning disorder, to rule out a hidden seizure disorder, to provide a baseline for future evaluation, and to better ensure the safety of a trial of medication which may precipitate a seizure (Whitsell, 1969).

Screening Tests for School Readiness

Screening tests to assess school readiness and to detect potential learning disabilities can be administered in the early school years. Three examples of screening tests are the Meeting Street School Screening Test (MSSST), the Preschool Readiness Experimental Screening Scale (PRESS), and the School Readiness Survey.

MSSST

The MSSST is designed for the early identification of children (5 to 6 years old) with learning disabilities in the areas of language and visual-perceptual-motor control. It requires 20 minutes to complete.

For further information write: The Meeting Street School, 333 Grotto Avenue, Providence, RI 02906.

PRESS

The PRESS is a simplified screening scale to assess maturational level. It does not estimate intellectual capacities. Most children 5 years of age should be able to complete the test without difficulty. It consists of a series of questions to test areas such as knowledge of colors and numbers and ability to draw. Coordination, comprehension, performance during testing, and personal-social maturity are noted. A 10-point scoring system includes three divisions to indicate school readiness, borderline school readiness, or inadequate school readiness. It can be completed in 2 to 3 minutes while performing the physical examination. For specific test information, the reader is referred to the article written by W. B. Rogers Jr. and R. A. Rogers listed in the references.

SCHOOL READINESS SURVEY

It is designed for children between 4 to 6 years of age. It can be administered and scored by parents with school supervision. For test materials write: Consulting Psychologists Press, Inc., 577 College Avenue, Palo Alto, CA 94306.

Speech and Language Assessment

Speech and language involve a complex series of interrelated developmental tasks: listening, speaking, reading, and writing.

HEARING ASSESSMENT

The ability to hear is critical for the development of speech, language, and learning. Early diagnosis of a hearing impairment is essential since even minimal loss may significantly affect the development of language. The response to frequencies of sound in the human ear ranges from 20 to 20,000 Hertz (cycles per second) with the speech range from 400 to 3000 Hertz (Vaughan, 1975).

Conductive hearing loss. Conductive hearing defects are most often secondary to problems in the external or middle ear that impair the normal conduction of sound to the inner ear. The primary effect of the conduction loss is a reduction in the sound without distortion of clarity. The Weber test lateralizes to the poor hearing ear and the Rinne test is negative. An audiogram confirms the hearing loss. These are the most common hearing impairments in children. The impairment is often mild and responds to medical or surgical intervention.

Sensorineural hearing loss. In children, it is generally inherited and can be produced by diseases of the inner ear or of the eighth cranial nerve. The principal result is that the sounds are distorted, making discrimination difficult. Only certain frequencies may be involved, and the child may respond to most sounds at ordinary levels of loudness. The high frequencies tend to be more affected than the low tones unless there is severe involvement which then causes both high and low tones to be impaired. The Weber test lateralizes to the good ear and the Rinne test is positive. An audiogram is performed to verify the clinical assessment. The impairment is rarely responsive to treatment, and generally it is a greater handicap to communication than conductive defects.

High-risk indicators for hearing loss

1. Parental concern about hearing problems such as paying little attention to parental requests
2. Family history of congenital hearing impairment or hearing loss before 50 years of age without obvious cause
3. History of infectious episodes in the early months of pregnancy such as rubella or syphilis
4. History of birth with any orofacial deformity, including ear anomalies, birth trauma, birth anoxia, kernicterus (bilirubin above 20 mg/dl), care in the newborn intensive care unit, birth weight under 1500 grams, or multiple congenital anomalies
5. History of fluid accumulation in the middle ear, treatment with ototoxic drugs such as kanamycin, streptomycin, or neomycin in infancy, or chronic nasal obstruction
6. Environmental history of continuous loud noise

Development of hearing responses. The following are normal developmental hearing responses to sound (Downs, 1972; Lillywhite, 1970):

Age	*Hearing Response*
Birth to 4 months	Startle reflex, blinking of eyes; orienting or localizing response by eye movements toward direction of sound occurs in prone position around 12 weeks and in the upright position between 12 and 18 weeks.
4 months	Widening of the eyes; slight turning of the head in the direction of the sound; quieting, listening posture
6 months	Turning of the head toward the sound but may not yet recognize that the sound source is below or above
8 months to 12 months	Turns head 45° or more in direction of sound; usually determines whether sound source is above or below; automatic and rapid localization of sound achieved by end of the first year

Age	*Hearing Response*
12 to 36 months	Rapid development of speech and language patterns based on hearing input; imitation of sounds and syllables progressing to ability to shape sounds closer and closer to adult patterns; increasing refinement of listening skills so by age 3 basic auditory attentional skills mastered and selective listening skills developed

Hearing screening. Suggested guidelines for hearing screening:

1. In a well child without any of the high-risk indicators, administer at least once during the first year, and then yearly.
2. In a child with some high-risk indicators, refer the child for a hearing evaluation and follow regularly.
3. In a child who has an ear infection or who has been treated with a known ototoxic drug, administer as part of the follow-up plan.

A child with a high-frequency loss may be regarded as hearing normally. Such a child may respond to lower frequency sounds including soft environmental noise, soft speech in the lower frequencies, and may partially compensate for the high frequency loss by reading lips or using context clues. Hearing losses can also vary in accordance with an associated upper respiratory infection or exacerbation of allergic symptoms. Be wary that normal audiograms recorded when the child is free of symptoms do not guarantee normal hearing at other times.

For best results:

1. Test infants between feedings
2. Test older infants and toddlers with sound stimuli that are interesting and familiar such as jingle bells, spoons, or tissue paper
3. Use more than one stimuli in a particular range if the child does not respond to the first noisemaker. The lack of response may be due to disinterest with the particular sound.
4. Check the squeeze toy for air flow to prevent a positive response from the air flow rather than the sounds

NEWBORN TO 3 MONTHS. Screening results during this age period are limited and may be inaccurate. Reflexive auditory responses do not eliminate the presence of mild, moderate, and even moderately severe bilateral hearing loss. Central auditory impairments which may later retard language growth and speech development may also be present with reflexive auditory responses (Lillywhite, 1970). Infants who are at high risk for auditory disorders should be referred to an audiologist for a more precise evaluation.

3 MONTHS TO 12 MONTHS. Observations are made of the child's ability to localize the source of the sound. A response indicates only that a child is not deaf; it does not indicate how well the child hears.

Technique. The hearing response is tested in a quiet room with the child seated on the parent's lap, supported under the arms, and held so the infant has freedom for head movement. Two examiners are required. The first examiner visually distracts the child with a silent bright-colored toy, while the other examiner delivers the sounds with the noisemaker as softly as possible on one side 18 to 24 inches out of the child's field of vision. The first examiner observes for a response. If the child does not react, increase the loudness of the noisemaker. The test is repeated on the other side. The first responses are the most consistent.

Test stimuli. Environmental sound stimuli are the most satisfactory. Examples are the crinkle of cellophane or tissue paper, the soft scrape of a spoon in a cup, squeeze toys, and small bells.

1 TO 3 YEARS. The child's activity level and alertness are increased so special care must be taken to keep the noisemakers out of the field of vision.

Technique. Two examiners may be needed. With the child in the parent's lap the child is either visually distracted or allowed to play with the toys. The second stimulus is delivered to the right and left ears. Noisemakers of known frequency and intensity are used. Test materials can be measured at most speech and hearing departments and electronic laboratories.

Test stimuli. In addition to noisemakers listed previously, speech signals may be used as test items; examples are softly voicing syllables such as "puh," "baa," "bu," "ga," or sounds such as "s" and "sh."

Indications for referral. A child should be referred for further evaluation if the following occur:

1. Failure to respond
2. Inconsistent responses
3. Any doubt on the part of the examiner

Referral of a deaf child before the age of 9 months or 1 year is critical to provide every opportunity for the child to develop normal speech (Fry, 1966).

3 YEARS AND OLDER. The principal screening procedure is pure-tone audiometry. The normal hearing response is a positive response at 20 decibels or less in frequencies between 400 and 3000 Hertz. Numerous sources are available which describe the screening audiometry technique. Several resources (Lillywhite, 1970; Caulfield, 1976) are listed at the end of this chapter. Children with hearing losses of 20 db or more in one or more frequencies should be referred for further evaluation by an audiologist.

DEVELOPMENT OF LANGUAGE (LENNEBERG, 1966, P. 222; MARGE, 1972)

Age	Language Development
Birth to 6 months	Emergence of cooing, babbling, chuckling
6 to 12 months	Babbling, production of sounds such as "ma" or "da"; repetition of sounds common; vocal play
12 to 18 months	Appearance of first words; ability to follow simple commands; responsive to "no"
18 to 21 months	Vocabulary of about 20 words at 18 months to about 200 words at 21 months; understands simple questions; forms two-word phrases

Age	Language Development
24 to 27 months	300 to 400 word vocabulary; forms two- to three-word phrases; uses prepositions and pronouns
30 to 33 months	Fastest increase in vocabulary; forms three- to four-word sentences; use of grammar sounds like language heard in environment, but many utterances are unlike adult grammar
36 to 39 months	Vocabulary of 1000 words or more; well-formed sentence structure using complex grammatical rules, even though certain rules have not yet been fully mastered; grammatical mistakes are less common; about 90 percent comprehensibility
40 to 60 months	Correct usage of sounds and language of adults in environment

ARTICULATION

Oral communication requires precise articulation of the written language. By 24 months of age all the vowels are present, while the consonants continue to develop in an orderly sequence until the child is 8 years and older. Table 1 lists the sequence of consonant development in speech.

SCREENING TESTS FOR SPEECH AND LANGUAGE DEVELOPMENT

Caution should be exercised when using screening tests, and the results should be judiciously interpreted and generalized. Selected screening tests are presented here.

Denver Articulation Screening Examination (DASE)—2½ to 6 years. This is a screening tool for use by personnel other than

Table 1
The Development of Consonants in Children's Speech[a]

Consonant	Age 2	Age 3	Age 4	Age 5	Age 6	Age 7
/p/	I	F				
/b/	I	F				
/d/	I			F		
/h/	I					
/w/	I					
/m/	I&F					
/n/	I	F				
/t/		I&F				
/k/		I		F		
/g/		I		F		
/f/		I	F			
/l/			I		F	
/y/			I			
/j/			I		F	
/ng/			F			
/v/				I	F	
/th/(voiceless)				I	F	
/s/				I		F

Source: From H. F. Gofman and B. W. Allmond: Learning and Language Disorders in Children. Part I: The Preschool Child, in L. Gluck (ed.): *Current Problems in Pediatrics*,
August 1971. Copyright © 1971 by Year Book Medical Publishers, Inc., Chicago. Used
by permission.

[a]This table indicates the age by which approximately 90 percent of children produce each
consonant in words with reasonable consistency. *I* indicates that the consonant is produced in
the initial position in syllables; *F* indicates that the consonant is produced in the final position in
syllables.

therapists. It is basically a word imitation test of 22 items complete
with pictures. In this test the examiner says the word and asks the
child to repeat it. Test materials are available from: LADOCA
Project and Publishing, Inc., 51st Avenue and Lincoln Street,
Denver, CO 80216.

**Denver Developmental Screening Test (DDST)—1 month to 6
years.** This is a test for overall development and includes limited
screening sections for receptive and expressive language development. Refer to Chapter 25, The Neuromuscular System, for more
information on the DDST. Test materials available from LADOCA
Project.

Developmental Profile—birth to 12½ years. This is a reliable over-all screening of child development, utilizing a structured interview method. The communication scale is designed to assess the expressive and receptive language skills of the child. Test materials are available from: Psychological Development Publications, 7150 Lakeside Drive, Indianapolis, IN 46278.

Peabody Picture Vocabulary Test. This is a test of the child's single word receptive vocabulary. The child is required to point to one of four drawings in response to the examiner's stimulus word. Test materials available from: American Guidance Service, Inc., Publisher's Building, Circle Pines, MN 55014.

Photo Articulation Test. This is a test of the child's ability to articulate consonants. The examiner points to a picture and the child is asked to name it. The examiner listens for the child's articulation of the consonant which is presented in three different positions. Test materials available from: King Co. Publishers, 2414 W. Lawrence Avenue, Chicago, IL 60625.

Sequenced Inventory of Language Development (SILD)—Birth through 3 years. This diagnostic tool allows the examiner to assess systematically the child's language skills and to estimate the child's level of receptive and expressive language functioning (Barnard, 1974). Test information is in the publication: D. L. Hedrick and E. M. Prather, *Sequenced Inventory of Language Development* (Seattle: University of Washington Press, 1970).

Verbal Language Development Scale—1 month to 15 years. This test assesses the development of the child's speech and language using the informant interview method. It is an extension of the communication section of the Vineland Social Maturity Scale by Edgar A. Doll. Test materials available from: American Guidance Service, Inc., Publishers Building, Circle Pines, MN 55014.

INDICATIONS FOR REFERRAL

Parental concern is the primary indication for referral. In addition, Lillywhite recommends referral to a speech pathologist or audiologist for detailed evaluation for the following conditions*:

---

*From V. C. Vaughan and R. J. McKay, *Nelson Textbook of Pediatrics*, 10th ed., © 1975 by W. B. Saunders Company, Philadelphia.

1. If the child is not producing any intelligible speech by age 2
2. If speech is largely unintelligible after age 3
3. If there are many omissions of initial consonants after age 3
4. If there are no sentences by age 3
5. If sounds are more than a year late in appearing, according to expected developmental sequence
6. If there is an excessive amount of indiscriminate, irrelevant verbalizing after 18 months
7. If there is consistent and frequent omission of initial consonants at any age
8. If there are many substitutions of easy sounds for difficult ones after age 5
9. If the amount of vocalizing decreases rather than steadily increases at any period up to age 7
10. If the child uses mostly vowel sounds in his speech at any age after 1 year
11. If word endings are consistently dropped after age 5
12. If sentence structure is consistently faulty after age 5
13. If the child is embarrassed and disturbed by his speech at any age
14. If the child is noticeably nonfluent (stuttering) after age 5
15. If the child is distorting, omitting, or substituting any sounds after age 7
16. If the voice is a monotone, extremely loud, largely inaudible, or of poor quality
17. If the pitch is not appropriate to the child's age and sex
18. If there is noticeable hypernasality or lack of nasal resonance
19. If there are unusual confusions, reversals, or telescoping in connected speech
20. If there are abnormal rhythms, rate, and inflection after age 5

The referral information should include impression of the child's mental status, developmental progress, emotional maturity, past illnesses, physical problems, and family and environmental factors (Lillywhite, 1970).

Resources. Help can be found at speech and hearing clinics affiliated with a university or college, community centers, medical centers, child guidance centers, child development programs, special education departments of public schools, or certified speech and hearing specialists in private practice. A Certificate of Clinical Competence from the American Speech and Hearing Association held by a speech and hearing specialist attests to adequate training and experience. The annual directory of the American Speech and Hearing Association lists the certified status of the members. Copies of the directory can be obtained from: American Speech and Hearing Association, 9030 Old Georgetown Road, Washington DC 20014.

ILLINOIS TEST OF PSYCHOLINGUISTIC ABILITIES (ITPA)—2 YEARS 4 MONTHS TO 10 YEARS 3 MONTHS. This is a common test used by speech and language specialists. It is a diagnostic test of specific cognitive abilities used to identify areas of difficulty in communication and to provide the basis for developing a remedial program. It tests the receptive, expressive, and organizing processes in the acquisition and use of language. Results are categorized according to the learning problem the child demonstrates, such as academic (reading, writing, arithmetic), nonsymbolic (perceptual-expressive), or symbolic (linguistic difficulty in the reception or idea expression) (Conway; 1977).

Academic Evaluation

BEHAVIOR

A description of the child's behavioral response to a new situation and to a comfortable situation provides insights into the child's ability to master the academic tasks of learning to read, to write, and to spell. Observations are made of the child's attention span and concentration while engrossed in a task, and in free play. Gofman and Allmond (1970, p. 40) state that

> Before a child is required to begin the task of learning to read, write and spell he should at least:
> be intelligible to his teacher and classmates when he talks;
> be able to follow oral directions made up of at least 3 different commands;

be able to listen to a story and tell about the events in logical sequence;
be able to copy simple geometric shapes such as a circle, square, cross;
be able to sit still and attend for at least 15 minutes; and
be able to accept limits and tolerate some frustrations and delayed
gratification.

CENTRAL NERVOUS SYSTEM

Optimum learning and language development requires intact visual-motor, auditory-vocal, tactile-kinesthetic processes, and a knowledge of two-dimensional spatial relationships. For example, intact visual-motor processes enable a child to transfer the word "pad" from the chalkboard onto paper by using the following skills (Gofman, 1971):

1. The ability to see the word on the chalkboard
2. The ability to visually discriminate the word form from the figure-background
3. The ability to develop a visual memory for forms, letters, the correct sequence of letters and eventually of entire words so a "p" always looks like a "p" to the child
4. The ability to develop a feel for the spatial orientation of forms and letters so the child knows the configuration of "p" as well as the sequence of "p-a-d" in the traditional left-right order.

EDUCATIONAL TESTING

Teachers are central figures in the entire evaluation-remediation process. The goal of the teacher's evaluation is to provide an educationally usable assessment of the child's areas of strengths and weaknesses. Standard tests used are:

- Durrell Analysis of Reading Difficulty. Materials available from: Harcourt Brace Jovanovich, Test Department, 757 Third Avenue, New York, NY 10017.
- Grays Oral Reading Test. Materials available from: Bobbs-Merrill Co. Inc., Indianapolis, IN.
- Monroe Reading Achievement Test. Materials available from: Houghton Mifflin Co., 777 California Avenue, Palo Alto, CA.

Graded reading paragraphs and spelling lists adapted from the California State Series Spelling List are included below. Observations are made of the child's ability to recognize words, comprehend words and paragraphs, decipher the sound or spelling of unknown words, discriminate sounds and letters, and write the letters of the alphabet.

I. Graded Reading Paragraphs*

MY	DOG	SEE	BOY

1.** A little girl had a pet cat. The cat liked to sit in the sun. It played with a red ball. One day the cat ran away. The little girl saw it and said, "I see you."

2. My friend lives in a new house. She goes to a new school. I am going to sleep at her house tomorrow. She has a big doll to play with. We will have fun.

3. My daddy bought a new car. We will drive it to the country to visit my cousins next week. They asked us to come on Saturday. I hope they like our new red car. We think it is beautiful.

4. Six boys went on a vacation together. They went fishing in a blue boat. One boy caught a big fish. The others did not catch a thing. They decided to go home.

5. A man built a house in the woods. It was almost winter before it was finally finished. He couldn't make up his mind about the furnace. Should he use gas or electricity? Which would you choose?

6. Ann and Bert decided to plant a garden. Their father declared it an excellent project. He advised them to start with a strip of ground by the fence. They worked hard and by the end of summer they had fresh beans, onions, peas, and cabbage for the table.

7. The Indians and the first white settlers knew how to conserve

---

*From H. F. Gofman and B. W. Allmond: Learning and Language Disorders in Children. Part II: The School-Age Child, in L. Gluck, ed.: *Current Problems in Pediatrics*, September 1971. Copyright © 1971 by Year Book Medical Publishers, Inc., Chicago. Used by permission. Adapted from California State Series Spelling List.

**The number of the paragraph and of the spelling list indicates the grade appropriate for mastery of these reading paragraphs and spelling words.

our natural resources. They took from nature only what was necessary for their food, clothing, and shelter. Recently we have come to realize that these resources are becoming scarce. Conservation is a national responsibility.

8. Have you chosen your vocation yet? Long ago man had little choice. His job was to provide food, clothing, and shelter for his family. Today there are many special skills required to keep our present economy going. A person is happier and more prosperous if he has chosen his vocation carefully. There are many people ready to help you if you ask their advice.

II. Graded Spelling List*

1	2	3
all	mother	teacher
bird	little	come
let	run	get
home	house	Saturday
she	bring	daddy
tell	dress	until
pin	cows	brother
was	letter	told
out	ran	ask
girl	school	every

4	5	6
many	young	lace
does	building	cart
head	hair	driving
bring	interesting	habit
where	report	ruler
water	class	knee
horse	read	lemon
wanted	receive	bandage
please	Monday	tramp
think	knew	motor

---

*From H. F. Gofman and B. W. Allmond: Learning and Language Disorders in Children. Part II: The School-Age Child, in L. Gluck, ed.: *Current Problems in Pediatrics*, September 1971. Copyright © 1971 by Year Book Medical Publishers, Inc., Chicago. Used by Permission. Selected from California State Series Spelling List.

7	8
chew	sold
pity	curious
flames	lovely
cough	shoot
spite	studying
view	believe
suddenly	between
tale	whom
crime	probably
organization	eight

Psychological Evaluation

An evaluation with a sensitive, astute psychologist provides insights into the child's learning style and coping behavior.

TESTS

A standard intelligence test is administered to evaluate the child's language skills, manipulative abilities, eye-hand coordination, memory, and visual and auditory attention. Examples of tests commonly used in standard evaluations are:

- Bayley Scales of Infant Development (2 to 30 months of age)
- Cattel Infant Intelligence Scale (up to 2½ years of age)
- Stanford-Binet Intelligence Scale (2 to 16 years of age)
- Wechsler Intelligence Scale for Children—Revised (WISC-R) (6 to 16 years of age)

Additional tests are done by the psychologist to verify the suspected areas of difficulty. For example, paper and pencil skills are evaluated by tests such as:

- Bender Visual Motor Gestalt Test. Tests the child's ability to combine more than one geometric figure in a contiguous order
- Boehm Test of Basic Concepts (BTBC). Tests the child's mastery of concepts considered necessary for achievement in the early school years

- Developmental Test of Visual Motor Integration (BEERY). Given to children who are unable to do the Bender test
- Frostig Developmental Test of Visual Perception. Tests the visual perceptual functions in children from 4 to 8 years

Evaluation of Family Interaction

A sensitive interview with the entire family should explore the dynamics of their interactions and the effects of the child's difficulties on the family. This provides a context with which to understand the child and family. Psychiatric consultation may be indicated in cases where questions exist about the emotional stability of the child and family interactions.

RESOURCES

Resources for family therapists or psychiatric referrals include family therapy centers affiliated with a university or college, community centers, medical centers, or family therapists in private practice.

Commonly Used Terms

AGNOSIA. The inability to interpret sensory input.

APHASIA. Impairment of the ability to use or understand oral language; usually associated with an injury or abnormality of the speech centers.

ASTEREOGNOSIS. A form of agnosia in which there is an inability to recognize objects or their forms by touch.

AUDITORY RECEPTION. Auditory decoding of words spoken by another person.

AUDITORY SEQUENCING. The ability to recall details in correct order, such as correctly repeating digits.

AUDITORY DISCRIMINATION. The ability to detect similarities and differences in sound stimuli.

DYSARTHRIA. The inability to intelligibly articulate speech sounds; usually due to central nervous system impairment in speech/motor musculature.

DYSDIADOCHOKINESIS. The inability to perform repetitive fine motor movements such as finger tapping.

DYSGRAPHIA. The inability to perform handwriting skills in an organized and legible manner.

DYSKINESIA. Impairment of the power of voluntary movements which manifests itself in fragmented, poorly coordinated and sequenced movements.

DYSLEXIA. The inability to read or to understand printed symbols, visually or orally; used when neurological dysfunction is suspected.

DYSLALIA. Functional impairment of speech due to defective speech organs.

ECHOLALIA. An involuntary, parrotlike dysfunction manifested in repetition of words or phrases spoken by another, without understanding the meaning of the language.

FIGURE-GROUND DISCRIMINATION. The ability to select a specific configuration from the total input of incoming stimuli by sorting out the important features, figures, and characteristics.

INTELLIGENCE QUOTIENT (IQ). The score obtained using the MA/CA formula: 100 X (Mental-Age/Chronological-Age).

LATERALITY. Internal awareness of the two sides of the body and their distinctness; frequently refers to the establishment of one dominant side, such as lefthandedness.

MINIMAL BRAIN DYSFUNCTION. Descriptive term for a child of average intelligence who has learning disabilities resulting from a possible minimal insult to the central nervous system; differentiated from major brain dysfunctions such as epilepsy or cerebral palsy.

PERSEVERATION. The continued repetition of words or motions that is no longer appropriate.

READING DISABILITY. The inability to read at a level that corresponds to the child's measured intellectual capacity and estimated reading level by about a year or more.

RECEPTIVE LANGUAGE. Ability to understand spoken, written, or sign language through listening, reading, and observing.

WORD-ATTACK SKILLS. A child's approach to unfamiliar words by a phonetic approach or contextual clues to arrive at the correct pronunciation.

MANAGEMENT

Depending on the available resources, time, and level of skill and knowledge, the nurse practitioner may be the primary coordinator of the evaluation and management. The primary goals in developing the management plan are to increase the child's self esteem and to continue the successful education of the child. The educational psychologist and the teacher in special education are responsible for developing a specific program of management and treatment for the learning problem.

The nurse practitioner may be the best person to explain the problem to the parents and to assist them in providing an atmosphere which is conducive and supportive of the child's best development.

Communication With the Family

The family with a learning disabled child requires a tremendous amount of continuing support and guidance. The parents need help with anxieties, misunderstandings, and fears about the child's school difficulties. They also need encouragement to verbally express their anger, frustration, and disappointment. Results of the evaluation may initially be difficult to grasp. Clarification of the parent's interpretation of the findings is essential. They may need further guidance in accepting and planning for the child.

Communication With School Personnel

Communication with school personnel is vital and must be done directly and tactfully. Sharing findings about the child's level of functioning and special needs in educational usable terms enables the school personnel to make the appropriate decision about special programs. Visits to the school may be valuable.

Medication

For the learning disabled child with symptoms of hyperactivity, treatment with a stimulant drug such as dextroamphetamine sulfate or methylphenidate may be useful. Medication, however, has not been found helpful in children who do not exhibit hyperactive behavior. For more information, refer to Hyperactivity, this chapter.

COMMON CLINICAL PROBLEM

Hyperactivity

ASSESSMENT

Hyperactivity is best described by a pattern of behavior in which the child demonstrates increased motor activity, short attention span, poor concentration, and impulsivity. The child is emotionally labile, easily distracted by visual and/or auditory environmental stimuli regardless of the environment, prone to mood swings, and temper outbursts. Symptoms of hyperactivity are sometimes accompanied by learning difficulties and "soft" neurologic signs. It is seen more frequently in males than females. The documentation of the symptoms requires careful history taking of development and observation of the child in a variety of situations. Information from both teachers and parents is essential.

MANAGEMENT

Medication. The use of stimulant drugs in the treatment of hyperactivity is controversial; however, most experts agree that a child with persistent hyperactivity and a short attention span is likely to benefit from treatment with stimulants (Council of Child Health of the American Academy of Pediatrics, 1975). Dextroamphetamine sulfate (Dexedrine) and methylphenidate (Ritalin) are the two most commonly used medications in the control of hyperkinesis. Both drugs can reduce inattention and hyperactivity, and therefore increase the ability to attend in the home and the school setting. Close monitoring and evaluation of effectiveness of the drugs are essential.

METHYLPHENIDATE (RITALIN).   It is most commonly used. The daily dose should not exceed 60 mg. If a definitive response does not occur after 1 month, the drug is discontinued. Side effects include insomnia, anorexia, increased blood pressure; initial period of irritability, tearfulness, and increased sensitivity to outbursts of aggressiveness, periods of extreme fearfulness, and an increased incidence of seizures. Recent studies have indicated that long-term treatment on high doses of methylphenidate causes a slowing of weight and height gain in children (Safer, 1973). Compensatory rebound has been observed when the medication was discontinued for several months (Safer, 1975).

DEXTROAMPHETAMINE SULFATE (DEXEDRINE).   It is available in a long-acting preparation that enables a child to take the drug once a day. Side effects include a high incidence of insomnia and anorexia.

Dietary management.   A popular but controversial method of treating hyperactivity is the use of a salicylate-free diet (Feingold, 1975; Silver, 1975). Artificial food color, flavors, and the salicylates that normally occur in certain foods are eliminated. For more information the reader is referred to Chapter 28, Allergies.

Long-term management.   There are no simple solutions to this problem. A total management plan should include an eclectic approach: medication if it works, parental counseling regarding behavior modification techniques, communication and intervention with school personnel, and support for the child.

Resource Information

Information for parents is available from these organizations:

1. Association for Children with Learning Disabilities, 5225 Grace Street, Pittsburgh, PA 15236.
   Write for: Becker, W. *Parents are Teachers.* Urbana, Illinois: Research Press, 1971. ($3.75)

2. *Closer Look.* (national information center for the handicapped. A project of the U.S. Department of Health, Education and Welfare Office of Education, Bureau of Education for the Handicapped). Box 1492. Washington DC 20013.

3. *The Orton Society, Inc.* (organization dedicated to informing public and professionals about speech and language disabilities), 8415 Bellena Lane, Towson, MD 21204.

4. Quebec Association for Children with Learning Disabilities, P.O. Box 22, Montreal 29, P.Q.
   Write for: Golick, M. *A Parent's Guide to Learning Problems.* ($0.50)

5. Science Research Associates, Inc., 259 East Erie Street, Chicago, IL 60611.
   Write for: Van Riper, C. *Helping Children Talk Better.* Chicago: Science Research Associates, 1951.

References

Abramowicz, M. *The Medical Letter* 19:53–54, July 1, 1977.

Barnard, K. and H. Douglas, editors. *Child Health Assessment Part 1: A Literature Review.* Bethesda, MD.: U.S. Department of Health, Education, and Welfare, 1974.

Brown, M. S. "Testing of a Young Child for Articulation Skills—Detecting Early Danger Signs." *Clin Pediatr* 15:639–644, July 1976.

Caulfield, C. "Hearing Screening in Children: A Self-Study Guide for Nurse Practitioners." *Nurse Practitioner* 1:22–27, March–April 1976.

Conway, B. L. *Pediatric Neurologic Nursing.* St. Louis: Mosby, 1977.

Council on Child Health of the American Academy of Pediatrics. "Medication for Hyperactive Children." *Pediatrics* 55:560–562, April 1975.

Downs, M. and H. Silver. "The A.B.C.D.'s to H.E.A.R." *Clin Pediatr* 11:563–565, October 1972.

Feingold, B. "Hyperkinesis and Learning Disabilities Linked to Artificial Food Flavors and Colors." *Am J Nurs* 75:797–803, May 1975.

Fry, D. B. "The Development of the Phonological System in the Normal and the Deaf Child." In F. Smith and G. A. Miller, *The Genesis of Language.* Cambridge, Mass.: M.I.T. Press, 1966. Pp. 187–206.

Gofman, H. F. and B. W. Allmond. "Learning and Language Disorders in Children, Part I: The Preschool Child." In L. Gluck, editor, *Current Problems in Pediatrics*, August 1971.

Gofman, H. F. and B. W. Allmond. "Learning and Language Disorders in Children Part II: The School-Age Child." In L. Gluck, editor, *Current Problems in Pediatrics*, September 1971.

Hedrick, D. L. and E. M. Prather. *Sequenced Inventory of Language Development*. Seattle: University of Washington Press, 1970.

Huessy, H. R. and A. Cohen. "Hyperkinetic Behaviors and Learning Disabilities Followed Over Seven Years." *Pediatrics* 57:4–10, January 1976.

Lenneberg, E. H. "The Natural History of Language." In F. Smith and G. A. Miller, *The Genesis of Language*. Cambridge, Mass.: M.I.T. Press, 1966. Pp. 219–252.

Lenneberg, E. H. *Biological Foundations of Language*. New York: Wiley, 1967.

Lillywhite, H. S., N. B. Young, and R. W. Olmstead. *Pediatrician's Handbook of Communication Disorders*. Philadelphia: Lea & Febiger, 1970.

Marge, M. "The General Problem of Language Disabilities in Children." In J. V. Irwin and M. Marge, editors, *Principles of Childhood Language Disabilities*. New York: Appleton-Century-Crofts, 1972. Pp. 75–98.

McElroy, C. *Speech and Language Development of the Preschool Child: A Survey*. Springfield, Ill.: Thomas, 1972.

Meier, J. H. *Development and Learning Disabilities: Evaluation, Management, and Prevention in Children*. Baltimore: University Park Press, 1976.

Rogers, M. "Early Identification and Intervention of Children with Learning Problems." *Pediatric Nursing* 2:21–26, January–February 1976.

Rogers, W. B. Jr. and R. A. Rogers. "A New Simplified Preschool Readiness Experimental Scale (The Press)." *Clin Pediatr* 11:558–562, October 1972.

Safer, D. J. and R. P. Allen. "Factors Influencing the Suppressant Effects of Two Stimulant Drugs on the Growth of Hyperactive Children." *Pediatrics* 51:660–667, April 1973.

Safer, D. J., R. P. Allen, and E. Barr. "Growth Rebound After Termination of Stimulant Drugs." *J Pediatr* 86:113–116, January 1975.

Silver, L. B. "Acceptable and Controversial Approaches to Treating the Child with Learning Disabilities." *Pediatrics* 55:406–415, March 1975.

Taichert, L. *Childhood Learning, Behavior, and the Family*. New York: Behavioral Publications, 1973.

Templin, M. "Development of Speech." *J Pediatr* 62:11–14, January 1963.

The Elementary and Secondary Act Amendments of 1969: Title VI, the Education of the Handicapped Act, April 13, 1970, pp. 91–230.

Vaughan, V. C. and R. J. McKay, editors. *Nelson Textbook of Pediatrics*, 10th ed. Philadelphia: Saunders, 1975.

Waechter, E. and F. Blake. *Nursing Care of Children*, 9th ed. Philadelphia: Lippincott, 1976. Pp. 625–645.

Whitsell, L. "Learning Disorders as a School Health Problem." *Calif Med* 111:433–445, December 1969.

27

Genetics

Up to 5 percent of all births in the United States involve physical or mental defects of varying severity. Birth defects may be inherited, may result from environmental factors, or may reflect a combination of both heredity and environment. Expanding knowledge of human genetics makes it possible now to identify carriers of defective genes, to predict the potential for transmitting defective genes, and to determine the presence or absence of defects in the fetus for a growing list of inherited disorders. Nurse practitioners need to understand basic patterns of genetic inheritance, the objectives of genetic counseling, and the indications for referring families for genetic counseling.

ASSESSMENT

Basic Patterns of Genetic Inheritance

CHROMOSOMES

The nucleus of every cell in the human body contains 46 chromosomes (23 pairs). Chromosomes are composed of linear structures which carry the genetic material, deoxyribonucleic acid (DNA), or genes. Before fertilization the gametes (egg and sperm cells) undergo a process of cell division resulting in separation of each pair of chromosomes. The mature gametes, therefore, each contain a set of 23 chromosomes which combine when fertilization occurs to provide the zygote with 46 chromosomes. Forty-four chromosomes are referred to as autosomes and the other two are the sex chromosomes. Chromosomal errors can occur, particularly during formation of reproductive cells, and as a result the zygote may contain chromosomes in abnormal number, structure, or arrangement (e.g., Down's Syndrome).

GENES

Genes are the functional hereditary units which transmit all the inherited characteristics from parents to children. There are thousands of genes on each chromosome, and each individual gene determines a specific hereditary characteristic. The genes, like the chromosomes, exist in pairs, one contributed by the mother and one by the father. The two genes in a pair work together to determine the outcome of a specific hereditary trait. The two members of each gene pair may carry similar or different instructions regarding the trait which they determine. If the members of a pair are the same, the person is *homozygous*. If the members of a gene pair supply different instructions, the person is said to be *heterozygous* for that trait. In this case the specific trait is determined by only one member of the pair, and the gene that is expressed is called *dominant*. The gene that is not expressed is called *recessive*. Most traits require the interaction of many gene pairs, but for some only a single pair is involved.

MUTATIONS

DNA is remarkably precise in duplicating or copying itself for transmission of genetic blueprints to the next cell or next generation. However, there are times when a slight error in replication results in a mutant gene and an altered *genotype* (basic genetic constitution) or an altered *phenotype* (observable appearance of the organism). Unless the mutation is harmful enough to be lethal, the mutant DNA material will also be faithfully transmitted through countless generations.

Table 1
Autosomal Dominant Inheritance

Parents	Children
Dn[a]	Dn (disease state)
nn	Dn (disease state)
	nn (normal)
	nn (normal)

[a] D = dominant faulty gene; n = normal gene.

AUTOSOMAL DOMINANT INHERITANCE

Genetic defects caused by dominant inheritance are relatively rare and occur when one parent carries a dominant gene for the disease and expresses the disease him or herself. The other parent almost always is free of the same pathologic trait. In such a family there is a 50 percent chance that each offspring will manifest the defect. See Table 1. Some cases of autosomal-dominant defects occur as new mutations. In other words, the parents are unaffected, but a mutation has occurred in the germ cell of one parent which causes the defect in the child. The parents in this case have no significant risk of producing further affected offspring, but the affected child carries a 50 percent chance of transmitting the defect to each of his or her children.

Examples of pathologic conditions inherited as dominant traits are achondroplasia (dwarfism), diabetes insipidus, ectodermal dysplasia, Huntington's chorea, neurofibromatosis, osteogenesis imperfecta, tuberous sclerosis, and polydactyly.

AUTOSOMAL RECESSIVE INHERITANCE

Genetic disorders caused by recessive inheritance occur when each parent carries the harmful recessive gene. Both parents are usually unaffected although genotypically abnormal. Each child of such parents has a 25 percent risk of manifesting the disease, a 25 percent chance of not inheriting the gene from either parent, and a 50 percent chance of receiving only a single defective gene and becoming a carrier. See Table 2. Other possibilities for combinations

Table 2
Autosomal Recessive Inheritance

Parents	Children
Nr*a*	NN (normal)
Nr	Nr (heterozygous: carrier state)
	Nr (heterozygous: carrier state)
	rr (homozygous: disease state)

a N = normal dominant gene; r = recessive faulty gene.

Table 3
Possible Combinations of Dominant and Recessive Inheritance

Parents	Children
1. NN*a*	NN (normal)
Nr	Nr (heterozygous: carrier state)
	NN (normal)
	Nr (heterozygous: carrier state)
2. Nr	Nr (heterozygous: carrier state)
rr	Nr (heterozygous: carrier state)
	rr (homozygous: disease state)
	rr (homozygous: disease state)
3. NN	Nr (heterozygous: carrier state)
rr	Nr (heterozygous: carrier state)
	Nr (heterozygous: carrier state)
	Nr (heterozygous: carrier state)

a N = normal dominant gene; r = faulty recessive gene.

of recessive and dominant genes and their probable outcomes are illustrated in Table 3. Examples of diseases inherited as autosomal recessive traits are adrenogenital syndrome, albinism, Tay-Sachs disease, cystinuria, deaf-mutism, cystic fibrosis, galactosemia, microcephaly, and phenylketonuria.

X-LINKED INHERITANCE

Normal females have two X chromosomes. Normal males have one X and one Y chromosome. The X chromosome carries many genes related to inherited traits other than sex. The Y chromosome seems

Table 4
X-Linked Inheritance: Female Transmission

Parents	Children
Xx^a	XY (normal son)
XY	XX (normal daughter)
	Xx (carrier daughter)
	xY (affected son)

^{a}X = faulty gene on X chromosome; X = normal chromosome; Y = normal chromosome.

to have no other function except for determining masculinity. Consequently, in the male, the genes on the X chromosome are not matched by corresponding genes on the Y chromosome. Therefore a defective gene on the X chromosome, even if recessive, can manifest itself since there is no normal gene on the Y chromosome to mask its effects. In females, a recessive faulty gene might be masked by a dominant normal gene on the other X chromosome.

The most common X-linked abnormalities occur when the mother carries a faulty gene on one of her X chromosomes. In this case each son has a 50 percent risk of inheriting the gene and manifesting the disease. Each daughter has a 50 percent chance of becoming a carrier capable of transmitting the disease to *her* sons. See Table 4.

If a male with a pathologic gene on his X chromosome and a normal female produce offspring, all sons will be normal having received a normal X chromosome from their mother. All the daughters will appear normal but will carry the faulty recessive gene on one of their X chromosomes. See Table 5. These

Table 5
X-Linked Inheritance: Male Transmission

Parents	Children
XX^a	XY (normal son)
xY	XY (normal son)
	Xx (carrier daughter)
	Xx (carrier daughter)

^{a}X = faulty gene on X chromosome; X = normal chromosome; Y = normal chromosome.

daughters then transmit the gene to their offspring as illustrated in Table 4.

Examples of disorders transmitted by X-linked inheritance are agammaglobulinemia, color blindness, diabetes insipidus, Duchenne type muscular dystrophy, and* hemophilia.

MULTIFACTORIAL INHERITANCE

There are genetic disorders which result from the combined interaction of multiple genes and environmental factors. Patterns of transmission are complicated, but it is known that the probabilities of recurrence are quite low. With one affected child, chances of another having the same defect are 5 percent or less. Examples of conditions resulting from multifactorial inheritance are cleft lip and palate, pyloric stenosis, congenital dislocation of the hip, club-foot, spina bifida, hydrocephalus, diabetes mellitus, and asthma.

Prenatal Diagnosis of Genetic Defects

AMNIOCENTESIS

Amniocentesis is the transabdominal withdrawal of amniotic fluid from the uterus during pregnancy. The prenatal diagnosis of many inherited defects is possible by subjecting the amniotic fluid to tissue culture, biochemical analysis, and chromosomal analysis.

Indications for amniocentesis. When the following situations exist, amniocentesis may be indicated:

1. Parental concern over known possibility of occurrence of a serious genetic abnormality
2. Parents who have given birth to a child with a chromosomal disorder
3. Parents who are known carriers for chromosomal, genetic, or X-linked diseases
4. Women over 35 years of age
5. Parents who have had a child with a neural tube defect

Procedure. Between the thirteenth to fifteenth week of pregnancy, under local anesthesia, approximately 10 to 12 cc of amniotic fluid is aspirated from the uterus. Before inserting the needle the physician determines fetal and placental position by palpation, ultrasound, and sometimes X-ray. Analysis of the fluid takes 3 to 4 weeks.

Risks. Even in experienced hands there are risks which include:

1. Direct damage to the fetus
2. Placental puncture and hemorrhage with secondary damage to the fetus
3. Stimulation of premature labor
4. Amnionitis
5. Maternal sensitization to fetal blood

It is suggested that amniocentesis be reserved for those cases in which the estimated value of the findings will outweigh the risks.

MANAGEMENT

Genetic Counseling

GOALS OF GENETIC COUNSELING

Genetic counseling aims to:

1. Provide individuals and families with sufficient and correct medical information about a specific disorder so they can understand the nature of the disorder
2. Provide guidelines for action so individuals and families can use the information wisely in making decisions about future offspring
3. Assist parents to deal with the impact of the information and to guide them toward effective coping
4. Reduce the number of affected individuals

PROCESS OF GENETIC COUNSELING

1. Data collection includes an accurate medical history, detailed family pedigree, and laboratory data obtained from clinical procedures (e.g., dermatoglyphics, chromosome analysis).

2. Once the nature of the defect is established, predictions on the probability of recurrence of a given abnormality in the same family can often be made using the basic laws governing heredity and knowledge of the frequency of specific birth defects in the general population.

3. The genetic counselor (physician, nurse, geneticist) then provides this information to the individuals and families concerned. The manner in which the information is delivered is crucial and demands effective communication skills with sensitivity to the psychologic impact on the family. Repeated conferences for reinterpretation and support are usually necessary.

INDICATIONS FOR REFERRAL FOR GENETIC COUNSELING

The nurse practitioner has the responsibility to refer individuals and families for genetic counseling. Referrals are indicated in the following situations:

1. A family which has a child with a congenital malformation or a group of congenital anomalies

2. A family which has one or more children who are mentally retarded

3. A family in which a medical problem has affected more than one member

4. A family in which a previously diagnosed condition is known to be genetic in origin

5. A child who "doesn't look right" or has delayed or abnormal development

6. Parents of children who have died at birth for unknown reasons

7. Related couples who want to know the risks of having defective children

8. Individuals concerned about exposure to environmental agents that may cause abnormalities
9. Couples seeking advice prior to marriage
10. Individuals with known defects who desire information
11. Individuals or families who have received genetics information but are not comfortable with it

Resource Information

Genetic counseling units have been established in many medical centers and teaching hospitals. Current information about specialized genetics services is available in the "International Directory of Genetic Services," published by: The National Foundation/March of Dimes, Box 2000, White Plains, NY 10602. Local March of Dimes chapters can provide information on available local services and written material for families.

References

Reisman, L. E. and A. P. Matheny. *Genetics and Counseling in Medical Practice.* St. Louis: Mosby, 1969.

Sahin, S. T. "The Multifaceted Role of the Nurse as Genetic Counselor." *Am. Journal of Maternal Child Nursing* 1:211–216, July–August 1976.

Scipien, G. M., editor. *Comprehensive Pediatric Nursing.* New York: McGraw-Hill, 1975.

Selwyn, A. *Genetic Counseling.* White Plains, N.Y.: The National Foundation/March of Dimes.

Vaughan, V. C. and R. J. McKay, editors. *Nelson Textbook of Pediatrics,* 10th ed. Philadelphia: Saunders, 1975.

Waechter, E. H. and F. G. Blake. *Nursing Care of Children,* 9th ed. Philadelphia: Lippincott, 1976.

Winchester, A. M. *Genetics: A Survey of the Principles of Heredity,* 4th ed. Boston: Houghton Mifflin, 1972.

28

Allergies

Allergy is one of the most common and complex entities encountered in the health care of children. Depending on the source, the incidence of allergy in the pediatric population has been estimated at 10 to 20 percent. Management of the allergic child is shared with the primary care physician with appropriate referrals to an allergist. The nurse practitioner can obtain the history, perform the physical examination, initiate diagnostic procedures, follow through with treatments, and counsel the child and parents.

ASSESSMENT

History

PRESENT HISTORY

Obtain information pertaining to the area of involvement following suggestions contained in Chapter 13, Assessment of Presenting Symptom. In addition, obtain information on colic, spitting-up, vomiting, diarrhea, constipation, and skin problems. Obtain information on frequency of upper or lower respiratory infections:

night or seasonal coughs; infections of the ears; allergies of the skin, eyes, or gastrointestinal systems; and the time of day and season of the year that symptoms are worse. Additional information regarding the environment can be found in this chapter, Environmental Control.

PAST HISTORY

Obtain information on gastrointestinal disturbances or skin problems in infancy. Obtain information on communicable diseases and immunizations.

NUTRITION HISTORY

Obtain a detailed diet history. See Chapter 6, Nutrition History. Be aware of cultural differences. Emphasis is placed on identifying foods which contain additives and preservatives. For more information, see this chapter, Diet Control.

FAMILY HISTORY

Obtain information about any family members with rashes, migraine headaches, hay fever, asthma, gastrointestinal disturbances, eye problems (such as itching, crusting of lids), food allergies, and food habits of the mother (excessive eating of a particular food during pregnancy can sensitize an unborn infant by transplacental transfer).

Physical Examination

Multiple involvement of organs is the common pattern for allergies.

SKIN

Observe for pallor, dryness, lichenification, and rashes.

EYES

Inspect for discharges; scleral redness; conjunctival swelling, redness, or tiny, grainy, palpebral conjunctival papules (cobblestoning); periorbital swelling; crusting of lashes; and discoloration below the eyes (allergic shiners).

EARS

Inspect tympanic membranes for retraction, scarring, and evidence of serous otitis media; observe for crusting or discharge behind the ears or in the auditory canals.

NOSE

Inspect nasal mucosa and turbinates for color, swelling, redness, dryness, bogginess, and pallor. Inspect for discharges noting color, consistency, and crusting.

MOUTH

Inspect for mouth breathing, malocclusion, and jaw deformity.

THROAT

Inspect for postnasal drip noting color and consistency; elongated pale uvula; lymphoid hyperplasia of the postpharyngeal wall; and enlarged tonsils or tonsillar tags.

LUNGS

Auscultate for rhonchi, rales, and expiratory wheezing.

ABDOMEN

Auscultate for increased bowel sounds (some gastrointestinal allergies present first with symptoms of an upper respiratory infection).

Differentiation Between Allergies and Upper Respiratory Infections

It is frequently difficult to distinguish between upper respiratory symptoms due to allergies and upper respiratory symptoms due to an infectious process. The distinction is important to make since treatment will differ as well as plans for long-term health maintenance care (e.g., the child with symptoms on an allergic basis is a safe candidate for routine immunizations; the child with an upper respiratory infection is not). Table 1 outlines features useful in differentiating the two conditions.

Table 1
Differentiation Between Allergies and Upper Respiratory Infections

Features	Allergies	Upper Respiratory Infections (Common Cold)
Onset	Sudden	Gradual
Attacks	Multiple, recurrent, or constant	Occasional, free of symptoms between colds
Symptoms	Sneezing, nasal itchiness, stuffy nose, irritative cough, seasonal or perennial	Nasal symptoms progress to chest and cough; duration less than 2 weeks
Fever	No	Maybe
Nasal discharge	Thin, watery, profuse	Thin to thick, maybe mucopurulent
Nasal mucosa	Pale, greyish pink, boggy, moist, swollen	Red and swollen
Exposure to infection	No	Yes
Exposure to environment	Yes	No
Associated allergies or family history	Yes	Not necessarily
Eosinophilia more than 10 percent	Usually	No

Definition of Allergy

Allergy means increased sensitivity to a substance which in ordinary amounts would cause no problem in most people (e.g., egg sensitivity, pollen sensitivity). The allergic disorders of children include a large, dissimilar group of conditions which have in common immunologic hypersensitivity of the child to molecular substances foreign to the child. These foreign molecules serve as *antigens* which, when they produce symptoms in the susceptible individual, are designated as *allergens*. When a particular allergen is absorbed by the body, it eventually comes in contact with lymphocytes which produce allergy antibodies or *reagin*, probably IgE, which react specifically with it. These allergy antibodies become attached to mast cells and basophils, cells which are rich in histamine and other mediators of the allergic reaction. On re-exposure to the allergen the allergen comes in contact with the antibody on the cell surface resulting in the release of the mediators. This produces an irritation in the susceptible tissues (e.g., the nose, the bronchial tubes, the skin).

Basic Principles

The development of allergic symptoms depends on inheritance, the nature of the allergen, and the degree, duration, and nature of the exposure. Some basic principles are as follows:

- Sensitivity usually occurs only after repeated exposure to the substance.
- Allergic individuals may be sensitive to more than one allergen.
- The tendency to be sensitized or allergic to some foreign substance is usually inherited.
- An individual who has inherited the tendency may develop sensitivities to different allergens at different age periods. The previous sensitivities may remain or may be lost.
- Allergic persons who tolerate some exposure to their allergens without developing symptoms are considered to be in allergic equilibrium or allergic balance, that is, the amount of allergens

taken in is balanced by the individual's "tolerance" or "resistance." Nonallergic factors may place an additional burden on such persons and thus disturb allergic equilibrium. Respiratory infections, such as common colds, may increase the total load to a point beyond a person's tolerance and thus upset what was previously a balanced allergic state. Fatigue, emotional tensions, excitement, exertion, cold foggy weather, and many other factors may also increase the burden, upset the balance, and allow an allergic attack to develop.

HOW ALLERGENS ENTER THE BODY

In order of frequency they enter via:

1. Ingestion, as foods, drinks, and drugs
2. Inhalation, as dust, pollens, and fumes (air pollution and cigarette smoke)
3. External contact, as clothes, cosmetics, and industrial products
4. Injection, as drugs and sera

FACTORS WHICH INCREASE ALLERGIC REACTIONS

Seasons. The seasons and allergens which cause increased reactions are:

- Winter—animals, house dust, and molds; food allergies are worse in winter.
- Spring—pollen of trees and grasses
- Summer—air pollution, grass pollens, insect bites, sun, and poison oak or ivy
- Fall—pollen of ragweed, and molds

Weather. High fronts can cause an increase in asthma, sinusitis, and rhinitis. Prophylactic decongestants should be increased at this time.

Emotions. Emotional disturbances usually play a part but do not cause allergic attacks.

Time of day. When the condition is worse in the morning, suspicion should develop that the allergen is in the bedroom.

ALLERGY IN INFANCY

Predisposing factors. Factors that predispose to the development of hypersensitivity in the infant include:

1. Heredity or the atopic hypersensitivity (see this chapter, Definition of Allergy). The most common allergic conditions in infancy are atopic dermatitis, gastrointestinal disturbances, and nasal sniffles.
2. The state of the digestive tract. The digestive tract has not fully matured and is more permeable which permits the assimilation of undigested food proteins.
3. The nature of the diet. Foods are the most common and most important allergens in infancy. Milk is the most common, followed by eggs, orange juice, wheat, corn, and beef.
4. The environment. Less common than food as a factor, an infant may be allergic to both food and environmental allergens.
5. Infection. Infection is a provocative agent not a primary allergen. Gastrointestinal infection serves to increase the permeability of the gut to undigested proteins which may induce sensitivity.

Familial incidence. The probabilities of inheriting allergic problems are as follows:

1. If neither parent has allergies, the children have less than a 10 percent chance of having an allergic problem.
2. If one parent has a history of allergies, 50 percent of the offspring may eventually manifest allergies.
3. If both parents are allergic, the incidence rises to 75 percent.

ALLERGY IN CHILDHOOD

Predisposing factors. Factors which predispose to allergic problems in childhood are similar to those in infancy including a history of infantile allergic problems. Environmental factors are the leading cause of allergic conditions in childhood.

Signs and symptoms. Signs and symptoms suggestive of allergic diseases are:

1. Tension-fatigue syndrome. This includes extreme fatigue, lassitude, listlessness, and irritability; facial pallor without anemia; and circles of discoloration under the eyes, "allergic shiners." In most cases the allergens are pollens, environmentals, and foods.
2. Recurrent otitis media and recurrent serous otitis media. See this chapter, Allergic Serous Otitis Media, or Chapter 18, Serous Otitis Media.
3. Upper respiratory symptoms. These include:

   - Features of the tension-fatigue syndrome
   - "Allergic salute." Itching of the nose and rubbing of the nose upward which may lead to a crease across the nose just above the tip
   - Excoriated nares and sometimes epistaxis caused by excessive nose picking
   - Rhinorrhea with a seromucoid discharge
   - Postnasal mucous discharge which may cause elongation of the uvula leading to a tickling cough followed by a productive cough
   - Nasal congestion leading to mouth breathing with pursing of the lips, facial deformity, and malocclusion

4. Recurrent laryngitis. Occurs with sudden onset usually at night; may be present with crowing respirations and, at times, suprasternal retractions
5. Lower respiratory tract. Allergic bronchitis is the commonly observed form of allergic pulmonary disease. Bronchial asthma and status asthmaticus are less frequent.
6. Skin disturbance. Urticaria occurs infrequently in children during the prepubescent period but increases in girls at menarche. Whealing of insect bites is often mistaken for urticaria.
7. Atopic dermatitis. See this chapter, Common Clinical Problems

MANAGEMENT

Immunotherapy

Immunotherapy consists of diagnostic skin testing and hyposensitization. It is usually managed by an allergist.

INDICATIONS FOR IMMUNOTHERAPY

Referral is made when children have severe and persistent allergic reactions (e.g., severe asthma). The decision for referral is generally made collaboratively with a physician. Mild cases are often treated successfully using environmental control and, at times, dietary measures.

DIAGNOSTIC SKIN TESTING

Techniques commonly used for skin testing are the scratch test, patch test, and intradermal test. Skin testing can be helpful in some cases (e.g., severe atopic dermatitis, asthma) and can provide additional data to consider in the overall assessment of the child.

Positive tests.   These are only clues to the allergens and must be interpreted cautiously since they are not always reliable.

Negative tests.   These do not always prove a substance harmless; the final answer depends on a therapeutic trial by removal of the suspected allergen through diet and environmental control.

Skin testing for food allergies.   This is believed to be unreliable possibly because digestive breakdown products of whole food are the true sensitizers, whereas extracts of naturally occurring foods are used in skin testing. Skin testing of a food when there is a clinical history of marked sensitivity to that food is dangerous and should not be done. An example is egg white which is a very antigenic material and even in minute quantities can induce violent reactions.

HYPOSENSITIZATION

This consists of a series of injections of extracts of specific antigens to which the child is sensitive and which cannot otherwise be controlled. Its value is limited mainly to atopic disorders and to severe bee sting allergy. The injections begin with a very dilute solution and are increased at 50 percent strength once or twice a week until a top dose is reached and then maintained. Injections may be given at regular intervals throughout the year or prior to the season associated with greatest symptoms.

Diet Control

Evaluation of data from the physical examination and a carefully taken diet history may provide sufficient evidence to warrant removing a suspected allergen (e.g., milk) from a child's diet. This simple form of diet control, in addition to symptomatic treatment, may be all that is necessary in most mild allergic problems. However, in the treatment of more severe cases, it may be necessary to follow a more stringent regimen.

INDICATIONS FOR USE OF AN ELIMINATION DIET

The indications for proceeding with an elimination diet are:

1. A history of food allergies
2. Failure to control symptoms with immunotherapy and environmental control
3. A recurrence of symptoms not attributed to a reaction to hyposensitization or an infraction of environmental control
4. A history of nasal polyps
5. A history of recurrent otitis media
6. A history of aspirin intolerance. Many food additives and preservatives contain salicylates.

HISTORY

A detailed diet history remains one of the chief tools in searching for a food offender. The diet history should include:

1. Foods eaten daily (consider cultural differences) and food excesses
2. Any unusual foods eaten recently and family food disagreements
3. Previous food intolerances, intense food dislikes, frequency of questionable foods
4. Foods that contain additives or preservatives. See next section, Elimination Diets.

PROCEDURE FOR AN ELIMINATION DIET

The procedure is as follows:

1. A diary of each food, beverage, or medication which is ingested at meals or between meals without alteration in customary patterns is to be recorded for 7 to 10 days.
2. Constituents of all home-prepared foods must be listed as well as ingredients of all packaged foods. Concealed foods may be included in prepared products (see Table 2).
3. Symptoms are also recorded for 7 to 10 days. By correlating symptoms with the information in the diary, the nurse practitioner frequently can determine the elimination diet suitable for the particular case, for example milk-free, salicylate-free, or others. See next section, Elimination Diets.
4. The elimination diet is initiated.
5. Two weeks following the start of an elimination diet, the client is interviewed and the diet is reviewed. Improvement can be expected within 2 to 3 weeks if the correct food has been eliminated.
6. Two weeks later another interview and review are conducted.
7. If symptoms have not subsided, the program is abandoned and another diet regimen is implemented.
8. If the diet is successful in eliminating symptoms it should be

Table 2
Eggs as an Example of Concealed Foods

Eggs occur in the following:
    Eggs, eggnogs, and other egg drinks
    Custard, puddings of various types
    Ice cream and sherbet
    Mayonnaise, hollandaise, and tartar sauce
    Egg noodles
    Cakes and cookies made with eggs
    Pastries and bakery goods
    Pancakes, waffles, muffins, sweet rolls
Eggs may be found in:
    Soups: for clarifying
    Baking powder: some brands
    Coffee: eggs and eggshells can be used for cleaning
    Root beer: for foaming
    Candies: for glazing jelly beans and some chocolate candies
    Meats: egg is used as a binding agent in many prepared meats
    Salad dressings: many contain eggs

continued for at least 2 months before attempting additions of new foods to the diet.

9. New foods can then be added individually every 5 to 7 days.

10. If symptoms return, the food should be discontinued.

11. If the second attempt at introducing the food is not successful, the food should be permanently excluded from the diet.

12. This procedure is repeated with other foods, each one taken individually, until a well-balanced and varied diet is provided for the client.

13. The diet diary should be continued for a few months, if possible, in the event of a recurrence of symptoms.

14. All labels, especially of prepared foods, must be read carefully.

15. Home-prepared foods are preferable because the ingredients can be controlled.

16. Absolute adherence to the diet is imperative. If undesirable weight loss occurs, more of the prescribed carbohydrates,

sugar, fats, and oils must be taken. This may require eating 4 to 5 meals a day.

17. Caution should be taken not to place a child on a nutritionally deficient diet for long periods of time when no specific results have been obtained.

ELIMINATION DIETS

Examples of some elimination diets follow.

Elemental diet. This is recommended for children who have been tried on other diets without success and for children who have a serious or life-threatening disease in which it is urgent that the role of food hypersensitivity be determined as soon as possible. Vivonex (Eaton Laboratories), a mixture of synthetic amino acids, simple sugars, safflower oil, vitamins, and minerals is used. This is given for 2 weeks unless symptoms completely disappear before that time. If the symptoms persist unchanged during this time, hypersensitivity to ingested foods can generally be ruled out. Once symptoms have completely cleared, additional foods may be added, one every second day (Gellis, 1976. p. 662).

Hypoallergenic diet. If the history does not suggest a specific food as an allergen this diet may be recommended to start the elimination diet. After the first 2 weeks of using this diet different foods are slowly started and reassessed. See Table 3.

Milk-free diet. See Table 4. This diet is recommended for children with sensitivities to milk or penicillin (milk can be contaminated with penicillin via treatment of cow's udders; natural cheeses which contain mold may cross-react with penicillin) or as a trial in a child with a history of recurrent serous otitis.

Salicylate-free diet. This diet is recommended for clients who are allergic to aspirin and foods containing natural salicylates (see Table 5), or who have a history of nasal polyps. Feingold (1975, p. 797) has reported that hyperactive children and possibly those with learning disabilities are helped with this diet.

Table 3
Hypoallergenic Diet for Infants and Young Children
(Foods Permitted)

Food Category	Specific Foods
Milk	Soy formulas: Mull-Soy, Neo-Mull-Soy (Borden) Sobee, Prosobee (Mead Johnson) Isomil (Ross) Soyalac (Loma Linda)
Cereals	Rice, oat, corn, barley, rye, poi
Breads	Rye, Rye-Krisp, Baltic rye
Vegetables	Beets, carrots, broccoli, asparagus, peas, green beans, white and sweet potatoes, yams; soups made from these vegetables
Fruits	Apples, pears, plums, bananas, apricots, grapes; juices of these fruits
Meats	Lamb, pork, veal, capon, tom turkey and rooster (young fryers and roasters) (no hens or hen turkeys)
Desserts	Fruits listed and their gelatin products
Spreads	Oleomargarine (most have additives and milk); jellies of the listed fruits
Vitamins, synthetic	Tri-Vi-Sol, Poly-Vi-Sol, Decca-Vi-Sol (Mead Johnson)

Source: From H. I. Lecks, "Allergic Gastrointestinal Disease," in S. S. Gellis, and B. M. Kagan: *Current Pediatric Therapy* 7, © 1976 by the W. B. Saunders Company, Philadelphia.

RESOURCES FOR DIET ASSISTANCE

Further diet assistance can be obtained from the following sources:

1. Ralston Purina Co., 1 Checkerboard Square, St. Louis, MO.
2. Department of Dietetics, University of Michigan, Ann Arbor, MI 48109.
3. Dietary Department of Massachusetts General Hospital, 32 Fruit Street, Boston, MA 02114.

Some allergy cookbooks are the following:

1. Conrad, M. L. *Allergy Cooking.* New York: Pyramid Publishing Co., 1968.
2. Emerling, C. G. and E. D. Jonekers. *The Allergy Cookbook.* Garden City, N.Y.: Doubleday, 1969.
3. Little, B. *Recipes for Allergies.* New York: Grosset and Dunlap, paperbook #1868, 1971.

Table 4
Milk-Free Diet

Foods Allowed	*Foods Not Allowed*
Milk substitutes: soy milk formulas, Mocha Mix, Coffee Rich	Milk—fresh, dry, evaporated
	Yogurt
Unprocessed mature cheese such as cheddar and parmesan	Cream cheese, cottage cheese, cheese snacks, processed cheese
Eggs	
Oils, lard, chicken and bacon fat, pure vegetable margarines (diet margarine, Willow Run, Nucoa)	Butter, cream, most margarines, foods dipped in butter or margarine for frying
Meats and fish	Meat with milk sauces, gravies, processed or packaged meats, sausages, frankfurters
All vegetables, cooked without milk or butter	Instant mashed potatoes
All fruits and fruit juices	
Breads and cereals containing wheat, rye, corn, rice, oatmeal, semolina, tapioca	Bread containing milk; check commercial and baby cereals and teething biscuits
Breads (Hillbilly by Colonial, Longhorn and Dark Hollywood by Wonder, water bagels)	
Fruit jellies, gelatin, pastry made with water (milk substitutes are not generally suitable for use in cooking)	All pastries, puddings, cakes, custards, biscuits, commercial packaged products, ice cream and sherbet, "milk" chocolate, muffins, sweet rolls, pancakes, cookies
Jam, honey, syrup, sugar, water ices, peanut butter, nuts	
Meat and vegetable soups	All soups containing milk
Tea, coffee, carbonated beverages, cocoa powder	Check chocolate and caramel flavorings
Herbs and seasonings	Check commercial dressings and mayonnaise

Table 5
Salicylate-Free Diet

Foods Allowed	Foods Not Allowed
Grapefruit, lemon, pears, bananas, dates, limes, figs, papayas, melons, and pineapple	Almonds, apples, apricots, blackberries, cherries, currants, gooseberries, grapes or raisins, nectarines, oranges, peaches, plums or prunes, raspberries, strawberries, cucumbers and pickles, tomatoes
All vegetables except cucumbers and tomatoes	
All meats, except those artificially flavored, such as frankfurters, bologna	
All fish except fish sticks	Ice cream, oleomargarine, gin and all distilled beverages except vodka, cake mixes, bakery goods (except plain bread), jello, candies, gum, frankfurters, cloves, mint flavors, jam or jelly, lunch meats (salami, bologna, etc.), licorice
Eggs	
Milk and milk products—may have Brockmeyer's vanilla or carob ice cream	
Pure maple syrup, all vegetable oils, distilled white vinegar, salt, pepper, and sugar	
	Breakfast cereals with artificial color or flavoring
	Wine and wine vinegars, all tea, diet drinks and supplements, cider and cider vinegars, Kool-aid and similar beverages, soda pop (all soft drinks)
Butter or Willow Run margarine	
Plain bread, rice, potato	
Bisquick mix	
	Flavorings (omit artificially flavored and colored foods, drinks, and drugs)
Coffee, 7-Up, water, milk	
	Drugs–all medicines containing aspirin, such as Bufferin, Anacin, Excedrin, Alka-Seltzer, Empirin, Darvon Compound
Drugs—Tylenol for fever or pain	
	Perfumes
	Toothpaste and tooth powder (a mixture of salt and soda can be used), oil of wintergreen, lozenges, mouthwash.

Source: From B. F. Feingold, *Introduction to Allergy,* 1973. Courtesy of Charles C Thomas, Publisher, Springfield, Ill.

Environmental Control

INDICATIONS

Those children in whom environmental control should be instituted include those with:

1. Positive skin test findings for environmental allergens
2. Pollenosis. Most pollen-sensitive children also react to environmental factors.
3. A strong history of atopic allergy in the parents
4. A clinical history of significant allergy symptoms (nasal, bronchial, atopic dermatitis)

GENERAL CONSIDERATIONS

General considerations related to environmental control are as follows:

- The child with an hereditary atopic constitution may react to every potential allergen in the environment.
- Food sensitivity is rarely observed without inhalant allergy, either to environmentals, pollens, or both.
- Environmental control includes elimination (avoidance) of inhalants such as pollens, dust, animal dander, and fumes (air pollution, cigarette smoke, and wood-burning fires); and all environmental factors found within the home, the school, and places visited. See Table 6.
- Control of the home should not be restricted to the child's room; all rooms including the basement and garage must be considered.
- The emotional upheaval caused by the removal of a pet must be tempered by the fact that the child's allergic symptoms can serve as an even greater potential for causing emotional disturbances.
- Failure to exercise environmental control is one of the most frequently encountered reasons for the failure of immunotherapy in the treatment of allergic diseases.

Table 6
Commonly Encountered Environmental Factors

Items	Where Found
Grass pollens	
Weed pollens	
Tree pollens	
Cotton linters	Not the same fibers used in cotton cloth. Linters are used in cotton wadding or batting to make pads, cushions, comforters, mattresses, upholstery and some varnishes.
Feathers and down	Pillows, down cushions, couches, and other upholstered articles, birds, sleeping bags
Coconut fiber	Tropical furniture, doormats, gymnasium mats, mattresses, box springs
Cat hair	Cats, toy animals, "imitation" furs, some fur caps, ear muffs, slippers, gloves
Cattle hair	Rugs, rug pads, blankets, carpet padding
Dog hair	Dogs—all dogs produce dander.[a]
Goat hair	Mohair, angora, cashmere, alpaca
Hog hair	Rug and carpet pads, hair brushes, furniture stuffing, mattresses, auto cushions
Horse hair	Horses, carpet padding, some blankets, some antique furniture
Rabbit hair	Fur coats, trimmings sold under trade name Coney or Lapin, toy animals, fabrics, some felts
Hemp	Rope, carpet pads, used as sisal in mattresses and box springs, rugs
Kapok	Kapok is a plant fiber used in cushions, mattresses, sleeping bags, pillows, upholstery
Wool	Raw wool and coarse woolens of all kinds should be avoided. Avoid wool blankets and knitting with wool yarn.
Flaxseed	Some cereals, laxatives, wave sets, paints, varnishes, linseed oil, furniture stuffings
Jute	Carpet pads, carpet backing, burlap, gunny sacks, crocus cloth, "Polynesian" articles such as grass skirts, handbags, place mats, cushions
House dust	A mixture of all the above agents. In addition, it in itself has factors that cause allergy. Control of the above factors in part controls the potency of house dust.

[a]The belief that hairless dogs are not allergenic is a myth. It is the dander and not the hair that is allergenic. There is no difference among species of dogs.

Table 6. (*Continued*)

Items	Where Found
Orris root	All ladies' and men's cosmetics, talcum, dusting powder, perfume, deodorants, gin factories, bakeries, toothpaste and powders
Pyrethrum	Insect sprays (almost all—check label)
Vegetable gums	Mucilage, bakery products
Acacia gum	
Karaya gum	In denture adhesive—check labels; also in cream cheeses
Tragacanth gum	Confections, gum drops, pastries and pies
Molds (fungi and mildew)	Dark, damp, cool places as shower stalls, bathrooms, cabinet under sinks, refrigerators, basement, windows, eaves of houses; also in the air and in cheeses. Check around for musty (mildew) odors. Clean thoroughly and spray repeatedly with Lysol

Source: From B. F. Feingold, *Introduction to Clinical Allergy*, 1973. Courtesy of Charles C Thomas, Publisher, Springfield, Ill.

HOW TO "DESENSITIZE" A ROOM

Ordinary house dust is a mixture of many things. See Table 6. Practically everything that can wear out can produce dust. A dust-free environment for even part of a 24-hour period will be substantially beneficial for the dust-sensitive child. This is usually the bedroom where the most concentrated amount of time is spent. Suggestions that follow for a bedroom can be applied to other rooms.

1. All clothes are kept in closets, never lying about the room. Closet and all other doors are kept closed. The closet should be cleaned well before clothes are placed inside. Some authorities prefer the closets emptied and sealed with clothes stored elsewhere.
2. No ornately carved furniture, books, or bookshelves should be in the room.

3. Upholstered chairs are replaced with rubberized canvas or plastic chairs.

4. Wood or linoleum floors (no rugs) are permitted. The walls should be scrubbed initially and the floor waxed.

5. No fabric toys or stuffed animals are permitted. Toys may be of wood, plastic, or metal. They may be stuffed with polyesters or old nylons as these are washable.

6. No pennants, pictures, or other dust-catchers are permitted on the walls.

7. The beds are made with allergen-proof encasings for pillows, mattress, and box springs. Allergen-proof pillow and mattress casings can be obtained from: Allergen-Proof Casings, Inc., 1450 E. 363rd St., Eastlake, OH 44094. The mattress and pillow covers are vacuumed frequently. Fuzzy blankets, quilts, and comforters are avoided. Washable cotton or synthetic blankets are best. The blankets are washed every 4 to 6 weeks. Blanket covers should be of sheeting or washable fabrics. No mattress pad is used on the bed. Dreft or White King D detergents may be used in the washing machine.

8. No kapok, feather, or foam rubber pillows are used. Dacron or other synthetics are substituted. Foam rubber grows mold, especially in a damp area.

9. Air-conditioning window units or central air conditioning may be installed. Windows are kept closed, especially in summer. No electric fans are used.

10. Roll-up, washable, cotton or synthetic window shades are installed. No venetian blinds should be used.

11. Easily washed cotton or fiberglass curtains are used and washed daily. No draperies are used.

12. In houses with forced hot air, a centrally installed electrostatic air filter may be used or a filter of damp cheesecloth is put over the air inlet and changed weekly.

13. Newly developed products, such as Allergex, which inhibit dust formation on furniture, rugs, drapes, and blankets may be used. These products immobilize old dust, retard the formation of new dust, and are applied with simple spray equipment.

14. The room should be damp mopped and dusted, including all

parts of the bed, daily with a thorough and complete cleaning once a week.

15. Clothes and shoes are brushed before storing in this room. They may carry pollens and dusts. Other clothes are aired before storing.

16. All dogs, cats, birds, and other pets are removed from the house.

17. No insect sprays or powders are used. Odoriferous substances, such as camphor, tar, and room deodorants, should be avoided.

Parents who are faced with the rigorous task of desensitizing a room need help and support from health personnel. They need to be encouraged and reassured that their difficult task will afford relief of symptoms for an ill child.

HUMIDITY IN THE HOME

Proper humidification of inhaled air is extremely important to the function of the lungs; and humidified air combats the allergic effect of house dust. A relative humidity of 50 percent has a lethal effect on nearly all infective bacteria and viruses. Efficient functioning of the cilia is dependent on optimal humidity (45 to 50 percent). Ideally the entire house should be humidified, but it is needed most in the bedroom. It is not necessary to have the child's room dripping with moisture to produce the desired conditions. In regions where humidity is not too low, no provision for added moisture is necessary. In dry climates, additional moisture can be added to the room by placing a container of water with a large exposed surface in the room. When a vaporizer is used, the concentration of moisture should be checked. Excessive moisture, particularly over prolonged uninterrupted periods, predisposes to the growth of molds which can complicate the clinical picture.

Pharmacologic Therapy

DRUG THERAPY

Drug therapy is no substitute for prevention. In most allergic conditions drug therapy is a relatively secondary aspect of the treatment. Treatment of allergic illnesses by drugs is managed in close collaboration with a physician; however, the nurse practitioner must know the implications of these drugs as applied to allergic diseases.

Antihistamines. Antihistamines are used for acute rhinorrhea, allergic rhinitis, hay fever, and pruritus; and they may be used as a preventive for the rhinorrhea preceding asthma attacks but are not used once wheezing is established. Effective use of antihistamines depends on achieving a balance between the desired histamine antagonism and the undesirable side effects of which sedation and drying are the most notable. Susceptibility to the side effects varies among clients, and generally, many different preparations are tried before the most effective one is found. Some clients have a prolonged and significant therapeutic effect from low dosages but experience associated sedative symptoms; others tolerate and need much higher quantities. The side effects may subside with continued use, while effectiveness persists. On the other hand some clients will benefit from alternating use of different groups of antihistamines from week to week. A therapeutic effect occurs within 30 minutes with a duration of 3 to 6 hours, but a prolonged effect (8 to 12 hours) can be obtained from sustained release preparations.

PRESCRIPTION PREPARATIONS. Some frequently used antihistamines are:

1. Benadryl (diphenhydramine hydrochloride). Benadryl is not for use in premature or newborn infants.
2. Pyribenzamine (tripelennamine)
3. Actidel (triprolidine)

OVER-THE-COUNTER (OTC) PREPARATIONS. Commonly used OTC antihistamine preparations containing chlorpheniramine in various amounts and some combinations are Alleroid, Contac, Coricidin, Dristan, Novahistine, and Chlor-Trimeton.

Antitussives. These drugs are contraindicated for the treatment of bronchial allergies because they suppress the cough and may aggravate the condition. Coughing is the major mechanism for removing bronchial secretions and mucous plugs.

Barbiturates. These drugs are contraindicated in the treatment of bronchial allergies because they depress the respiratory center and may aggravate the condition.

Bronchodilators. See Sympathomimetics.

Corticosteroids. The most common use of steroids is to bring an end to status asthmaticus in infants or in severe asthma in children. The dangers lie in reliance on steroids as a substitute for a thoughtful and searching program of conventional management of childhood allergies and the side effects of steroids.

INJECTABLE STEROIDS. These are not recommended for children because of the risk of retardation of bone development and growth.

OPHTHALMIC STEROIDS. These are not used topically to treat minor disorders of the eye because they are potentially toxic agents.

OTIC STEROIDS. These are not recommended because of their potential sensitizing effect.

TOPICAL STEROIDS. Topical steroids are of undisputed value as anti-inflammatory and antipruritic agents. Topical steroids are useful in the treatment of small, localized patches of dermatitis; however, those containing parabens as a preservative may cause contact dermatitis. Application of topical antibiotics, especially neomycin, with or without steroids is not recommended. The risk of sensitization is very great. The steroids offer no protection against the development of such sensitivities.

The "use" test. The "use" test should be employed when using topical ointments which may contain known sensitizers. Before applying a cream or ointment to a large area, apply the medication to an area the size of a dime and watch for several hours for signs of primary irritation (Gellis, 1973, p. 715).

Preparations. Some topical steroid preparations which are recommended are triamcinolone acetonide (Aristocort, Kenalog), flurandrenolide (Cordran), and fluorometholone (Oxylone). Some which do not contain parabens are dexamethasone (Decadron), and fluocinolone (Synalar).

Decongestants. See Sympathomimetics.

Expectorants. Expectorants are given to aid in the liquefaction and mobilization of the bronchial secretions. Expectorants are commonly combined with bronchodilators. The most important expectorant is water.

WATER. Adequate hydration increases the watery secretions in the bronchioles which thins mucous secretions. This thinning allows for easier removal of mucus and decreased formation of mucous plugs. Effective delivery of water to the lungs depends on adequate oral intake. Additional benefit may be gained from vaporizers and cool-mist humidifiers.

PREPARATIONS. Drugs included in this group are potassium iodide, glyceryl guaiacolate (Robitussin), and iodinated glycerin (Organidin).

Opiates. See Barbiturates.

Sedatives. See Barbiturates. They have no place in routine treatment of children. If there is a specific indication for sedation a nonbarbiturate sedative may be safer to use (e.g., chloral hydrate).

Sympathomimetics. These drugs include bronchodilators and decongestants. They produce dilation of the air passages and tend to correct the edema of the mucous membranes. They are used in the treatment of allergic rhinitis and bronchial allergies. Children with asthma who take these medications must concurrently increase their fluid intake.

PREPARATIONS. The two sympathomimetics used most often in the treatment of asthma are epinephrine and ephedrine. Both drugs have side effects of tachycardia, sometimes mild muscular incoordination, and stimulation of the central nervous system. These side effects are sometimes perceived by the child as feelings of anxiety which engender further anxiety. A word of explanation to the child that these sensations are normal, and that they mean the medicine is taking effect is indicated. Epinephrine is the most physiologic sympathomimetic. The therapeutic effects are felt in about 15 to 20 minutes after an injection. Ephedrine is the most commonly used sympathomimetic sometimes in combination with aminophylline or theophylline, a sedative, and an expectorant. Benefits from ephedrine may be delayed 45 minutes or more.

Ephedrine compounds.   Some frequently used ephedrine compounds are:

1. Theophylline, ephedrine sulfate, and hydroxyzine hydrochloride (Marax)
2. Theophylline, ephedrine sulfate, and phenobarbital (Tedral)

Combined with antihistamines.   Preparations which contain these drugs in combination with antihistamines are:

1. Triprolidine hydrochloride and pseudoephedrine hydrochloride (Actifed Syrup)
2. Brompheniramine maleate, phenylephrine hydrochloride, and phenylpropanolamine hydrochloride (Dimetapp Elixir)
3. Phenylpropanolamine hydrochloride, pheniramine maleate, and pyrilamine maleate (Triaminic Syrup)

Eye preparations.   Decongestant eye preparations are phenylephrine hydrochloride (Neo-Synephrine) and Visine and Vasocon-A.

Nasal sprays and nose drops.   Sympathomimetic amines are used topically as nasal sprays and nose drops. Used in this form vasoconstriction and relief of swelling is much more dramatic and rapid than in the systemic use of these amines. However, there is often a rebound vasodilation occurring an hour or so after the use of the topical agents, and long-term use should be avoided because of the hazard of resulting atrophy of mucosal tissues. There is little justification for their use in children. A commonly used preparation is phenylephrine (Neo-Synephrine).

Nebulizers. These are aerosol inhalators which contain isoproterenol, a bronchodilator. They are used in some cases of bronchial allergies. Nebulizers have been associated with worsening of symptoms; use or misuse has also been associated with sudden death, either from toxicity or from sudden severe bronchospasm. They may be used by an older, more stable child. They are more effective when used very early in the development of an asthmatic paroxysm rather than later in the attack. It is important that the parents and the care provider know exactly how it is to be used, and that the use is reasonably monitored. There is no justification for their use in young children.

Tranquilizers. These agents should be used in the allergic child only for those who present serious neurotic traits or other behavior disturbances with anxiety or hyperactivity as outstanding features.

TOPICAL THERAPY

Baths. For treatment of a widespread dermatitis, baths are antipruritic and mildly anti-inflammatory. The tub is half filled with lukewarm water and the child is bathed for 15 to 30 minutes.

COMMON PREPARATIONS. Common bath preparations are:

1. Water alone
2. Linit starch, half a box to one tub. This is used for generalized dermatoses.
3. Aveeno colloidal oatmeal. This is used in the treatment of widespread poison ivy or oak dermatitis, diaper rash, atopic dermatitis, and contact dermatitis. One cup is added to a tub of warm water once or twice daily. For infants, 1 or 2 tablespoonfuls are added to the bathinette. The oilated type is not used for treatment of acute oozing dermatitis.
4. Soyaloid colloidal bath. This is a colloidal soya protein complex with 2 percent polyvinylpyrrolidone. It is very valuable for the treatment of diaper dermatitis, poison ivy or poison oak, and sunburn. One packet is dissolved in a tub of warm water, or 2 to 3 tablespoonfuls to each gallon of warm water for an infant's bath.

LUBRICATING BATHS.   These baths are useful for treatment of dry or pruritic skin as in atopic dermatitis. They can also be used after showering or sponge bathing, and also for general cleansing of the skin. Some lubricating baths are Alpha-Keri, Domol, Lubath, and Nutraspa.

Lotions.   Lotions are suspensions of a powder in liquid. As the liquid evaporates, a coating of powder remains on the skin surface. Evaporation cools the surface and the powder soothes, protects, and dries the skin. Lotions are useful in the treatment of acute dermatitis but must be avoided on oozing surfaces and in hairy or intertriginous areas. They are most often applied with fingers, gauze, or with a small paint brush, in which case they should be dispensed in a widemouthed bottle. They are applied evenly and removed by soaking, not by peeling, the dried material from the skin. If used for more than 3 or 4 days, shake lotions may cause chapping. The "caine-type" anesthetic lotions should be avoided because of potential sensitivity.

PREPARATIONS.   Some commonly used lotions are:

1. Aveeno Lotion. In acute and subacute dermatoses, Aveeno Lotion forms a flexible adherent coating which does not crack or flake off.
2. Calamine Lotion USP. Calamine lotion is inexpensive and has a wide and well-deserved reputation. Its disadvantages are that it tends to dry and to cake, especially in the presence of oozing.
3. Cetaphil Lotion. Cetaphil Lotion is a lipid-free lotion used commonly for atopic dermatitis. It is used as a waterless cleaner, for the relief of itching, and as a vehicle for various active ingredients, especially hydrocortisone.
4. Cordran Lotion. Cordran Lotion (flurandrenolide) is easy to apply and useful in acute and subacute dermatoses. It is rather expensive.
5. Kenalog Lotion. Kenalog Lotion (triamcinolone acetonide) is very effective for seborrheic dermatitis on the face and in the intertriginous areas.

Occlusive dressings.   Occlusive dressings are very effective in the treatment of chronic dermatitis, such as atopic dermatitis. Treatment usually is overnight for a period of 8 to 12 hours. No more than 10 percent of the body should be treated at any one time, since significant systemic absorption may occur, especially with the fluorinated corticosteroids. Complications include an objectionable odor, folliculitis, sweat retention, secondary irritation, and infection. Late sequelae may include atrophy and striae.

METHODS.   Some methods for applying occlusive dressings are as follows:

1. Topical steroids are covered with a thin plastic film followed by a covering of stockinette, cotton glove, stocking, T-shirt, pair of shorts, or Ace bandage.

2. Cordran tape is useful for the treatment of small and medium-sized lesions of chronic dermatoses. Before application the area must be cleansed gently to remove scales, crusts, dried exudate, and any traces of medications. Dry the skin thoroughly and apply the tape smoothly against the skin, usually leaving it in place for about 12 hours.

Open wet dressings (compresses and soaks).   Open wet dressings, the mildest form of topical therapy, cool the skin by evaporation, relieve itching, and clean the surface by loosening and removing crusts and debris. Used on acute blistered dermatitis, open wet dressings often may be the only treatment possible. The treatment ordinarily has a duration of 30 minutes to 1 hour, three to four times daily. Ordinary tap water is used and it is not necessary to sterilize the water or the dressings. The solution is kept at room temperature and mixed immediately before each treatment. It is not kept overnight, since it may become unstable and more concentrated on standing.

METHOD.   The method for applying wet dressings is as follows:

1. Kerlix gauze, plain gauze without absorbent cotton, thin white handkerchiefs, any soft cotton cloth, or strips of bed linen are used with a solution. See following section for solutions.

2. The dressings are moistened in the solution and applied, wet but not runny, flat and smooth against the skin of the affected area. They are left uncovered. One layer is usually sufficient. The fingers are wrapped separately; the arms and legs are wrapped so that the elbows and knees can bend. No more than

one third of the body is covered at a time, and chilling is avoided. The child must be comfortable during treatment and positioned so some form of play activity is possible.

3. When evaporation begins to dry the cloth, after 5 to 10 minutes, the entire dressing is removed, resoaked, and reapplied to the inflamed area. The solution is never poured directly over the dressings.

4. After treatment, the skin is dried by patting with a towel or washcloth. At this time a lotion or other medication may be applied.

5. Wet dressings are usually discontinued after 36 to 48 hours; if they are continued longer than this, drying of the skin can result.

SOLUTIONS. Solutions commonly used for open wet dressings include:

1. Water alone

2. Burow's solution. A 1:20 solution (i.e., 1 tbsp to 1 quart) is prepared by mixing one packet of powder or one tablet in 1 quart of tap water. The more concentrated solutions indicated on the package directions may be irritating. Burow's solution is mildly astringent and antiseptic and leaves a fresh, dry feeling.

3. Dalibour solution. The contents of one powder packet are dissolved in 1 quart of water, making a 1:16 solution.

4. Silver nitrate. A 0.1 percent to 0.25 percent solution for infected or ulcerated skin is used. Stains are removed by painting the skin with tincture of iodine, washing off, and rubbing with hypertonic saline.

5. Soyboro powder packets. One packet of powder in a quart of tap water provides a soothing and cleansing wet dressing combining Burow's solution with a soya protein complex. This preparation is highly acceptable to clients.

Prophylaxis of Allergy in Infancy

Onset of symptoms in a child of allergic parents may be significantly delayed by advising the following measures:

1. Breast feeding
2. Artificial feeding with soy formula
3. Exclusion of milk, citrus, eggs, beef, and wheat for the first 9 to 12 months
4. Introduction of new foods to the diet every 7 days, keeping a careful history of reactions
5. Exclusion of pets from the environment
6. Avoidance of feathers, jute, and Kapok in home furnishings
7. Filtration of heating outlet in child's room

While this subject is debatable, these measures can be practiced without risk and give the parent and primary health provider alternative approaches to the problem.

Psychologic Aspects of Allergy

Each client presenting with a complaint must be evaluated from an organic standpoint and on a psychologic basis. Psychiatric factors related to allergic diseases have been frequently misinterpreted and have led to much misinformation. When symptoms of allergy and of nervous tension are present, there are four major theoretical possibilities:

1. The allergy may cause the behavioral symptoms. For example, children with hay fever may misbehave and be resistant to normal discipline; the dyspnea of severe bronchial asthma is a frightening experience. Often relief from symptoms will greatly improve the behavior.
2. A psychic illness associated with a state of nervous irritability may accentuate the allergic symptoms. Psychic factors as well as weather changes, infection, and endocrine disturbances act as aggravating, secondary, or precipitating factors in the production of allergic symptoms. Commonly there will be a flare-up of allergic diseases following periods of stress. Immunologic and pharmacologic management alone will fail unless the psychologic aspects are considered.
3. The two conditions may have nothing other than a coincidental relationship. For example, it is not necessary to be emotionally unstable to have hay fever.

4. Both conditions may be due to some third factor or combination of factors. A genetic predisposition to both allergies and tensional stress merits consideration.

Results of studies (Patterson, 1972) have shown:

1. That there is not an allergic personality pattern
2. That chronically ill children with any major illness present with similar neurotic problems
3. That maternal rejection is no different in allergic illness than with other medical problems
4. That methodologic problems, lack of standardization of techniques of allergic and psychiatric treatment, and insufficient follow-up have hampered the meaningful interpretation of research results in this field

Counseling

The nature of allergic illness is both crisis-ridden and chronic, frequently producing anguish and stress within the family. Parental concerns which are most frequent are: contagiousness, disfigurement, malignancy, and inheritance. Reassurance plays an important role in the successful outcome of the therapeutic program. The nurse practitioner can be of great assistance to the child and to the family in the following ways:

• Be sure that the child and parents know exactly what is expected of them and give them explicit written directions.
• Explain the many aspects of the illness such as genetic basis, day-to-day management, psychologic factors, and prognosis.
• Explain that the amount of relief from symptoms is often in direct proportion to the thoroughness with which the allergens are removed from the environment or diet.
• Teach them safe and appropriate use of medications and when to seek medical assistance.
• Be aware that ideal situations may be recommended but that many families are unable to follow through with directions because of lack of understanding, lack of motivation, or pressures within the family.

- Recognize the difficulties faced and the impact on the family. Help them to find a level of symptom which is tolerable for the child that can be tolerated by the entire family.
- Maintain good communications. Be available to work with them when they encounter behavioral and discipline problems with the allergic child.
- Help them to recognize when hospitalization of the child is necessary.
- Keep informed of the hospitalized child's progress and relate the progress to the parents.
- Help parents to seek help from local agencies for counseling, household help, or financial aid.
- Visit the home to evaluate the physical and emotional climate or request help from the public health nurse agency.
- Act as liaison to the school for interpreting symptoms and treatment as necessary.

COMMON CLINICAL PROBLEMS

Allergic Skin Disorders

ALLERGIC DERMATITIS

Assessment. Allergic dermatitis is dermatitis that is caused by increased IgE antibodies (atopic reagins) as a result of hypersensitivity to specific allergens such as pollens, environmentals, and foods. The types of allergic dermatitis are atopic dermatitis and contact dermatitis.

The term "eczema" is used in a variety of ways in relation to skin disorders. Some use it to mean allergic dermatitis; some to mean atopic dermatitis; and others to mean any dermatitis or dermatosis. Eczema is a descriptive term and should be applied when describing the typical rash of atopic dermatitis. See this chapter, Atopic Dermatitis.

CLINICAL FINDINGS. The symptoms of allergic dermatitis are as follows:

1. Acute form: erythema, edema, oozing, and crusting vesiculation

2. Chronic form: dryness, scaliness, *hyperkeratosis* (thickening of the keratinized layer of the skin, the stratum corneum), and *lichenification* (thickening of the skin with exaggeration of its normal markings so that striae form a crisscross pattern; it is a response to chronic rubbing and scratching)

3. Both forms: pruritus. This is the most important single nonspecific factor that leads to histopathologic changes in the skin. Some individuals have a low threshold of tolerance, scratch easily, and traumatize the skin; to others the intensity of itching depends on the intensity of the allergic reaction, or even the emotional state of the individual.

SECONDARY INFECTION. Secondary infection of dermatitic skin may be subtle and easily overlooked. Children with atopic dermatitis are particularly likely to develop secondary pyogenic infection. Often the dermatitis is improved following childhood communicable diseases. It will recur after convalescence from the secondary disease; the reason is not known. Infants with allergic dermatitis are very susceptible to infection with herpes virus (see Chapter 29, Viral Infections) and vaccinia virus. Strict avoidance of individuals with either herpes or recent vaccination is necessary. *Neither children with dermatitis nor their siblings should be vaccinated for smallpox.*

LABORATORY FINDINGS. Those common to the diagnosis of allergic dermatitis are:

1. Atopic reactivity (increased IgE antibodies). These are generally found on skin testing.

2. Eosinophilia. More than 10 percent is common in association with allergic dermatitis. (Eosinophilia is the accumulation of unusual numbers of eosinophil cells in the blood or in nasal or ear secretions.)

3. Streptococci or staphylococci. These are commonly revealed on cultures of the skin.

Management. Most of the management of children with allergic dermatitis can be assumed by the nurse practitioner. Consultation is recommended for severe or complicated cases and when corticosteroids are indicated. Referral to a specialist is recommended for management by immunotherapy. See this chapter, Immunotherapy. Treatment may also include diet and environmental control, prevention of pruritus, and topical and systemic therapies.

DIET AND ENVIRONMENTAL CONTROL. See this chapter, Diet Control, and Environmental Control.

PREVENTION OF PRURITUS. Measures that help to prevent scratching and further itching are as follows:

1. Fingernails are cut short; elbows are splinted as needed; and the bed is covered with a thick plastic sheet to prevent rubbing.
2. Cotton clothing and socks are worn; wool is an irritant.
3. Exposure of the child to heat, cold, wind, moisture, sunlight, physical effort, or emotional disturbances is avoided as possible.

TOPICAL TREATMENT. (See this chapter, Pharmacologic Therapy.) Topical treatment is managed as follows:

1. Cool compresses or soaks are helpful for small areas of involvement.
2. Tepid baths are used for generalized involvement. Given two to four times daily for 10 to 20 minutes, the times are reduced as the condition improves. Cetaphil Lotion may be used following the baths.
3. Topical steroids may be used for small areas of involvement. The "use" test is employed.
4. General use of soap and water is avoided. Dehydration of the skin tends to improve allergic dermatitis; overhydration to make it worse. The use of a waterless cleanser such as Cetaphil Lotion is recommended.
5. Lotions, oils, or greasy ointments should not be used on the affected areas. These can cause increased itchiness and redness.

SYSTEMIC TREATMENT. (See this chapter, Pharmacologic Therapy.) Systemic treatment is managed as follows:

1. Pruritus and/or burning pain are reduced with aspirin, usually in combination with antihistamines. "Caine" anesthetics may produce further sensitization.
2. Secondary infection is handled with antibiotics.
3. Sedation can be achieved with antihistamines.
4. Severe and extensive cases are treated with corticosteroids.

COUNSELING. Parents should be reminded that these children need care and affection. They should be played with, held, and cuddled. For further counseling measures see this chapter, Counseling, and Psychological Aspects of Allergy.

ATOPIC DERMATITIS, INFANTILE

Assessment. Infantile atopic dermatitis is a form of allergic dermatitis. Its onset is commonly associated with the introduction of new foods to the diet, especially milk and eggs, but it may be due to environmentals such as wool, dust, and others. It is uncommon in breast-fed babies. See this chapter, Milk Allergy.

INCIDENCE. Infantile atopic dermatitis rarely appears before 6 weeks of age, more often after 2 or 3 months of age. There is a strong familial history.

CLINICAL FINDINGS. The rash of atopic dermatitis develops in the following pattern:

1. The initial lesion is a small erythematous, papular patch over one or both cheeks.
2. There is intensification of the redness, coalescence of lesions, and development of minute vesicles which give the skin a ground-glass appearance.
3. Oozing and weeping of the lesions become pronounced and the drying exudate forms honey-colored crusts.
4. Excoriation which appears as denuded, raw, and bleeding patches results from itching, scratching, and rubbing.

Table 7

Distinguishing Characteristics of Atopic Dermatitis, Seborrheic Dermatitis, and Contact Dermatitis

	Atopic Dermatitis	Seborrheic Dermatitis	Contact Dermatitis
Age of onset	After 2 months	Any age	Any age
Family history of eczema or asthma	Positive	Negative	May be either
Cause	Allergenic	Nonallergenic	May be either
Clinical features	Erythema, edema, oozing, crusting, vesiculation, or lichenification	Erythema, yellowish, scaly lesions; may ooze and crust	Slight to intense erythema; vesicles, or bullae
Distribution	Cheeks, forehead, limbfolds; may extend to extremities and torso	Scalp, forehead, behind and in ears; chest, neck, and axilla	Exposed areas, regional areas, diaper area; may be unilateral
Pruritus	Marked	Mild	Slight to burning pain
Prognosis	May lead to severe dermatitis or asthma	Clears with treatment	Clears with treatment

5. Nodes near the affected areas may become enlarged. This may be due to an immune response; the nodes are neither tender nor suppurative.

6. Secondary infection of bacterial or viral origin may occur. It is usually low-grade; impetigo is the most common; upper respiratory infections are also common.

PROGRESSION OF THE DISEASE. The rash begins on the face and forehead but soon extends to the neck, the postauricular areas, and particularly to the bends of the arms (anticubital fossae) and the legs (popliteal fossae). With a more severe reaction, the torso or entire body may show involvement. The circumoral and periorbital regions, and diaper area may be free of rash. The disease may continue without remission for the first 2 years of life, or it may wax and wane with brief periods of clearing of the skin. As the second year approaches, the disease may clear spontaneously. If it continues, the lesions may lose their acute character and become a mixture of acute and chronic forms.

DIFFERENTIAL DIAGNOSIS. Skin disorders that resemble infantile atopic dermatitis (see Table 7) and must be ruled out include:

1. Contact dermatitis
2. Seborrheic dermatitis

Management. The treatment of infantile atopic dermatitis is essentially the same as that which is outlined for allergic dermatitis. See this chapter, Allergic Dermatitis, for indications for consultation and referral, prevention of pruritus, topical and systemic treatments, and counseling.

ATOPIC DERMATITIS, CHILDHOOD

Assessment. (See also this chapter, Allergic Dermatitis.) Atopic dermatitis which occurs beyond the age of 2 or 3 has a more chronic character. It may continue from infancy; however, infantile atopic dermatitis usually clears spontaneously by 2 years of age. It may be caused by environmental allergens and, sometimes, food. A history of familial allergens or infantile atopic dermatitis is common.

CLINICAL FINDINGS. The skin, which assumes chronic characteristics of the disease, appears as follows:

1. Lesions appear with scaling papules with crusted summits, hypertrophy, and lichenification.
2. The skin may become leathery, fissured, and striated.
3. A greyish discoloration of the involved area is frequently observed.
4. Scratch marks capped with crusted blood are present.
5. Itching may become intolerable. Itching is caused by obstruction of the sweat glands and occurs in any situation which causes increased sweating.

PROGNOSIS. Atopic dermatitis is subject to remission and may reappear at pubescence, adolescence, and/or young adulthood.

Management. The treatment of atopic dermatitis is essentially the same as that for allergic dermatitis. See this chapter, Allergic Dermatitis, for indications for consultation or referral, prevention of pruritus, topical or systemic treatment, and counseling.

CONTACT DERMATITIS

Assessment. (See also this chapter, Allergic Dermatitis.) Contact dermatitis can be classified as:

1. *Nonallergic or irritant.* This form is induced by any substance that is irritating to the skin. The mechanism is either mechanical or chemical. Any part of the body may be affected, and the intensity of the skin reaction depends on the strength of the irritant and the duration of the exposure. The skin response is immediate with no history of previous exposure.
2. *Allergic.* This is a manifestation of the delayed type of hypersensitivity. The latent period, the period of no reactivity, may extend to weeks or longer.

ETIOLOGY. Contact dermatitis can be induced by anyone holding the child, through bedding or floor material, or from such items as plastic toys or foods. See below, Suggested Contactants. A careful history of exposure to offending agents is taken.

CLINICAL FINDINGS. Common positive signs of contact dermatitis in infancy are involvement of only one cheek, or involvement of knees, anterior surfaces of legs, anterior abdomen, and chest (from crawling on floor). Other signs are as follows:

1. Lesions may range from slight erythema to intense redness, through various degrees of inflammation, and from vesiculation to bullae.
2. Pruritus, at times burning and painful, may be evident.
3. Hypertrophy, hyperplasia, and lichenification may be present.
4. Regional distribution can be a clue.

SUGGESTED CONTACTANTS. Some regional areas with suggested contactants (adapted from Feingold, 1973, p. 132) are:

1. Forehead. Hat bands
2. Eyes. Eyedrops
3. Eyelids. Fingernail polish, hair dyes, rinses, shampoos, cosmetics of all kinds
4. Ears. Perfumes, shafts of eyeglass frames (postauricular eruption)
5. Nose. Eyeglass frames
6. Face and neck. Smoke of burning poison oak or ivy; aerosol sprays, paint sprays, dusts, and pollens
7. Neck. Scarves, coat, permanent press garments
8. Apex of the axilla. Antiperspirants, deodorants, clothing, fabric dyes, and permanent press materials
9. Arms. Lateral surfaces from leaning on plastic, lacquered or varnished table or desk tops, or chromium trim on tables. Forearm from ladies purses. Whole arm from clothes lining; inner aspect of arm from upholstered material.
10. Body. Girdles, bras, garter belts, cosmetics, suntan lotions, or pollens (the exposed parts of the body)

11. Ano-genital region. Suppositories, contraceptives, douches, rectal and vaginal discharges, perfumes, soaps, bubble bath, and detergents

12. Legs (lateral surfaces). Floor covering

13. Feet. Shoes, the glue and dye; foot powders and deodorants

Management. Rapid clearing of the skin usually follows elimination of the offending contactant. Patch testing is limited to children for whom the elimination of the suspected items has not been successful. Further treatment of contact dermatitis is essentially the same as that which is outlined for allergic dermatitis. See this chapter, Allergic Dermatitis, for indications for consultation or referral, prevention of pruritus, topical or systemic treatment, and counseling.

Bites of Arachnids and Insects

Insects attack by direct bites, penetrating stings, injected venom, or tunnel-like burrows. The skin reaction to the bite itself is due to hypersensitivity and is species specific. There may be an immediate or delayed response. The first step in diagnosis is to determine if the eruption is an expression of a systemic disease such as varicella, response to allergens, or is an insect bite. Clues come from careful history, geography, season, and knowledge of the environment. Distribution of the lesions is a clue; mosquito, gnat, fly, flea, and hornet bites appear on exposed parts of the body; body parasites establish themselves in covered areas; different insects can have identical appearing lesions.

BITES OF ARACHNIDA

The class Arachnida includes spiders, scorpions, mites, and ticks.

Black widow spider bite

ASSESSMENT. Black widow spider venom is neurotoxic, causing ascending paralysis and destruction of peripheral nerve endings. These spiders like dark places such as wood piles and latrines; they may bite on genitalia or buttocks. The black widow spider has a red hourglass configuration on its abdomen.

Clinical findings. These include:

1. Local reaction. Pin-prick sensation is felt at the instant of the bite followed by a dull pain. Two puncture points will be surrounded by redness and edema.

2. Early systemic reactions. Child may feel comfortable in the period immediately following the bite until abdominal rigidity, becoming boardlike, develops in 15 to 30 minutes.

3. Later systemic reactions. Manifestations are weakness, tremor, sweating, and salivation. Skin becomes extremely sensitive. Excruciating pain develops in limbs. Bradycardia and feeble pulse follow. Child may groan persistently and have expiratory grunt. Temperature and blood pressure are often elevated. Stupor, delirium, and convulsions may occur especially in small children. Death can occur if treatment is delayed.

MANAGEMENT. Treatment is carried out collaboratively with a physician. It consists of the following:

1. Local. Local treatment is usually ineffective and unnecessary, although the child may be made comfortable if the area is cleansed with antiseptic and ice is applied. *Do not apply tourniquet or attempt to remove venom by incision and suction.* The child should be hospitalized or taken to a medical facility as quickly as possible.

2. Supportive. Prolonged warm bath and injections of calcium gluconate and barbiturates are given immediately and prn to control muscle pain. Venom can cause respiratory paralysis, and these drugs are respiratory depressants.

3. Antivenom. Symptoms usually subside within 3 hours following injection. The dose for adults and children is the entire contents of a restored vial (2.5 ml) of antivenin. Without fail, test for equine serum hypersensitivity. Antivenin may be given intravenously in 10 to 50 ml of saline solution over a 15-minute period. It is the preferred route in severe cases, or when the child is under 12 years, or is in shock.

4. Prevention. Area may be sprayed with Malathon.

Brown recluse spider bite

ASSESSMENT.   Venom is necrotoxic and, in severe cases, hemo-lytic. This spider is also called house spider and has a violin-shaped configuration on its back.

Clinical findings.   Symptoms are as follows:

1.   Local reaction. Mild stinging is felt at instant of bite. Erythem-atous vesicle develops with ischemic center.
2.   Intermediate local reaction. Mild to severe pain develops in 2 to 8 hours.
3.   Later local and systemic reactions. Star-shaped area develops in 3 to 4 days which changes to deep purple eschar, firm to the touch. Within 2 weeks the area becomes depressed leaving a disfiguring scar. Generalized reactions may occur such as fever or scarlatiniform rash. Hemolysis can occur and be fatal.

MANAGEMENT.   Treatment is managed collaboratively with a physician as follows:

1.   Local. Mild local symptoms do not require treatment at the site.
2.   Supportive. If the child reports to a physician within 24 hours, administration of parenteral antihistamine and a steroid may limit the effect of necrotoxin to the surface of the bitten area, may prevent fatal systemic reactions, and may minimize depth of the disfiguring scar.

Scorpion bite

ASSESSMENT.   A wound is caused by the sting. Venom consists of neurotoxin, cardiac toxin, and agglutinins. The scorpion is often seen and should be caught for identification whenever feasible.

Clinical findings.   Symptoms are as follows:

1.   Local reaction. A sharp pain followed by local "pins-and-needles" sensation is felt. No swelling or discoloration is seen.
2.   Systemic reaction. Itching of the nose, mouth, and throat de-velops, with speech impairment if no immediate first aid mea-sures have been given. Numbness and weakness generally occur in affected limb. Lymphangitis and lymphadenitis may

be observed proximal to the wound. Severe reactions are characterized by involuntary twitching progressing to muscular spasms with pain, nausea, vomiting, and convulsions. Symptoms may last through 48 hours. If not fatal in 3 hours, prognosis is optimistic. Fatalities are frequent in children under 3 years.

MANAGEMENT. Treatment should be started instantly as follows:

1. Local, at site

   • An icebag is applied locally or the bitten extremity is immersed in ice water.
   • A tourniquet is applied (with momentary releases). This will slow down the absorption of the toxin. The wound should not be incised nor suction applied. The body is kept warm. Opiates are not given. Injections of barbiturates or calcium gluconate solution may be given to control convulsions.

2. Antivenom. Antevenin is particularly indicated for children. (A specific antivenom for southwest scorpions is prepared by Laboratories Myn, Av. Coyoacan 1707, Mexico 12, D.F.)

Chigger (mite) bites

ASSESSMENT. The usual mite is the almost invisible red larva of the "harvest mite" or "red bug." They abound in tall grass, decaying matter, and underbrush. They adhere to clothing, and finally attach themselves to areas covered by clothing or near hair follicles or sweat glands. They pierce the skin, suck off tissue juices, and fall off. They may be identified with a hand lens as tiny red dots.

Clinical picture. The symptoms are intense itching; formation of a macule, papule, vesicle, or wheal, 1 to 2 cm in diameter; secondary infection as a result of scratching.

MANAGEMENT. This consists of reducing the itching and prophylaxis against bacterial infection. See this chapter, Pharmacologic Therapy. Treatment consists of the following measures:

1. Itching is reduced with starch baths, calamine lotion, topical anesthetics, and the use of oral antihistamine with aspirin.

2. Tension is relieved and sleep is supported with a mild barbiturate.
3. Infection is prevented with bacitracin or neomycin ointments.
4. Insect-repellent agents are sprayed on clothing and skin to safeguard the individual who has to go through mite-infested areas.

Tick bites

ASSESSMENT. The Wood Tick, the Eastern Tick, and the Lone Star Tick cause toxic manifestations. They live on dogs or in the woods. They climb up clothing and attach themselves to the neck for a meal. At times the bite can be painful; usually the child is unaware.

Clinical findings. These are:

1. Local reaction. The lesion at the site of attachment becomes red and indurated. Petechial hemorrhages may be noted. The tick may be attached.
2. Systemic reaction. The child experiences flaccidity and a slowly ascending motor and sensory paralysis, which can culminate fatally. Removing the tick reverses the symptoms.

Complications. A rare complication of tick bite is Rocky Mountain Spotted Fever. A rickettsial infection, it is transmitted by the bites of certain species of ticks if they themselves are infected. It occurs in late spring and early summer. The incubation period is 2 to 14 days. Any child who becomes ill with fever and chills after a known tick bite should be observed for a macular skin rash which will occur 2 to 4 days after the prodromal symptoms.

MANAGEMENT. See this chapter, Pharmacologic Therapy. Treatment consists of the following measures:

1. The tick is removed (do not crush) with a forceps after the application of alcohol or oil. Incomplete removal can lead to the formation of a nodule requiring surgical incision.
2. The locale is treated as necessary for itching or pain.

3. Appropriate emergency and supportive treatment is given for paralysis.

BITES OF SIPHONAPTERA

The insect order Siphonaptera includes human and dog fleas.

Assessment. Bites are in a zigzag pattern. Lesions are usually found on the arms or legs or in areas where the clothing fits tightly. Diagnosis of papular urticaria from flea bites is confirmed by:

- Seasonal incidence
- Distribution of lesions
- Presence of household pets
- Abatement of eruptions when child is removed from suspected source.

CLINICAL FINDINGS. Symptoms are as follows:

1. The lesions appear grouped in an irregular pattern producing itching and papular urticarial eruptions, some with a central punctum.
2. The lesions are 3 to 10 mm in size and are often excoriated from scratching.
3. The secondary infection is often impetigo.

Management. See this chapter, Pharmacologic Therapy. Treatment consists of the following measures:

1. Itching is relieved with cool, wet compresses; applications of topical steroid or spray; and oral antihistamines and aspirin.
2. Secondary infections require topical antibiotic ointment.
3. Hyposensitization may be instituted for repeated attacks of papular urticaria.
4. Pets are dusted with flea powder and given flea collars.
5. Residual insect sprays are used for severe household infestations.

STINGS OF HYMENOPTERA

The insect order Hymenoptera includes hornet, honey-bee, wasp, and yellow jacket.

Assessment. The yellow jacket is more likely to produce anaphylaxis, followed by bee, wasp, and hornet stings. Only female Hymenoptera sting, and only the honey bee has a barbed stinger which it is unable to withdraw, leaving a portion of the venom sac at the site. (This should not be picked off with a forceps, but should be flicked off, to keep the venom from being squeezed further into the bite.) Wasp, hornet, and yellow jacket stings are frequently infected by bacteria. Severe reactions are more likely to occur in persons over 30 years of age. August is the month in which the greater number of reactions occur. Reactions are as follows:

1. Local reaction. This consists of sharp pain, local edema, redness with later induration, and itchy swelling for days. A detached "stinger" can be identified sometimes as a black dot at the center. When the bite is on loose tissue such as the eyelid, the edema and redness may be very pronounced.
2. Systemic reaction. These symptoms are generally present within 15 minutes of the sting, and almost always within 1 hour. In decreasing order of frequency they are: dyspnea, weakness, feelings of anxiety, nausea, abdominal cramps, loss of consciousness, and anaphylactic shock.

Management. This may consist of treatment of anaphylaxis or mild reaction, and prevention.

TOXIC REACTION. The treatment is that for anaphylactic shock and is managed collaboratively with a physician. See Chapter 30, Anaphylaxis. When the lesion is on an extremity, a tourniquet should be applied proximally to slow absorption. The stinger should be picked off except for the honey bee which should be flicked off. Ice will slow absorption and should be applied. A soluble antihistamine should be injected also to prevent further absorption. The child should be removed to a medical facility.

MILD REACTION. Local applications of alcohol, ice, or a 10 percent solution of ammonia may relieve pain temporarily and calm a frightened child. Uncomfortable and persistent itching is treated with aspirin in combination with an antihistamine.

PREVENTION. Preventive measures (adapted from Patterson, 1972, p. 326) include the following:

1. Shoes should be worn out-of-doors at all times.
2. Dark clothing should be avoided; white is preferred.
3. Clothes should fit close to the body. Insects can become trapped in loose-fitting clothing.
4. Scented soaps or cosmetics should be avoided.
5. Insect feeding grounds (flower beds, fields of clover, garbage, and orchards with ripe fruit should be avoided).
6. Automobile windows should be closed. Aside from the possibility of actually being stung, stinging insects in a car can arouse such terror in a sting-sensitive driver as to make him or her an irresponsible driver.
7. If it is necessary to dispose of garbage, the area should first be sprayed with an effective, rapid-acting insecticide.
8. Wasp or hornet nests or bee hives noted in the vicinity of the home should be destroyed by a professional exterminator.
9. A survival kit should be available. Every child known to be exquisitely sensitive to insect stings should carry a survival kit and be taught to use it immediately after a sting. The kit contains: a) a tourniquet, b) 25 mg tablets of ephedrine combined with an antihistamine, c) alcohol sponges, d) a syringe with attached needle containing 1:1000 epinephrine solution. The child should wear a Medic-Alert tag identifying him or her as allergic to insect stings.

URTICARIA

Assessment. Urticaria is a mechanism of hive formation: tissue fluid leaks into tissues and causes raised, edematous areas. They seem to be expressions of sensitivity to an irritant or allergen of some sort, although this cannot always be identified. There is a familial factor. Skin tests are generally of little value. These children do not usually have eosinophilia and sometimes give no other signs of being allergic. Chronic urticaria is not associated with atopy and may not have an allergic etiology.

CLINICAL FINDINGS. The wheals are of variable sizes. They are usually multiple and may be painful or stinging. They may change in size and shape within hours or may lie in deep tissue layers of the skin and cause large areas of swelling in such parts as the face (angioedema), an extremity, the back, the throat, or the scrotum.

CAUSATIVE AGENTS. These are as follows:

1. Alcohol
2. Allergies
3. Cancers, lymphomas, and leukemias (rare)
4. Cosmetics, soaps, and lotions
5. Foods (strawberries, spicy foods, peanuts, butter, and dairy products)
6. Insect bites (mosquito bite)
7. Low-grade infection (strep throat, cystitis)
8. Medications (long-lasting penicillin, sulfas, antibiotics, aspirin)
9. Sunlight, extremes of heat or cold, emotions, and exercise

TYPES OF URTICARIA. These include:

1. Angioedema. This presents as subcutaneous edema. It is seen on the eyes, the cheeks, the ear lobes, and the genitalia and may lead to anaphylaxis.
2. Papular urticaria. This is seen on the extensor muscles of the arms and legs or on the trunk. It comes seasonally and is due to insect bites.
3. Erythema multiforme. It is an allergic reaction. It forms papules and is bullous.

Management. Systemic and long-term treatment is managed collaboratively with a physician. Treatment consists of the following:

1. Local
   - Calamine lotion is applied. Topical antihistamines, such as Caladryl, are never applied because they are potent sensitizers.
   - Lukewarm or cool water is helpful. Extremes of hot and cold are avoided.

- Starch baths may be given.
- Antihistamines and aspirin are given for itching.
- If infection is the basic cause, the urticaria will disappear as the infection is treated.

2. Systemic. Treatment is for anaphylaxis. See Chapter 30, Anaphylaxis.

Food Allergies

Food allergy occurs more frequently in infants and children than in adults. It is believed that the frequency of food allergy in children is due to incompletely digested food protein which passes into the circulatory system. Food allergies should be suspected in cases of urticaria, angioedema, suspected gastrointestinal allergy, unexplained and sporadic respiratory allergies, and atopic dermatitis.

TYPES OF REACTIONS

The two types of reactions to food allergies are described as follows:

1. The rapid appearance of symptoms which appear within a few minutes after the offending food is eaten; a reaction may occur before the food is swallowed. Fish and seafoods, berries (especially strawberries), nuts, and sometimes egg white are the most common offenders.
2. A delayed reaction in which hours or, rarely, a day or more elapse between ingestion of the allergen and the appearance of the symptoms.

COMMON FOOD ALLERGENS

Foods which are commonly responsible for allergic reactions are wheat, corn, milk, eggs, beef, white potato, orange, pork, chocolate, and legumes. Almost all foods may be responsible for allergic reactions. Although reactions to chocolate are observed, this is not a strong antigen and does not deserve the reputation it has as a very common cause of food allergy.

FACTORS IN DIAGNOSIS OF FOOD ALLERGY

Factors that should be considered in diagnosing food allergy are:

1. Quantitative factor. Small amounts of food can be tolerated without difficulty whereas larger amounts will precipitate symptoms.
2. Degree of cooking. Rare-cooked or raw foods are more allergenic.
3. Cumulative factor. The child may react if allergenic foods are eaten on successive days.
4. Cyclic factor. After a reaction there may be a refraction period during which ingestion of the allergen will not provoke symptoms.
5. Multiplicity factor. A reaction may occur if several foods to which child is allergic are eaten at the same time, but not if eaten separately.

GASTROINTESTINAL ALLERGIES IN INFANCY

Assessment. Many infant feeding problems can be attributed to allergy. Milk is the primary offender; other common allergens are egg, wheat, and citrus. This disturbance occurs mainly in artificially fed infants, and rarely in breast-fed infants. However, if large amounts of one food such as orange juice or eggs are ingested by the mother, the allergen can be transmitted via the breast milk to the child. A careful diet history and behavioral history are taken. Food allergies should be suspected in infants with signs and symptoms that do not clear in a reasonable length of time.

CLINICAL FINDINGS.   Infants may show these signs:

1. Irritability and fussiness
2. Crying and pain which is spasmodic and similar to colic
3. Spitting up
4. Loose stools
5. Constipation

PROGNOSIS.   In some infants this problem will abate after the first or second year. In others the area of involvement may change to problems of the skin, respiratory tract, or ear. If symptoms appear in later life, consideration is given to the possibility that the identical allergens are the cause.

Management. The goals of management include:

1. Removal of the offending food (see this chapter, Diet Control). This usually brings quick relief.
2. Substitution of commercial cow milk formula with soy milk formula. All soy milk formulas contain corn oil (a known sensitizer) except Neo-Mull-Soy (Borden), and I-soyalac (Loma Linda).
3. Control of the mother's diet if allergy is suspected in the breast-fed infant.
4. Consideration of environmental factors if the infant fails to respond to dietary changes.

MILK ALLERGY

Assessment. See also Chapter 21, Malabsorption: Disaccharide Deficiencies. Milk intolerance occurs in 0.3 to 7 percent of all children. In infancy milk intolerance is attributed to the increased permeability of the gut which permits passage of undigested proteins into the serum. The cow milk protein, casein, found in commercially prepared infant formula and fresh cow milk, is the sensitizing agent. Contamination of milk with extraneous substances such as fodder containing grasses and pollens can be a factor in cow milk. Breast milk is not allergenic; however, foods eaten by the mother, especially egg, may be excreted in the milk to produce symptoms in allergic children.

CLINICAL FINDINGS. Milk intolerance symptoms may include:

1. Frequent loose stools, colic, and gas
2. Frequent upper respiratory infections, especially serous otitis media
3. Skin manifestations such as allergic dermatitis
4. Allergic rhinitis or bronchial asthma in older children

PROGNOSIS. Milk allergy may subside at about 2 to 3 years of age. Children with early milk allergy may develop other manifestations of allergy in later life, and the former intolerance should be a consideration in the diagnosis.

Management.   Milk intolerance in infancy is managed by the elimination of all milk products from the diet.

INFANCY.   These measures should be taken:

1. Cow milk or cow milk formula is substituted with breast milk or soy milk formula. See also this chapter, Gastrointestinal Allergies in Infancy.
2. If soy is not tolerated, meat-base formula (MBF, Gerber) can be substituted. Because of cross reactivity between beef and milk, meat-base formula may not be tolerated.
3. When the infant starts to eat solid foods, a diet is followed which excludes wheat, eggs, fish, milk, and beef for at least 9 to 12 months. At that time, these foods may be started very slowly introducing one food at a time in small, increasing amounts.

CHILDHOOD.   A milk-free diet is followed being careful to read labels of all foods not prepared at home. It is recommended that foods be home prepared. See Table 4, Milk-Free Diet.

Ocular Allergies

ACUTE ALLERGIC CONJUNCTIVITIS

Assessment.   Allergic conjunctivitis is one of the most common forms of eye allergy. The airborne allergens induce immediate reactivity. A swab of eye scrapings may show marked eosinophils.

TYPES OF ALLERGIC CONJUNCTIVITIS.   These include:

1. Atopic. The usual causes are pollens, dust, animal hair, and occasionally foods.
2. Drug. The most common offenders are atropine and neomycin.
3. Vernal. It occurs in spring and summer in older children and adolescents.

CLINICAL FINDINGS. These include acute and chronic symptoms. Acute symptoms which are almost always bilateral and rarely occur as an isolated event, include:

1. Marked injection and redness of the conjunctivae
2. Edema of the mucosa and profuse tearing, at first watery but may later become mucopurulent
3. Intense itching, burning, rubbing, and occasional pain of varying degrees.
4. Edema and pallor of the nasal mucosa.

Chronic symptoms are:

1. Itching and burning
2. Photophobia and dryness

Management. Generally, a search is made for the causative agents through smears and conjunctival scrapings. The child is placed on broad-spectrum antibiotics or sulfonamides while awaiting the results of the cultures.

MEDICATIONS. Drugs used in treatment are as follows:

1. Topical medication (drops) may be given as often as every 2 hours for severe reactions. The usual frequency is every 4 hours.
2. In young children eye ointment is easier to apply with less chance of overdosage. Older children tolerate drops during the day.
3. Antihistamines afford some relief in mild cases. Failure to respond to antihistamines suggests an infection.

COUNSELING. The parents are taught the correct procedure for instilling topical eye medications. Explanations are provided about the causative agent, expected results of medication (see Chapter 16, The Eye), handwashing techniques to decrease contagion, and symptoms of increased severity of the disorder, such as fever, increased discharge, keratitis, and erythema.

Respiratory Allergies

ALLERGIC RHINITIS

Assessment. In infancy allergic rhinitis may be due to hypersensitivity to food caused by reaginic antibody, IgE, or occasionally to inhalant factors. After 1 or 2 years it can be traced to environmental factors as dust, feathers, animal danders, house plants, or molds. When the symptoms persist throughout the year, the condition is known as allergic rhinitis; when the symptoms occur seasonally from pollens, the condition is known as "hay fever." The symptoms are sometimes worse in the winter when the child spends more time indoors.

CLINICAL FINDINGS. These include acute symptoms as well as other more chronic signs.

Acute symptoms are:

1. Stopped-up, itchy nose
2. Paroxysms of sneezing
3. Irritating, watery, nasal discharge
4. Conjunctivitis
5. Possible sore throat, hoarseness, and thirst
6. Irritable and short-tempered disposition
7. Possible headache

Chronic signs are:

1. The "allergic salute" and "allergic shiner"
2. Thicker nasal discharge. Some children may develop nasal polyps in later childhood.
3. Swollen and pale nasal mucous membranes which may partially or completely block the passages
4. Red and excoriated nares
5. Thickened nasal sinuses
6. Inflammatory sinusitis with a purulent discharge due to complication with bacterial infection
7. Conjunctivae may show evidences of chronic irritation such as itchiness and dryness

SKIN TESTING. Testing for food allergens is unreliable. Testing for pollens and environmentals is reliable and may be instituted if the history so indicates.

Management. Initially the treatment is aimed at making the child comfortable; later the offending allergens may be sought by skin testing and hyposensitization may be instituted. Diet and environmental control may be instituted.

MEDICATIONS. Decongestants are given to relieve swelling and to promote drainage. Antihistamines are given to relieve itching. Antibiotics are given to treat chronic infections. Sometimes this will interrupt the vicious cycle of allergic reaction and infection. Applications of corticosteroids may be used to treat nasal polyps.

SURGICAL INTERVENTION. Chronic infections or polyposis may be indications for surgical intervention as follows:

1. Chronic ear infection may need myringotomy.
2. Chronically infected tonsils and adenoids may be removed, but this is done only when all other methods fail to control the obstructions or infections.
3. Nasal or sinus polyps may be removed.

HAY FEVER

Assessment. The name hay fever is a legacy from earlier times. "Fever" was a term for illness, and "hay" pointed to the relationship to grasses and harvesting. It is an allergic (reaginic antibody, IgE) reaction to one or more inhalants, typically very small windborne pollens. The condition is known as "hay fever" when pollens are in the air. When the symptoms persist throughout the year, the condition is called allergic rhinitis.

INCIDENCE. Hay fever usually starts in late childhood or early adolescence. Skin lesions of atopic dermatitis usually fade away at about the time hay fever begins. Offending pollens, early in the spring, are mainly from birches, oak, alders, and hazels. Grass pollens are less time-related. One may have symptoms from timothy, redtop, orchard, sweet vernal, blue grass, Russian thistle, sugar-beet, and ragweeds. Ragweed is the primary offender in the eastern and midwestern United States and occurs in the autumn. Pollens tend to be thrown off on sunny days and are carried miles by the wind. Many children have their worst symptoms after sundown.

CLINICAL FINDINGS. The symptoms are usually of an acute nature such as:

1. Stopped-up, itchy nose
2. Paroxysms of sneezing
3. Irritating, watery, nasal discharge
4. Congested and tearing conjunctivae
5. Hoarseness and thirst, possible sore throat
6. Irritable disposition
7. Possible headache
8. Possible cough
9. Bronchitis or asthma

SKIN TESTING. This is usually reliable for pollen.

Management. This is directed initially at easing the discomforts of the ailment. Environmental control may be instituted. Later skin testing may be done followed by hyposensitization.

MEDICATIONS. Decongestants are given to relieve swelling and to promote drainage. Antihistamines are given to relieve itching. Systemic antibiotics or sulfonamides are used to treat secondary infections.

PREVENTION. Preventive measures which are also part of the treatment are as follows:

- The child should be kept indoors in the evenings, on windy days where possible, and when the pollen count is especially high.
- Windows that face the winds should be kept closed.
- The child's room should be air-conditioned using a fine-meshed, "anti-allergy" air filter.

- Automobile rides, especially to the country, should be avoided.
- Open land near the home should be cleared of suspected weeds, grasses, and plants.
- Written notes should be kept of the dates of onset and subsidence of hay fever symptoms in the child. The pattern after 1 or more years will be a valuable clue to the caretaker.

ALLERGIC BRONCHITIS

Assessment. In allergic bronchitis the tracheobronchial mucous membrane is chronically sensitized and irritated by continued exposure to molds, pollens, danders, and dusts. The irritated membranes are more readily invaded by bacteria, and the lower respiratory infection is difficult to cure. Sometimes an upper respiratory infection will trigger the bronchial symptoms. If it becomes chronic, permanent bronchial damage may result leading to bronchiectasis.

CLINICAL FINDINGS. Symptoms and signs are:

1. Cough, the most prominent sign, that tends to be worse at night
2. Malaise and loss of appetite
3. Wheezing or rhonchi
4. Sibilant or musical rales

DIFFERENTIAL DIAGNOSIS. Because the cough is the most distinctive feature of allergic bronchitis it may be confused with other diseases. These diseases should be ruled out:

1. Acute bronchitis. Cough with sudden onset and fever, wheezing, and sibilant rales is not necessarily associated with allergies. This illness may develop following flu or similar virulent respiratory tract infection and may last a week or more or may exhibit other features (including X-ray changes) indicative of bronchopneumonia.
2. Chronic bronchitis. This manifests with a persistent dry cough without malaise or fever, with the chest negative on physical or X-ray examination.

3. Chronically infected tonsils, adenoids, or nasal sinuses. Postnasal drip is a symptom.
4. Pertussis cough. This is a paroxysmal cough not always terminated with a distinctive "whoop."
5. Cystic fibrosis cough. This is paroxysmal with wheezing from viscid mucus in the tracheobronchial tree.

Management. Treatment is managed collaboratively with a physician and is directed at:

1. Correcting the obstruction. This should not be achieved by suppressing the respiratory center and the cough reflex or by drying the mucosa. For these reasons sedatives, antitussives, and antihistamines are contraindicated. The medications of choice are bronchodilators and decongestants (sympathomimetics), epinephrine and ephedrine, and expectorants which will liquefy the secretions. See this chapter, Pharmacologic Therapy.
2. Humidifying the home. See this chapter, Humidity in the Home.
3. Keeping child moderately active if afebrile. Moving about and breathing more energetically help to free the mucus from the bronchial tract.
4. Cautioning against smoking to older children and adolescents with a tendency to allergic bronchitis.
5. Eventually identifying and removing allergens through environmental and diet control.

BRONCHIAL ASTHMA

Assessment. Bronchial asthma is the extreme form of bronchial allergy. The interaction of the antibody IgE with a specific allergen induces the release of histamine and SRS-A (Slow-Reacting Substance, which is a strong contractor of bronchial smooth muscle equal to that of histamine but with a more prolonged action). These induce tissue changes resulting in edema, stimulation of glands to increase mucus secretion, and bronchospasm.

INCIDENCE. The condition begins at any age although less often in infancy. Bronchospasm in infancy is usually secondary to infection rather than to an allergic reaction. It is variable in frequency and duration. Children may have only one or two attacks a year associated with an upper respiratory infection during hay fever season. Others may have it often, usually irregularly.

ETIOLOGY. Contact with or exposure to known or suspected allergens that enter the body through the respiratory system can cause asthma. Allergens may be pollen, dust, smoke or fumes, mold, animal danders, or a drug or food taken internally. Asthma may be brought on by upper respiratory viral infections (respiratory syncytial virus). Asthma attacks brought on by weather changes (cold, wind), excitement, or psychologic factors are sometimes referred to as "intrinsic" or "nonallergic."

CLINICAL FINDINGS. The signs and symptoms are as follows:

1. The attack may be preceded by rhinitis, sneezing, or coughing, or may begin abruptly (this suggests an inhalant as the allergen). It may occur at night.
2. The attack may occur as intense, sudden, paroxysmal episodes of dry, irritating cough, wheezing, and dyspnea. The bronchospasm causes airway obstruction and interference with respiration, particularly expiration which is prolonged.
3. Wheezing may be audible. Those who have continuous wheezing which is refractory to medication are in "status asthmaticus," a medical emergency.
4. Epigastric pain may be present, or the child may have anorexia, nausea, and vomiting. Often gastrointestinal symptoms can be indicative of food allergy.
5. The child is anxious and may be more comfortable in a sitting position.
6. Low fever, headache, malaise, and irritability are nonspecific symptoms often found.
7. The child who has had asthma a long time may exhibit emphysematous or barreled-shaped chest with widened anteroposterior diameter.

LABORATORY FINDINGS. Common findings are as follows:

1. Eosinophilia can often be demonstrated in the peripheral blood, nasal secretions, and sputum.

2. Polymorphonuclear leukocytosis may be present with infection.
3. Pulmonary function studies will disclose diminished maximal breathing capacity and timed vital capacity.
4. There may be an increase in serum P_{CO_2} and bicarbonate level and a decreased pH in severe asthma indicating respiratory acidosis.

DIFFERENTIAL DIAGNOSIS. These diseases may occur in children who have asthma as well:

1. Spasmodic croup. This disturbance is in the larynx rather than in the bronchi and bronchioles. See Chapter 18, Croup Syndrome.
2. Cystic fibrosis. See this chapter, Allergic Bronchitis.
3. Foreign body in lungs. The chest signs resemble asthma but are typically one-sided, have a sudden onset, and the aspirated object will show in the chest X-ray if it is opaque.
4. A semihysterical behavior pattern with hyperventilation (breathing shallowly and rapidly with excessive anxiety)
5. Mediastinal lesions. These may compress the trachea or bronchi.

Management. Asthma is managed collaboratively with a physician.

ACUTE ATTACK. During the acute attack attention is paid to environment, diet, medication, and counseling.

Environment and diet.

1. The child is placed on bed rest, if possible, in an allergen-free room with optimal humidity of 35 to 50 percent. See this chapter, Humidity in the Home.
2. Cold foods or drinks are avoided since changes in temperature aggravate allergic reactions.

Medications. See this chapter, Pharmacologic Therapy.

1. Bronchodilators (sympathomimetics) are given as soon as possible to relax the smooth muscle of the bronchioles and relieve the spasm. They may be given orally, by injection, by nebulizer,

or in some cases sublingually. Initially with wheezing the child may receive one to two doses of aqueous epinephrine at 20- to 30-minute intervals.

2. Expectorants should be administered separately. Water as an expectorant is superior. Without adequate fluid intake the various expectorants are ineffective.

Medications contraindicated. Among these are:

1. Antihistamines. Valueless and contraindicated, the atropine-like action of the antihistamines has a drying effect on secretions which leads to further airway obstruction. Prophylactic administration of antihistamines is used in children in whom an asthmatic episode is commonly preceded by acute rhinorrhea. In these children prompt use may prevent the asthmatic paroxysm.

2. Barbiturates and sedatives. In general these should be avoided because of their depressant effect on the respiratory center.

3. Cough mixtures. They are not recommended. In such mixtures one constituent counteracts the effect of another.

4. Aerosol inhalation preparations. They have no application to symptoms unless the condition is complicated by chronic pulmonary changes. In asthma care must be taken in the use of these preparations to avoid the induction of bronchospasm. Instructions must be read carefully before advising the use of these medications.

Counseling. A severe paroxysm of asthma may be anxiety provoking to both child and parents. Some parents and some caretakers may overdramatize the occasion. The caretaker must discern whether parents reflect a warm and insightful manner or whether a program of education as to the child's real needs is indicated. When a child is hospitalized, the continued presence of a member of the family may allay anxiety. If conflicts and anxieties in the family perpetuate the child's asthmatic paroxysms, psychiatric consultation should be sought.

LONG-TERM MANAGEMENT. This includes:

1. Environmental and diet control. See this chapter, Diet Control, Environmental Control.

2. Immunotherapy as necessary

3. Psychotherapy as needed

Psychologic aspects of asthma

Effect on the child and family. Williams (1975) has investigated the impact of asthma on the child and family.

> *Behavioral disturbances in the child, the mother-child and family relationships, and family social structure were studied in a representative sample of the whole range of asthmatic children and compared with a control group of normal children.*
>
> *Behavioral disturbances occurred more frequently and at a statistically significant level only in the small group of children with severe and continuing asthma. These children were those with severe chronic airway obstruction as assessed physiologically and also had the most severe allergic manifestations.*
>
> *The predominant mother-child relationship was an overconcern to protect the child's health in those children with continuing asthma at 14 years of age.*
>
> *The families of the very severely affected group of children exhibited evidence of more stress than other families.*
>
> *Socioeconomic conditions were not significantly different in any group of asthmatic children compared with the control group. (Williams, 1975, p. 51)*

Working with the child and family. The parents as well as the child require repeated and comprehensible information about etiologic, clinical, and therapeutic aspects of asthma. Parents need instruction to develop in their child with asthma an increasing responsibility for self-care and to promote the goal of raising the child as normally as possible. Appropriate activities with other children and regular schooling are essential. The primary caretaker should inquire about how the various family members react and relate to the asthmatic child and pay attention to the healthy siblings' common feelings of resentment, anxiety, and overconcern regarding their ill brother or sister. Finally, one must call attention to parental attitudes of overprotection, lenient discipline, rejection, or neglect which may endanger the child's personality development as well as the asthmatic condition.

The long-range management of childhood asthma requires a close working relationship between the primary provider, the allergist, and the psychiatrist (or other mental health worker) regarding those children where psychosocial factors significantly contribute to the course of asthma.

Sports and asthma. There is no justification for keeping the child with asthma from participating in school or in competitive athletics (Cropp, 1975). Regular participation in sports is extremely important for the physical and emotional development of children. Since exercise-induced asthma can be prevented effectively in most asthmatics by the administration of isoproterenol aerosol or selected oral bronchodilators shortly before exercise, these attacks do not have to be feared. Sports which elicit no or relatively mild exercise-induced asthma should be encouraged. Year round swimming, skiing, and touch-football are well tolerated by asthmatic children. Physical education teachers and coaches should be advised to include asthmatic children in all sports activities and should permit the children to premedicate themselves prior to exercise. The choice and use of medications should be under the direction of a physician.

Referral for psychosocial evaluation. Referral for psychosocial evaluation of a family with an asthmatic child is indicated in the following situations:

1. Children in whom emotional factors seem to be of precipitating and aggravating importance
2. Children whose asthma perpetuates individual and family psychopathology and maladaptation
3. Behavioral problems in a child seemingly unrelated to his/her asthma (Mattsson, 1975)

RESOURCE INFORMATION

Pamphlets for families about asthma can be obtained by writing to: Mead-Johnson Laboratories, Evanston, IL 47721, or Cooper Laboratories, Inc., Wayne, NJ 07470. Information about a camp developed for asthmatic children can be obtained by writing or calling:
Camp Broncho Junction, 810 Atlas Building, Charleston, WV 25301.

ALLERGIC SEROUS OTITIS MEDIA ("ALLERGIC EAR")

Assessment. See Chapter 18, Serous Otitis Media. Allergic serous otitis media is most commonly secondary to obstruction of the eustachian tube caused by edema and lymphoid hyperplasia of the upper respiratory tract on an allergic basis. Less commonly it occurs in response to a primary allergic reaction of the mucosal lining of the middle ear.

SIGNS AND SYMPTOMS. Children who have a strong family history of allergy; those who have any of the classical allergic symptoms and signs (rhinitis, "allergic shiners," "allergic salute") and exhibit the following findings most likely have "allergic ear." Symptoms of hearing loss, fullness or crackling in the ears, tinnitus, vertigo, or earaches are noted. Hearing loss is the most common and may be responsible for delayed speech development or short attention span.

The tympanic membranes are often tan, yellow, or varying shades from amber to dark blue. The surface may be dull, shiny, or waxy. The drums are often retracted, but sometimes are flat or bulging. Bubbles or fluid levels may at times be seen through the drums.

Management. See Chapter 18, Serous Otitis Media. In addition to symptomatic medication there are three methods. These are:

1. Environmental control
2. Diet control
3. Immunotherapy. This is used only if the problem is seasonal or if it is perennial and nonresponsive to home and diet changes.

Resource Information

Additional resources include the following:
1. Somekh, E., *A Parent's Guide to Children's Allergies.* Springfield, Ill.: Thomas, 1972.
2. Allergy Rehabilitation Foundation, Inc., 805 Atlas Building, Charleston, WV 25301.

References

Aas, K. *The Allergic Child.* Springfield, Ill.: Thomas, 1971.

Cropp, G. D. A. "Exercise-Induced Asthma." *Pediatr Clin North Am* 22:63–76, February 1975.

Feingold, B. F. *Introduction to Clinical Allergy*. Springfield, Ill.: Thomas, 1973.

Feingold, B. F. "Hyperkinesis and Learning Disabilities Linked to Artificial Food Flavors and Colors." *Am J Nurs* 75:797–803, May 1975.

Frazier, C. A. *Insect Allergy: Allergic and Toxic Reactions to Insects and Other Arthropods*. St. Louis: Warren H. Green, 1969.

Gellis, S. S. and B. M. Kagan. *Current Pediatric Therapy*. Philadelphia: Saunders, 1976.

Glaser, J. and D. E. Johnstone. "Prophylaxis of Allergic Disease in the Newborn." *JAMA* 153:620–622, October 1953.

Halpern, S. R. et al. "Development of Childhood Allergies in Infants Fed Cow's Milk." *J Allergy Clin Immunol* 51:139–151, March 1973.

Johnstone, D. E. and A. M. Dutton. "Dietary Prophylaxis of Allergic Disease in Children." *N Engl J Med* 274:715–719, March 1966.

Kempe, C. H., H. K. Silver, and D. O'Brien. *Current Pediatric Diagnosis and Treatment*, 4th ed. Los Altos, CA: Lange Medical Publications, 1976.

McGovern, J. P., T. J. Hayward, and A. A. Fernandez. "Allergy and Secretory Otitis Media." *JAMA* 200:124–128, April 1967.

Mattsson, A. "Psychologic Aspects of Childhood Asthma," *Pediatr Clin North Am* 22:77–88, February 1975.

Miller, J. B. *Food Allergy, Provocative Testing and Injection Therapy*. Springfield, Ill.: Thomas, 1972.

Patterson, R. *Allergic Diseases: Diagnosis and Management*. Philadelphia: Lippincott, 1972.

Rapaport, H. G. and S. M. Linde. *The Complete Allergy Guide*. New York: Simon and Schuster, 1970.

Rapp, D. J. and I. F. Fahey, "Allergy and Chronic Secretory Otitis Media," *Pediatr Clin North Amer* 22:259–264, February 1975.

Rudolph, A. M., editor. *Pediatrics*, 16th ed. New York: Appleton-Century-Crofts, 1977.

Shirkey, H. C., editor. *Pediatric Therapy*, 5th ed. St. Louis: Mosby, 1975.

Tuft, L. and H. L. Mueller. *Allergy in Children*. Philadelphia: Saunders, 1970.

Vaughan, V. C. and R. J. McKay, editors. *Nelson Textbook of Pediatrics*, 10th ed. Philadelphia: Saunders, 1975.

Waechter, E. H. and F. G. Blake. *Nursing Care of Children*, 9th ed. Philadelphia: Lippincott, 1976.

Williams, H. E. and K. N. McNicol. "The Spectrum of Asthma in Children," *Pediatr Clin North Am* 22:43–52, February 1975.

29

Infectious Disease

Infection is the largest single cause of illness in infants and children. A complete understanding of infectious disease requires basic knowledge of immunologic principles, infectious agents, the infectious process, epidemiology, manifestations of infection, treatment, control of infection, and preventive measures. Such complete information is beyond the scope of this chapter and is available in major pediatric texts. The purpose of this chapter is to provide information which will assist the nurse practitioner to assess and to identify common infectious diseases to obtain appropriate medical consultation and intervention and to provide adequate counseling for home management. Discussions of respiratory, urinary tract, gastrointestinal, and skin infections are found in the corresponding chapters. Neonatal sepsis is presented in Chapter 4 and immunizations are discussed in Chapter 2.

ASSESSMENT

History

PAST HISTORY

Obtain information on past infections, communicable diseases, immunodeficiency states, and immunization status.

PRESENT CONCERN

See Chapter 13, Assessment of Presenting Symptom. What is the age of the child? Does the child look sick? Obtain a chronologic history of the signs and symptoms, exposures (other family members, schoolmates, neighbors, babysitters), what treatment has been tried, and what the parent thinks it is (older parents and grandparents remember polio and pertussis). If a rash is present, where did it begin, where did it spread, what does it look like, and does it itch? Inquire as to recent travel to other countries or geographic areas.

Physical Examination

- A thorough general physical examination is performed. See Chapter 1, Child Health Assessment.
- Age and general appearance of the child are clues to potential seriousness or toxicity. Fever and/or infection in any site in an infant under 4 months of age is serious. Sepsis, meningitis, and bacterial diarrheas must be considered.

MANAGEMENT

General Measures

Specific treatment measures exist for bacterial infections and are discussed in subsequent sections. Infectious diseases, whether of bacterial or viral origin, are usually associated with a variety of constitutional symptoms: fever, upper respiratory symptoms (cough, rhinorrhea, sore throat), anorexia, headache, malaise, irritability, pain, generalized aching, and rash. The provision of symptomatic relief is accomplished by the following general measures.

FEVER (SEE CHAPTER 13, FEVER)

1. Antipyretic medication
2. Tepid sponge baths
3. Liberal fluid intake
4. Rest and limited activity

UPPER RESPIRATORY SYMPTOMS (SEE CHAPTER 18, THE RESPIRATORY SYSTEM)

1. Liberal fluid intake
2. Cool mist vaporizers
3. Decongestants
4. Warm gargles, saline mouth and throat irrigations, cool liquids, and soft foods for sore throat
5. Petrolatum jelly to protect skin around the nares
6. Cough preparations are generally ineffective and are contraindicated in infants and young children

GENERALIZED ACHING AND MALAISE

1. Rest and limited physical activity
2. Warm baths
3. Body massage
4. Cold compresses for headache
5. Analgesic medication

ANOREXIA

1. Small, frequent feedings of favorite foods and liquids
2. A relaxed attitude about oral intake. Forcing foods and fluids is usually counterproductive.

RASH

1. Proper hygiene and bathing to reduce incidence of secondary infection

2. Cool baths, local applications of calamine lotion, and mild anesthetic ointments or systemic antihistamines to relieve pruritus

3. Fingernail care, including frequent cutting and cleaning, to reduce effects of scratching. Gloves or mittens may be used at night in younger children.

4. Saline mouthwashes if mucous membranes are involved

Isolation

The prevention of the spread of communicable infectious diseases is attempted through various isolation techniques. Whether or not the child is isolated in the hospital or at home depends on the specific disease, the severity of symptoms, the home environment including the presence of susceptible persons, and the ability of the parents to carry out the necessary procedures. Isolation measures are as follows.

STRICT ISOLATION

A private room is necessary; door must be kept closed. Gowns, masks, and gloves must be worn by all persons entering the room. Hands must be washed on entering and leaving the room. Articles must be discarded or wrapped before being taken out for disinfection.

RESPIRATORY ISOLATION

A private room is necessary; the door must be kept closed. Gowns and gloves are not necessary. Masks must be worn by all susceptible persons entering the room. Hands must be washed on entering and leaving the room. Articles contaminated with secretions must be disinfected.

ENTERIC PRECAUTIONS

A private room is necessary for children only. Gowns and gloves must be worn by all persons having direct contact with the client.

Masks are not necessary. Hands must be washed on entering and leaving the room. Special precautions are necessary for articles contaminated with urine and feces. Articles must be disinfected or discarded.

SECRETION PRECAUTIONS, LESIONS

Private room, gowns, masks, gloves are not necessary. Hands must be washed before and after contact with client. Articles: double bagging technique used for soiled dressings and equipment.

SECRETION PRECAUTIONS, ORAL

Private room, gowns, masks, gloves are not necessary. Hands must be washed before and after client contact. Articles: disposable handkerchiefs are discarded in bags which should be sealed before being placed in the trash (Brunner, 1974, pp. 820–822).

COMMON INFECTIOUS DISEASES

Bacterial Infections

CELLULITIS

Assessment. Cellulitis is an infection of the skin that involves both the dermis and subcutaneous tissues. See Chapter 15, The Skin, for a discussion of impetigo and furunculosis. In children it is caused by *Staphylococcus aureus*, group A beta-hemolytic streptococci, or *Hemophilus influenzae* and is frequently an infection secondary to impetigo or other local skin lesions. Since it is a deeper infection than impetigo, it is less apt to be communicable, but more apt to lead to septicemia.

CLINICAL PICTURE. The affected area is warm, tender, erythematous, swollen, and indurated. Fever, malaise, and lymphadenopathy are present. Lymphangitis ("streaking") may be seen on the extremities.

LABORATORY. Needle aspiration of the lesion is done for culture and gram stain.

Management. Specific treatment is appropriate systemic antibiotic therapy. Additionally, application of warm compresses and immobilization (if the lesion is on an extremity) are recommended. If the organism is streptococcal, family members should be examined to detect carriers.

DIPHTHERIA

Assessment. This is an acute infectious disease caused by *Corynebacterium diphtheriae* which produces a virulent exotoxin. It is characterized by sore throat and formation of a membrane that may cover the tonsils, pharynx, and larynx. The membrane is the result of necrotic epithelial cells and inflammatory exudate coagulating on the surface of the affected structures.

EPIDEMIOLOGY

Mode of transmission. Transmission is by direct contact via coughing, sneezing, and talking with a person who has the disease or is a healthy carrier.

Incubation period. It is 2 to 4 days with a range from 1 to 6 days.

Period of communicability. It is variable; 2 to 4 weeks in untreated individuals; 1 to 2 days in treated persons.

Population at risk. This depends on the immune status of the population. Infants born of immune mothers are relatively immune for about 6 months. Where children are routinely immunized the incidence is predominantly in adults whose immune levels have diminished with time. Recent outbreaks have occurred among poor populations without adequate access to health care services. Crowding enhances spread.

Seasonal patterns. It is most common in the autumn and winter months in temperate zones.

CLINICAL PICTURE. Signs and symptoms vary with the site of localization.

Nasal diphtheria. The major symptom is unilateral or bilateral nasal discharge, serous at first and then serosanguinous and mucopurulent, which excoriates the anterior nares and upper lip. Systemic symptoms are slight. A membrane may be visible on the nasal septum.

Tonsillar and pharyngeal diphtheria. Malaise, anorexia, sore throat, and low-grade fever precede the formation of the membrane (white to grey-green in color) which may involve both tonsils, pharynx, soft palate, and uvula. Swelling of the neck may result from marked lymphadenopathy. Pulse rate is rapid. Mild cases last about a week, then the membrane sloughs off and recovery ensues. Severe cases involve severe toxemia and may lead rapidly to prostration, stupor, coma, and death within 6 to 10 days.

Laryngeal diphtheria. It is often associated with severe pharyngeal diphtheria but occurs alone as well. It is the most dangerous form. It resembles croup or acute laryngitis. Fever, hoarseness, and cough may be followed by airway obstruction, congestion, and edema, with inspiratory stridor, retractions, dyspnea, and cyanosis. The membrane may progress down into the tracheobronchial tree and contribute to airway obstruction. If pharyngeal diphtheria is present, the course involves both obstruction and toxemia.

LABORATORY. The diagnosis is confirmed by culture of the organism from the nose and throat. The swab must be rubbed firmly over the lesions and, if possible, inserted under the membrane.

COMPLICATIONS. Up to 50 percent of cases develop myocardial involvement within 2 weeks after onset since the toxin has an affinity for heart muscle. Nervous system complications (neuritis) occur less frequently and as late as 6 weeks after onset. Soft palate paralysis is the most common but usually subsides completely.

Management. Management includes medication therapy, supportive care, care of exposed individuals, and preventive measures.

MEDICATION. Medication therapy includes:

1. Diphtheria antitoxin. This must be given as soon as possible to neutralize the toxin while it is still circulating. Once toxin becomes fixed to tissues, antitoxin has no effect. Hypersensitivity to horse serum must be determined before therapy is begun. By the second to third day after onset, the fatality rate rises sharply if antitoxin is not given.

2. Antibiotic therapy. This is given as a supplement to antitoxin therapy. Antibiotics act against the organism and decrease the numbers of people who remain carriers after recovery. Penicillin and erythromycin are used.

3. Diphtheria toxoid. Adequate immunity does not develop in many persons recovering from diphtheria. A Shick test should be performed and, if positive, immunization with diphtheria toxoid is indicated. A negative Shick test indicates immunity to diphtheria toxin.

COUNSELING FOR HOME CARE

Supportive care. Severely ill children are hospitalized. Complete bed rest is of particular importance for at least 12 days in all children with diphtheria because of the possibility of myocarditis. Diet should be high carbohydrate as blood sugars are frequently low. Other supportive measures are presented earlier in this chapter under General Measures.

Isolation. Strict isolation is required and is continued following completion of antibiotic therapy until two or three successive nose and throat cultures taken at least 24 hours apart are negative.

EXPOSED CONTACTS. All contacts and household members should be isolated until nose and throat cultures and Shick tests are performed.

- Contacts with negative cultures and negative Shick tests are immune and uninfected and need not be isolated.
- Contacts with positive cultures and negative Shick tests are considered carriers and should be treated with antibiotics.
- Contacts with positive cultures and positive Shick tests should be treated with diphtheria antitoxin and antibiotics.

- Contacts with negative cultures and positive Shick tests should receive active immunization (Krugman, 1977, p. 24).
- Previously immunized children should be given diphtheria toxoid boosters.
- Persons who completed the primary series more than 10 years previously should also receive a booster.

PREVENTION. Active immunization. See Chapter 2, Immunizations.

MENINGITIS, BACTERIAL

Assessment. Bacterial meningitis is an acute infection of the meninges following invasion of the spinal fluid by a variety of bacteria. It is a serious disease with etiology, morbidity, and mortality dependent on the age of the child, the causative agent, the severity of the illness, and the rapidity with which effective treatment is begun.

ETIOLOGY. Causative organisms vary with age. In the neonate the most common causes are enteric organisms: *Escherichia coli* and group B streptococci. In infants and young children the three most common causes are *Hemophilus influenzae, Neisseria meningitidis,* and *Diplococcus meningitidis.*

EPIDEMIOLOGY

Mode of transmission. Neonatal meningitis reflects the environment of the fetus and newborn infant (e.g., a maternal infection, exposure in the nursery from equipment or unrecognized infection in other infants or personnel). In infants and children the route of infection is most often via the blood stream, the result of bacteremia due to invasion of bacteria in another part of the body. Infections in the region of the brain (otitis media, mastoiditis, sinusitis, facial infections) may also spread by direct extension. Meningococcal meningitis begins in the nasopharynx, and transmission occurs by droplet spray from the mouth or nose of healthy carriers or those with a mild URI caused by the meningococcal organism.

Other factors. Seasonal patterns exist with *H. influenzae* meningitis as the incidence of upper respiratory infections is greatest in the autumn and winter. Any situation leading to high incidence of URIs will increase the incidence of meningitis (e.g., crowding, ill health, malnutrition). Only meningococcal meningitis occurs in epidemic form.

CLINICAL PICTURE. Presentation of this disease varies with age and with the type of organism.

Neonates. Unfortunately, the clinical signs in neonates are vague and nonspecific, and the process is insidious. The infant may look well at birth but within a few days may appear to be "doing poorly." Fever may or may not be present. The infant may manifest poor tone, poor sucking with feeding difficulties, vomiting, poor cry, irritability, and either drowsiness or hyperactivity and jitteriness. The fontanelle may be full, tense, or bulging. Other meningeal signs may be absent. See Chapter 25, Meningeal Signs. Jaundice, if present, is associated with sepsis, and if sepsis is suspected, meningitis must also be considered. See Chapter 4, Sepsis in the Newborn. If the diagnosis is not established the mortality is high (65 to 75 percent). Neurologic sequelae (hydrocephalus, brain damage) occur frequently if the infection is detected late in its course.

Infants. The classical presentation of meningitis is rarely seen in infants from 3 months to 2 years of age, although the incidence is highest in this age group. Any unexplained febrile illness should arouse suspicion of meningitis. A previous respiratory or gastrointestinal infection may be present. The infant may become increasingly irritable. Fever, anorexia, vomiting, drowsiness, and high-pitched cry are common. Convulsions may occur. The fontanelle may be bulging, but if the infant is dehydrated or the fontanelle has closed, this sign may not be seen. Nuchal rigidity, and Kernig's and Brudzinski's signs may be difficult to elicit in this age group.

Older children. The classic picture begins usually with fever, chills, vomiting, severe headache, and stiff neck. Irritability, convulsions, stupor, and coma may occur. Meningeal signs are present consistently and as nuchal rigidity progresses opisthotonos may develop. Photophobia, blurred vision, and papilledema may be present.

Meningococcemia. Children with meningococcal meningitis have sudden onset of high temperature and frequently demonstrate a petechial rash. See Table 1. The presence of a rapidly developing petechial rash associated with a shocklike, toxic state in children between 3 months to 6 years indicates fulminant meningococcemia and represents a *true medical emergency.*

LABORATORY. Definitive diagnosis is made by examination of cerebrospinal fluid (CSF). The characteristic findings include:

- Cloudy appearance
- Increase in white cells (polymorphonuclear leukocytes). Cell count is usually well over 1000/cu mm (Krugman, 1977, p. 159).
- Decreased glucose. Blood glucose is obtained for comparison with CSF glucose.
- Increased protein
- Culture and smear positive for a pathogenic causative organism. The organism can also be recovered from blood, nasopharynx, and, in the case of meningococcemia, the petechiae.

COMPLICATIONS. Complications have been reduced since the advent of antimicrobial therapy, but if early treatment is not initiated, the danger of complications remains. Hydrocephalus, cerebral edema leading to permanent damage to cranial nerves and other structures, subdural effusions, peripheral circulatory collapse, shock, and respiratory failure are most common. Persistent fever may be due to brain abscess, drug reaction, or continued sepsis.

Management. Whatever work setting the nurse practitioner is in, protocols for prompt referral and priority service should be established with appropriate medical sources. Bacterial meningitis is a medical emergency. At the first suspicion of meningitis the nurse practitioner must refer to the physician. The child is hospitalized immediately.

MEDICATION. Antibiotic therapy depends on the causative agent and on the age and weight of the child. Weights should be obtained early. Consult a pediatric text for full discussion of the acute care of the child with meningitis.

Table 1

Differential Diagnosis of Common Exanthematous Diseases

Disease	Incubation Period	Prodrome	Exanthem	Other Characteristic Signs
Measles	9–14 days	3–4 days of malaise, fever, conjunctivitis, cough, and coryza	Reddish-brown or purple-red maculopapular rash appearing first on face, hairline, forehead, and neck (confluent); and proceeding to trunk, extremities, and feet (discrete). Duration of rash is 5–7 days. Desquamation may occur but not on hands and feet.	Koplik's spots (bluish-white dots with red areola) appear about 12 hours before the rash on buccal mucosa and sometimes on labial mucosa. They usually fade and disappear by the second day of the rash. They are pathognomonic for measles.
Rubella	14–21 days	Usually none	Pink-red maculopapular, discrete rash appearing first on face and neck and rapidly progressing to trunk and extremities. Lasts 3–5 days with earliest lesions fading first so that on the third day the face and neck may be clear. No desquamation.	Lymphadenopathy with post-auricular or occipital nodes is characteristic.
Scarlet fever	2–4 days (range: 1–7 days)	12 hours to 2 days with abrupt onset of fever, sore throat, vomiting, headache, chills, and malaise	Bright red, punctate lesions that blanch on pressure. Rough, sandpaperlike texture. Appears within 12–48 hours of fever, first on the flexor surfaces and	Tonsils and pharynx are beefy red and may have exudate. Tongue has a white coating which peels off as the papillae become red and swollen, and assumes the

Disease	Incubation	Fever	Rash	Characteristics
			rapidly becomes generalized. Most intense on neck, axillary, inguinal, and popliteal folds. The face is smooth, red, and flushed, with circumoral pallor. Duration is approximately 7 days, followed by desquamation, including hands and feet.	"strawberry tongue" appearance. Petechiae may be present on pharynx and palate. Pastia's sign (hyperemic lines on flexor surfaces at wrists, elbows, and groin) are characteristic.
Roseola (exanthem subitum)	10–14 days	3–4 days of high fever and irritability. Fever may go to 40°C.	Rose-pink, maculopapular, discrete rash may begin on chest and trunk, then spread to face and extremities. Duration from several hours to 2 days. Rash immediately follows the rapid fall of temperature to normal levels.	May be first seen with a febrile convulsion. Cervical and occipital lymph nodes are enlarged.
Erythema infectiosum (Fifth's disease)	6–14 days	None	Rash erupts in three stages: 1. Bright red, confluent, maculopapular rash on face, especially cheeks, with circumoral pallor 2. Discrete maculopapular rash on upper and lower extremities 3. After the rash has subsided (a week or more), it tends to recur following a variety of skin irritants.	"Slapped cheek" appearance in an otherwise well child; lacelike appearance as the rash fades

Continued on next page

Table 1 (Continued)

Disease	Incubation Period	Prodrome	Exanthem	Other Characteristic Signs
Meningococcemia	Variable depending on primary infection.	24-hour period of fever, vomiting, irritability, nuchal rigidity, bulging fontanelle	Rash is maculopapular but becomes petechial and purpuric. Distribution is variable.	Petechial rash associated with meningeal signs suggests meningococcemia. See text, Meningococcemia.
Enteroviral infections (ECHO and Coxsackie)	Variable but usually brief	Variable; can be absent or include 3–4 days of fever, irritability	Rash resembles the rubella rash, is maculopapular, discrete, and generalized.	Concurrent family illness, gastroenteritis, and local epidemics are commonly associated. Incidence highest in summer and fall. See Chapter 18, The Respiratory System.
Varicella (Chicken-pox)	14–16 days (range: 11–20 days)	Usually none. Adolescents may have 1–2 days of fever, headache, and malaise.	Fever, malaise, and rash appear simultaneously. Rash rapidly evolves from macules to papules to vesicles to crusts. Lesions are centripetal in distribution, profuse on trunk, and occur in successive crops over a 3–5 day period. Lesions in all stages are present simultaneously. Lesions are present on scalp, hairline, and mucous membranes. All lesions eventually crust and dry up.	Rash is pruritic.

Source: Based on information from S. Krugman, et al, *Infectious Diseases of Children*, 6th ed., (St. Louis: C. V. Mosby, 1977).

COUNSELING. During the acute process and the long-term follow-up period, both child and family require support and teaching. Bacterial meningitis is a frightening diagnosis, and parents will have realistic fears about the outcome.

- Teaching should include discussion of the disease process and symptoms and care of the child at home during the convalescent period: restoring resistance to infection, adequate nutrition, health maintenance care, resumption of school and recreational activities, and follow-up procedures.
- Follow-up should include careful developmental appraisals every few months for a year to identify any residual damage. Vision, hearing, and cognitive evaluations should also be performed (Conway, 1977, p. 300).

EXPOSED CONTACTS. In cases of meningococcal meningitis household and intimate contacts may be carriers or may develop infection. Sulfonamides are given to such contacts prophylactically if the organism is sensitive to sulfa. Contacts should be observed for fever or illness and cultured at the first sign of disease. School contacts do not require antibacterial therapy unless an epidemic situation exists.

PREVENTION. Meningococcal polysaccharide vaccines effective against two serogroups (A and C) of meningococcal disease are licensed for selective use in the USA. They have been given routinely to military recruits since 1971. Routine use in civilians is currently not recommended because of insufficient data. There is no vaccine for serogroup B which currently causes the majority of cases (Krugman, 1977, p. 494).

PERTUSSIS (WHOOPING COUGH)

Assessment. Pertussis is an acute infection of the respiratory tract caused by *Bordetella pertussis*. It is characterized by a prolonged period of respiratory symptoms progressing to repetitive paroxysms of coughing that often end with a spasmodic inspiratory whoop and, frequently, vomiting.

EPIDEMIOLOGY

Mode of transmission. Direct contact with an infected person via coughing, sneezing, or talking is the most common mode of spread.

Incubation period. It is from 5 to 21 days but almost uniformly within 10 days.

Period of communicability. This extends from 7 days after exposure to 3 to 4 weeks after onset of paroxysms. Most spread occurs during the catarrhal period.

Population at risk. Little to no immunity is transferred via the placenta. Thus, infants and children under 4 years are most susceptible and the disease is most serious in infants under 1 year. Severe attacks can occur in elderly people. Pertussis is highly contagious for unimmunized individuals. Attack rates in unimmunized family contacts are up to 90 percent on exposure to an index case in the family. Morbidity and mortality are higher in females. Naturally acquired immunity is highly effective.

Seasonal patterns. There is less seasonal variation than for other respiratory infections as it maintains a high incidence during spring and summer.

CLINICAL PICTURE. The complete course lasts 6 to 8 weeks and includes three stages.

Catarrhal stage. Symptoms of an upper respiratory infection are present, and pertussis may not be suspected until the cough continues to worsen rather than to improve during the second week.

Paroxysmal stage. The coughing paroxysms (bursts of short, rapid coughs on one expiration; red or cyanotic face; sudden inspiration with whoop; dislodgement of mucous plug, and vomiting) are exhausting and anxiety producing and may be precipitated by a variety of stimuli (movement, swallowing, speech, pressure on the trachea). The paroxysms occur from four to five times a day in mild cases to 40 or more in severe cases. This stage may last from 4 to 6 weeks.

Convalescent stage. Whooping and vomiting gradually diminish, and the cough becomes less severe although it persists for 2 or 3 weeks.

LABORATORY. Although the paroxysmal episode and whoop are seldom mistaken, earlier diagnosis may be possible if there is a history of contact with a known case and isolation of the organism from the nasopharynx. White blood count is very high with predominant lymphocytosis.

COMPLICATIONS. Pneumonia is a common complication and is responsible for significant mortality in children under 3 years of age. Hemorrhages (nose bleeds, conjunctival hemorrhage), hernia, rectal prolapse, and trauma to the tongue may result from increased pressure during paroxysms. Intracranial hemorrhage is rare. Nutritional disturbances, malnutrition, and weight loss secondary to exhaustion and vomiting are not infrequent. Neurologic complications are serious and include encephalopathy, brain damage related to asphyxia from severe paroxysms, and seizures.

Management. Small infants or those with severe disease and frequent exhaustive paroxysms require hospitalization where equipment for oxygen therapy, suctioning, and resuscitation is available and where continuous nursing surveillance is possible.

MEDICATION. Medication therapy includes:

1. Pertussis immune globulin. This is recommended for all children under 2 years and for older children with severe cases. Its efficacy is questioned but some beneficial effect may occur.
2. Pertussis vaccine. This is not of value once symptoms have begun.
3. Antibiotics. These are not effective in shortening the paroxysmal stage or in modifying the severity of the disease but can eliminate the organism and decrease contact spread.

COUNSELING FOR HOME CARE. Mild cases can be cared for at home.

Supportive care. The child should rest in bed as tolerated. Stimuli that precipitate paroxysms must be kept to a minimum: activity, excitement, smoke, and sudden changes in temperature. Small frequent feedings are indicated and re-feeding after vomiting is recommended as another paroxysm is less likely at that time.

Isolation. Respiratory isolation is required for the period of communicability. Since family members have high attack rates, no infant under 2 years of age should be brought into the household.

EXPOSED CONTACTS. In small infants pertussis immune globulin may be attempted as soon after exposure as possible but the preventive effects are questionable. Erythromycin is also recommended for 5 to 7 days. Once the full incubation period has passed, active immunization should be instituted. Pertussis in adults is usually a mild to moderate disease and incidence is low. Thus, pertussis vaccine is not routinely given to persons over 6 years of age.

PREVENTION. Active immunization. See Chapter 2, Immunizations.

SCARLET FEVER (SCARLATINA)

Assessment. Scarlet fever is an infection caused by an erythrogenic toxin-producing group A hemolytic streptococcus in an individual who does not have antitoxin antibodies. The toxin produces a characteristic rash.

EPIDEMIOLOGY

Mode of transmission. Spread is through direct contact with airborne droplets from the respiratory tract of a symptomatic or asymptomatic individual.

Incubation period. It is 2 to 4 days with a range of 1 to 7 days.

Period of communicability. This is variable but is greatest during the acute respiratory illness until a day or 2 after the start of antibiotic therapy.

Population at risk. Streptococcal infections are uncommon in children under 2 years of age. Incidence is highest in children 6 to 12 years of age.

Seasonal patterns. It is more common during winter and early spring in temperate areas.

CLINICAL PICTURE. Table 1 describes the clinical features of several exanthematous diseases, including scarlet fever.

LABORATORY. Throat culture is obtained for group A hemolytic streptococci. During convalescence antistreptolysin (ASO) titer will rise.

COMPLICATIONS. Complications occur when the streptococcal organism enters adjacent tissues or the blood stream and establishes metastatic lesions. Early complications usually result from delayed diagnosis and treatment. Common ones include cervical adenitis, otitis media, and sinusitis. More infrequent complications are pneumonia, mastoiditis, osteomyelitis, and septicemia. Late sequelae are rheumatic fever and acute glomerulonephritis (Krugman, 1977, p. 347).

Management. The child can usually be cared for at home.

MEDICATION. Penicillin is the drug of choice. Erythromycin is used if allergy to penicillin exists. Treatment must continue for a minimum of 10 days to eradicate the organisms. Even though the child appears well in 3 to 4 days, the importance of the full course of medication must be emphasized. If family disorganization or lack of comprehension raise questions about the reliability of medication administration, parenteral therapy is indicated.

COUNSELING FOR HOME CARE

Supportive care. See this chapter, General Measures. Bed rest used to be mandatory and is still recommended during the febrile period. The difficulties of imposing bed rest on a young child who feels well are obvious, and often the child becomes more restless than if allowed some natural activity. Thus, bed rest should not be insisted upon as the child feels better. Parents should be prepared for the period of skin desquamation.

Isolation. Respiratory isolation for 1 day after the start of treatment is recommended. The child may return to school upon clinical recovery but not less than 7 days from onset.

Follow-up. The child should be seen within 2 to 4 weeks and examined for signs of rheumatic fever (careful cardiac examination) and glomerulonephritis (urine specimens).

EXPOSED CONTACTS. Prevention of streptococcal infection in exposed susceptible contacts is desirable, but the guidelines are unclear. It is advisable to obtain throat cultures on intimate household contacts. Contacts with a previous history of rheumatic fever should receive penicillin prophylaxis.

TETANUS (LOCKJAW)

Assessment. Tetanus is an acute infection caused by the virulent toxin produced by *Clostridium tetani*. The organism enters through a break in the skin, and the toxin travels and binds to central nervous system tissue causing tonic muscular spasms, stiffness of skeletal muscles (especially the jaw), and convulsions.

EPIDEMIOLOGY

Mode of transmission. The organisms are found in soil; horse, cattle, and sheep manure; and street dust. Spread is through direct or indirect contamination of an obvious or unrecognized wound. Puncture wounds, scratches, burns, crushing injuries, and the umbilicus of the newborn are favorable portals of entry.

Incubation period. It is variable; from 1 to 2 days to 5 to 12 days to longer periods.

Period of communicability. None.

Population at risk. All unimmunized persons are susceptible and no lasting immunity results after an attack of the disease. Maternal transfer of passive immunity to the infant is of short duration.

CLINICAL PICTURE. The minor local wound usually shows nothing unusual. The onset is insidious and initial symptoms are muscle stiffness in the neck and jaw. There is difficulty in opening the mouth and difficulty in swallowing. Within 24 hours the disease becomes full-blown with generalized muscle rigidity. Various stimuli (lights, sounds, movement) initiate paroxysmal spasms which become frequent and painful as the disease progresses. During spasms trismus (lockjaw), risus sardonicus (sardonic grin caused by distortion of face), and opisthotonos are marked. In fatal cases, death usually results from respiratory failure within 3 to 4 days.

LABORATORY. No specific laboratory procedures are generally useful, and the diagnosis is made primarily on clinical grounds.

COMPLICATIONS. In persons who survive, pulmonary complications may occur from laryngospasm, respiratory obstruction and asphyxia, or tracheostomy. Seizures may result in tongue lacerations or thoracic vertebral fractures. Malnutrition may also occur. Long-term sequelae are not common.

Management. The child with tetanus requires hospitalization, and meticulous nursing and medical care. See major texts for full discussion. Control of muscular spasms, antitoxin and antimicrobial therapy, wound care, respiratory care, and general supportive care are required.

ANTITOXIN THERAPY. This is the most specific therapy, and human Tetanus Immune Globulin (TIG) is the recommended agent. If human globulin is not available, tetanus antitoxin is used after determining hypersensitivity to horse serum.

COUNSELING. In the United States the incidence of tetanus in children is extremely rare, and the nurse practitioner may never have occasion to support a family affected by this serious disease. If the situation does occur, support appropriate to the care of a critically ill child is required. In children who survive, the convalescent period may be lengthy but is usually uneventful in terms of complications.

PREVENTION. See Chapter 2, Immunizations. Active immunization, when achieved and maintained, effectively prevents tetanus.

TUBERCULOSIS

Tuberculosis is a serious infectious disease, still widespread throughout the world, which can cause major and chronic disability among the population. It is a complicated entity, and for a complete discussion the reader is referred to major texts listed at the end of this chapter. The purpose of this section is to present a brief description of the disease in children and to consider management procedures for the most common clinical situations the nurse practitioner encounters in practice; specifically, the infant or child with a positive tuberculin test and the child who has been exposed to active tuberculosis.

Assessment. Tuberculosis is caused by the bacilli *Mycobacterium tuberculosis* and *M. bovis*.

EPIDEMIOLOGY

Incidence. In 1973 the new active case rate in the United States was 14.8/100,000. In 1974 over 30,000 cases were reported (Krugman, 1977, p. 390).

Characteristics of the tubercle bacillus. The bacillus is unique in several ways. It is capable of survival for long periods of time in the environment and is resistant to drying although sunlight and ultraviolet light will destroy it. Once bacilli enter the body, they "escape body defenses by taking up sequestered positions deep in the tissues where they remain inactive for years but are able to revive and produce new disease in favorable circumstances" (Waechter, 1976, p. 469). This ability to remain dormant accounts in large part for the insidious nature of tuberculosis.

Mode of transmission. An adult or adolescent with active pulmonary tuberculosis is the usual source of infection in children. Coughing and sneezing spray droplets which are inhaled into the lungs. Transmission depends on the number of bacilli discharged into the atmosphere, and this depends on the number of organisms in the sputum, the amount of sputum, the frequency of the cough, and conscientiousness in hygiene while coughing. Also, the frequency and intimacy of exposure affect transmission. Children rarely transmit the disease.

Predisposing factors. Only a small percentage of persons infected with tubercle bacilli develop overt disease. Factors affecting host resistance and the degree of illness include:

1. Numbers of tubercle bacilli and virulence
2. Possible genetic factors
3. Age (increased morbidity and mortality in adolescent girls)
4. Nutrition
5. General state of health
6. Intercurrent infections (e.g., measles)
7. Physical and mental stress (e.g., chronic fatigue)
8. Environmental and socioeconomic circumstances (e.g., poverty, crowding, poor sanitation)
9. Administration of immunosuppressive and corticosteroid drugs
10. Cellular immunity

Incubation period for primary tuberculosis. It is 4 to 8 weeks with a range of 2 to 10 weeks.

PATHOGENESIS. The infection begins with local disease at the portal of entry and in the regional lymph nodes draining the area of primary focus. This is called the *primary complex*. The lung is the most common portal of entry. The bacilli multiply in lung parenchyma and create a small area of inflammatory exudate. Almost immediately some bacilli are carried through the lymphatic system to the regional lymph nodes. As bacilli multiply and die a change occurs in tissue reaction to the bacilli, and hypersensitivity develops. This takes about 4 to 8 weeks (which is when the tuberculin test will convert to positive). As hypersensitivity and acquired resistance develop, the primary lesion becomes encapsulated and walled off and may resolve or calcify over a period of months. "A healed primary complex results and the child acquires only a positive tuberculin reaction and perhaps some spots of calcification . . . visible on x-ray" (Waechter, 1976, p. 470). If this result does not occur, the infection may remain, and any of the following outcomes are possible:

1. Persistence of indolent lesions
2. Extension of the local site with progressive destruction of tissue
3. Erosion of bronchial walls and subsequent pulmonary complications
4. Widespread hematogenous spread (miliary TB) or establishment of localized lesions at distant sites
5. Subsequent re-activity of the lesion
6. Re-infection, endogenous or exogenous (Vaughan, 1975, p. 628)

TUBERCULIN TESTING. The tuberculin test measures the presence or absence of delayed hypersensitivity to the protein portion of the tubercle bacillus.

Tuberculin material. Two types are available: old tuberculin (OT) and purified protein derivative (PPD). Both materials are effective, but question about the variable potency of different batches of OT has resulted in the widespread use of PPD.

Methods of testing

1. Intradermal test (Mantoux). If done properly this is the most accurate and reliable test. Old tuberculin or PPD is injected intradermally into the volar surface of the forearm. The dose is 0.1 ml of the desired concentration (strength). First strength is used if an individual is thought to be highly sensitive; intermediate strength is the standard; and second strength is used to exclude the diagnosis if a negative reaction occurs with intermediate strength.
2. Multiple puncture tests (Heaf test, Tine test, Applitest, Monovacc). The exact amount of tuberculin is difficult to mea-

sure. These tests are suitable for mass screening but should not be used for making specific diagnoses. Positive reactions should be confirmed via Mantoux testing.

3. Jet injection test. A jet gun deposits PPD intradermally under high pressure.

Interpretation of standard-dose tuberculin tests. Tests are read 48 to 72 hours after administration.

1. Intradermal and jet injection tests. Erythema without induration is not significant. Induration is measured at the maximum transverse diameter. Reactions of 4 mm or less are negative; 5 mm to 9 mm are doubtful and a repeat test is done at a different site. If still doubtful and the child has close contact with a person with active tuberculosis, or has clinical or X-ray evidence of disease, the results should be treated as positive. Ten mm or more is a positive reaction, and the test is not repeated for confirmation.

2. Multiple puncture tests. Induration is measured using the diameter of the largest single reaction. If the reaction consists of discrete papules, the individual diameters should not be added together. Reactions of less than 2 mm are negative; 2 mm to 4 mm are doubtful and Mantoux testing is done. Reactions of 5 mm or more indicate a positive test which may be confirmed by Mantoux testing.

Unreliable tuberculin testing. Negative test results in the presence of the disease may occur in the following situations:

1. Children on immunosuppressive drugs
2. During the 4- to 8-week incubation period of primary tuberculosis infection
3. For up to 4 weeks after onset of measles or following measles immunization

Significance of positive tuberculin test. A positive test indicates that the individual has been infected with the tubercle bacillus and is allergic or hypersensitive to its protein. It does not prove the presence of active infection. After identification of tuberculin sensitivity, procedures are required to:

1. *Locate, if possible, any and all lesions.*
2. *Determine whether infection is active, quiescent, or healed.*
3. *Detect any tuberculosis contacts (Vaughan, 1975, p. 628).*

Therefore, in the child with a positive tuberculin skin test the procedures instituted by the nurse practitioner include:

1. Referral to the physician
2. Chest X-ray to detect evidence of pulmonary infection. If the X-ray is positive, efforts to recover the tubercle bacilli are made (cultures of sputum, gastric contents, spinal fluid, urine).
3. Careful history of all contacts to determine exposure to active tuberculosis.

Management

ACTIVE TUBERCULOSIS.   Children with positive skin tests and demonstrable active lesions are treated with antimicrobial drugs and general supportive measures. Isoniazid, rifampin, streptomycin, and para-aminosalicylic acid are the more frequently used drugs. See major references for full discussion.

PREVENTION OF PROGRESSIVE TUBERCULOSIS.   In children with positive skin tests and no clinically demonstrable disease, prophylactic treatment with isoniazid (INH) for 1 year is indicated in the following cases:

1. Children under 4 years of age with positive skin tests.
2. Any child who has recently converted from a negative to a positive skin reaction.
3. Any child with a positive skin test and a known exposure to active tuberculosis.
4. Any child with inactive primary tuberculosis who has never been treated.

CONTACTS.   Members of the household and other close associates of a person with active tuberculosis should be skin tested. Those with positive reactions are treated. Those with negative skin tests are re-tested in 6 weeks and at least every 3 months for the duration of the contact. Isoniazid may be recommended regardless of tuberculin status. Infants should be removed from contact with the infected person until at least 6 months after all cultures are reported as negative.

CASEFINDING. Tuberculin testing is an essential aspect of preventive child health care. The first test is usually made when the child is between 9 and 12 months of age and yearly or every other year thereafter. Adults who have consistent contact with children (e.g., school personnel, babysitters) should be tested routinely.

VACCINATION. Bacillus Calmette-Guerin (BCG) is used in many areas of the world to produce active artificial immunity to tuberculosis. The immunity is variable and not complete but lasts several years and does provide protection. The efficacy of the vaccines currently available is thought to be about 75 percent (Rudolph, 1977, p. 478). BCG vaccination results in hypersensitivity to tuberculin which may last for several years. Thus the value of skin testing in the diagnosis of tuberculosis is lost. It is felt that in the United States, where incidence of tuberculosis is low, the importance of tuberculin test sensitivity is greater in terms of diagnosing infection than in the provision of artificial immunity. Exceptions might be individuals who are at increased risk because of repeated exposure (e.g., infants of mothers with tuberculosis) and persons in groups with high incidence of tuberculosis (e.g., drug addicts, alcoholics, migrant workers). "It is recommended that those who have been vaccinated with BCG be re-tested periodically with tuberculin and the reactions recorded so that comparisons can be made that will be helpful in differentiating subsequent changes" (Rudolph, 1977, p. 478). Since there is associated risk of tissue necrosis in this situation, it is not a procedure that the nurse practitioner would institute without physician consultation.

Viral Infections

HEPATITIS

Assessment. Viral hepatitis is a clinical condition commonly found in the United States. Up to 70,000 cases are reported each year but the real incidence is likely 10 times that figure. There are two types of viral hepatitis which show many similarities and some differences. Table 2 compares the major features of each type.

CLINICAL PICTURE. The prodromal period may resemble a respiratory or gastrointestinal infection. Then, during this preicteric phase, symptoms of fever, malaise, anorexia, nausea, vomiting, headache, and abdominal pain are common. Arthralgia may be present. If the individual smokes, lack of taste for cigarettes occurs. The liver may be enlarged and tender. These symptoms usually begin 4 to 5 days before the appearance of jaundice (icteric phase). During the icteric phase the urine becomes darker and the stools lighter in color. Jaundice of sclera and skin may last from a few days to as long as a month. In moderate to severe cases, significant weight loss may occur. The vast majority of individuals have an uneventful recovery and complete regeneration of liver cells is observed after 2 or 3 months (Krugman, 1977, p. 99). Children usually have milder disease than adults and are less likely to develop jaundice.

LABORATORY. Abnormal liver function and other laboratory tests are presented in Table 2.

COMPLICATIONS. In severe cases acute hepatic failure may develop. If drowsiness occurs after the onset of jaundice, it indicates possible pre-hepatic coma and the individual must be hospitalized. Chronic infection may lead to cirrhosis.

DIFFERENTIAL DIAGNOSIS. Before the appearance of jaundice, infectious mononucleosis, acute appendicitis, salmonellosis, shigellosis, and influenza may be considered.

Management

COUNSELING FOR HOME CARE. Most children can be cared for at home, and the treatment is entirely symptomatic and supportive. Adequate rest and a well-balanced, calorically sufficient diet are the two most appropriate measures to aid in regeneration of damaged liver tissue. Restriction of fat intake is not necessary. Vitamin supplements, particularly B complex, are recommended.

Table 2
Hepatitis A and Hepatitis B: Comparison of Major Features

Features	Hepatitis A	Hepatitis B
Synonym	Infectious hepatitis	Serum hepatitis
Incubation period	15–40 days	50–180 days
HB Ag (Australia antigen in blood)	Absent	Present in incubation period
Age group	Usually children and young adults	All age groups
Mode of transmission	Primarily fecal-to-oral route; some parenteral spread (blood products); contaminated water, food, infected shellfish	Primarily parenteral (transfusion of blood or blood products, drug inoculation); some nonparenteral (body fluids of infected persons)
Seasonal	Fall and winter predominantly but also throughout the year	Any season
Onset	Usually acute	Usually insidious
Fever	Common; precedes jaundice	Less common
Jaundice	Rare in children; more common in adults	Rare in children; more common in adults
Severity	Usually mild	Often severe
Abnormal SGOT	Transient; 1–3 weeks	More prolonged; 1–8 months
Thymol turbidity	Usually elevated	Usually normal
IgM levels	Usually increased	Usually normal
Virus excretion		
Blood	Present during late incubation period and early acute phase	Present during late incubation period and acute phase; may persist for months and years
Feces	Present during late incubation period and acute phase	Probably present but no direct proof
Value of gamma globulin prophylaxis	Good	Uncertain
Immunity		
Homologous	Present	Present
Heterologous	None	None

Source: Adapted from S. Krugman, et al, *Infectious Diseases of Children*, 6th ed., (St. Louis: C. V. Mosby, 1977), p. 101; and D. H. Carver and D. S. Y. Seto, "Hepatitis A and B," *Pediatr Clin North Am* 21:674, August 1974.

ISOLATION

Hepatitis A. The virus is excreted in the feces as early as 2 weeks before onset and into the early part of the icteric phase. Therefore, enteric precautions are required during the acute illness and at least 1 week after the onset of jaundice. See this chapter, Enteric Precautions. A single room with private bath is recommended for any person with the disease.

Hepatitis B. Infectivity is present in persons with acute hepatitis during the latter part of the incubation period and during the acute phase of the infection. It is also present in persons who are healthy chronic carriers. Enteric precautions are required during the acute illness. The virus may be present in the blood for variable and long periods of time and careful screening of blood donors is imperative.

PREVENTION AND PROPHYLAXIS

Hepatitis A. Gamma globulin is effective in prevention and/or modification of hepatitis A when given during the incubation period. See Table 3. Family members and other intimate contacts should receive injections of gamma globulin preferably within 1 week of exposure. Even if a clinically inapparent infection results, it is believed that such persons do not contribute to transmission of the disease (Rudolph, 1977, p. 528). Protection with gamma globulin is also recommended for persons who will experience prolonged exposure (e.g., travel to endemic areas).

Hepatitis B. Specific hepatitis B immune globulin (HBIG) is being evaluated and has proven efficacious for the prevention or modification of hepatitis B infection (Krugman, 1977, p. 113). Gamma globulin has had variable and inconsistent effectiveness in the prevention of hepatitis B but should be used if HBIG is not available. Screening of blood donors and the appropriate care of equipment used to break the skin (syringes, needles, stylets) are the best preventive measures.

Active immunization. An experimental inactivated hepatitis B vaccine has been tested in animals and found effective. Studies are continuing to evaluate its use in humans (Krugman, 1977, p. 116).

Table 3

Gamma Globulin in Prophylaxis of Viral Diseases for Exposed Susceptibles

Disease	Indication	Dosage	Efficacy
Measles	Close contact within 5 days	0.04 ml/kg 0.25 ml/kg	Modification Prevention (recommended for high risk patients only)[a]
Hepatitis A (infectious hepatitis)	Close contact (preferably within 1 week of exposure)	0.02 ml/kg	Modification (to anicteric, mild disease)
	Anticipated travel to endemic areas	0.02 ml/kg per months of exposure (up to 0.12 ml/kg for 6 months at which time a repeat dose is recommended)	Modification (to anicteric, mild disease)
Varicella	Close contacts at high risk (within 3 days)	0.6–1.2 ml/kg[b] for patients on corticosteroids for various diseases, on immunosuppressive drugs, with leukemia or other disseminated malignancies, or impaired delayed hypersensitivity	Possible modification

Source: Reprinted with permission from J. W. Graef and T. E. Cone, *Manual of Pediatric Therapeutics*, (Boston: Little, Brown, 1974), p. 190.

[a]When gamma globulin is indicated it should be given as soon as possible following exposure. It is of no proved value in the prophylaxis of rubella and mumps. In posttransfusion hepatitis hyperimmune gamma globulin, when available, may be beneficial.

[b]Zoster immune globulin (ZIG), if available, is preferable. Request should be directed to the CDC, Atlanta, Georgia or regional representative. Convalescent plasma also may modify the illness, if given immediately after exposure.

HERPES SIMPLEX

Assessment. Herpes simplex viruses are common infectious agents which cause a variety of clinical diseases. Primary infection occurs in susceptible persons and usually is inapparent. If clinical disease occurs, it can affect the skin, mucous membranes, eyes, genitals, or brain. In newborns who contract the disease from herpes vaginitis in the mother, herpes simplex is a very serious, disseminated disease with a high mortality.

PRIMARY INFECTION. Gingivostomatitis is the most common primary infection in children.

Epidemiology. The mode of transmission is thought to be by direct body contact and introduction of the virus through a break in the skin (e.g., kissing a teething baby). The incubation period is from 2 to 12 days. It is more common in overcrowded environments.

Clinical picture. Onset is abrupt with fever, irritability, anorexia, and sore mouth. The gums are red, swollen, and bleed easily. Multiple small vesicles appear on the palate, tongue, buccal mucosa, and gums which rupture and become white ulcerations. Eating and swallowing are painful. Symptoms usually subside within 10 days.

RECURRENT INFECTION. After the primary infection antibodies develop, but this disease is unusual in that the virus remains dormant in the host and can be reactivated when the body is under stress. Reinfections are localized and commonly take the form of "cold sores," "fever blisters," or "canker sores."

COMPLICATIONS. Herpes stomatitis, if severe, may result in dehydration. Children with atopic dermatitis who develop eczema herpeticum can have very serious disease.

Management. The child with herpes stomatitis is severely uncomfortable for several days (3 to 4) and presents a challenge to parents who want to provide relief. Treatment is supportive with primary attention to care of the mouth. Cool liquids and soft, bland foods are offered. Citrus juices are avoided. Oral hygiene with mouth washes and rinses is indicated. Analgesics may relieve the pain. Infants should be watched carefully for signs of dehydration. Older children will probably not take sufficient food or fluid, but parents can be reassured that they will soon recover. Secretion precautions are indicated.

Care of recurrent lesions is also symptomatic. Petroleum jelly is soothing and protective and is used if lesions appear at corners of the mouth and tend to crack and bleed.

HERPES ZOSTER (SHINGLES)

Assessment. Herpes zoster is caused by varicella-zoster virus and is thought to be a reactivation of a latent virus after an attack of chickenpox. It is characterized by pain and crops of vesicles confined to an area of distribution of one of the spinal or cranial sensory nerves.

EPIDEMIOLOGY. It is spread by direct contact with infected vesicle fluid. It is not as contagious as chickenpox but is communicable for 5 to 7 days after the vesicles appear. It is uncommon in children under 10 years of age and incidence increases with age.

CLINICAL PICTURE. The individual usually has pain along the involved dermatone. Malaise and fever may occur. Then, within a few days the first vesicles develop. The vesicles may be itchy. Successive crops of vesicles continue to appear for 1 to 4 days. The vesicles erupt and crust over and skin clears within 1 to 2 weeks.

Management. No specific therapy is available. Wet compresses or calamine lotion may soothe the lesions. Aspirin is given for pain.

ISOLATION. Contact with lesions is to be avoided until all lesions have crusted and dried. Some also recommend respiratory isolation.

EXPOSED CONTACTS. Susceptible individuals will develop varicella (chickenpox). If susceptible high-risk individuals (e.g., infants, immunosuppressed persons) are exposed to herpes zoster,

Zoster Immune Globulin given within 72 hours of exposure can prevent varicella (Rudolph, 1977, p. 880). See Table 3.

INFLUENZA

Assessment. Influenza is an acute disease of the respiratory tract caused primarily by influenza viruses A, B, and C. Mutant strains of influenza virus A have recently caused pandemics of the disease: Asian strain in 1957 and Hong Kong strain in 1968–69. Since the viruses have this ability to change their dominant antigenic properties, cyclic epidemics can be expected. This factor mitigates against simple influenza immunization programs.

EPIDEMIOLOGY

Mode of transmission. The virus is spread by airborne droplet and direct contact.

Incubation period. The incubation period is from 1 to 2 days.

Period of communicability. Infected persons are communicable from the first to the fifth day of the disease, including the incubation period.

Population at risk. Since mutant strains of influenza virus A occur at intervals, new groups of susceptible hosts accumulate during these intervals. When major antigenic changes occur, susceptibility is universal. Between epidemics, smaller outbreaks occur in new young susceptible children and in others who escaped the previous epidemic.

Seasonal patterns. Epidemics of influenza A occur during the winter months every 2 to 3 years.

CLINICAL PICTURE. The onset is rapid with chills, fever, headache, generalized aches and pains, malaise, anorexia, and prostration. Vomiting and diarrhea may be the major symptoms in young children. A hacking cough and rhinitis may develop. The eyes may be painful. The lungs are clear, but severe infections may involve the lower respiratory tract and cause pneumonia. Uncomplicated cases usually clear in 3 to 4 days.

Management. Treatment is entirely symptomatic. See this chapter, General Measures. Effective isolation is largely impractical in epidemic situations.

PREVENTION. Available influenza vaccine for viruses A and B is recommended for children who are at risk because of chronic illness (cardiac, pulmonary). Adverse reactions are less common now as the vaccines are more purified. The emergence of new strains of virus renders old vaccines ineffective and the difficulties in developing and testing new vaccines continue to be problematic (Krugman, 1977, pp. 489–492).

MEASLES (RUBEOLA)

Assessment. Measles is a highly contagious disease of childhood which can cause severe morbidity and serious complications.

EPIDEMIOLOGY

Mode of transmission. It is spread by respiratory droplets and by contact with articles freshly contaminated by secretions from the nose, throat, mouth, and eyes.

Incubation period. It is 9 to 14 days.

Period of communicability. Children are contagious for at least 7 days after onset of the first symptom.

Population at risk. Unimmunized persons are at risk. In crowded urban areas infants and preschool children have the highest incidence. In less populated areas school age children have the highest incidence. Infants under 4 to 5 months of age whose mothers had measles rarely contract the disease because of passive immunity transmitted via the placenta. Infants of mothers who never had measles are susceptible. In underdeveloped countries severe measles epidemics still occur. One attack of measles infection generally produces permanent immunity.

Seasonal patterns. Peak incidence occurs during winter and spring months. In the past epidemics occurred at 2- to 3-year intervals as new groups of susceptibles developed. Since introduction of measles vaccine in 1963, epidemics have declined, but concern presently exists over inadequate levels of immunization in some population groups. See Chapter 2, Immunization Levels.

CLINICAL PICTURE. Approximately 9 to 10 days after exposure the prodrome begins with fever, malaise, cough, coryza, and conjunctivitis. These symptoms increase in severity, peak on the fourth day coincident with the appearance of the rash, and persist until the second or third day of the rash. See Table 1 for description of the rash and Koplik's spots. During this period the child may be extremely uncomfortable and look miserable. Fever may be high; cough and coryza are severe. The conjunctivae are swollen and inflamed and photophobia may result. Nausea, vomiting, headache, and myalgia are common. In uncomplicated measles the temperature falls by the third day after onset of the rash, other symptoms begin to subside, and within a few days the child feels well. Fever that persists may indicate complications.

LABORATORY. Measles HI titer, if performed, will demonstrate a rise in antibodies by the second day of the rash.

COMPLICATIONS. Complications result from extensive viral inflammation and/or secondary bacterial infection. Otitis media is one of the most common complications. Other respiratory complications include mastoiditis, pneumonia (leading cause of fatality), and laryngotracheobronchitis. Acute encephalitis, a serious complication, occurs in about 0.1 percent of cases (or one in 2000 to 3000 cases), and mortality or severe sequelae are frequent.

Management

COUNSELING FOR HOME CARE

Supportive care. Treatment is symptomatic. Bright lights should be avoided if photophobia is present. Warm water is used to cleanse the eyes. See this chapter, General Measures.

Isolation. Respiratory and discharge precautions are recommended from the onset of the catarrhal stage through the third day of rash. Isolation may also serve to prevent exposure of the infected child to secondary bacterial infection.

Return to school. The child may resume school attendance upon clinical recovery and at least 5 days after appearance of rash.

EXPOSED CONTACTS

Active immunization. Measles vaccine given within 24 hours of exposure can prevent infection.

Passive immunization. Gamma globulin given within 5 days after exposure can modify or prevent measles in susceptible persons. See Table 3. Modified measles usually results in lasting immunity so the recommendation is to give a modifying dose of gamma globulin to susceptible persons of all ages. Complete protection is indicated for infants and children with chronic illness because of the dangers of severe complications. Subsequently, normal infants should receive active immunization at 15 to 18 months of age or at least 2 to 3 months after gamma globulin injection. High-risk, chronically ill children can best be protected by active immunization of their regular contacts.

PREVENTION. Active immunization can effectively prevent measles. See Chapter 2, Immunizations.

MONONUCLEOSIS, INFECTIOUS

Assessment. Infectious mononucleosis is an acute infectious disease occurring primarily in adolescents and young adults, caused by the Epstein-Barr virus (EBV).

EPIDEMIOLOGY

Mode of transmission. The virus is not very contagious and is spread through oropharyngeal secretions and intimate contact (e.g., kissing).

Incubation period. Eleven days is average with a range of 4 to 14 days.

Period of communicability. This is uncertain since the source and time of contact are usually unknown, but it is probably only during the acute illness.

Population at risk. Adolescents and young adults are most susceptible. EBV infections occur in infancy and childhood but are likely to be mild and unrecognized.

CLINICAL PICTURE. The illness is generally benign. Onset is abrupt or insidious with mild symptoms of headache, malaise, and fatigue. Fever rises gradually and may persist. Sore throat occurs by the end of the first week, and the tonsils are enlarged, reddened, and covered with a shaggy membrane. The membrane peels off in 5 to 8 days. Lymphadenopathy and splenomegaly are common. Erythematous maculopapular skin rash, hepatomegaly, jaundice, pneumonitis, and CNS involvement are less frequent manifestations of the disease. Most cases clear by the end of the third week although weakness and fatigue may persist for several weeks.

LABORATORY. Blood smear will show atypical lymphocytes accounting for more than 10 percent of the field. Leukocyte count may be markedly elevated. Heterophile antibodies appear in blood serum by the end of the first week of illness and persist for variable periods of time. Liver function tests are often abnormal. A rapid slide test (MONO spot) has been developed which detects antibody and is a valuable diagnostic aid.

COMPLICATIONS. Severe cases may be associated with severe dysphagia, dyspnea, myocarditis, hepatitis, hemolytic anemia, and CNS involvement. Rarely, rupture of the spleen occurs.

Management

MEDICATION. Corticosteroids are used in severe and toxic cases to relieve symptoms. They are not recommended for routine cases.

COUNSELING FOR HOME CARE

Supportive care. Symptomatic treatment is indicated. See this chapter, General Measures. Bed rest with gradual increase in activity is recommended. Social contact may resume after the acute phase. Strenuous physical activity is contraindicated while the spleen remains significantly enlarged.

Isolation. None is required.

MUMPS

Assessment. Mumps (epidemic parotitis) is caused by a virus that has affinity for glandular and nervous tissue.

EPIDEMIOLOGY

Mode of transmission. Intimate contact is required with spread occurring through droplets of saliva.

Incubation period. It is usually 16 to 18 days but may be up to 3-1/2 weeks.

Period of communicability. It is less communicable than measles, pertussis, and chickenpox. The period of infectivity is uncertain but may be from 6 days prior to 9 days after the appearance of parotid swelling. In persons with inapparent infections, virus has been recovered in saliva between the fifteenth and twenty-fourth days after exposure.

Population at risk. The disease is endemic in urban populations at all times and individuals of all ages are susceptible. The highest incidence is in unimmunized children between 5 and 15 years. One attack usually results in lifelong immunity.

Seasonal patterns. It has year round occurrence but is more prominent in winter and spring months.

CLINICAL PICTURE. Mild cases may not have a prodrome. When a prodrome exists, it consists of fever, headache, anorexia, malaise, and muscle pain. Within 24 to 48 hours local pain around the ear and jaw develops. This is followed by swelling of the parotid gland which reaches maximum size in 1 to 3 days. One or both parotid glands may be involved. Twenty-five percent have unilateral parotitis. The ear lobe is distorted upward and outward by the swelling. Pain and tenderness may be severe. Other glands (submaxillary, sublingual) also may swell. The swelling gradually subsides over a period of 3 to 7 days. This is the "classic" case, but there is much individual variation in the clinical signs and symptoms.

Epididymo-orchitis.   This is a common manifestation (20 to 30 percent) in adolescent and adult males. The orchitis is usually unilateral and develops within the first 2 weeks of the infection. Testicular swelling may occur as the only manifestation of mumps. The inflammation and swelling subside as the fever disappears. Some testicular atrophy occurs in about half the cases (Krugman, 1977, p. 184). Complete atrophy of both testicles is so rare that the concern about sterility and sexual impotence has no basis.

Meningoencephalitis.   This occurs in over 10 percent of cases. It may be the only clinical expression of mumps, but it usually follows parotitis by 3 to 10 days. The signs and symptoms of fever, headache, nausea and vomiting, nuchal rigidity, and Kernig's and Brudzinski's signs are similar to aseptic meningitis and usually clear entirely. Rarely a secondary encephalitis develops after the mumps, and paralysis, particularly of cranial nerves, may occur along with drowsiness and coma.

LABORATORY.   Mumps antibody can be identified most reliably by the complement fixation test.

COMPLICATIONS.   Complications are rare but include deafness, usually unilateral (once in every 300 to 400 cases); postinfectious encephalitis with serious sequelae; myocarditis, pancreatitis, hepatitis, neuritis, and arthritis.

Management

COUNSELING FOR HOME CARE

Supportive care.   Citrus fruits and fluids should be avoided. Pain may be relieved by aspirin, codeine, and warm or cold compresses. See this chapter, General Measures.

Isolation. Respiratory precautions are recommended until swelling subsides, but the value of isolation is questionable.

Return to school. Children may return to school after the first week of the illness.

EXPOSED CONTACTS. Mumps immune globulin and ordinary gamma globulin are not efficacious in protecting exposed susceptibles. There is no evidence that vaccination with live attenuated vaccine will protect exposed susceptibles but there is no contraindication to its use in this group.

PREVENTION. Active immunization. See Chapter 2, Immunizations.

POLIOMYELITIS

Assessment. Poliomyelitis is a viral infection (enterovirus) that used to be widespread throughout the world. There are three types of virus: Type 1 is the most virulent; Types 2 and 3 are less virulent. Prior to polio vaccine most of the population were exposed to the virus through contact with the wild natural polio virus strains. It is primarily a mild, nonspecific febrile illness or a completely asymptomatic infection, but occasionally a severe paralytic form occurs which can leave lifelong sequelae or can cause death. With the advent of poliovirus vaccine, it has become a preventable disease.

EPIDEMIOLOGY

Mode of transmission. Polio virus is a wild virus that circulates in the population and multiplies in the human intestinal tract. Direct contact via the fecal-oropharyngeal route is the principal mode of spread.

Incubation period. The average is 7 to 10 days with a range of 5 to 35 days from the time of exposure to the onset of CNS symptoms. Minor illness has an incubation period of 3 to 5 days.

Period of communicability. Virus is present in throat, blood, and feces 3 to 5 days after exposure and is excreted in the stools in large concentration for 6 to 8 weeks after onset of abortive, nonparalytic, and paralytic infections.

Population at risk. Young children are especially susceptible. See Chapter 2, Oral Poliovirus Vaccine.

Seasonal patterns. The summer and early autumn months have the greatest incidence.

CLINICAL PICTURE. Exposure of a susceptible person to polio virus results in one of the following responses listed in order of frequency:

1. Asymptomatic infection
2. Abortive poliomyelitis. A picture of fever, sore throat, headache, nausea and vomiting, and abdominal pain lasting 24 to 72 hours represents the entire course of the disease and never is identified as polio.
3. Nonparalytic poliomyelitis. The above symptoms may be more severe. Pain and stiffness occur in the neck, back, and legs.
4. Paralytic poliomyelitis. Minor illness occurs as described above (abortive illness) and may be followed by 1 to 7 days of feeling well. Then symptoms return accompanied by weakness and paralysis in one or more muscle groups. Respiratory difficulties may occur from a variety of causes. Site of paralysis depends on the area of the CNS affected as follows:

   • Spinal form affects muscles supplied by motor neurons in the spinal cord.
   • Bulbar form affects muscles supplied by the cranial nerves or the medulla which are concerned with respiration and circulation.
   • Encephalitic form affects higher cortical centers.

Once the fever subsides, the spread of weakness and paralysis stops. Spontaneous improvement will occur but if full muscle power has not returned by 18 months to 2 years, the residual is usually permanent. Consult major references for a full discussion of the manifestations and management of this disease.

Management. There is no specific treatment. Abortive and non-paralytic cases are treated symptomatically at home.

COUNSELING FOR HOME CARE

Isolation. Enteric precautions are recommended for several weeks.

Return to school. Return to school is permitted 1 week after onset of symptoms or after defervescence, whichever is longer.

EXPOSED CONTACTS. See Chapter 2, Oral Poliovirus Vaccine. Protection of susceptible individuals during polio outbreaks can be enhanced by avoiding:

1. Visits to families and communities where the disease is prevalent
2. Overexertion and chilling
3. Fruits and vegetables that have not been thoroughly washed
4. Tonsillectomy and other operations in the nasopharynx and mouth
5. Unnecessary injections and routine immunizations with other than poliovirus vaccine

PREVENTION. Active immunization. See Chapter 2, Immunizations. The virus serotype should be identified and the corresponding monovalent vaccine given on a community-wide basis to all persons over 2 months of age.

ROSEOLA (EXANTHEM SUBITUM)

Assessment. Roseola is an acute, benign viral infection of infants and young children. It is the most common exanthem in infants between 6 months and 2 years of age.

EPIDEMIOLOGY

Mode of transmission. Contact is probably respiratory, but the pattern is unclear.

Incubation period. It is probably between 10 to 15 days.

Period of communicability. The degree of contagiousness is unclear. Transmission to siblings and other close contacts is rare.

Population at risk. Ninety-five percent of cases occur in children between 6 months and 3 years of age.

Seasonal patterns. It occurs year round with peak incidence in spring and autumn.

CLINICAL PICTURE. The onset is sudden with an abrupt rise in temperature to high levels (40 to 41°C). Initial presentation may be with a febrile convulsion. Anorexia, irritability, and mild pharyngitis may be present. After 3 to 4 days of high fever, the temperature rapidly falls and coincides with the appearance of the rash. See Table 1 for description of the rash. Occipital and postauricular lymph nodes are commonly present. A feature of the disease is the lack of physical findings sufficient to explain the fever. The child looks alert and nontoxic in spite of the high fever. Recovery is uneventful and complete.

COMPLICATIONS. Febrile convulsion is the most common complication.

Management

COUNSELING FOR HOME CARE. Treatment is symptomatic. See this chapter, General Measures. Parents need support to survive the anxiety of 3 to 4 days of unresponsive fever. No isolation is necessary. Permanent immunity results from the attack.

RUBELLA (GERMAN MEASLES)

Assessment. Rubella is a common viral infection characterized by mild constitutional symptoms, a 3-day rash, and lymphadenopathy. It is of note, primarily, because of its severe effects in the fetus if contracted by a susceptible pregnant woman during the first trimester.

EPIDEMIOLOGY

Mode of transmission. The infection spreads directly by airborne droplets or by contact with infected persons.

Incubation period. Incubation period is 14 to 21 days.

Period of communicability. Rubella is communicable from 7 days before to about 5 days after the rash. Greatest communicability is 3 days before the rash.

Population at risk. Unimmunized persons are susceptible. The infection is rare in infancy and uncommon in preschool children. Highest incidence occurs in school age children, adolescents, and young adults. In the United States 80 to 85 percent of women of childbearing age are immune. The fetus of a susceptible mother is at greatest risk.

Seasonal patterns. It is endemic in populated areas. Most cases occur during the spring months in temperate zones.

CLINICAL PICTURE. Often the infection goes unnoticed. If there is a prodrome, it consists of mild catarrhal symptoms (fever, malaise, sore throat, coryza). Typically the first manifestation is postauricular, occipital, and posterior cervical adenopathy. The rash usually appears shortly after lymph nodes become enlarged and tender. See Table 1 for description of the rash. Women may experience polyarthralgia or polyarthritis, but this is uncommon in children. As the rash fades, complete recovery follows.

LABORATORY. Rubella infection is confirmed by virus isolation or by rising titers of rubella antibody in the serum (rubella HI antibody test). Antibody is usually detectable by the third day of the rash.

COMPLICATIONS. Complications are very rare in postnatally acquired rubella but arthritis, encephalitis, and purpura have occurred.

CONGENITAL RUBELLA SYNDROME. The risks of rubella syndrome following maternal rubella are not clear but are thought to be significant: 30 to 50 percent if contracted during the first 4 weeks of gestation; 25 percent during the first 5 to 8 weeks; 8 percent during the first 9 to 12 weeks. Overall risk in the first trimester is 20 percent (Krugman, 1977, p. 284). Manifestations of congenital rubella include growth retardation, eye defects, congenital heart disease, deafness, CNS defects, mental retardation, thrombocytopenic purpura, bone defects, and others. Infants who survive remain infective for many months (up to and beyond 18 months) and present hazards to susceptible caretakers.

Management

COUNSELING FOR HOME CARE

Supportive care.   The disease is usually so mild that symptomatic treatment is not necessary.

Isolation.   None is required except that women in the first trimester of pregnancy should not be exposed.

Return to school.   Quarantine is not usually imposed.

PREGNANT WOMEN EXPOSED TO RUBELLA.   See Chapter 2, Rubella.

PREVENTION.   Active immunization. See Chapter 2, Immunizations.

VARICELLA (CHICKENPOX)

Assessment.   Varicella is a highly contagious disease caused by the varicella-zoster virus (see this chapter, Herpes Zoster). The characteristic feature is the generalized, pruritic, vesicular rash.

EPIDEMIOLOGY

Mode of transmission.   Direct contact with persons infected with varicella and herpes zoster is the predominant mode. Respiratory spread also occurs.

Incubation period.   It is 14 to 16 days with a range of 10 to 21 days.

Period of communicability. Transmission occurs from 1 day before the rash until 5 to 6 days after onset of the rash when all vesicles have crusted.

Population at risk. Highest incidence is in children between 2 and 8 years, but all ages are susceptible. It is much more severe in adults. Maternal passive protection exists for the first few months of life.

Seasonal patterns. There is a higher incidence during the winter and spring.

CLINICAL PICTURE. The rash is generally the first symptom. See Table 1 for description of the rash. Fever, headache, malaise, and anorexia parallel the severity of the rash. Once an individual lesion dries, a crust forms and falls off within 5 to 20 days, depending on the extent of the lesion. Usually there is no scarring but lesions that become secondarily infected (usually by vigorous scratching with dirty fingernails) may leave permanent scars.

COMPLICATIONS. Complications are not common in children. Secondary bacterial skin infections occasionally lead to impetigo, furunculosis, cellulitis, erysipelas, or conjunctivitis. Children with leukemia or on immunosuppressive medications may develop encephalitis, pneumonia, or disseminated varicella.

Management

COUNSELING FOR HOME CARE

Supportive care. Care of the skin is paramount. Itching may be relieved by cornstarch baths, systemic antipruritic medication such as diphenhydramine (Benadryl) and topical lotions (calamine). See this chapter, General Measures. Occurrence of secondary skin infection can be reduced by bathing with soap and water, changing bed linens and clothes frequently, keeping fingernails short and clean, and using mittens while the child sleeps.

Isolation. The child should be kept at home until the vesicles have dried. Respiratory and secretion precautions are advised.

Return to school.   Return to school is permitted not sooner than 7 days after onset.

EXPOSED CONTACTS.   In most instances exposure occurs before the disease is detected. Due to its inevitability and benign nature, protection or isolation of healthy susceptible contacts is not warranted. Infants and high-risk children require strict protection from exposure. If exposure occurs Zoster Immune Globulin given within 3 days of exposure is effective in modifying varicella. See Table 3.

PREVENTION.   Active immunization. Efforts are underway to develop a live attenuated varicella vaccine.

Parasitic Infections

Infections caused by parasites (helminths, protozoans) are less common in the United States than in tropical and subtropical parts of the world, but they do occur, especially with the increase in intercontinental travel. Children are affected more frequently than adults. Prevalence varies with climate, sanitation, and socioeconomic conditions. Information on some of the most common parasitic diseases is briefly presented in Table 4. For more extensive discussion, including specific medical treatment, refer to major pediatric texts listed in the References.

ENTEROBIASIS (PINWORMS)

Assessment.   See Table 4.

Management

MEDICATION.   Since the infection is so easily transmitted, many physicians recommend medication for the entire family. The following medications are commonly used:

1. Pyrantel pamoate (Antiminth). 11 mg/kg orally in a single dose. Maximal dose is 1 gm. It comes in suspension form. Side effects may be nausea, vomiting, and abdominal cramps.

2. Pryvinium pamoate (Povan). 5 mg/kg orally in a single dose and repeated in 2 to 3 weeks. It comes in suspension form. Stool becomes red. Vomiting and abdominal cramps may occur.

3. Piperazine citrate (Antepar). 65 mg/kg orally for 7 days. It is given in the morning before breakfast. It comes in syrup, wafer, and tablet forms. Vomiting, diarrhea, and visual disturbances have been reported.

COUNSELING FOR HOME CARE

Hygienic care. Eradication is difficult because of the ease of reinfection and transmission. Some authorities recommend vigorous hygienic measures such as daily boiling of bed linens, underwear, and pajamas, and thorough vacuuming. Such measures are probably of little value, but scrupulous parents may feel better carrying out such a regimen. The most reasonable and effective means of reducing infection is personal hygiene including handwashing and fingernail cleaning and cutting.

Supportive care. Most parents react with shock and revulsion when told their child has "worms." Mothers often feel it must be a reflection of their mothering abilities and become defensive. The nurse practitioner can allay guilt and support parents by explaining the benign nature of pinworms, the high incidence in young children, and the causative factors. Reassurance is necessary that it occurs in all types of families and has no stigma attached.

Venereal Diseases

GONORRHEA

Assessment. Gonorrhea is an acute infectious bacterial disease caused by *Neisseria gonorrhoeae*. It is the most frequently reported communicable disease in the United States and it is estimated that there may be upwards of 2 million cases per year. An alarming increase in cases is occurring in the 10- to 19-year-old age group.

Table 4
Common Parasitic Infections

Disease and Name of Parasite	Mode of Transmission	Mechanism of Infection	Clinical Findings	Diagnosis	Comments
Protozoan infections:					
Amebiasis (*Entamoeba histolytica*)	Cysts contained in human feces are ingested via contaminated food or water.	Cysts deposit in colonic mucosa causing ulcers. Ulcers cause erosion of blood vessels and also permit amebae to enter the portal system and invade the liver.	Many are asymptomatic or have mild symptoms. Diarrhea, abdominal pain, and dysentery occur. May develop liver abscess.	Stool reveals cysts or trophozoites (vegetative stage of the amebae).	Children in institutional settings are especially vulnerable. Food handlers must use careful handwashing. In environments with unsanitary conditions, do not eat raw food or drink water without precautions.
Giardiasis (*Giardia lamblia*)	Cysts contained in human feces are ingested via direct contact or contaminated food and water.	Trophozoites inhabit the duodenum, upper jejunum.	May be asymptomatic. May have anorexia, nausea, flatulence, abdominal pain. In severe cases, protracted mucous diarrhea, fever, weight loss, and malabsorption can occur.	Diarrheal stool reveals trophozoites. Formed stool reveals cysts.	See Amebiasis, above. Sanitary disposal of feces is important.
Helminthic infections:					
Ascariasis (Roundworm; *Ascaris lumbricoides*)	Ingestion of ova contained in soil contaminated with human feces via dirt, food, water.	Ova hatch in small intestine. Larvae penetrate bowel wall, enter portal system, migrate to the liver and eventually the	May be asymptomatic. May have abdominal distress, malaise; cough during the lung stage. Pneumonia and	Detection of ova in stool. Eosinophilia is marked during migration.	Common in Gulf Coast states, Ozark area, and southern Appalachia. Stress sanitary disposal of feces.

Disease (organism)	Transmission	Life cycle / Pathology	Clinical features	Diagnosis	Comments
		lungs. From the lungs they ascend to the oropharynx and are swallowed. Thus the adult worm inhabits the jejunum.	intestinal obstruction can occur in severe cases.		
Enterobiasis (Pinworm: *Enterobius vermicularis*)	Ova are swallowed either after the child scratches the anal area and transfers fingers to mouth, or by inhalation of ova while handling contaminated bed linens or clothing.	Mature worms inhabit the large intestine and the female migrates to the anus and lays eggs on the perianal and perineal skin.	Nocturnal perianal pruritus. Usually no systemic symptoms, although irritability, anorexia, and loss of sleep can occur. Girls have vulvitis, vaginitis.	Scotch tape test. Press clear tape on perianal skin, transfer tape to glass slide, and observe ova under a microscope.	Up to 30% of children in the United States have pinworms. See text, this chapter, for management.
Hookworm (*Necator americanus*)	Eggs passed in infected feces develop into larvae in the soil. Larvae penetrate human skin, usually through bare feet.	From the skin they enter the blood stream and then pass through the lungs, ascend to the pharynx, and are swallowed. The adult worms attach to intestinal villi and feed on blood.	Small infestations may be asymptomatic. May have dermatitis of feet, cough, fever, abdominal pain, diarrhea. Chronic and large infestations may lead to anemia, iron deficiency, malnutrition.	Detection of ova in stool. Elevated eosinophilia.	Prevalent in the southern United States. Stress sanitary disposal of feces. Encourage wearing of shoes.
Trichinosis (*Trichinella spiralis*)	Ingestion of infected pork, insufficiently cooked.	Larvae emerge in small intestine, mature, and burrow into intestinal wall. New larvae are produced and migrate throughout the body and invade striated muscle.	During the intestinal phase, gastroenteritis is seen. subsequently periorbital and facial edema, headache, fever, conjunctivitis, photophobia, severe muscle pain and tenderness may develop. Cardiac and CNS symptoms may also develop.	History of eating raw or partially cooked pork. Muscle biopsy. Serologic tests. Marked eosinophilia.	In the United States, meat is *not* inspected for this worm. Cook pork thoroughly.

EPIDEMIOLOGY

Mode of transmission. Sexual contact with an infected person is the primary mode of transmission. Newborn infants become infected while passing through the birth canal of an infected mother.

Incubation period. The incubation period is short, 3 to 5 days.

Communicability. The organisms are deposited on a mucosal surface (genitourinary, rectal, oral), colonize, and survive until treated. Communicability is high.

Population at risk. All persons are at risk. There is no permanent immunity after an infection. One to two percent of cases occur in children under 14 years of age, and sexual abuse of young children must be considered. The incidence in men, according to reported cases, is three times greater than in women, but this is explained by the fact that the symptoms in men are more overt and result in the seeking of medical care. Approximately 10 to 40 percent of men may be asymptomatic. On the other hand, over 80 percent of women are asymptomatic.

Seasonal patterns. It is more prevalent during the summer, for unknown reasons.

CLINICAL PICTURE. Clinical presentation differs in men, women, and newborns.

Male. Two days to 2 weeks after contact, there is sudden onset of burning on urination and a profuse purulent discharge from the urethra. The infection may spread and involve the posterior urethra (cloudy urine), prostate (retention of urine, pain, fever), and/or the epididymis (pain, tenderness, swelling, possible sterility). If treated, it usually subsides within 24 hours. Proctitis and oropharyngitis may also be primary signs of infection.

Female. Early signs in the symptomatic female are dysuria and purulent vaginal discharge. The infection may spread from the cervix to the fallopian tubes and cause acute salpingitis (pelvic inflammatory disease). Symptoms are fever, chills, severe bilateral lower abdominal pain, nausea, and vomiting. Sterility may occur. These symptoms must be distinguished from acute appendicitis.

Newborn. Instillation of 1 percent silver nitrate solution into the eyes of newborns at birth has greatly reduced infection, but failures do occur. Gonococcal ophthalmia may affect one or both eyes. Symptoms begin 2 to 7 days after delivery and include mild conjunctivitis followed by serosanguinous or purulent discharge. The eyelids are edematous and, if untreated, corneal ulceration, iritis, and permanent eye damage may occur.

LABORATORY. There is no serologic test available. Gram stain smears can be used as adjuncts to cultures. Cultures are confirmatory. Specimens are obtained from cervix, urethra, rectum, pharynx. All persons should also have serologic test done for syphilis.

COMPLICATIONS. Dissemination via hematogenous spread may occur and the most common manifestations are skin lesions, arthritis, and tenosynovitis in adolescents and adults; meningitis, sepsis, and arthritis in the newborn.

Management

MEDICATION. The "single shot" therapy is the method of choice in gonorrhea. Antimicrobial agents are used, but the gonococcus has been developing progressive resistance to the majority of effective antimicrobials, especially penicillin. As a result, it is necessary to give extremely large single doses of antibiotic (4.8 million units of aqueous procaine penicillin G, IM; or 3.5 gm of ampicillin, orally), and there is danger that the era of single dose therapy is ending. This would greatly hinder control programs (Grossman, 1974, p. 108). Probenecid (a renal tubular blocking agent) is given with the antibiotic to delay urinary excretion of the antibiotic and to enhance its effectiveness.

FOLLOW-UP. Cultures are done as follows:

1. Male. Seven days after treatment
2. Female. Seven to fourteen days after treatment

EXPOSED CONTACTS. All exposed contacts should be cultured for the presence of gonorrhea, but the problems of identification of all contacts are obviously enormous. Sex education of individuals, in schools, communities, and via the communications media and laws permitting treatment of minors can assist but, in fact, gonorrhea remains epidemic in our current society. See Chapter 10, Health Care of the Adolescent. Gonorrhea cultures should be considered as part of routine health maintenance screening in pubertal males and females.

SYPHILIS

Assessment. Syphilis is a systemic infectious disease caused by the spirochete *Treponema pallidum*. It is the sixth most frequently reported infectious disease in the United States, but since only 12 percent of cases are reported, the actual incidence is thought to be approximately 140,000 cases annually. As a result of the increased incidence of acquired syphilis, the incidence of congenital syphilis is also rising and has doubled in the last 10 years.

EPIDEMIOLOGY

Mode of transmission. Acquired syphilis is spread primarily by close sexual contact between an infective lesion and a break in the skin or mucous membrane of the genitalia, anus, mouth, or other parts of the recipient. Congenital syphilis is acquired by transplacental spread from an infected mother to the infant in utero after the fourth month of pregnancy.

Incubation period. Within 10 to 90 days after acquired syphilitic infection (average is 21 days) the characteristic lesion, chancre, appears at the site of contact.

Communicability. Communicability exists while moist lesions are present and, if untreated, during primary, secondary, and latent syphilis. Late lesions are thought to be noninfectious. "After an infection has been present more than 4 years, it is rarely communicable" (Krugman, 1977, p. 315).

Population at risk. Children and adults of all ages are susceptible to acquiring syphilis. The fetus of the infected pregnant woman is at high risk. Having syphilis once does not prevent second attacks.

CLINICAL PICTURE

Acquired syphilis. In *primary syphilis* the primary lesion (chancre) is a painless, indurated, eroded ulcer often found on the glans penis, labia, vagina, cervix, anus, rectum, or mouth. Chancres are frequently accompanied by hard, nonfluctuant, painless, enlarged regional lymph nodes (bubo). The chancre disappears with or without treatment within 3 to 5 weeks and is followed by the manifestations of *secondary syphilis*. These include a generalized, painless, nonpruritic, macular, papular or pustular rash usually involving the palms and soles; condylomas of the anogenital area; mucous patches in the mouth; general malaise, fever, and alopecia. These symptoms may last from a few days to a year. If untreated, the disease progresses to the stage of *latent syphilis*. There are no symptoms during this stage; the disease is hidden and may remain so for the life of the individual. However, untreated syphilis that reaches this stage may result, 15 or 20 years later, in the serious and widespread CNS and vascular complications of late syphilis including neurosyphilis, paresis (with minor to major personality changes), tabes dorsalis, blindness, and cardiac disease.

Congenital syphilis. Severely affected fetuses die in utero or shortly after birth. In infants who appear normal at birth, the first signs are:

1. Rhinitis (snuffles) appearing in the first week of life or up to the third month which is persistent, severe, often blood-tinged, and often associated with laryngitis.
2. Rash which is usually diffuse, symmetric, copper-colored, maculopapular, and most prominent on the face, palms, and soles.
3. Bone lesions which are the most common single finding. X-rays show multiple bone involvement, and areas of destruction and growth disturbance (Grossman, 1974, p. 122).

Other features of congenital syphilis are fissures and mucous patches around the lips, nares, and anus; jaundice; anemia; generalized glandular involvement; hepatomegaly; splenomegaly; malnutrition; weight loss; pneumonia; nephrotic syndrome; and meningovascular involvement. If treatment is given during the first few months of life, complete recovery usually occurs.

If undetected or insufficiently treated the manifestations (stigmata) of late congenital syphilis include:

1. Hutchinson's teeth (upper central incisors are peg-shaped and notched) and other tooth deformities
2. Interstitial keratitis (intense inflammation of the cornea, scarring, and potential blindness)
3. Eighth nerve deafness
4. Clutton's joints (synovial effusions of knees)
5. Saddle nose

LABORATORY. Diagnosis is made using the following methods:

1. Dark-field examination. Microscopic examination of exudate from a lesion or rash reveals the organism. This technique is effective only during primary, secondary, early congenital, or infectious-relapse syphilis.
2. Serologic tests.

   • Venereal Disease Research Laboratories (VDRL), Kline, Kahn, and others are screening tests that will detect reagin (antibody thought to be the product of interaction between *Treponema pallidum* and body tissues). They are not specific for syphilis and do not become positive until 1 to 3 weeks after the primary lesion.
   • Fluorescent Treponemal Antibody Absorption Test (FTA-ABS) is a specific test and is used almost universally since it can detect syphilis in the early stages and gives few false readings.

Management

MEDICATION. Penicillin is the preferred treatment for all stages and manifestations of syphilis.

FOLLOW-UP. After treatment, persons with primary and secondary syphilis should have periodic VDRL tests for at least a year as the VDRL becomes negative 6 to 12 months after primary syphilis and 1 to 2 years after secondary syphilis.

EXPOSED CONTACTS. These persons should be examined and screened for syphilis. A VDRL should be part of routine health maintenance visits during adolescence. Pregnant women routinely have a VDRL test during pregnancy, but if a woman is considered high risk for contracting syphilis after the fourth month of pregnancy, a repeat VDRL is indicated.

Recurrent Infections

PRIMARY IMMUNODEFICIENCY DISEASE

Assessment. Children with primary immunodeficiencies affecting cell-mediated immunity or antibody-mediated immunity usually present between the ages of 2 months and 2 years with increased numbers of infections which are unusually severe. These children also never seem to completely recover from one infection before the next one begins. They appear to be "sick all the time." Table 5 shows the common clinical signs and symptoms in such children. It is important to obtain a detailed history of all infections, the intervals between infections, environmental factors (e.g., exposure to sources of infection), and parental expectations and ideas about illness in their children. Some parents may have unrealistic notions and fears about childhood illness and may think their child is chronically sick when, in fact, the child is experiencing the normal number of routine infections.

LABORATORY. If suspicion of primary immunodeficiency disease exists, diagnostic tests include:

1. Complete blood count with total lymphocyte count. Normal lymphocytes number 1200 or more. If the lymphocyte count is less than 1200, cellular immune deficiency is likely.
2. Quantitative immunoglobulins

Table 5
Common Clinical Findings in Children with Primary Immunodeficiency Disease

Common Symptoms	Less Common Symptoms	Occasional Symptoms
Recurrent respiratory infections	Chronic pneumonitis or bronchiectasis	Pneumocystis carinii pneumonia
Recurrent bilateral otitis media	Irritability and pallor Pyoderma	Nonspecific skin rashes, hair loss, and eczema
Unusually severe bacterial infections (sepsis and meningitis)	Lack of lymph nodes and tonsils Oral apthous ulcers	Severe viral disease Arthritis
Recurrent diarrhea		Enlarged liver and spleen
Fungal skin infections (thrush)		Enlarged lymph nodes Increased or decreased white blood cell count, decreased platelets, and anemia
Developmental retardation and failure to thrive		

Source: Reprinted with permission from: E. H. Waechter and F. G. Blake, *Nursing Care of Children*, 9th ed., (Philadelphia: J. B. Lippincott, 1976), p. 301.

Management. The child with primary immunodeficiency disease needs specialized care by qualified physicians. It is the nurse practitioner's responsibility to consider these deficiency diseases in the child with recurrent infections and obtain medical consultation.

Resource Information

The most up-to-date information on infectious diseases is available from: Center for Disease Control, Atlanta, GA 30333; (404) 633-3311.
See Chapter 2, Resource Information.

References

American Academy of Pediatrics. *Report of the Committee on Infectious Diseases*, 18th ed. Evanston, Ill., 1977.

Brunner, L. S. and D. S. Suddarth. *The Lippincott Manual of Nursing Practice.* Philadelphia: Lippincott, 1974.

Carver, D. H. and D. S. Y. Seto. "Hepatitis A and B." *Pediatr Clin North Am* 21:669–681, August 1974.

Conway, B. L. *Pediatric Neurologic Nursing.* St. Louis: Mosby, 1977.

Gardner, P., S. Breton, and D. G. Carles. "Hospital Isolation and Precaution Guidelines." *Pediatrics* 53:663–673, May 1974.

Graef, J. W. and T. E. Cone. *Manual of Pediatric Therapeutics.* Boston: Little, Brown, 1974.

Grossman, M. and D. J. Drutz. "Venereal Disease in Children." In I. Schulman, editor, *Advances in Pediatrics* 21:97–137. Chicago: Year Book Medical Publishers, 1974.

Krugman, S., R. Ward, and S. L. Katz. *Infectious Diseases of Children,* 6th ed. St. Louis: Mosby, 1977.

Murray, J. D., et al. "Acute Bacterial Meningitis in Childhood: An Outline of Management." *Clin Pediatr* 11:455, August 1972.

Rudolph, A., editor. *Pediatrics,* 16th ed. New York: Appleton-Century-Crofts, 1977.

Smith, D. H., et al. "Bacterial Meningitis. A Symposium." *Pediatrics* 52:586, October 1973.

Vaughan, V. C. and R. J. McKay, editors. *Nelson Textbook of Pediatrics,* 10th ed. Philadelphia: Saunders, 1975.

Waechter, E. H. and F. G. Blake. *Nursing Care of Children,* 9th ed. Philadelphia: Lippincott, 1976.

Wilson, H. D. and H. F. Eichenwald. "Sepsis Neonatorum." *Pediatr Clin North Am* 21:571–582, August 1974.

30

Emergencies

A medical emergency is any situation which requires immediate medical attention to preserve life or health or to alleviate suffering. Many medical conditions require prompt but not immediate attention and are better considered situations of urgency rather than emergency. Care must be taken not to abuse the term to expedite the treatment of conditions which do not warrant emergency care.

Anticipating all presentations of medical conditions requiring immediate attention is not possible. This chapter includes a brief discussion of problems most likely to present as emergencies. In many situations the threat to life and limb will be obvious: for example, coma, major trauma, hemorrhage, and near drowning. The nurse practitioner serves as an intermediate care provider until the child arrives at a health care facility or until the emergency is resolved. Management of these conditions by the nurse practitioner will usually involve "first aid," that is, nonsurgical and nonpharmacologic intervention designed to help the child until more sophisticated care is available. Some situations, such as sudden upper airway obstruction and cardiac arrest warrant more vigorous intervention and the use of emergency techniques.

ASSESSMENT

The first step in emergency care is accurate assessment. Different aspects of the child's condition are assessed in order of priority as

947

expeditiously as possible. The coexistence of concomitant serious conditions must be considered

History

Determine if the child is in immediate jeopardy. If so, proceed to appropriate supportive and emergency measures. If not, proceed to elaborate on the history. Be alert to contributory factors and openminded about the possible causes of the immediate problem. Often overlooked is the possibility of poisoning, infection, or nonaccidental injury.

TELEPHONE

The person who calls the health care facility for help is often frantic and upset and needs a calm approach and clear, simple directions. Obtain the following information as soon as possible:

1. Name of the caller and relationship to the child
2. Phone number where the caller can be reached
3. Location of the child

Ask the following questions to assess the seriousness of the child's condition:

1. What is the child's age?
2. Is the child having difficulty breathing?
3. Is the child unconscious?
4. What has already been done for the child?
5. When did the emergency occur and exactly how did it happen?
6. What symptoms does the child have? For example, rapid pulse, rash, or fever?

Physical Examination

The nurse practitioner must be alert to the signs which indicate a serious or potentially serious condition. Presentation of the signs listed in Table 1 warrants immediate referral to a physician. Evaluate in order of priority:

1. The cardiorespiratory system: cardiac and respiratory rates, adequacy of ventilation, skin color, blood pressure, degree of agitation, and hemorrhage. With acute airway obstruction, respiratory movement may be exaggerated. With carbon monoxide poisoning, the child may be bright red rather than blue. Agitation may be a sign of carbon dioxide retention.
2. The neurologic system: state of consciousness, orientation, localizing neurologic signs.
3. The rest of the child: state of hydration, urinary output, other injuries.

MANAGEMENT

Emergency First Aid

Institute necessary life-saving measures:

1. Assure adequate airway, respiration, and circulation
2. Control hemorrhage
3. Immobilize injured parts
4. Relieve pain
5. Provide for the child's comfort, with caution to avoid worsening the child's condition

Emergency Techniques

CARDIOPULMONARY RESUSCITATION (CPR)

A precise description of CPR techniques is beyond the scope of this chapter. The American Heart Association offers courses in basic

Table 1
Signs Which Indicate Need for Physician Referral

Signs	Condition
Absent or poor chest movements and breath sounds, weak or absent pulses and heart sounds, marked bradycardia or tachycardia, cyanosis or pallor, loss of consciousness, fixation of pupils	Cardiopulmonary arrest
Poor skin turgor, dry mucous membranes, sunken eyes, sunken fontanelle, tachycardia, tachypnea, hypotension, shock, oliguria	Dehydration
Coma, convulsions, aberrant behavior, pinpoint pupils	Drug abuse
Tachycardia, hypotension; pale, ashen appearance; cold, sweaty skin; pale, cold extremities; weak, thready pulse; oliguria, anxiety, agitation, anxiousness, restlessness	Hypovolemic shock
Rising pulse rate, restlessness, increased retractions, cyanosis	Hypoxia
Bulging fontanelle, prominent veins, nausea, vomiting, headache, papilledema	Increased intracranial pressure
Irritability, bulging fontanelle, severe headache, projectile vomiting, stiff neck, positive Brudzinski, positive Kernig, lethargy, focal neurologic signs, convulsions, petechial or purpuric rash	Meningitis
Rapid onset of fever, headache, lethargy, tachycardia, petechial rash, shock	Meningococcemia
Restlessness, irritability, nasal flaring, intercostal retraction during inspiration, flaring of lower rib margins, absent breath sounds over involved areas, or noisy breath sounds with rales, sitting with head forward, mouth open and drooling	Respiratory distress
Early signs: hyperventilation, depressed level of consciousness, warm flushed skin, decreased urine output, fever, chills, normal blood pressure	Septic shock
Late signs: hypotension, tachycardia, cold clammy skin with peripheral mottling and cyanosis, marked lethargy, oliguria to anuria	

Source: Compiled from D. Pascoe and M. Grossman, *Quick Reference to Pediatric Emergencies* (Philadelphia: Lippincott, 1973); J. W. Graef and T. E. Cone, Jr., editors, *Manual of Pediatric Therapeutics* (Boston: Little, Brown, 1974).

and advanced resuscitation. Annual review is recommended. Basic points will be reviewed here:

Airway. Extend the head to raise the tongue out of the pharynx. Remove foreign matter, dentures, and vomitus from the airway. The Heimlich maneuver (rapid compressions of the upper abdomen by the resuscitator) should be used to remove material that the resuscitator cannot reach. Emergency tracheotomy may be necessary.

Breathing. Inflate the lungs with air or oxygen by breathing mouth-to-mouth or mouth-to-nose or by using bag or mask devices. In infants, puffs of air from the cheeks into the mouth is sufficient insufflation. Observe for good thoraco-abdominal motion. Breathe at the following rates (Brown, 1976, p. 23):

- 40 breaths per minute for infants
- 30 breaths per minute for preschoolers
- 20 breaths per minute for school age children

Circulation. *Infants:* Support the back of the thorax with both hands and compress the midsternum with the thumbs. Coordinate lung inflation and heart compression with 1-respiratory inflation/3-heartbeats. (The heart rate should be 80 to 120 beats per minute.) *Older children:* Support the back with a board or place the child on the floor. Compress the lower sternum with the heel of the hand. Coordinate lung inflation and heart compression with 1-respiratory inflation/4-to-5-heartbeats. (The heart rate should be 60 to 80 beats per minute.)

HEIMLICH MANEUVER

The Heimlich maneuver is used to dislodge a foreign body impacted in the hypopharynx, larynx, or trachea. The rescuer should first attempt to retrieve the foreign matter from the victim's mouth, taking care not to push it deeper. If unsuccessful, the rescuer then grasps the victim from behind, clenching the palms of the hands together over the upper abdomen in the midline. The rescuer then compresses the victim's abdomen with a *quick upward thrust*. The thrust is repeated as necessary. The thrusting movement is *NOT* a punch, bearhug, or squeeze (Block, 1976). If the object is not dislodged, an emergency tracheotomy should be performed.

TRACHEOTOMY

Tracheotomy may be necessary in cases of laryngeal spasm or edema, epiglottitis, foreign body in the larynx, or crushing injury to the larynx. A vertical incision over the cricothyroid membrane will allow for the widening of the incision with a blunt instrument or fingers. The incision should be kept open with lateral traction on its edges, and, if necessary, used to inflate the victim's lungs. Tracheotomy equipment should be a part of every resuscitation cart.

Emotional Support of the Family

Health personnel should be sensitive to parental feelings of guilt, helplessness, and responsibility for the emergency. Parents need a warm smile and gentle touch. During the crisis, parents should be informed of the child's progress. Adjustment to the reality of the crisis usually evolves through the following stages:

1. *Emotional shock.* The nurse practitioner must not assume that the parents' or child's comprehension of what is said is complete or accurate.
2. *Denial.* The nurse practitioner may find the parent or child acting in a manner inconsistent with the gravity of the situation.
3. *Anger.* The child or parent may react emotionally or even physically to those attempting to help.
4. *Resignation.* Often, only at this state of adjustment will the family or child begin to develop rapport with the health team.
5. *Integration.* The family will often begin to seek the real causes of shock or loss, and the nurse practitioner may find it possible to enlighten the family about prevention of accidents and illness.

Emotional Support of the Child

Support of the child in a situation of acute emotional stress requires an understanding of the particular fears of children with regard to threatened loss of life, limb, or love. Children fear bodily harm and loss of control.

The child's anxiety response is influenced by developmental maturity, previous medical experiences, and parental reaction to the situation.

INFANTS AND TODDLERS

Loss of the parent is feared. The child may cry, cling to the parent, avoid eye contact, and be restless and combative. The following may decrease anxiety:

1. Permission for the parents to remain with the child
2. Inclusion of the parents in treatment procedures when appropriate
3. Reassurance to the child that the parents will return as soon as the procedure is completed
4. The presence of an object which the child associates with the parent

PRESCHOOL THROUGH SCHOOL AGE CHILDREN

The major fear is of pain or bodily harm. The child may protest, scream, clench the teeth, reach for parent, and be combative. The following may decrease anxiety:

1. Address the child at eye level
2. Encourage the child to verbalize fears
3. Allow the child to play with equipment and materials prior to use
4. Allow the child to sit up rather than lie down for procedures whenever possible
5. Allow the expression of pain
6. Reward bravery and accept fear

Legal Aspects of Emergency Care

All states protect the health professional who renders "roadside" emergency care from liability except in cases involving the utmost negligence.

Any unconscious victim is assumed to consent to lifesaving treatment. If a child needs emergency treatment, and no guardian is available to give consent, care should be given anyway with careful documentation in the medical record to substantiate the necessity of emergency treatment.

If a guardian refuses to provide consent for lifesaving treatment (e.g., blood transfusion), authorization by a superior court magistrate can and should be obtained. A parent does not have the right to jeopardize the life of the child for religious or philosophical reasons. The aid of law enforcement officers may be necessary to ensure the provision of such care to the child.

In the absence of consent by a guardian who may reasonably be expected to give consent once contacted, one should not render more than care of the emergency problem. When such consent cannot be obtained by a reasonable effort, arrangements should be made for temporary custody of the child, usually through an agent of the local social services welfare department.

COMMON CLINICAL PROBLEMS

Amputation

Amputation of an extremity or bodily appendage calls for prompt action to preserve the severed member, preferably on ice, and rapid transfer of it and the child to a health care facility with the capacity to perform anastomosis.

Anaphylaxis

ASSESSMENT

Anaphylaxis is the sudden, lifethreatening reaction to an antigen, which may be injected, ingested, or inhaled. The reaction is mediated through the release of histamine, bradykinin, and other vasoactive substances. The reaction may encompass pruritis, urticaria, agitation, bronchospasm, edema, and cardiac arrest.

MANAGEMENT

Emergency treatment. Steps include:

1. Administration of aqueous epinephrine 1:1000, subcutaneously in a dose of 0.01 ml/kg, up to 0.5 ml. Repeat every 20 minutes as necessary. Corticosteroids and antihistamines may also be indicated.
2. Emergency tracheotomy may be necessary to relieve airway obstruction from laryngospasm. Have equipment ready.
3. Restriction of the blood return from the site of injected antigen with a tourniquet and ice. Immediately transport the child to a hospital.

Preventive measures

1. Identify and avoid known allergens in a hypersensitive individual. Obtain a history of reactions to drugs and other foreign substances such as insect stings, and record clearly on the front of the child's chart.
2. When practicable, administer medications orally rather than parenterally to reduce the likelihood of anaphylaxis.
3. Desensitize individuals who have experienced systemic reactions to allergens such as insect stings. Observe the child receiving a desensitization injection for 15 to 20 minutes following the injection. See Chapter 28, Insect Bites, for specific preventive measures.
4. Recommend the use of a Medic Alert bracelet or wallet card which indicates the allergen.

Asphyxiation

ASSESSMENT

Asphyxiation is the consequence of being unable to breathe.

Etiology. The causes include airway obstruction (from food, crushing injury, acute laryngeal edema, laryngospasm, bronchospasm, epiglottitis, infectious laryngotracheitis (croup), lingual movement to the back of the pharynx in an unconscious person, and interference with oxygenation of blood in the lungs (carbon monoxide poisoning, acute pulmonary edema, shock, thermal injury to the lung, pneumothorax, flail chest).

Clinical findings. The presence of respiratory efforts depends on the etiology. Seesaw respiratory efforts indicate airway obstruction. Toxic causes and chest trauma are visually accompanied by hyperventilation with the aid of the accessory muscles of respiration. Agitation is usually present, although in its early stages, hypoxia may cause a euphoric indifference to the situation.

MANAGEMENT

Treatment must be swift and bold. The airway must be opened. See Emergency Techniques. Respirations if absent must be sustained artificially. Oxygen, if available, should be generously administered. Hospitalization is indicated for treatment of the basic illness. For developmental preventive counseling tips, see Chapter 9, Choking.

Bites

Bites by poisonous snakes, lizards, and spiders are mentioned mainly to condemn the use of the standard snake bite kit. Attempts to draw out the venom are ill advised. A tourniquet applied above and below the bite with periodic release and the application of a cold compress are in order until appropriate medical treatment (antivenins, corticosteroids, antibiotics) is available. Identification of the animal will aid in the antivenin selection. The prognosis for bites by rattlesnakes and copperheads is favorable; coral snake bites are much graver. For related information see Chapter 28.

Burns

ASSESSMENT

Burns may be thermal or chemical injuries, external or internal (lye ingestion, hot smoke inhalation, aspiration of hot liquid). Abuse is not an uncommon cause. Table 2 summarizes the burn hazards for children.

The history should provide information necessary for the nurse practitioner to reconstruct the incident. The explanation should be plausible, with respect to the child's development, the pattern of the burns, and the possibility of events happening as described.

Burn surface area.   This is estimated by the "rule of nines" (Table 3) or, preferably, with age-specific tables (see Figure 1). Palmar surface of hands at all ages represent 1 percent of the body surface area.

Burn depth.   Burns are rated by degree:

First degree: epidermis not irreversibly damaged. No blistering. Erythematous. Painful.

Second degree: epidermal necrosis. Blistering. Erythematous. Painful.

Third degree: dermis damaged irreversibly. Eschar formation. Painless.

Fourth degree: tissue damage extending to underlying organs and tissues. Eschar. Painless.

MANAGEMENT

First-degree burns respond well to cooling and to aspirin, which has analgesic and anti-inflammatory effects. More severe burns re-

Table 2
Burn Hazards of Children

Group	Type of Burn	Hazard	Time/Place
Infants and toddlers (6–24 mos)	Scalds	Playing underfoot in kitchen, overturning cups, pulling electric cords of coffee pots, frying pans; bath water too hot; parents (neglect/abuse)	Daytime/home
	Electric burns	Chewing extension cords	
Young child (2–6 yrs)	Flame burns	Playing with matches, climbing on stove, warming with heating source	Early morn/ kitchen, bedroom
	Scalds	Water too hot	
Older child (6–14 yrs)	Flame burns	Playing/working with gasoline, campfires, barbecues, chemistry sets, firecrackers, rockets, matches; reaching over stove, candles, making candles, "innocent bystander" (observing others play with fire or gasoline).	After school, holidays/ outdoors, indoors

Morn, eve/ kitchen; after school/yard |
| | Electric burns | Climbing around high-tension wires (usually fatal) | |
| All children | Flame burns | House fires; gas tank explosion during auto accident | Usually night; anytime |

Source: Adapted from material courtesy of Northern California Burn Council.

958

Table 3
Estimating Burn Surface Area Using the "Rule of Nines"

Age and Body Area	Percent of Total Body Surface Area
Over 12 years	
Head and neck	9%
Each upper extremity	9%
Anterior trunk	18%
Posterior trunk	18%
Each lower extremity	18%
Under 12 years	
Head and neck	9% *plus* 1% for each year under 12
Each upper extremity	9%
Anterior trunk	18%
Posterior trunk	18%
Each lower extremity	18% *minus* ½% for each year under 12

Source: Reprinted by permission from E. H. Waechter and F. G. Blake, *Nursing Care of Children*, 9th ed., (Philadelphia: Lippincott, 1976), p. 433.

quire expert medical evaluation. For preventive counseling tips, see Chapter 9.

Cardiac Arrest

ASSESSMENT

Cardiac arrest is the sudden cessation of cardiac function. The principal forms are ventricular fibrillation, asystole, and electromechanical dissociation. Causes include myocardial infarction, electrolyte abnormalities, and electrical shock. Relevant historical information includes the name of any medications the child has been taking as well as a search for an immediate insult.

Physical signs are those of asphyxia and absence of pulse and blood pressure. In electromechanical dissociation, organized electrical activity persists until the heart becomes too ischemic to generate it.

BURN SHEET

Name_____ Age_____ Number_____

Burn Record. Ages—Birth-7½   Date of Observation_____

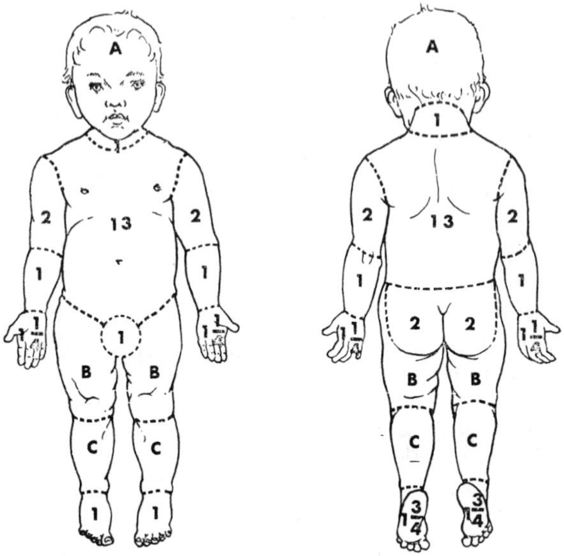

RELATIVE PERCENTAGES OF AREAS AFFECTED BY GROWTH			
Area	Age 0	1	5
A = ½ of Head	9½	8½	6½
B = ½ of One Thigh	2¾	3¼	4
C = ½ of One Leg	2½	2½	2¾

% BURN BY AREAS

Probable { Head_____ Neck_____ Body_____ Up. Arm_____ Forearm_____ Hands_____
3rd Burn { Genitals_____ Buttocks_____ Thighs_____ Legs_____ Feet_____

Total Burn { Head_____ Neck_____ Body_____ Up. Arm_____ Forearm_____ Hands_____
{ Genitals_____ Buttocks_____ Thighs_____ Legs_____ Feet_____

Sum of All Areas_____ Probably 3rd _____ Total Burn_____

FORM MD-8

Figure 30.1   Calculation of burn surface area. (Redrawn with permission from D. Pascoe and M. Grossman, *Quick Reference to Pediatric Emergencies*, Philadelphia: Lippincott, 1973.)

960

MANAGEMENT

Cardiopulmonary resuscitation must begin immediately. See this chapter, Cardiopulmonary Resuscitation.

Coma

ASSESSMENT

Coma has numerous causes, including uncontrolled diabetes mellitus, hypoglycemia, the postconvulsive state, electrolyte imbalance, infection of the central nervous system, cerebrovascular accident, head trauma, Reye's syndrome, hypoxia from hypoperfusion or asphyxia, and drug and poison ingestion. That someone is indeed comatose rather than sleeping or malingering may be determined by firm rubbing of the sternum with the examiner's knuckles.

MANAGEMENT

Until the child arrives at a hospital, attentions should be focused on the maintenance of vital bodily functions and prevention of aspiration of vomitus. Utmost care must be taken with the comatose trauma victim to prevent inadvertent injury to the spinal cord. Comatose diabetics may have injectable glucagon on their persons. Its use can only help.

Congestive Heart Failure

See Chapter 19, The Heart

Convulsions

See Chapter 25, The Neuromuscular System.

Epiglottitis

See Chapter 18, The Respiratory System

Eye Emergencies

See Chapter 16, The Eye.

Fractures

ASSESSMENT

Obtain history about the child's position prior to the injury, circumstances surrounding the injury, source of pain or tenderness, hearing or feeling of bone snap.

Clinical findings. The signs of a fracture include:

- Deformities such as angulation, crookedness, shortening or rotation of an extremity or an open wound over a bone
- Pain or tenderness to touch at the site of the expected fracture
- Shape and length differences of corresponding bone on the top sides of the child's body
- Swelling and discoloration of the overlying skin due to hemorrhage

Fractures of bones may have threatening aspects. Vertebral fractures may injure the spinal cord, especially when the child is being moved. Basilar skull fractures often result in hemorrhage into the middle ears, which is visible through the tympanic membrane. Parietal fractures may lacerate the middle meningeal artery resulting in intracranial hemorrhage. Rib fractures may perforate the lung or the chest wall, resulting in a pneumothorax. Almost any fracture may produce internal hemorrhage which is difficult to detect, especially in the thigh.

MANAGEMENT

Fractures should be splinted until definitive treatment is possible.

Frostbite

ASSESSMENT

Frostbite is the injury resulting from the freezing of tissue. The affected part will be numb, hard, and blue. Earlobes, nose, cheeks, hands, and feet are the areas most likely to suffer frostbite. Early signs of frostbite are shivering, numbness, and low body temperature. Progressive signs are drowsiness, apathy, loss of consciousness, and freezing of the extremities.

MANAGEMENT

"Frost nip" (mild skin blanching). Rewarm with a warm hand, blow through cupped hands, or place frost-nipped fingers in the armpit.

Deep frostbite. Rapidly rewarm the frostbitten areas in warm water bath with temperature between 40 to 42°C. Tetanus toxoid is recommended (*The Medical Letter,* December 3, 1976). Avoid rubbing the cold-injured part with the hands or with snow to prevent damaging thawing tissue irreparably. If there is a possibility that thawing could be followed by refreezing, do not thaw the frozen part to avoid further loss of tissue.

Hemorrhage

ASSESSMENT

Hemorrhage is significant if more than 20 percent of the total circulating blood volume (approximately 5 liters for the average adult male) is lost internally or externally (see Fractures). The signs and symptoms of massive bleeding are extreme paleness, rapid and weak pulse, thirst, restlessness, possibly tenderness over the affected area, and shock. Signs of internal bleeding are:

- Bright red blood in the urine (acute bleeding, infection, post trauma)
- Copious amount of bright red blood in the stools (lower bowel)
- Pink, foamy tinges of blood in vomitus (lung)
- Severe vaginal bleeding (menstrual bleeding, miscarriage, ruptured tubal pregnancy)
- Smokey appearance to the urine (bladder, kidneys, or urethra)
- Tarry stools (upper regions of the colon and small intestine)

MANAGEMENT

Immediate referral to a health care facility is warranted. During the interim, apply pressure. Properly applied pressure is preferable to a tourniquet because it permits perfusion of the rest of the extremity. The pressure bandage need not be sterile. Infection resulting from such treatment will usually be easier to treat than shock. For open wounds a tourniquet should be applied above the wound for no longer than 15 minutes at a time except in extreme circumstances. Do not overwarm the child or offer oral fluids.

Head Injury

ASSESSMENT

There are three types of head injuries:

- *Concussion* is the most common type of serious head injury. It is characterized by a transient loss of consciousness, amnesia for the event, and no structural brain damage.
- *Contusion* is a severe head injury in which there is structural damage to the brain including hemorrhage and swelling of the brain tissue. The immediate neurologic deficit depends on the area of the brain involved. Seizures may occur acutely or from residual damage after healing is complete.

- *Intracranial hemorrhage* is an accumulation of blood within the cranium. It may result from a seemingly insignificant head injury and may occur several weeks after the initial insult. Signs of intracranial hemorrhage include lethargy progressing to coma, focal neurologic deficits, pupillary dilation, intractable headache, nausea, emesis, bradycardia, hypertension, and even cardiorespiratory failure. Rapid onset of symptoms within hours to several days post injury is indicative of acute epidural hemorrhage. Slow onset of symptoms indicates chronic subdural hemorrhage.

History. Information to be obtained includes the following:

1. The child's age
2. What happened and exactly how it happened
3. The nature of the impact (Was it a massive force such as a moving vehicle or a fall from a considerable height?)
4. The child's behavior since the injury
5. State(s) of consciousness since the injury
6. Presence of a neurologic condition which may have contributed to the injury

Clinical evaluation. Consistent, repeated observation is the key to establishing the neurologic status of the child and determining the progress of the child's condition. Table 4 highlights the observations to be made at regular intervals and lists the abnormal responses.

Radiology. Whether or not to obtain skull X-rays is a diagnostic dilemma. Absence of radiographically visible fracture does not preclude a severe brain injury. Indications for obtaining a skull X-ray include a palpable deformity, a significant open scalp wound, a suspicion of the presence of other injuries in addition to the head injury, especially if abuse is suspected, and uncertainty about the severity of the injury.

MANAGEMENT

Superficial scalp injuries. Bring the edges together and apply pressure if the skull is not depressed. Raise the head and shoulders

Table 4
Clinical Evaluation of a Head Injury

Observation	Abnormal Response
Physical examination of the head	Swelling, depression, crepitus, scalp injury, bleeding
Level of consciousness	I. Alert; II. Arousable; III. Unarousable, normal reflexes; IV. Abnormal reflexes; V. No reflexes
Cardiovascular system	↑ Blood pressure, persistent bradycardia (below 60), Cheyne-Stokes respirations, central neurogenic hyperventilation (rapid, deep, regular), apnea
Pupillary response	Asymmetry of pupils, dilation of pupils
Optic disks	Retinal hemorrhage, papilledema (unusual before 6 hours)
Eye movements	No spontaneous movements in all fields of gaze
Tympanic membranes	Presence of blood
Spinal cord integrity	Babinski sign, altered sensation, increased or decreased deep tendon reflexes

if possible. Do not bend the neck since a fracture may be present. Gently cover the wound with a snug, preferably sterile dressing.

Suspected brain injury.   Ensure respiration and circulation. Maintain the child in the position in which found. Promptly obtain medical assistance, and request a spinal splint. Identify other injuries. Observe and record the extent and duration of unconsciousness. Do not give fluids by mouth. Keep the child warm. Hospital admission for observation and treatment is indicated for significant injury, including concussion.

Home observation.   The decision to observe the child at home will be influenced by all the following (Shillito, 1977):

1.   Emesis less than three times immediately after injury
2.   Short duration to no loss of consciousness
3.   Stability of vital signs

4. Stability or improvement of mental status and alertness
5. Negative neurologic examination
6. Responsive pupillary reaction
7. No evidence of penetrating skull injury, spinal fluid otorrhea or rhinorrhea, blood behind the ear drums, or bleeding from the external canals
8. Competency of parents

COUNSELING. If the decision is made to follow the child at home, parents are given specific instructions on the danger signals for which to observe. Rapid transportation to the hospital must be assured in anticipation of complications. An appointment to return is scheduled. For preventive counseling tips, see Chapter 9, Falls.

DANGER SIGNS. Parents are instructed to return the child immediately to the health care facility if any of the following occur (Shillito, 1977):

1. Excessive drowsiness (initially test at 15-minute intervals arousing the child by methods ordinarily used to awaken from a deep sleep)
2. Changes in vital signs: slowing of pulse, irregular respirations with short periods of apnea, increasing temperature
3. Persistent vomiting
4. Weakness on one side, limping
5. Worsening headache
6. Double vision
7. Difficulty speaking
8. Pupillary constriction or dilation or inequality
9. Convulsion
10. Appearance or progression of swelling beneath the scalp

Heat Stroke

ASSESSMENT

Heat stroke is an immediate life-threatening problem due to an accumulation of body heat and a disturbance of the sweating mechanism. It results in generalized cellular damage to the central nervous system, liver, kidneys, and the clotting mechanism.

Clinical findings include temperature of 41.1 to 41.7°C, profuse sweating (skin may be hot and dry), convulsions (about 60 percent of the cases), delirium to coma, ataxia, incontinence, hypotension, rapid pulse, shock, oliguria or renal failure, vomiting, diarrhea, and abdominal pain.

MANAGEMENT

Therapy. Rapidly cool the child by continuous sponging on the bare skin with cool water or immersing the child in cool water (do not add ice) until the temperature is sufficiently lowered (about 38.9°C). Obtain medical assistance. Treat shock. Administer oxygen.

Prevention. Advise parents about the following precautions:

1. During exercise cool off, rest, and drink fluids. Do not exercise in heavy-weight clothing.
2. During hot spells and when the humidity index exceeds 87 reduce activity. The humidity index is available from the local weather bureau.
3. During hot weather never leave the child alone in a car with inadequate ventilation, and ensure adequate hydration on car trips in hot weather also.
4. During hot weather slowly acclimate the body to the increased heat by gradually increasing periods of work or exercise.
5. During illnesses, particularly gastrointestinal illnesses, avoid heavy activity.

Infections

Infections of several types may present as medical emergencies. More complete discussion will be found in Chapter 29, Infectious Disease. Septic shock may result from infection with enteric bacteria, *Streptococcus pneumoniae, Streptococcus viridans,* usually through the mediation of endotoxins. Children without spleens, including those with sickle cell disease are at a high risk for *S. pneumoniae* and sepsis. Meningitis may present as intractable headache, coma, or shock. It may present atypically without fever, nuchal rigidity, or even without obvious abnormality of the cerebrospinal fluid.

Near Drowning

ASSESSMENT

Near drowning in fresh or salt water presents many of the same problems in emergency management. Deaths are caused by asphyxia and fluid aspiration or asphyxia and laryngospasm. Electrolyte concentrations are of little importance at the site of the accident and compensation usually occurs rapidly. For more information the reader is referred to standard pediatric texts.

MANAGEMENT

The cornerstone of emergency treatment is immediate, persistent cardiopulmonary resuscitation. Vomitus is often present in the hypopharynx, and the rescuer should search for it. Mouth-to-mouth resuscitation should begin in the water, with cardiac compression, if appropriate, performed out of the water. Hypothermia should be rapidly corrected. Emergency tracheotomy may be necessary if laryngospasm persists. See also Asphyxia, Cardiac Arrest, and Cardiopulmonary Resuscitation, this chapter. For water safety information and preventive counseling tips, see Chapter 9.

Resource information.   Water safety information can be obtained from these sources:

1.   Public Enquiries, National Center for Urban Industrial Health, 222 East Central Parkway, Cincinnati, OH 45202.
2.   American Red Cross Association: local chapter

Poisoning: Ingestion

ASSESSMENT

Poisoning may result from ingestion, inhalation, or contact. It should be considered whenever a child presents with otherwise inexplicable symptoms.

Epidemiology. Poisonings are complicated episodes involving a victim, a poison, and a location. The victim is most often a child under 5 years of age. The poison (a drug, home remedy, or household product) is often not in its usual place and occasionally not in the original container. Fifty percent of poisonings occur in the kitchen, 20 percent in the bathroom, and 10 percent in the bedroom. The ingestion often occurs when the environment is in upheaval due to cleaning, repairing, or moving or because the family is under stress (Pascoe, 1973).

The unknown poison. Poisoning is considered when the following conditions exist (Mofenson, 1974, p. 339):

- Abrupt onset of illness
- Child is between 1 to 4 years of age
- Previous history of ingestion
- Involvement of several organ systems which are inconsistent with a specific disease entity

When the poison is unknown the health care provider must depend on the child's signs and symptoms (odors, pupil evaluation, and skin evaluation are especially helpful) and laboratory evaluation to provide the clues to the poisonous agents.

To help in the recognition of emergency signs and symptoms, the reader is referred to Table 5 and to Table 6 which lists the combination of signs and symptoms (toxidromes) in children that are commonly encountered and the agents that can reproduce them.

MANAGEMENT

Telephone. The pertinent history must be obtained quickly to identify the ingested substance and to determine its potential toxicity so management can be quickly initiated. The steps are:

1. Obtain the following information:

   - Caller's name, address, and telephone number
   - Child's age and condition
   - Name of ingested substance if known (look at the label)
   - Amount ingested
   - Time of ingestion

2. Reassure the caller if the ingested substance is nontoxic. Refer to Table 7 for representative nontoxic commercial products.

3. If the toxicity is unknown, call the nearest Poison Control Center immediately and consult a toxicology text. See references listed under Resource Information, this section.

4. Use a toxicity rating scheme to aid in a decision to induce vomiting, lavaging, or instituting a specific treatment.

   Refer to Table 8 for a toxicity rating chart and to Table 7 for a listing of the representative commercial products in each toxicity class. Remove the gastric contents for toxicity ratings greater than two, unless a contraindication exists. Contraindications for the induction of emesis are:

   - A caustic substance (i.e., lye, acid)
   - A comatose or convulsing child
   - Petroleum distillates (i.e., kerosene, gasoline, lighter fluid, furniture polish) that do not contain a dangerous insecticide
   - Strychnine (may induce convulsions)

5. If treatment requires induction of emesis instruct the caller to induce vomiting as follows:

   - Give 15 ml of syrup of ipecac
   - Give 6 to 8 oz of water
   - Keep the child active
   - Closely monitor the child so the proper position is main-

Table 5

Emergency Symptoms and Signs Which May be Encountered in a Poisoning

ABDOMINAL COLIC
Black widow spider bite
Heavy metals
Narcotic depressant withdrawal

ATAXIA
Alcohol
Barbiturates
Bromides
Carbon monoxide
Diphenylhydantoin
Hallucinogens
Heavy metals
Organic solvents
Tranquilizers

BREATH ODOR
Acetone: acetone, alcohol (methyl, isopropyl), phenol, salicylates
Alcohol: alcohol (ethyl)
Bitter almonds: cyanide
Coal gas: carbon monoxide
Garlic: arsenic, phosphorus, organic phosphate insecticides, thallium
Oil of wintergreen: methyl salicylate

MOUTH

Salivation
Arsenic
Corrosives
Mercury
Mushrooms
Organic phosphate insecticides
Thallium

OLIGURIA-ANURIA
Carbon tetrachloride
Ethylene glycol
Heavy metals
Hemolytic poisons (naphthalene, plants)
Methanol
Mushrooms
Oxalates
Petroleum distillates
Solvents

PARALYSIS
Botulism
Heavy metals

Dryness
Atropine
Amphetamines
Antihistamines
Narcotic depressants

Petroleum: petroleum distillates
Violets: turpentine

COMA AND DROWSINESS
Alcohol—ethyl
Antihistamines
Barbiturates and other hypnotics
Carbon monoxide
Narcotic depressants (opiates)
Salicylates
Tranquilizers

CONVULSIONS AND MUSCLE TWITCHING
Alcohol
Amphetamines
Antihistamines
Boric acid
Camphor
Chlorinated hydrocarbon insecticides (DDT)
Cyanide
Lead
Organic phosphate insecticides
Plants (lily-of-the-valley, azalea, iris, water hemlock)
Salicylates
Strychnine
Withdrawal from barbiturates, benzodiazepine (Valium, Librium), meprobamate

Plants (coniine in poison hemlock)
Triorthocresyl phosphate

PULSE RATE
Slow
Digitalis
Lily-of-the-valley
Narcotic depressants

Rapid
Alcohol
Amphetamines
Atropine
Ephedrine

PUPILS
Pinpoint
Mushrooms (muscarine type)
Narcotic depressants (opiates)
Organic phosphate insecticides
Nystagmus on Lateral Gaze
Barbiturates
Minor tranquilizers (meprobamate, benzodiazepine)

Dilated
Amphetamines
Antihistamines
Atropine
Barbiturates (coma)
Cocaine
Ephedrine
LSD
Methanol
Withdrawal-narcotic depressants

Continued on next page

Table 5 (Continued)

RESPIRATORY ALTERATIONS		SKIN COLOR	
Rapid	*Slow or Depressed*	*Jaundice* (hepatic or hemolytic)	*Cyanosis*
Amphetamines	Alcohol	Aniline	Aniline dyes
Barbiturates (early)	Barbiturates (late)	Arsenic	Carbon monoxide
Carbon monoxide	Narcotic depressants (opiates)	Carbon tetrachloride	Cyanide
Methanol	Tranquilizers	Castor bean	Nitrites
Petroleum distillates		Fava bean	Strychnine
Salicylates		Mushroom	
	Paralysis	Naphthalene	*Red Flush*
Wheezing and Pulmonary Edema	Organic phosphate insecticides	Yellow phosphorus	Alcohol
Mushrooms (muscarine type)	Botulism		Antihistamines
Narcotic depressants (opiates)		*VIOLENT EMESIS OFTEN WITH HEMATEMESIS*	Atropine
Organic phosphate insecticides		Aminophylline	Boric acid
Petroleum distillates		Bacterial food poisoning	Carbon monoxide
		Boric acid	Nitrites
		Corrosives	
		Fluoride	
		Heavy metals	
		Phenol	
		Salicylates	

Source: Adapted with permission from H. Mofenson and J. Greensher, "The Unknown Poison," *Pediatrics* 54(3):340–341, September 1974. Copyright 1974, American Academy of Pediatrics.

Table 6
Diagnosis by Toxidromes

Poison	Toxidrome
Amphetamines	Excessive activity, argumentativeness, tremors, headache, diarrhea, dry mouth with foul odor, sweating, tachycardia, arrhythmia, dilated pupils
Aspirin	Vomiting, hyperpnea, fever
Atropine-like agents (LSD, STP, scopolamine)	Agitation, hallucinations, dilated pupils, beet-red color, dry skin, fever
Barbiturates and tranquilizers	Slurred speech, nystagmus, slightly constricted pupils, skin vesicles, ataxia, sleepiness, coma
Cyanide (insecticides, silver polish, seeds of apple, peach, apricot, plum, cherry)	Silver polish (bitter almonds) odor; GI, CNS, and respiratory symptoms; coma, convulsions, abnormal ECG, bradycardia, heart block, dilated pupils, protrusion of eyes
Heroin	Coma, depressed respirations, pinpoint pupils
Imipramine (tricyclate antidepressants)	Coma, convulsions, cardiac arrhythmias
Organic phosphates	Pinpoint pupils, salivation, lacrimation, pulmonary congestion, abdominal cramps
Phenothiazine	Uncoordinated spasmodic movements, tremor, ataxia, postural hypotension, rhythmic body movements

tained when vomiting occurs and the risk of aspiration is minimized.

- Repeat the 15 ml dose if vomiting does not occur in 15 to 20 minutes.
- If ipecac is unavailable, have the child drink a glass of water and then insert a finger down the throat or gently tickle the back of the throat with a spoon or similar blunt object. Do not use salt water because fatal salt poisoning can occur.

Table 7
Representative Commercial Products in Each Toxicity Class

Class 1
(Practically Nontoxic)
Abrasives
Candies
Candles
Chalk
Cosmetics (especially baby
  products, lipstick, rouge, eye
  makeup)
Crayons (marked AP or CP)
Fish bowl additives
Foods
Lead pencils
Modeling clay
Mucilage and pastes
Paint (latex)
Pure soaps
Putty
Sweetening agents (saccharin)
Toothpaste

Class 2
(Slightly Toxic)
Adhesives (most)
Ballpoint pen inks
Bleaches (less than 6% Na
  hypochlorite)
Bubble bath soaps (detergents)
Caps (toy pistol)
Cigarettes or cigars (tobacco)
Contraceptive pills
Cosmetics (most) (colognes,
  perfumes)
Dehumidifying packets
Deodorants
Deodorizers (spray and
  refrigerator)
Detergents (most—not electric
  dishwasher)
Fabric softeners
Incense

Inks (most)
Iodophil disinfectant
Lubricants (most)
Lubricating oils
Matches (book)
Mineral oil
Paint—indoor (less than 1% lead)
Phenolphthalein laxatives (Ex-Lax)
Polaroid picture coating fluids
Polishes (porcelain, some furniture)
Porous tip ink markers (felt tip
  markers)
Shampoos
Shaving creams
Soap products
Thermometer mercury
Vitamins with or without fluoride

Class 3
(Moderately Toxic)
Adhesives (rubber, linoleum,
  roofing, plastic cement)
Agricultural chemicals (many)
Antifreeze
Bleach (oxalate type and greater
  than 6% Na hypochlorite)
Brake fluids
Cleaners (window, stain removers)
Cosmetics (depilatories, permanent
  wave neutralizers, nail polish
  removers and enamel)
Disinfectants (bathroom, toilet,
  garbage can)
Indelible inks
Lighter fuels
Mothballs (most)
Motor fuels
Polishes (metal, wood, shoe, stove)
Preservatives (brush, canvas, roof)
Stain removers

Continued on next page

Table 7 (Continued)

Class 4 (Very Toxic)	Class 5 (Extremely Toxic)
Agricultural chemicals (many)	Drain and sewer cleaners (caustics)
Ammonia	Insecticides (some)
Bleach—commercial	Fireplace flame colors (blues and greens)
Degreasers (metal, etc.)	Fungicides (some)
Depilatories (some)	Herbicides (some)
Dishwasher granules—electric	Rodenticides (some)
Disinfectants (acid, alkali, halogen, pine oil, and phenolic types)	Class 6 (Super Toxic)
Drain cleaners (some)	Fungicides ⎤
Dry cleaner solvents (some)	Herbicides ⎟
Fire extinguisher liquid	Insecticides ⎬ a few
Leather dyes	Rodenticides ⎦
Moth repellents (naphthalene)	Botanicals (nicotine, strychnine)
Petroleum products (most)	Inorganic chemicals (cyanide, phosphorus, arsenic, thallium, fluoride)
Radiator cleaners	
Rust removers	

Source: From Mofenson, H. and J. Greensher, "The Unknown Poison," *Pediatrics* 54(3):338, September 1974. Copyright 1974, American Academy of Pediatrics.

6. Instruct the caller to bring the child, the container with the poisonous agent, and any vomitus to the closest emergency facility.

Health care facility. Management of ingestions at the health care facility requires prompt removal of the poisonous agent, administration of antidote, and provision of excellent supportive care. Removal of the toxic substance is done by the physician.

Specific antidotes. Few poisons have specific antidotes. Prompt use of the specific antidote and excellent supportive care are crucial and life saving. See Table 9 for a list of poisons and their specific antidotes.

Activated charcoal is highly effective in adsorption of unretrievable ingested toxins, except cyanide. A thin, pasty solution is prepared with 1 to 2 tablespoons of any USP activated charcoal product in 6 to 8 oz of water. Caution: activated charcoal binds ipecac.

Table 8

Definitions of Toxicity Rating: Toxicity Rating Chart

Signal Word[a]	Toxicity Rating or Class	Probable LETHAL DOSE (human) for 70-kg Man (150 lb)
No label	1 Practically nontoxic	Above 15 gm/kg—more than 1 qt
No label	2 Slightly toxic	5 to 15 gm/kg—between 1 pt and 1 qt
Caution	3 Moderately toxic	0.5 to 5 gm/kg—between 1 oz and 1 pt (or 1 lb)
Warning Danger	4 Very toxic	50 to 500 mg/kg—between 1 tsp and 1 oz
Poison Danger	5 Extremely toxic	5 to 50 mg/kg—between 7 drops and 1 tsp
Poison	6 Super toxic	Under 5 mg/kg—a taste (less than 7 drops)

Source: Reprinted with permission from H. Mofenson and J. Greensher, "The Unknown Poison," *Pediatrics* 54(3):337, September 1974. Copyright 1974, American Academy of Pediatrics.

[a]Based on Federal Insecticide, Fungicide and Rodenticide Act of 1947.

Table 9
Specific Antidotes

Poison	Antidote
Cyanide	Cyanide poison kit (contains amyl nitrite, sodium nitrite, sodium thiosulfate). Available from American Cyanamid Company and Eli Lilly and Company
Organic phosphates	Atropine sulfate Pralidoxime chloride (Protopam)
Narcotics	Naloxone hydrochloride (Narcan) 0.01 mg/kg IV
Methanol, ethylene glycol	Ethanol

Specific poisonous agents

COMMON POISONS. The clinical findings and management of specific poisons are summarized in Table 10. For a discussion of lead poisoning, the reader is referred to Chapter 29, The Neuromuscular System.

Counseling. For specific developmental preventive counseling tips, see Chapter 9.

Resource information

Reference texts

Arena, J. *Poisoning: Toxicology, Symptoms, Treatment*, 3rd ed. Springfield, Ill.: Charles C Thomas, 1974.

Driesbach, R. H. *Handbook of Poisonings*. Los Altos, CA: Lange Medical Publishers, 1974.

Gosselin, R. and H. Smith. *Clinical Toxicology of Commercial Products,* 4th ed. Baltimore: Williams & Wilkins, 1976. (Toxicity ratings are listed.)

Handbook of Common Poisonings in Children. U.S. Department of Health, Education, and Welfare, Public Health Service, 5600 Fishers Lane, Rockville, MD 20857, HEW Publication No. (FDA) 76-7004, 1976, $1.50.

Table 10
Common Poisonings

Poison	Symptoms	Treatment	Comments
Caustics (lye in washing powders, drainpipe cleaners, paint removers, Clinitest tablets)	Burning pain from mouth to stomach, difficulty swallowing, edema of mucous membranes, bloody vomitus, weak, rapid pulse, increased respirations	Emesis is not induced. Preferably milk or water is given. Olive oil may ease the pain. Esophagoscopy is indicated. Corticosteroids may be given to reduce inflammation and decrease scar tissue formation	
Petroleum distillates (kerosene, mineral seal oil, charcoal igniting fluid, turpentine, gasoline, naphtha, fuel oils, lubricating oils)	*Large ingestions:* pulmonary symptoms (cough, respiratory distress, pulmonary edema, cyanosis), central nervous system symptoms (irritability, lethargy progressing to coma, convulsions)	*Small ingestions:* emesis is not induced. *Large ingestions:* emesis is indicated in an alert child. Antibiotics are indicated in the treatment of secondary bacterial infections. Epinephrine is contraindicated due to cardiac sensitivity.	Emesis is indicated in large ingestions because toxic central nervous system or cardiac effects may be produced.

Iron	Vomiting, epigastric pain, diarrhea, weak, rapid pulse, pallor, cyanosis, coma, respiratory depression, and massive hemorrhage	Emesis is induced with ipecac syrup. Gastric lavage is also indicated using a concentrated solution of sodium bicarbonate, 5% disodium phosphate, or milk. Lab studies of blood levels are done. Deferoxamine may also be used.	Lethal dose is about 40 mg/kg of iron. Mortality is 30–50%.
Salicylates (aspirin, methyl salicylate, oil of wintergreen)	Rapid, deep breathing; vomiting; extreme thirst; profuse sweating; fever; confusion; severe circulatory collapse; oliguria or anuria; hemorrhage	Emesis or gastric lavage is performed immediately. Activated charcoal is used. Severe poisonings will require IV fluids with careful monitoring of urine output, metabolic and electrolytes status, and glucose.	Salicylates can be detected in urine using Phenistix or Nitrazine paper. Potential fatal serum levels are 100–150 mg/100 ml. One tsp of methyl salicylate equals 21 five-grain aspirin tablets.

POISON CONTROL INFORMATION

1. National Clearinghouse for Poison Control Centers
   U.S. Department of Health, Education, and Welfare, Public Health Service,
   5401 Westbard Avenue, Bethesda, MD 20016.
   Information available from the National Clearinghouse includes:
   Listing of Poison Control Centers
   Publication of Bulletin
   Publication of poison information cards—Poison Control Cards
2. Poisindex, Washington DC 20201.
   The Poisindex outlines the management of certain poisons on paper and
   microfiche.
3. Poison Information Centers
   - Baltimore, Maryland   301-528-7604
   - Boston, Massachusetts   617-734-6000
   - Denver, Colorado (largest)   303-629-1123
   - Detroit, Michigan   313-494-5711
   - Galveston, Texas   713-765-3332
   - New Mexico   505-843-2551
   - New York   516-542-2323
   - Pittsburgh, Pennsylvania   412-681-7423
   - Sacramento, California   916-453-3692
   - Salt Lake City, Utah   801-581-7503
   - San Diego, California   714-294-6000
   - Seattle, Washington   206-634-5252
4. Local poison control information center: call directory assistance.
5. National Poison Center Network, Children's Hospital of Pittsburgh, 125 De
   Soto Street, Pittsburgh, PA 15213.
   Available material: "Poison Treatment Chart" as a desk reference ($2.00) or as a
   wall chart ($1.00).

Poisonings: Plant

ASSESSMENT

The common house and garden plants which cause poisonings are
listed in Table 11.

MANAGEMENT

Treatment of plant poisonings is difficult due to the problems in
plant identification and inadequate experience with plant toxicity.

Plant ingestions should be considered as potentially toxic, and vomiting should be induced even prior to identification of the plant. References that are useful in plant identification and toxicity are listed in Resource Information at the end of this section. A local expert in plant identification is a valuable community resource.

Prevention. Instruct parents about these practical rules (*The Sinister Garden,* 1966, pp. 3–4):

- Eat only properly prepared foods from well-known sources.
- Learn to identify the poisonous plants in your neighborhood and home.
- Never chew on jewelry made from imported seeds or beans.
- Never eat any part of an unknown plant.
- Never use anything prepared from nature as a medicine or "tea."
- Supervise toddlers carefully in gardens, patios, and public parks.

Resource information
Reference texts
Kingsbury, J. *Poisonous Plants of the United States and Canada.* Englewood Cliffs, N.J.: Prentice-Hall, 1964.
The Sinister Garden: A Guide to the Most Common Poisonous Plants. New York: Wyeth Laboratories, Division of American Home Products Corporation, 1966.

Respiratory Arrest

ASSESSMENT

It is the cessation of effective ventilation. It can be caused by acute airway obstruction, central nervous system depression, or neuromuscular paralysis. Apnea and cyanosis are the cardinal signs of respiratory arrest.

MANAGEMENT

Pulmonary resuscitation is begun immediately. See this chapter, Cardiopulmonary Resuscitation.

Table 11
Poisonous Parts of Common House and Garden Plants

Plant	Toxic Part	Symptoms
Flower Garden Plants		
Autumn crocus (meadow crocus)	All parts	Vomiting, nervous excitement
Azalea	All parts	Produces nausea and vomiting, depression, difficult breathing; may be fatal
Bleeding heart (Dutchman's breeches)	Foliage, roots	May cause convulsions and difficult breathing when eaten in large quantities
Christmas rose	Rootstocks, leaves	Inflammation of skin, numbing of oral tissues, gastric distress and nervous effects
Daffodil	Bulb	Nausea, vomiting, diarrhea; may be fatal
Delphinium	Seeds, young plants	Stomach upset, nervous excitement or depression if eaten in large quantities; toxicity decreases with age of plant
Four-o'clock	Roots, seeds	The powdered root is an irritant to the skin, nose and throat
Foxglove	Leaves, seeds	One of the sources of the drug digitalis, used to stimulate the heart. In large amounts, the active principles cause dangerously irregular heartbeat and pulse, usually digestive upset and mental confusion. May be fatal.
Hyacinth	Bulb	Nausea, vomiting, diarrhea; may be fatal

Plant	Part	Effects
Iris (blue flag)	Underground stems	Severe, but not usually serious, digestive upset
Jonquil	Bulb	Nausea, vomiting, diarrhea; convulsions and death if eaten in large quantities
Larkspur	Seeds, young plants	Digestive upset, nervous excitement, depression; may be fatal
Lily-of-the-valley	Leaves, flowers	Irregular heart beat and pulse, usually accompanied by digestive upset and mental confusion
Monkshood	Roots, seeds, leaves	Digestive upset and nervous excitement
Morning glory	Seeds	Produce LSD-like effects and may cause mental disturbances when ingested in large quantities
Narcissus	Bulb	Nausea, vomiting, diarrhea; may be fatal
Oleander	Leaves, branches	Dizziness, nausea, irregular heartbeat; may be fatal
Peony	Roots	Juice can cause paralysis
Star-of-Bethlehem	Bulb	Vomiting and nervous excitement
Violet (pansy)	Seeds	In quantity, the cathartic effects can be serious to a child

House Plants

Plant	Part	Effects
Castor bean	Seeds	Burning of mouth and throat, excessive thirst, convulsions. One or two seeds are near the lethal dose for adults.
Dieffenbachia (dumbcane, caladium)	All parts	Intense burning and irritation of the mouth and tongue. Death can occur if base of tongue swells enough to block the air passage of the throat.
Jequirity bean	Seeds, especially orange spot	Stomach pains, irregular pulse, cold sweat. Usually fatal. Does not grow in the U.S., is used for native type jewelry and necklaces.

Table 11 (Continued)

Plant	Toxic Part	Symptoms
Mistletoe	Berries	Acute stomach and intestinal irritation with diarrhea and slow pulse; may be fatal
Mother-in-law	Leaves	Produces swelling of tongue
Poinsettia	Leaves	Severe irritation to mouth, throat and stomach; may be fatal
Rosary pea	Seeds	Stomach pains, irregular pulse, cold sweat; may be fatal
Ornamental Plants		
Daphne	Berries, bark, leaves	Upset stomach, abdominal pain, vomiting, bloody diarrhea, weakness, convulsions and kidney damage
Golden chain	Bean-like capsules in which seeds are suspended	Severe poisoning; excitement, staggering, convulsions, nausea and coma; may be fatal
Lantana (red sage, wild sage)	Green berries	Affects lungs, kidneys, heart and nervous system; grows in southern U.S. and in moderate climates; may be fatal
Magnolia	Flower	Headache and depression
Rhododendron (western azalea)	All parts	Nausea, vomiting, depression, difficult breathing, prostration and coma; may be fatal
Wisteria	Seeds, pods	Mild to severe digestive upset
Yellow jessamine	Berries	Digestive disturbance and nervous symptoms; may be fatal
Yew	All parts, especially seeds except fleshy red pulp of fruit	Convulsions with rapid death

Trees and Shrubs

Plant	Toxic parts	Symptoms
Apple	Seeds	Releases cyanide when ingested in large quantities; may be fatal
Black locust	Bark, sprouts, foliage, seeds	Children have suffered nausea, weakness and depression after chewing the bark and seeds
Cherry	Leaves, twigs, seeds	Contains a compound that releases cyanide when eaten; difficult breathing, excitement, paralysis of voice and prostration; may be fatal
Elderberry	All parts, especially roots	Nausea and digestive upset
Oak	Foliage, acorns	Affects kidneys gradually; symptoms appear only after several days or weeks; takes a large amount for poisoning.
Peach	Leaves, twigs, especially seeds	Contains a compound that releases cyanide when eaten; difficult breathing, excitement, paralysis of voice and prostration; may be fatal

Vegetable Garden Plants

Plant	Toxic parts	Symptoms
Potato	All green parts	Cardiac depression; may be fatal
Rhubarb	Leaf blade	Kidney damage. Large amounts of raw or cooked leaves can cause convulsions, coma, followed rapidly by death.
Tomato	Green parts	Cardiac depression; may be fatal

Wild Plants

Plant	Toxic parts	Symptoms
Baneberry	All parts	Stomach and intestinal irritation, spasms
Buttercup	All parts	Irritant juices may severely injure the digestive system

Continued on next page

987

Table 11 (Continued)

Plant	Toxic Part	Symptoms
Jack-in-the-pulpit	All parts	Intense irritation and burning of mouth and tongue
Jimson weed (thornapple)	All parts	Abnormal thirst, distorted sight, delirium, incoherence and coma; may be fatal
Marsh marigold (cowslip)	All parts	Irritation of oral tissues, digestive upset, diarrhea, respiratory depression and convulsions
Moonseed	Berries	Blue, purple color, resembling wild grapes; severe digestive upset and abdominal pain
Mushrooms (fly agaric, death cap, and several *Amanita*)	All parts	Stomach cramps, thirst, difficult breathing. Fatal. AVOID ALL WILD MUSHROOMS UNLESS POSITIVE OF THEIR IDENTITY.
Nightshade	All parts	Intense digestive disturbances and nervous symptoms; may be fatal
Poison hemlock	All parts	Digestive disturbances; may be fatal
Poison ivy, oak, sumac	All parts	Itching, burning, redness
Skunk cabbage	Leaves, rhizomes	Burning and swelling of mouth, tongue and throat; large quantities may cause stomach and intestinal irritation
Water hemlock (cowbane)	All parts	Diarrhea, convulsions; may be fatal

Source: Reproduced with permission of The National Association of Retail Druggists, Washington D.C.

Shock

ASSESSMENT

Shock is a generalized circulatory disorder characterized mainly by hypotension. It may be caused by hemorrhage, cardiac failure, dehydration, poisons (including bacterial endotoxin), adrenal insufficiency, anaphylaxis, hypoxia, and neurovascular derangement. Physical findings include rapid, weak pulses; diaphoresis; ashen color; oliguria; hypothermia; and altered sensorium. Prolonged shock can lead to irreversible organ damage.

MANAGEMENT

The immediate measures to reverse shock include specific therapy for the cause of the shock and assurance of perfusion of vital organs. The latter is aided by placing the child in a recumbent position, preferably with the head lower than the body. Administration of salt and fluids by mouth is to be done only in the extreme situation and with the utmost caution since the danger of loss of consciousness with subsequent aspiration of vomitus is high. Supportive measures include judicious administration of oxygen and maintenance of body temperature.

Syncope (Fainting)

ASSESSMENT

Syncope is a transient, usually sudden episode of unconsciousness, loss of body tone, and falling due to cerebral ischemia.

Etiology. Syncope is most commonly due to a sudden and marked fall in the blood pressure. Other causes include:

• Anemia
• Breathholding
• Cardiac causes (rare)

- Epilepsy (syncopal episode usually lasts longer than 30 seconds)
- Hyperventilation
- Hypoglycemia
- Hysteria

Clinical picture. Fainting is heralded by dizziness, feeling of weakness, numbness of the hands and feet, extreme pallor, nausea, sweating, coldness of the skin, and occasionally vision disturbances. Clonic movements may follow if the child remains unconscious longer than 20 seconds or if the child is positioned in a semi-erect posture.

MANAGEMENT

No specific management is indicated except to keep the child in a horizontal position or tilt the head downward at a 45° angle until recovery.

Trauma

Trauma is too extensive to discuss fully here. Refer to other appropriate references, including other chapters in this book, for further information. (See also Hemorrhage, Shock, Fractures.) Penetrating chest wounds bear specific mention. These may result in pneumothorax, with subsequent deflation of the lung. If only the chest wall is penetrated, compression of the chest followed by closure of the wound can reduce the degree of air accumulation in the pleural space. If the lung is also penetrated, air would be drained from the pleural space to prevent a tension pneumothorax, which is more serious. Internal injuries pose the additional hazard of lack of recognition and thus delay in treatment. Large amounts of blood may be lost into the chest, abdomen, and thigh almost imperceptibly. The abdominal viscera are poorly protected from blunt trauma, and their rupture should be considered following significant trauma. Even minor trauma can rupture an inflamed or swollen spleen.

References

Abramowicz, M., editor. *The Medical Letter* 18:105–108, December 3, 1976.

Abrams, M. "Introduction: Traumatic Injuries in Children." *Pediatric Annals* 5:10–11, October 1976.

American National Red Cross. *Advanced First Aid and Emergency Care.* 1973.

Arena, J. *Poisoning: Toxicology, Symptoms, Treatment,* 3rd ed. Springfield, Illinois: Thomas, 1974.

Arena, J. *The Treatment of Poisoning.* Summit, NJ: CIBA Pharmaceutical Company, 1977.

Block, C. R. and C. E. Block. "Help, My Child is Choking." *Pediatric Nursing* 2:48–49, September/October 1976.

Brown, W. "Emergency Management of the Injured Child." *Pediatric Annals* 5:22–34, October 1976.

Canright, P. and M. J. Campbell. "Nursing Care of the Child and His Family in the Emergency Department." *Pediatric Nursing* 3:43–45, July–August 1977.

Chinn, P. L. *Child Health Maintenance.* St. Louis: Mosby, 1974.

Corby, D. G. and W. J. Decker. "Management of Acute Poisoning with Activated Charcoal." *Pediatrics* 54:324–329, September 1974.

Cosgriff, J. H. Jr. and D. Anderson. *The Practice of Emergency Nursing.* Philadelphia: Lippincott, 1975.

DeAngelis, C. *Basic Pediatrics for the Primary Health Care Provider.* Boston: Little, Brown, 1975.

Dietz, P. E. and S. P. Baker. "Drowning Epidemiology and Prevention." *Am J Public Health* 64:303–312, April 1974.

Done, A. K. "Salicylate Intoxication: Significance of Measurements of Salicylate in Blood in Cases of Acute Ingestion." *Pediatrics* 26:800–807, November 1960.

Gellis, S., editor. *The Year Book of Pediatrics.* Chicago: Year Book Medical Publishers, 1977.

Goldberg, A. H. "Cardiopulmonary Arrest." *N Engl J Med* 290:381–385, February 14, 1974.

Graef, J. W. and T. E. Cone, Jr. *Manual of Pediatric Therapeutics.* Boston: Little, Brown, 1974.

Green, M. and R. J. Haggerty. *Ambulatory Pediatrics II.* Philadelphia: Saunders, 1977.

Hardin, J. and J. Arena. *Human Poisoning from Native and Cultivated Plants.* Durham, N.C.: Duke University Press, 1973.

Heimlich, H. J. "Update on the Heimlich Maneuver." *Emergency Medical Services.* Pp. 11–20, January–February 1977.

Lampe, K. F. and R. Fagerstrom. *Plant Toxicity and Dermatitis.* Baltimore: Williams & Wilkins, 1968.

Mayer, B., and N. Schlackman. "Organophosphates—A Pediatric Hazard." *AFP* 11:121–124, May 1975.

Mennear, J. H. "The Poison Emergency." *Am J Nurs* 77:842–844, May 1977.

Metropolitan Life Insurance Company. "Accidental Drownings by Age and Activity." *Statistical Bulletin* 58:2–4, May 1977.

Mofenson, H. and J. Greensher. "The Unknown Poison." *Pediatrics* 54:336–342, September 1974.

Pascoe, D. and M. Grossman, editors. *Quick Reference to Pediatric Emergencies.* Philadelphia: Lippincott, 1973.

Peterson, B. "Morbidity of Childhood Near-Drowning." *Pediatrics* 59:364–370, March 1977.

Phelan, W. "Camphor Poisoning: Over-the-Counter Dangers." *Pediatrics* 57:428–430, March 1976.

Prior, J. A. and J. S. Silberstein. *Physical Diagnosis,* 4th ed. St. Louis: Mosby, 1973.

Report of National Conference on "Standards for Cardiopulmonary Resuscitation and Emergency Cardiac Care." *JAMA* 227(suppl.):835–868, February 18, 1974.

Rudolph, A., editor. *Pediatrics,* 16th ed. New York: Appleton-Century-Crofts, 1977.

Rumack, B. H. and H. Matthew. "Acetaminophen Poisoning and Toxicity." *Pediatrics* 55:871–876, June 1975.

Shillito, J. Jr. "Head Injuries." In M. Green and R. J. Haggerty, editors. *Ambulatory Pediatrics, II,* Philadelphia: Saunders, 1977. Pp. 247–252.

The Sinister Garden: A Guide to the Most Common Poisonous Plants. New York: Wyeth Laboratories, Division of American Home Products Corporation, 1966.

Vaughan, V. C. and R. J. McKay, editors. *Nelson Textbook of Pediatrics*, 10th ed. Philadelphia: Saunders, 1975.

Waechter, E. H. and F. G. Blake. *Nursing Care of Children,* 9th ed. Philadelphia: Lippincott, 1976.

Wheatley, G. M. "Childhood Accidents 1952–1972: An Overview." *Pediatric Annals* 2:10–30, January 1973.

31

Sudden Infant Death Syndrome

Sudden Infant Death Syndrome (SIDS) remains one of the most perplexing and agonizing problems facing affected families and health care providers. The etiology of the syndrome and the identification of infants at risk are crucial areas in which knowledge is incomplete. In the past and, unfortunately, all too often in the present, the management of families who experience this tragedy has been insensitive, accusatory, and punitive. Information is presented here to assist the nurse practitioner in the supportive management and counseling of families who lose an infant to SIDS.

ASSESSMENT

Definition

SIDS is the sudden death of any infant or young child which is unexpected by history and in which a thorough postmortem examination fails to demonstrate an adequate cause for death.

Etiology

Although more than 70 theories of causation have been proposed to explain SIDS, the specific cause remains unknown, and there is no known way to prevent it. Several prominent theories are reviewed here since parents of young infants may query the nurse practitioner as to what causes SIDS and what can be done to prevent it.

DISPROVEN THEORIES

Theories that have been disproven or that have yielded insufficient proof include:

- Abnormalities in the myocardial conduction system
- Accidental suffocation by bedclothes. Even very young infants can clear their airways if obstructed by bedclothes.
- Allergic reactions or immunopathology. Hypersensitivity to cow milk, anaphylactic reactions to recent immunizations, and anaphylaxis to house dust or house mite have not been proven.
- Nutritional deficiency or infection per se
- Traumatic, endocrine, and toxic causes

CURRENT THEORIES

Theories currently mentioned and being studied include:
- Depressed CO_2 sensitivity which may fail to stimulate respiratory drive during periods of apnea or hypoxia
- Instantaneous interruption in central control functions for respiratory and/or cardiac action
- Nasal obstruction in infants who are obligate nose breathers (under 5 months of age) and who make no attempt to open their mouths to breathe (Shaw, 1970, p. 416)
- Neurologic problem in which the laryngeal sensory receptors, when stimulated by fluid or regurgitated gastric contents, reflexively inhibit breathing and cause respiratory arrest
- Oropharyngeal occlusion of airways during sleep as a result of

deep muscle relaxation of the tongue and soft palate, and displacement of a hypermobile mandible (Tonkin, 1975, p. 653)

- Respiratory instability and normal prolonged apneic periods occurring during REM sleep as a result of muscle relaxation (Steinschneider, 1972, p. 653)
- Viral infection affecting laryngeal nerves causing laryngeal spasm and sudden closure of the vocal cords during sleep (Bergman, 1972, p. 776)

Current research is also attempting to identify any predisposing characteristics that might indicate infants at risk to SIDS. The issue of apnea monitors arises in this regard. Interest in the use of apnea monitors for the prevention of SIDS stems from "(1) the observation that some otherwise healthy infants have prolonged sleep apnea during the critical age period for SIDS, and (2) the *hypothesis* that prolonged sleep apnea is part of the pathophysiologic process resulting in SIDS" (Steinschneider, 1976, p. 1). Since definitive research studies have not specified the cause of SIDS, there is no scientific justification for advocating the general use of home monitoring systems to prevent SIDS.

Incidence

It is estimated that SIDS claims from 8000 to 10,000 infants per year in the United States or between two and three infants per 1000 live births. It occurs most often between 2 to 4 months of age and is uncommon before 1 month and after 7 to 8 months of age. It occurs more frequently in males, in low-birth-weight infants, in twins, in low socioeconomic groups living in overcrowded conditions, and during times of the year when upper respiratory illnesses abound.

Clinical Picture

Most of these infants die at home, during the night while sleeping, silently, without struggle, and unobserved. Approximately one half have had symptoms of a cold in the week prior to death, but the other 50 percent have not. Parents or caretakers discover their presumably healthy infant lying lifeless in the crib, in a state of disarray, often with frothy, blood-stained fluid in the nose, mouth, and on the bedclothes. Thus begins the agonizing human experience of coping with the sudden and unexplained death of an infant.

MANAGEMENT

Management is aimed at preventing the potentially crippling psychologic effects of SIDS on parents and family members.

Immediate Management

THE GRIEF PROCESS

Acute grief reactions are intense and include predictable symptoms and behaviors. They may be more intense when the event is unexpected. Initial reactions include shock, denial, anger, guilt, emotional disintegration, and remorse. During the first few days after the death a sense of emotional numbness may develop with depression, insomnia, inability to carry on with daily routines, fatigue, anorexia, preoccupation with the lost child, and continued reexamination of what could or should have been done to prevent the tragedy. Feelings of disbelief may last for several weeks. As the acute stress abates, parents are able to talk about the experience and will be ready for more detailed information.

EMERGENCY ROOM CARE

1. When a dead infant arrives in the E.R., presume the parents innocent until proven otherwise. Accusations or implications of child abuse are devastating to these parents.

2. Provide a room and privacy for the family and explanations of what procedures are being carried out. Answer questions simply.

3. Offer emotional support and accept the anger expressed without retaliation. Knowing the "right words" is not as important as simply being there, communicating concern and involvement.

4. When SIDS is presumptively diagnosed, emphasize that it was not anyone's fault and could not have been prevented.

5. Obtain permission for an autopsy.

6. Before leaving the E.R. provide parents with printed material on SIDS. The pamphlets put out by the National Foundation for Sudden Infant Death, Inc., are most helpful. Have a supply on hand. See this chapter, Parent Groups.

7. Inform the family that arrangements for a home visit by a public health nurse (or other supportive professional) will be made within the following week.

AUTOPSY

Autopsy is necessary to confirm the diagnosis of SIDS and should be performed on all infants. Characteristic autopsy findings include congestion and edema of the lungs; intrathoracic petechial hemorrhages on the surfaces of the lungs, pericardium, and thymus; microscopic inflammatory changes in the respiratory tract; minor pharyngeal erythema. Autopsy results should be relayed to families within 24 hours.

LEGAL ASPECTS

In most jurisdictions, any unexplained death mandates an autopsy, but whether or not the procedure is mandatory, the death certificate should read, "sudden infant death syndrome." Procedures for death investigations vary from state to state and often cause untold trauma to grief-stricken families. An excellent model for a humane system exists in the state of Oregon. It is available from the Oregon State Deputy Medical Examiner, 301 N.E. Knott, Portland, OR.

Follow-Up Counseling

Nurses are frequently the most available and appropriate professionals to assist families through the grief process following SIDS. Such support and counseling may be required for long periods.

INTERVALS FOR VISITS

The first visit with the family is best accomplished in the family home within 1 week of the infant's death. During this and subsequent visits the objectives of care are to:

1. Provide emotional support during the grieving period
2. Listen empathetically
3. Provide information on SIDS to the family as they are ready for it
4. Anticipate normal grief reactions and reassure parents that their reactions are normal
5. Answer all questions asked by parents and give printed material on SIDS
6. Assist parents in dealing with siblings and relatives
7. Put parents in touch with parent groups and The National Foundation for Sudden Infant Death
8. Support the family during the pregnancy and infancy period of a subsequent child
9. Refer parents for psychiatric referral if abnormal reactions exist and persist

INDICATIONS FOR PSYCHIATRIC REFERRAL

1. Parent who shows no emotion
2. Parent who over-intellectualizes, e.g., is obsessed by the scientific details
3. Parent who persistently denies the infant's death
4. Continuing inability of parent to resume previous responsibilities and level of functioning

QUESTIONS MOST FREQUENTLY ASKED BY PARENTS

- What is SIDS?
- How can a healthy baby die so suddenly?
- Was it my fault?
- Did the baby suffocate in the bedding?
- Did the baby vomit and choke?
- Did the baby suffer?
- Why was there blood around the baby's nose and mouth?
- Could the baby have cried and I didn't hear?
- Was it something infectious?
- Should I have breast-fed the baby?
- What if we have another child? Could it happen again?

These and other questions are answered simply and directly in materials available from the National Foundation for Sudden Infant Death. See this chapter, Parent Groups.

SIBLINGS

Siblings also are affected by SIDS. Although the child's age and developmental level determine the concept of death and the nature of the mourning process, all siblings will normally experience guilt feelings about the loss of the infant. Toddlers may fear that a similar fate awaits them and may become clinging and demanding. A detailed explanation is inappropriate at this age, but love, attention, and reassurance that they are safe will promote a feeling of security.

Older children need encouragement to express what they are feeling, need explanations and facts geared to their level of understanding, and need reassurance that they were in no way responsible and that they are safe and loved. Regressive behavior, nightmares, bedwetting, difficulty at school, and depression might be anticipated and indicate presence of continued guilt and insecurity. Professional counseling may be required.

PARENT GROUPS

A significant source of comfort can be contact with other parents who have experienced and successfully coped with SIDS. Two major national organizations exist and can be contacted for local chapter resources.

1. National Sudden Infant Death Foundation (formerly The National Foundation for Sudden Infant Death), 310 S. Michigan Avenue, Chicago, IL 60604.
2. International Guild for Infant Survival, Inc., 6822 Brompton Road, Baltimore, MD 21207.

SUBSEQUENT CHILDREN

Parents are frequently concerned about whether or not to have a subsequent child. This decision should be deferred until the grief work involving the lost infant is successfully completed. The new child must *not* be considered a replacement child. The odds of having SIDS recur in the same family are essentially the same as in the general population.

When a subsequent pregnancy occurs and during the subsequent child's first year of life, parents will need continual support and counseling to master their fears and concerns. The pamphlet, "The Subsequent Child," by Carolyn Szybist, R.N., is most helpful in providing guidelines for this support. See this chapter, References.

Anticipatory Counseling

Occasionally new parents with their first, healthy newborn show exaggerated concern about their infant's well-being. Normal findings such as nasal congestion, sneezing, mucus, or noisy breathing during sleep result in the parent asking repeated questions without seeming to be satisfied with the answers. The nurse practitioner who identifies such a situation can simply say, "You seem worried about your baby's breathing. Is there any particular reason?" If the parent is vague about the reason for the concern, then ask, "Are you worried about crib death?" This often brings a rush of feelings and fears to the surface which have been occasioned by experiences with neighbors, relatives, or friends who have lost an infant to SIDS, or by media publicity. Once the unspoken fears are verbalized, teaching and reassurance are heard.

References

Beckwith, J. B. "The Sudden Infant Death Syndrome." *Curr Probl Pediatr* 3:3, June 1973.

Bergman, A. B. "Sudden Infant Death." *Nurs Outlook* 20:775–777, December 1972.

Bergman, A. B. "Sudden Infant Death Syndrome: An Approach to Management." *Primary Care* 3:1–8, March 1976.

Friedman, S. B. "Psychological Aspects of Sudden Unexpected Death in Infants and Children." *Pediatr Clin North Am* 21:103–111, February 1974.

Merritt, T. A., et al. "Sudden Infant Death Syndrome: The Role of the Emergency Room Physician." *Clin Pediatr* 14:1095–1096, December 1975.

Patterson, K. and M. R. Pomeroy. "Nursing Care Begins After Death When the Disease is: Sudden Infant Death Syndrome." *Nursing 74* 4:85–88, May 1974.

Rudolph, A. M., editor. *Pediatrics,* 16th ed. New York: Appleton-Century-Crofts, 1977.

Shaw, E. B. "Sudden Unexpected Death in Infancy Syndrome." *Am J Dis Child* 119:416–418, May 1970.

Steinschneider, A. "A Reexamination of 'the Apnea Monitor Business'." *Pediatrics* 58:1–5, July 1976.

Steinschneider, A. "Prolonged Apnea and the Sudden Infant Death Syndrome: Clinical and Laboratory Observations." *Pediatrics* 50:646–654, October 1972.

Szybist, C. *The Subsequent Child.* New York: National Foundation for Sudden Infant Death, Inc., 1972.

Tonkin, S. "Sudden Infant Death Syndrome: Hypothesis of Causation." *Pediatrics* 55:650–661, May 1975.

Valdes-Dapena, M. A. "Sudden, Unexpected and Unexplained Death in Infancy—A Status Report." *N Engl J Med* 289:1195–1197, No. 29, 1973.

32

Failure to Thrive

The problem of failure to thrive (FTT) is not uncommon in pediatric practice. The management of this condition is complex because of long-term involvement of health personnel needed for some of the more chronic causes such as socioeconomic instability and maladjustment in the parent-child dyad. Cases of this type are frequently seen by a physician-nurse practitioner team.

ASSESSMENT

Definition

In any child who consistently decelerates on the growth curve or who falls below the third percentile (-2-1/2 SD) a suspicion of FTT is considered. The above situations are monitored over a period of weeks or months depending on the age and the nutritional and developmental status of the child. Labels of FTT based on very short periods of observation are not substantial.

Establishing a Diagnosis

The following variables are considered in establishing a diagnosis (Rowe, 1977):

- There are frequent shifts in growth patterns in children.
- Length measurements are frequently inaccurate.
- Many large newborns do not remain large during the first 6 months of life.
- Acute and/or chronic illnesses influence growth patterns.
- Some racial groups have smaller bone structures and therefore weigh less.
- Growth charts may not be representative of the clinical population. For example, many growth grids used in the U.S.A. reflect measurements of white middle-class children. When comparing measurements of other racial and ethnic groups with these grids, discrepancies occur. The nurse practitioner should be aware of the representative population used in the growth grid in the health care agency.

Normal Growth Patterns

NEWBORNS

Newborns can normally lose up to 10 percent of their birth weight in the first few weeks of life through fluid losses: urination, defecation, respiration, and through normal decreased nutritional intake. If an infant has not regained its birth weight by 3 weeks of age, etiologies are investigated. Normally infants gain at a rate of approximately 175 to 245 grams a week (5 to 7 ounces), or 17 to 35 grams a day (1/2 to 1 ounce); 1 ounce equals approximately 35 grams.

INFANTS AND TODDLERS

Generally infants double their birth weight by 6 months of age and triple it by 12 months of age. However, it is the experience of many practitioners that infants achieve these levels well before 6 and 12 months of age. Toddlers quadruple their birth weight by 2 years of age.

CHILDHOOD

During the ages of 2 and 9 years the annual increase in weight averages approximately 2.6 kilograms (5 pounds).

The average child grows approximately 25.4 centimeters (10 inches) in the first year of life, 12.7 centimeters (5 inches) in the second year, 7.6 to 10.2 centimeters (3 to 4 inches) in the third year, and 5.1 to 7.6 centimeters (2 to 3 inches) per year until puberty (Kempe, 1976, p. 9).

A practical method to predict a child's approximate adult height is to double the child's height in inches at 2 years of age for males. For females the height at 2 is also doubled and 4 inches are subtracted.

The rate of growth after the first year of life reduces considerably and during childhood the rate is slow but steady. The nurse practitioner is referred to developmental texts for specific growth averages during childhood.

ADOLESCENCE

During adolescence a height spurt commences with females at approximately 9-1/2 years of age, peaking at approximately 12 years of age, and stops at approximately 14 years of age. The height spurt in boys commences at approximately 10-1/2 years of age, peaks at approximately 14 years of age, and stops at approximately 16 years of age (Tanner, 1962).

Etiology

Decreased nutritional intake, genetic short stature, and central nervous system deficits are the more frequent cause of FTT. When FTT is due to decreased caloric intake or to malabsorption, the weight decelerates more than the height, and the head circumference continues to accelerate.

When FTT is due to genetic short stature, the length decelerates more or equal to the weight, and the head circumference continues to accelerate.

When FTT is due to a central nervous system deficit or due to intrauterine growth retardation, weight, height, and head circumference decelerate.

Other etiologies are numerous but infrequent. See Table 1 for a complete list of the possible causes of FTT. In determining the possible etiologies the nurse practitioner:

- Obtains a health history
- Assesses the child's nutritional intake
- Assesses the parent-child relationship
- Collects a family history in reference to adult height and weight
- Performs a physical examination to rule out anomalies
- Assesses the child's development
- Obtains appropriate laboratory studies

History

PARENTAL CONCERNS

Elicit the parents' concerns about the child's condition. This provides the practitioner with clues to the parents' feelings and insight into the problem.

FEEDING

- Review current nutritional intake including frequency of feedings, amounts and types of foods, snacks, how the child is fed: bottle (propped or held), spoon, or self-fed.
- Investigate eating habits that are suggestive of emotional deprivation such as eating spoiled foods, garbage, and nonfood items (pica).

PRESENT AND PAST HEALTH

Obtain information on:

- Frequency and duration of acute illnesses
- Exposure to infectious diseases
- Fevers
- Frequency of hospitalizations
- Severe injuries
- Allergies
- Stool pattern, including frequency, consistency, and color
- Occurrence of vomiting, regurgitation, and rumination

PARENT-CHILD DYAD

Investigate with parents how they see the child in reference to:

- Difficulty with feedings, burping, vomiting
- General responses of the child to the parents: degree of cuddling, amount of crying, ability to be comforted
- Relation to other siblings, amount of rivalry
- Behavior suggestive of decreased stimulation: rocking, head banging, spinning
- Reaction to methods of discipline

PREGNANCY AND BIRTH

Determine:

- Age of parents
- Gravida and para of the mother
- If pregnancy was planned
- Trimester prenatal care was commenced
- Maternal nutrition during pregnancy
- Amount of smoking, drug, or alcohol use.

Table 1
Causes of Failure to Thrive

Socioeconomic
1. Poverty, unemployment
2. Drug, alcohol problems

Feeding problems
1. Organic abnormalities: cleft palate, mental retardation
2. Inadequate breast-feeding techniques or formula preparation

Maternal child deprivation

Low birth weight
1. Prematurity
2. Intrauterine growth retardation

Endocrine
1. Thyroid disorders
   Hypothyroid
   Hyperthyroid
2. Hypopituitarism
   Idiopathic
   Organic lesions in hypothalamus or pituitary
3. Adrenal Insufficiency
   Addison's Disease
   Adrenogenital syndrome (salt-losing form)
   Prolonged steroid therapy
   Hyperparathyroidism

Genetic
1. Trisomies

Respiratory
1. Asthma

Cardiovascular
1. Congenital heart defects

Gastrointestinal
1. Chronic diarrhea
2. Malabsorption syndromes
   Disaccharide deficiency
   Glucose-galactose malabsorption
   Celiac disease
   Disorders causing dysphagia, regurgitation, and vomiting: anatomic malformations, chalasia, pyloric stenosis

Renal
1. Chronic renal insufficiency
2. Renal tubular acidosis
3. Infections

1008

Table 1 (*Continued*)

Musculoskeletal and connective tissue abnormalities
1. Juvenile rheumatoid arthritis
2. Muscopoly saccharidosis
3. Myopathies
4. Hypophosphatasia
5. Pseudohypoparathyroidism

Neurologic
1. Tumors including diencephalic syndrome
2. Perinatal central nervous system trauma
3. Developmental disorders
4. Subdural hematoma
5. Idiopathic

Hematologic
1. Iron deficiency anemia
2. Hemaglobinopathies

Metabolic
1. Rickets
2. Hypercalcemia
3. Galactosemia
4. Hereditary fructose intolerance
5. Glycogen storage disease
6. Phenylketonuria

Chronic or recurrent infection
1. Intrauterine: rubella, cytomegalovirus, toxoplasmosis, syphilis
2. Frequent, minor infections
3. Immunodeficiency syndromes
4. Phagocytic disorders

Idiopathic short stature
1. Constitutional (familial) short stature
2. Delayed maturation and adolescence

Source: From D. S. Rowe, Unpublished material.

• Hospitalizations, illnesses including:

1. Infections: syphilis, rubella, toxoplasmosis
2. Toxemia
3. Hypertension
4. Anemia
5. Congenital heart disease
6. Renal disease

- Amount of emotional support given to the mother during pregnancy
- Gestation in weeks, birth weight and length, type of delivery, type of anesthesia, postpartum and neonatal course

DEVELOPMENT

Discuss milestones appropriate for age: head up prone, smiles responsively, rolls over, sits, walks, first words.

FAMILY

Discuss:

- Familial diseases: allergies, heart disease, anemia, epilepsy, diabetes, congenital malformations
- Heights, weights, and developmental history of all family members

GROWTH OF CHILD

Plot as many measurements as are available on the growth grid; discuss with parents their observations in reference to the child's height and weight as compared with peers.

SOCIAL

Discuss family unit, type housing, means of financial support, relatives and friends available for help, degree of marital cohesiveness.

REVIEW OF SYSTEMS

- Ear, nose: otitis media, chronic rhinorrhea
- Gastrointestinal (bowel movements: presence of mucus, blood, fat, foul odor); presence of vomiting, rumination, regurgitation
- Cardiorespiratory: shortness of breath, slow feeding, tiring easily with feeding, diaphoresis
- Neurologic: delayed developmental milestones

Physical Examination

In addition to a complete examination, the following areas are emphasized:

- Weight, height, and head circumference are accurately measured.
- As many measurements as are obtainable are plotted on the growth grid.
- The number of teeth are counted and correlated with the chronologic age.
- Intellectual development is correlated with age.
- Sexual development is correlated with age.
- There is thorough assessment of any physical defect.
- Complete neurologic exam is done.
- Complete developmental assessment is made.

Laboratory

Initial laboratory tests include:

- Complete blood count to rule out anemia, infection
- Creatinine, BUN to rule out impaired kidney function
- Serum electrolytes and CO_2 to rule out renal tubular acidosis
- Stool analysis for:
  1. Occult blood to rule out possible cow milk intolerance
  2. Ova and parasites
  3. Reducing substances and pH to rule out mono- and disaccharide deficiency
  4. Fat to rule out malabsorption
- Tuberculin test

  Other laboratory studies if indicated include:

- X-rays for bone age to help ascertain growth hormone deficiency
- Sweat chloride to rule out cystic fibrosis

- PBI and T4 to rule out hypothyroidism
- Buccal smear in short-stature children with delayed pubescence to rule out Turner's syndrome
- Seventy-two-hour stool fat analysis and stool trypsin to rule out malabsorption
- Liver function studies
- Upper GI series to rule out anatomic anomalies
- Lower GI series to rule out ulcerative colitis, Hirschsprung's disease
- Skull X-rays to rule out increased intracranial pressure, hematomas, tumor

While laboratory studies provide additional information in determining the etiology, the initial nutritional, developmental, family/psychosocial histories, and physical examination in many instances help to determine some of the more common etiologies.

Indications for Hospital Admission

Children are hospitalized with FTT for the following reasons:
- Child at risk nutritionally and needs immediate treatment
- Observation of parental-child interaction, infant behavior, feeding routines, clarification of nutritional intake
- Performance of complex diagnostic procedures
- Observation of weight gain if any when removed from the home
- Interrupt dysfunctional parent-child relationship if evident
- Provide respite for caretakers

Common Problems with Short-Term Hospitalization (Rowe, 1977)

- Multiple caretakers in the hospital are frequently confusing to the parents.
- It is difficult to consistently observe mother-infant interaction and feeding techniques in a busy hospital.

- Occasionally hospital staff are unfriendly or punitive toward parents.
- Diagnostic procedures interfere with feeding routines and nurturing.
- It may be difficult for parents to visit the child in the hospital due to lack of transportation, baby-sitting problems at home, and lack of financial resources.
- Parents may feel threatened if the child improves clinically.

MANAGEMENT

Specific management depends on the results of the history, observations of the parent-child relationship, physical examination, and laboratory studies.

Ambulatory

If no organic cause for FTT is found, the initial steps in management are to provide adequate calories and to measure the child's caloric intake. If the nurse practitioner has any confusion about the oral intake a 3-day dietary history is written by the parent at home. The nurse practitioner discusses with parents feeding difficulties such as regurgitation, chalasia, and vomiting and advises frequent burping and sitting up after feeding.

The nurse practitioner establishes a therapeutic milieu where parents can discuss their own frustrations and feelings in reference to the child. Home visiting is performed to further assess parent-child interaction and feeding routines. Follow-up is provided on abnormal laboratory studies.

Hospital

Oral intake is more accurately monitored in the hospital than in the home. Depending on the cause of FTT support services if needed can be instituted by social service. After a period of observation on a therapeutic nutritional regime, the following conclusions are drawn:

- Adequate intake with normal weight gain indicates past history of inadequate feeding with decreased calorie intake due most commonly to dysfunctional parent-child relationship.
- Adequate intake with no weight gain indicates possible malabsorption problem, chronic infection, kidney malfunction and psychosocial problems.
- Inadequate intake with no weight gain indicates possible anatomic abnormalities: cleft palate, micrognathia, tracheo-esophageal fistula, congenital heart disease, neurologic disorder.

Follow-Up Care

FTT children generally require long-term follow-up. It is helpful for these clients to see the same health professionals for ambulatory management after hospital discharge. Other personnel helpful in providing support services are the public health nurse, community agencies with programs for children with congenital defects, and day-care nurseries for role modeling and respite services for the parents.

ROLE OF THE NURSE PRACTITIONER

Organic etiology. The nurse practitioner:

- Provides psychologic support and counsel in helping the family cope with the child
- Monitors compliance with the management plan
- Assesses the need for additional health education and support services

Nonorganic etiology. The nurse practitioner:

- Establishes a therapeutic, nonthreatening, long-term relationship with the family
- Intervenes and reverses the faulty parent-child relationship by:

1. Nurturing the parents
2. Acting as a nonthreatening role model in demonstrating how to care for the child
3. Developing a nonpunitive approach in teaching nutrition, stimulation, and play
4. Helping the family to understand their stresses and to seek solutions

COMMON CLINICAL PROBLEM

Failure to Thrive (FTT) Due to Maternal Deprivation

ASSESSMENT

Definition. The concept of maternal deprivation has evolved over a period of years. Originally it was felt to be the cause of failure to thrive in children who were receiving institutionalized care. Gradually the concept of maternal deprivation has been expanded to include any situation in which there is insufficient interaction, be it physical or emotional between the child and the mother figure. The term maternal deprivation denotes caretaker be they female or male. Children react to this lack of interaction in various ways:

- Slow or very irregular growth patterns
- Lack of responsiveness to the environment
- Delayed emotional development
- Lack of weight gain
- Autistic behavior. See Chapter 5, Assessment of Parent-Child Interaction.

Psychodynamics. An understanding of the underlying factors is essential for adequate management of the problem.

MATERNAL. Implicit in the way women respond to the needs of their children is the way in which they themselves were nurtured as children. Normally the mother or maternal figure nurtures and cultivates in the child a responsiveness, closeness, and sense of trust in human beings. Women lacking in adequate emotional support and nurturing during their childhood emerge into adulthood with a severe lack of self-esteem and with a failure to establish and to maintain satisfying relationships with those people who are close to them. Hence, their inability to adequately care for and to nurture their own children. Frequently they are also isolated and without satisfying recreational outlets or emotionally supportive peer relationships. The pregnancy most often is unplanned. Frequently they are chronically depressed and are burdened by stresses: financial, marital, and emotional. They have difficulty recognizing the needs of their infants and have problems in performing adaptive mothering behaviors which support maternal infant bonding, such as smiling, cooing at the infant, maintaining eye contact, holding the infant close, and formulating adequate feeding routines. See Chapter 5, Assessment of Parent-Child Interaction. Many mothers are easily frustrated by the infant's response to their mothering which may not always be positive. For example, some infants may continue to cry when held or may regurgitate frequently.

PATERNAL. Fathers or parental figures are usually unsympathetic and not understanding of the mother's social and psychologic situation. They offer the mother little physical and emotional support.

FAMILY. There are usually family stresses including: unemployment, financial or marital problems, transient family members, chronic illness, drug or alcohol use, depression.

History. In considering maternal deprivation as a cause of FTT, the following information is obtained:

PAST HISTORY. Discuss: general health during pregnancy, trimester at which care was first obtained, if pregnancy was planned, emotional support received by mother during pregnancy, if therapeutic abortion was considered, illnesses, hospitalizations, injuries during pregnancy, length of labor, type of delivery, anesthesia, rooming-in in hospital, when mother first began to care for the baby in the hospital.

NUTRITION. Discuss: type and amount of foods, difficulties in feeding routines as perceived by parents, child's reaction to food, difficulties with swallowing, sucking, regurgitation, vomiting; type and consistency of bowel movements.

FAMILY. Discuss: current support measures available to mother, current familial stresses: financial, social, unemployment, use of drugs, alcohol, illness in family.

Observation of maternal child interaction. Observe if the mother or maternal figure holds the child close to her body, if there is eye contact, if the mother smiles or plays with the child; ask the mother if she has any complaints about the child: cries too much, dirty, bad; ascertain if the mother has time for herself away from the infant; changing diapers, bathing the baby; ascertain if the mother is an able historian in reference to the child's daily routine.

Observation of infant behavior. Observe if the infant cuddles toward the mother and gives responses either verbally or facially when stimulated; observe the child's response toward food; observe if the child looks to the parent for comfort and security in stressful situations; ascertain the child's general developmental status.

Physical examination. In addition to a complete physical examination, a developmental assessment is done to determine the degree of social interaction and covert developmental delays.

Behavioral manifestations. Authorities cite various behavioral manifestations in FTT children. Growth retardation is strongly associated with disturbances in eating and abnormalities in sleeping and elimination with the most noticeable differences in eating behaviors: less regular meals, small amount of food served at mealtimes, and meals more often skipped (Pollitt, 1976). Children are understimulated and retarded in motor and social skills and show little differentiation between strangers and caretakers (Rhymes, 1966). Evidence exists which shows environmental deprivation, marital instability, and a high proportion of mothers with character disorders (Fischoff, 1971, p. 209). There is an increased incidence of FTT in abused and premature children (Fanaroff, 1972). Infantile posture in FTT children due to sensory deprivation is occasionally observed. In this posture, the elbow joints are flexed 90° or more, the humerus is abducted and rotated outward, the hands are pronated and positioned at the side of the head (Kreiger, 1967, p. 335).

Response of mother to infant. The nurse practitioner recognizes maternal behaviors that signal rejection of the infant:

- Holds infant away from own body
- Avoids eye contact
- Seldom coos or talks with infant
- Plays roughly with infant and holds body parts without proper support
- Makes negative comments about infant
- Has difficulty understanding needs of infant. See Chapter 5, Manifestations of Maladaptions of Mothers to Infants.

Home visit. The purpose of the home visit is to:

- Assess maternal child interaction over a longer period of time than is permissible in an office visit
- Observe feeding techniques
- Assess the home environment in reference to safety, availability of infant care items (sleeping area, toys, utensils for feeding, bathing)
- Discuss with other family members their availability to support parents
- Continue to develop a relationship based on nurturing and the establishment of trust
- Act as a nonthreatening role model, in reference to age-appropriate play activities, stimulation, feeding techniques, nutrition, development of mothering behavior.

MANAGEMENT

Hospitalization. FTT children with suspicion of psychosocial causes are admitted to the hospital for the following:

- To perform further diagnostic tests to determine if organic etiology is also present
- To allow for possible weight gain away from the home environment
- To obtain further social and psychologic assessment of the family milieu
- To explore family stresses
- To provide respite for the family
- To assess family's ability to care for the child
- To provide role modeling in caring for and nurturing the infant
- To encourage the parents to become active in the child's care and to support them in their attempts at parenting
- To explore with the family community resources for support after hospitalization
- To offer an on-going therapeutic regimen for the family

Role of the nurse practitioner. The long-term follow-up demands active participation of the nurse practitioner in all areas of management.

IN-PATIENT. During hospitalization the nurse practitioner is involved in the hospital conferences with the family and helps plan for the child's discharge by formulating a plan for care, implementing the follow-up, and establishing the family with available community services.

COUNSELING. To promote a feeling of acceptance and self-worth in mothers of FTT infants, the nurse practitioner listens and exhibits sincere interest in the mother as a person. In order not to intimidate the mother, the nurse does not act as an authority figure on any aspect of child care. The primary focus of the nurse's role is to nurture the mother. It is in this consistent and therapeutic contact that the mother is able to form a trusting relationship with the nurse and therefore begins to develop a positive self-image. In discussing feeding and play regimens, the nurse assumes a role of collaboration with the mother where ideas and suggestions are mutually discussed and accepted or discarded. The mother is encouraged to find solutions to her questions and is praised for any attempt at communication however slight. The nurse assesses the

mother's understanding of age-appropriate nutritional requirements and play activities. The nurse discusses the child's physical
and emotional needs and together with the mother outlines ways to
meet these needs.

The nurse initiates discussion around the mother's past experience in nurturing and in her own relationship with her mother.
The nurse discusses current stresses in the mother's life and helps
to formulate possible solutions. Acceptance of the mother's feelings
both positive and negative toward the child is necessary.

In all discussions the nurse acts as a trusted friend teaching by
role modeling and suggestions about child caring rather than by
threatening, didactic instruction. Social service is involved in counseling when needed for further support and for psychologic evaluation.

HOME VISIT.   In the management of any complex health problem adequate reversal of negative trends cannot be accomplished
without reinforcement of positive aspects of the office visit through
follow-up home visits. In FTT due to maternal deprivation the
consistency of a limited number of caretakers is desirable to aid the
mother in establishing a relationship. Therefore it is advisable to
have the home visiting done by a person who will be involved with
the mother on a long-term basis. The goals of home visiting are
discussed under Assessment.

ROLE MODELING.   To help the mother or parent figure become more nurturing the nurse is a role model in projecting a
nurturing, caring, and supportive behavior toward the child in a
manner that is nonthreatening to the mother. Although the child is
the object of the discussions, the main focus of attention continues
to be the mother, and she is encouraged and supported in whatever
response she makes toward the child.

Projecting a nurturing behavior encompasses a variety of actions:

- Feeding: holding the infant close, positive eye contact, smiling
  and cooing
- Stimulation: initiating verbal behavior, repeating the child's
  sounds, stroking and touching the child, providing age-
  appropriate visual stimulatory objects
- General care: inadvisability of propping the bottle, importance

of maintaining routine feeding times, asking for support when needed

Role of the family. Improved interactions between mother and child cannot be accomplished without the inclusion of other family members into the management milieu. If they are unable to accompany the mother on ambulatory visits, or if they are not available during home visits, it is advisable to:

- Encourage their direct participation in providing support to the mother
- Discuss possible stressful situations in the family that may hinder adequate establishment of maternal-child bonding
- Offer resources in reference to further discussion of family or interpersonal stresses

Community. Community agencies assist parents in helping to further establish an identity, to cope with the demands of living, and to provide occasional respite from parenting. The goals of referral are to:

- Offer the mother other therapeutic relationships where she can discuss her fears and feelings
- Offer her a constructive outlet to enhance her feelings of self-worth in areas such as job training, part-time and volunteer work, and school

Agencies helpful in accomplishing some of these tasks are:

- Talk or crisis lines where parents can call at any hour for support and counsel
- Local child abuse councils
- Parent discussion groups at local health centers or hospital clinics
- Adult education
- Child development classes
- Local community agencies that are advocates for increased funding for day care, support for single parenting
- Day-care nurseries

References

Barnard, M. and L. Wolf. "Psychosocial Failure to Thrive." *Nurs Clin North Am* 8:557–565, September 1973.

Barbero, G. and C. Shaheen. "Environmental Failure to Thrive: A Clinical View." *J Pediatr* 71:639–644, November 1967.

Durand, B. "Failure to Thrive in a Child with Down's Syndrome." *Nurs Res* 24:272–285, July–August 1975.

Fanaroff, A., et al. "Follow-Up of Low Birth Weight Infants: The Predictive Value of Maternal Visiting Patterns." *Pediatrics* 49:289–290, February 1972.

Fischoff, J., et al. "A Psychiatric Study of Mothers of Infants with Growth Failure Secondary to Maternal Deprivation." *J Pediatr* 79:209–215, August 1971.

Green, M. and R. J. Haggerty. *Ambulatory Pediatrics II*. Philadelphia: Saunders, 1977.

Graef, J. W. and T. Cone, Jr. *Manual of Pediatric Therapeutics*. Boston: Little, Brown, 1974.

Harrison, L. L. "Nursing Intervention with the Failure to Thrive Family." *The American Journal of Maternal Child Nursing* 1:111–116, January 1976.

Hufton, I. and R. K. Oates. "Failure to Thrive: A Long-Term Follow-Up." *Pediatrics* 59:73–77, January 1977.

Johnson, P. "Role of the Pediatric Nurse Practitioner in Early Recognition of Failure-To-Thrive Infants Due to Maternal Deprivation." Unpublished masters thesis, University of California, San Francisco, 1976.

Kempe, C., et al. *Current Pediatric Diagnosis and Treatment*. Los Altos, CA.: Lange Medical Publications, 1976.

Kennedy, J. "The High-Risk Maternal-Infant Acquaintance Process." *Nurs Clin North Am* 8:549–556, September 1973.

Krieger, I. and D. A. Sargent. "A Postural Sign in the Sensory Deprivation Syndrome in Infants." *J Pediatr* 70:332–339, March 1967.

Leonard, T. "Failure to Thrive in Infants: A Family Problem." *Am J Dis Child* 111:600–612, June 1966.

McMillan, J. A., et al. *The Whole Pediatrician Catalogue*. Philadelphia: Saunders, 1977.

Money, J. "Dwarfism, Questions and Answers in Counseling." *Rehabilitation Literature* 28:134–138, May 1967.

Pollitt, E. "Behavioral Disturbances Among Failure to Thrive Children." *Am J Dis Child* 130:24–29, January 1976.

Pollitt, E., et al. "Psychosocial Development and Behavior of Mothers of Failure to Thrive Children." *Am J Orthopsychiatry* 45:525–537, 1975.

Rhymes, J. P. "Working with Mothers and Babies Who Fail to Thrive." *Am J Nurs* 66:1972–1976, September 1966.

Rowe, D. S. Unpublished material, February 1977.

Smith D. and R. Marshall. *Introduction to Clinical Pediatrics.* Philadelphia: Saunders, 1972.

Tanner, J. M. *Growth at Adolescence.* Oxford, England: Blackwell Scientific Publications, 1962.

Warshaw, J. B. and R. Mauy. "Identification of Nutritional Deficiencies and Failure to Thrive in the Newborn." *Clinics in Perinatology* 2:327–344, September 1975.

33

Child Abuse

The possibility of child abuse was considered in 1940 when John Coffey, M.D., noted frequent associations of chronic subdural hematomas in infants with multiple fractures of the long bones (Rudolph, 1977, p. 828). National attention was brought to the issue of child abuse by C. Henry Kempe, M.D., in 1962 when he invented the phrase "battered child syndrome." Since then, the public has become increasingly aware of the phenomenon of child abuse as one of the major causes of death and permanent disability in children.

The assessment and management of this complex problem requires an understanding of the psychodynamics of child abuse and the development of a therapeutic, nonthreatening relationship with the family. Occasionally the decision is made that the child's welfare is more secure away from the family. However, the focus is to have the child reunited with the family after rehabilitation has begun.

The nurse practitioner is an integral part of the multidisciplinary team approach to the assessment and long-term management of child abuse. The nurse offers psychosocial support to the parents, acts as a role model for nurturing the child, and investigates community support services for the family.

ASSESSMENT

Incidence

The first nationwide analysis, reported in February 1977, for the Department of Health, Education and Welfare, estimated that more than a million children in the U.S. are victims of physical abuse or neglect each year. Minimally, at least 2000 children die annually from circumstances associated with abuse or neglect. In addition to the fatalities that occur a large number of abused and neglected children suffer permanent physical, neurologic, and emotional retardation.

Epidemiology

Children below the ages of 3 years are the most frequent victims of abuse. Women are more frequent abusers than men because they are usually the primary caretakers. Men abuse more severely and are involved in sexual abuse. Occasionally other relatives and friends commit abuse.

Abuse occurs in all races and socioeconomic classes, but statistics report a higher incidence in lower socioeconomic classes. However, these clients use facilities where reporting is routinely done, in contrast to private physicians where only approximately 2 percent of all cases are reported.

Psychodynamics

SOCIAL

There is usually a crisis which precipitates the abusive occurrence. The crisis is in line with a long series of frustrations and inabilities to cope such as living in poverty, marital disharmony, single parent, heavy drug and alcohol use, isolation, unemployment, too many children, and chronic illness. Occasionally the crisis may be a relatively minor event, but one that carries enough force to result in the abuse of a child. Occasionally, the injury is premeditated.

PARENTS

A large portion of abusive parents were themselves abused as children. Other traits include early marriages, unwanted pregnancies, social and emotional isolation, and lack of supportive relationships with spouses.

Parents exhibit a lack of trust toward other people and see the child as the person who can provide the love, support, and nurturing they lack in their own lives. They may also exhibit feelings of anger, ambivalence, and rejection toward the child.

It has been estimated that 10 percent of abusive parents are psychotic or seriously disturbed (Joyner, 1973, p. 806). Generally, parents have little self-esteem and are in need of constant reassurance.

Abusive parents usually visit several health care agencies for treatment and initially may bring in the child for minor complaints before abuse is commenced. They usually demonstrate little concern about the injury and understand little in reference to the child's development. Generally, they have poor impulse control.

CHILD

The child is singled out as someone who is different. Although it is common for several children in one family to be abused, there is usually one child who is more abused than others. This child is quite possibly chronically ill, was premature at birth, is hyperactive, and generally more difficult to manage.

Abused children show a high degree of ability, in reference to their age, in caring for the parent and in responding to the parents' need for nurturing. Occasionally, abused children show overall poor hygiene. They sometimes exhibit unusual fear and will not look at the parents for reassurance in unfamiliar situations.

Approach to Interviewing the Parents

An attitude of empathy is necessary in interviewing parents of children with suspected nonaccidental injuries. Knowledge of social and psychological dynamics of child abuse helps the interviewer to develop an objective, nonpunitive approach toward the parents.

It is not relevant to obtain an admission from the parents if abuse took place and who committed it. As an ego defense to the guilt, fear, and inadequacy they feel, parents frequently use the mechanisms of denial and projection in child abuse situations. Antagonizing the parents with interrogating questions will create further denial, hostility, and an inability to establish a relationship of trust with the health team.

If the facts surrounding the injury are confusing to the interviewer it is best to assume that for whatever reasons, there is, or has been, a family or social crisis. The expression of a sympathetic attitude and recognition that the parents have been trying to do their best in the worst of circumstances focus attention on the parents' needs and problems and avoids discussing the child and the injuries (Kempe, 1972, p. 7). This course of action begins the therapeutic and supportive relationship that must be established if meaningful interventions are to be produced. A therapeutic interview allows the parents to maintain their sense of ego esteem.

Depending on the parent's response and attitude, the interviewer proceeds to gain insight into the family situation, possible stressful occurrences, degree of isolation felt by the parents, and availability of support measures. If the parent is hostile, distrustful, or resentful to the interviewer, it is best to discuss this with the parent using "I feel that you are very angry" language. The interviewers maintain a calm attitude and let the parents know of their desire to help and to be supportive.

Some parents will deny that there are any problems. In this situation after initial attempts to establish rapport have failed, it is best not to proceed further and to allow the parent time with the denial mechanism.

Hospitalization is approached from the standpoint of observation of the child and the necessity to perform other diagnostic procedures. The best time to discuss the suspicion of child abuse is debatable. This situation depends on the attitude of the parents, the degree of injury, and the possibility that the parents might leave with the child. In·many instances the parents are informed after the child is admitted into the hospital. If rapport has been established with the parents in the emergency room, occasionally they are told at that time. In telling the parents a simple statement is best: "I am required by law to report suspected cases of child abuse to the proper agency." Further explanations are given to the parents about the usual follow-up procedures when appropriate.

If there is any reason to believe that the parents will leave with the child, a police hold is obtained for a period of 72 hours, by calling the local child protective agency or, if at night or on weekends the local police department. If the parent attempts to leave with the child, he or she should not be stopped, and the police should be called immediately.

History

Investigate circumstances surrounding the injury, past history of accidents or similar injuries, other agencies used in the care of the child, accidents with siblings, time of occurrence of injury, and time of arrival at the health agency; there is usually a long delay between the two in child abuse cases. Also inquire about number of people in the family, support measures for child care, recent family stresses, or financial burdens.

Physical Examination

A complete physical examination is done including:

- Skin: observe for abrasions, burns, belt marks, bites
- Eyes: perform funduscopic examination
- Abdomen: palpate for tenderness, organomegaly
- Extremities: observe for symmetrical movements, full range of motion exercises

Common Clinical Findings

- Skin: burns, old scars, ecchymosis, soft tissue swelling, human bites
- Fractures: skull, rib, limb, presence of old fractures on X-rays, epiphyseal separations
- Subdural hematomas
- Intestinal injuries
- Trauma to genitals
- Growth retardation
- Poor hygiene
- Whiplash: shaken infant syndrome caused by manual shaking of trunk or extremities resulting in intraocular and intracranial hemorrhage (Caffey, 1974, p. 396)

Rare Injuries

- Subgaleal hematomas caused by pulling of braids or hair (Kempe, 1975, p. 1265)
- Tear of mouth mucosa caused by forceful feeding (Kempe, 1975, p. 1265)
- Traumatic pancreatic cysts and rupture of liver caused by abdominal blows (Kempe, 1975, p. 1265)
- Hypernatremic dehydration in older children in instances where a psychotic parent withholds water to decrease bed wetting (Kempe, 1975, p. 1265)

Laboratory

- Full body X-rays
- Complete blood count
- Urinalysis
- Electrolytes
- Toxicology screen

Differential Diagnosis

- Accidental trauma
- Rare bone diseases: osteogenesis imperfecta
- Scurvy
- Rickets
- Syphilis of infancy

Risk Screening

See Tables 1, 2, 3, and 4.

Table 1
Observations of Parents-To-Be in Physician's Office or Prenatal Clinic

1. Are the parents overconcerned with the baby's sex?
2. Are they overconcerned with the baby's performance? Do they worry that he will not meet the standard?
3. Is there an attempt to deny that there is a pregnancy (mother not willing to gain weight, no plans whatsoever, refusal to talk about the situation)?
4. Is this child going to be one child too many? Could he be the "last straw"?
5. Is there great depression over this pregnancy?
6. Is the mother alone and frightened, especially by the physical changes caused by the pregnancy? Do careful explanations fail to dissipate these fears?
7. Is support lacking from husband and/or family?
8. Where is the family living? Do they have a listed telephone number? Are there relatives and friends nearby?
9. Did the mother and/or father formerly want an abortion but not go through with it or waited until it was too late?
10. Have the parents considered relinquishment of their child? Why did they change their minds?

Source: Reprinted with permission from C. H. Kempe, "Approaches to Preventing Child Abuse," *American Journal of Disease in Children* 130:941–947, 1976; copyright 1976, American Medical Association.

Table 2
Observations to be Made at Postpartum Check-ups and Pediatric Check-ups

1. Does the mother have fun with the baby?
2. Does the mother establish eye contact (direct en face position) with the baby?
3. How does the mother talk to her baby? Is everything she expresses a demand?
4. Are most of her verbalizations about the child negative?
5. Does she remain disappointed over the child's sex?
6. What is the child's name? Where did it come from? When did they name the child?
7. Are the mother's expectations for the child's development far beyond the child's capabilities?
8. Is the mother very bothered by the baby's crying? How does she feel about the crying?
9. Does the mother see the baby as too demanding during feedings? Is she repulsed by the messiness? Does she ignore the baby's demands to be fed?
10. What is the mother's reaction to the task of changing diapers?
11. When the baby cries, does she or can she comfort him?
12. What was/is the husband's and/or family's reaction to the baby?
13. What kind of support is the mother receiving?
14. Are there sibling rivalry problems?
15. Is the husband jealous of the baby's drain on the mother's time and affection?
16. When the mother brings the child to the physician's office, does she get involved and take control over the baby's needs and what's going to happen (during the examination and while in the waiting room) or does she relinquish control to the physician or nurse (undressing the child, holding him, allowing him to express his fears, etc)?
17. Can attention be focused on the child in the mother's presence? Can the mother see something positive for her in that?
18. Does the mother make nonexistent complaints about the baby? Does she describe to you a child that you don't see there at all? Does she call with strange stories that the child has, for example, stopped breathing, turned color, or is doing something "on purpose" to aggravate the parent?
19. Does the mother make emergency calls for very small things, not major things?

Source: Reprinted with permission From C. H. Kempe, "Approaches to Preventing Child Abuse," *American Journal of Disease in Children* 130:941–947, 1976; copyright 1976, American Medical Association.

Table 3
Positive Family Circumstances

1. The parents see likeable attributes in the baby and perceive him as an individual.
2. The baby is healthy and not too disruptive to the parents' life-style.
3. Either parent can rescue the child or relieve one another in a crisis.
4. The parents' marriage is stable.
5. The parents have a good friend or relative to turn to, a sound "need-meeting" system.
6. The parents exhibit coping abilities, ie, the capacity to plan, and understand the need for adjustments because of the new baby.
7. The mother is intelligent and her health is good.
8. The parents had helpful role models when they grew up.
9. The parents can have fun together and with their personal interests and hobbies.
10. The parents practice birth control; the baby was planned or wanted.
11. The father has a steady job. The family has its own home, and living conditions are stable.
12. The father is supportive of the mother and involved in the care of the baby.

Source: Printed with permission from C. H. Kempe. "Approaches to Preventing Child Abuse," *American Journal of Disease in Children* 130:941–947, 1976; copyright 1976, American Medical Association.

Table 4
Special Well-Child Care for High-Risk Families

1. Promote maternal attachment to the newborn.
2. Phone the mother during the first two days at home.
3. Provide more frequent office visits.
4. Give more attention to the mother.
5. Emphasize nutrition.
6. Counsel discipline only for accident prevention.
7. Emphasize accident prevention.
8. Use compliments rather than criticism.
9. Accept phone calls at home.
10. Arrange for regular home visits by a public health nurse or a lay health visitor.

Source: Reprinted with permission from C. H. Kempe, "Approaches to Preventing Child Abuse," *American Journal of Disease in Children*, 130:941–947, 1976; copyright 1976, American Medical Association.

MANAGEMENT

Reporting

It is mandatory that all cases of suspected abuse and neglect in the U.S. be reported to the proper authorities. Physicians commonly report child abuse but in various states paraprofessional or lay persons can also report. All persons reporting child abuse are immune from court action for civil liability. Failure to report suspected cases can result in prosecution.

Generally, cases are reported to child protective agencies of the local or state government. The objectives of this agency are to prevent and to investigate child abuse and to provide social services to help rehabilitate abusive parents. It also refers those cases to juvenile court when parents are unable or unwilling to use the help offered by the agency. Occasionally cases are reported to the local police department, but most authorities recommend reporting to the child protective agency. Their approach is less punitive and more psychotherapeutically oriented. The agency is called first, and a written report follows in 24 to 48 hours.

LEGAL DEFINITIONS

1. A dependency hearing (petition) is a legal maneuver that permits the child protective agency to request temporary custody of the child. If the petition is granted, the child becomes a ward of the state, and the court can insist that the parents undergo a rehabilitation program before the child is returned to the home. The case is reviewed in 6 months.

2. Placement is when a ward of the court is placed in a foster home due to the parents' inability to care for the child. The goal is eventual re-uniting of the family, after rehabilitation is evident.

Goals of Management

- Protection of the child
- Support and rehabilitative regimes for parents and caretakers
- Returning the child to the home when it is judged safe
- Eliminating social ills from society that contribute to child abuse

Hospitalization

Placing the child in the hospital even for minor suspicious injuries accomplishes several objectives. It gives the health professional time to investigate the family's psychologic milieu, methods of functioning with one another, and current life stresses. It also separates the family and the child which is therapeutic in that it gives the family a rest and it protects the child.

During hospitalization, the parents' attitudes are continuously assessed for their desire and cooperation in participating in the care plan. If they exhibit symptoms of psychosis or extreme neurosis, a psychiatric evaluation is made.

Role of the Health Care Team

Management of child abuse is provided by a multidisciplinary team involving physicians, nurses, social workers, and protective service agencies. Other disciplines are involved as needed including a psychiatrist, lawyer, and community representatives.

The role of the team is to develop a therapeutic relationship with the family, to evolve a care plan for the protection of the child, to rehabilitate the abusive caretakers as much as possible, and to provide consistent follow-up care.

The protective services agency and public health nurse or nurse practitioner remain involved with the family after hospital discharge to assess the continued potential for abuse and to provide therapeutic and emotional support.

Follow-Up Care

The child is returned to the home when:

- The family crisis is resolved and future episodes are handled more therapeutically.
- The parents exhibit a positive, caring attitude toward the child.
- Consistent nurturing is provided for the parents to help improve their self-esteem.
- Parents demonstrate the willingness and knowledge to use available support services in the community.
- A routine follow-up plan is determined.

Community Services

In some cities, depending on funds available, there are sheltered residencies where parents are rehabilitated through behavior modification techniques, role modeling, and educational experiences (Fontana, 1976, p. 760). Other services include:

- Lay community workers offer nurturing, friendship, and support to the family for several months
- Crisis nurseries offer intermittent respite from child care
- Parents Anonymous offers 24-hour counsel and support
- Day-care centers offer child care skills and parent-child nurturing
- Health visitors—this concept involves trained lay people working with health professionals, who assure that basic health needs of all children are met during the first 4 years of life. They are also alert for symptomatology of child abuse (Kempe, 1976, p. 943).

References

Caffey, J. "The Whiplash Shaken Infant: Manual Shaking by the Extremities with Whiplash-Induced Intracranial and Intraocular Bleedings, Linked with Residual Permanent Brain Damage and Mental Retardation." *Pediatrics* 54:396–403, October 1974.

Caipoli, J. and C. Newberger. "Optimism or Pessimism for the Victim of Child Abuse." *Pediatrics* 59:311–312, February 1977.

Fontana, V. J. and E. Robinson. "A Multidisciplinary Approach to the Treatment of Child Abuse." *Pediatrics* 57:760–764, May 1976.

Graef, J. W. and T. E. Cone. *Manual of Pediatric Therapeutics*. Boston: Little, Brown, 1974.

Green, F. C. "Child Abuse and Neglect: A Priority Problem for the Private Physician." *Pediatr Clin North Am* 22:329–339, May 1975.

Joyner, E., et al. "Symposium on Child Abuse." *Pediatrics* 51:771–812, April 1973.

Kempe, C. H. and R. E. Helfer. *Helping the Battered Child and His Family*. Philadelphia: Lippincott, 1972.

Kempe, C. H. "Family Intervention: The Right of all Children." *Pediatrics* 56:693–694, November 1975.

Kempe, C. H. "Uncommon Manifestations of the Battered Child Syndrome." *Am J Dis Child* 129:1265, November 1975.

Kempe, C. H. "Approaches to Preventing Child Abuse." *Am J Dis Child* 130:941–947, September 1976.

Kempe, C. H., and J. Hopkins. "The Public Health Nurse's Role in the Prevention of Child Abuse and Neglect." *Public Health Currents* 15:1–4, May 1975.

Kempe, C. H., et al. *Current Pediatric Diagnosis and Management*. Los Altos, CA.: Lange Medical Publications, 1976.

Newberger, E. "Knowledge and Epidemiology of Child Abuse: A Critical Review of Concepts." *Pediatric Annals* 5:140–144, March 1976.

Rudolph, A. M., editor. *Pediatrics*, 16th ed. New York: Appleton-Century-Crofts, 1977.

Wolf, P. H. "Mother-Infant Interactions in the First Year." *N Engl J Med* 295:999–1001, October 1976.

Appendix

Table 1
Weights and Measures—Metric System

Mass

1000	grams	=	kilogram	$(kg)^a$
1.0	gram^a	=		(g)
0.001	gram	=	milligram	$(mg)^a$
10^{-6}	gram	=	microgram	$(\mu g)^a$
10^{-9}	gram	=	nanogram	(ng)
10^{-12}	gram	=	picogram	(pg)

Capacity

1000	cubic centimeters	=	liter	$(1)^a$
100	cubic centimeters	=	deciliter	(dl)
10	cubic centimeters	=	centiliter	(cl)
1.0	cubic centimeter^a	=	milliliter	(ml, cc)
0.001	cubic centimeter	=	microliter	(μl)
			cubic millimeter	(cmm)

^{a}Commonly employed units.

Table 2
Metric and Apothecaries' Equivalents[a]

1 milligram	=	1/65	grain	(1/60)
1 gram	=	15.43	grains	(15)
1 kilogram	=	2.20	pounds	[avoirdupois]
1 milliliter	=	16.23	minims	(15)
1 grain	=	0.065	gram	(60 mg)
1 ounce	=	31.1	grams	(30)
1 minim	=	0.062	ml	(0.06)
1 fluid ounce	=	29.57	ml	(30)
1 pint	=	473.2	ml	(500)
1 quart	=	946.4	ml	(1000)

[a]Figures in parentheses are approximate values and are *not* used in compounding prescription orders.

Table 3
Household Measures

Measure	Approximate Metric Equivalents
1 drop[a]	1/20 ml
1 teaspoon[b]	5 ml
1 dessertspoon	8 ml
1 tablespoon	15 ml
1 wineglass	60 ml
1 glass	250 ml

[a]The USP does not sanction the prescribing of doses in drops. An official standardized USP dropper is available for those who wish to use it. If it is necessary to prescribe oral medications in "drop dosage," the pharmacist should be instructed to mark the medicine dropper to deliver the desired amount of drug or to supply a calibrated dropper.
[b]The size of the household teaspoon varies considerably, and a given teaspoon will yield different volumes of medicine. The USP specifies that for household purposes an American standard teaspoon may be regarded as containing 5 ml.

Table 4
Celsius (Centigrade) and Fahrenheit Temperatures

Centigrade (Celsius)	Fahrenheit
0	32
36.0	96.8
36.5	97.7
37.0	98.6
37.5	99.5
38.0	100.4
38.5	101.3
39.0	102.2
39.5	103.1
40.0	104.0
40.5	104.9
41.0	105.8
41.5	106.7
42.0	107.6

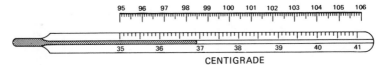

To convert degrees F. to degrees C.
  Subtract 32, then multiply by 5/9
To convert degrees C. to degrees F.
  Multiply by 9/5, then add 32

Table 5
Conversion Table for Pediatric Weights
(Pounds to kilograms)

Pounds→	0	1	2	3	4	5	6	7	8	9
0	0.00	0.45	0.90	1.36	1.81	2.26	2.72	3.17	3.62	4.08
10	4.53	4.98	5.44	5.89	6.35	6.80	7.25	7.71	8.16	8.61
20	9.07	9.52	9.97	10.43	10.88	11.34	11.79	12.24	12.70	13.15
30	13.60	14.06	14.51	14.96	15.42	15.87	16.32	16.78	17.23	17.69
40	18.14	18.59	19.05	19.50	19.95	20.41	20.86	21.31	21.77	22.22
50	22.68	23.13	23.58	24.04	24.49	24.94	25.40	25.85	26.30	26.76
60	27.21	27.66	28.12	28.57	29.03	29.48	29.93	30.39	30.84	31.29
70	31.75	32.20	32.65	33.11	33.56	34.02	34.47	34.92	35.38	35.83
80	36.28	36.74	37.19	37.64	38.10	38.55	39.00	39.46	39.91	40.37

90	40.82	41.27	41.73	42.18	42.63	43.09	43.54	43.99	44.45	44.90
100	45.36	45.81	46.26	46.72	47.17	47.62	48.08	48.53	48.98	49.44
110	49.89	50.34	50.80	51.25	51.71	52.16	52.61	53.07	53.52	53.97
120	54.43	54.88	55.33	55.79	56.24	56.70	57.15	57.60	58.06	58.51
130	58.96	59.42	59.87	60.32	60.78	61.23	61.68	62.14	62.59	63.05
140	63.50	63.95	64.41	64.86	65.31	65.77	66.22	66.67	67.13	67.58
150	68.04	68.49	68.94	69.40	69.85	70.30	70.76	71.21	71.66	72.12
160	72.57	73.02	73.48	73.93	74.39	74.84	75.29	75.75	76.20	76.65
170	77.11	77.56	78.01	78.47	78.92	79.38	79.83	80.28	80.74	81.19
180	81.64	82.10	82.55	83.00	83.46	83.91	84.36	84.82	85.27	85.73
190	86.18	86.68	87.09	87.54	87.99	88.45	88.90	89.35	89.81	90.26
200	90.72	91.17	91.62	92.08	92.53	92.98	93.44	93.89	94.34	94.80

Table 6

Conversion of Pounds and Ounces to Grams

Pounds	Ounces 0	1	2	3	4	5	6	7	8	9	10	11	12	13	14	15
0	—	28	57	85	113	142	170	198	227	255	283	312	340	369	397	425
1	454	482	510	539	567	595	624	652	680	709	737	765	794	822	850	879
2	907	936	964	992	1021	1049	1077	1106	1134	1162	1191	1219	1247	1276	1304	1332
3	1361	1389	1417	1446	1474	1503	1531	1559	1588	1616	1644	1673	1701	1729	1758	1786
4	1814	1843	1871	1899	1928	1956	1984	2013	2041	2070	2098	2126	2155	2183	2211	2240
5	2268	2296	2325	2353	2381	2410	2438	2466	2495	2523	2551	2580	2608	2637	2665	2693
6	2722	2750	2778	2807	2835	2863	2892	2920	2948	2977	3005	3033	3062	3090	3118	3147
7	3175	3203	3232	3260	3289	3317	3345	3374	3402	3430	3459	3487	3515	3544	3572	3600
8	3629	3657	3685	3714	3742	3770	3799	3827	3856	3884	3912	3941	3969	3997	4026	4054
9	4082	4111	4139	4167	4196	4224	4252	4281	4309	4337	4366	4394	4423	4451	4479	4508

	0	1	2	3	4	5	6	7	8	9	10	11	12	13	14	15
10	4536	4564	4593	4621	4649	4678	4706	4734	4763	4791	4819	4848	4876	4904	4933	4961
11	4990	5018	5046	5075	5103	5131	5160	5188	5216	5245	5273	5301	5330	5358	5386	5415
12	5443	5471	5500	5528	5557	5585	5613	5642	5670	5698	5727	5755	5783	5812	5840	5868
13	5897	5925	5953	5982	6010	6038	6067	6095	6123	6152	6180	6209	6237	6265	6294	6322
14	6350	6379	6407	6435	6464	6492	6520	6549	6577	6605	6634	6662	6690	6719	6747	6776
15	6804	6832	6860	6889	6917	6945	6973	7002	7030	7059	7087	7115	7144	7172	7201	7228
16	7257	7286	7313	7342	7371	7399	7427	7456	7484	7512	7541	7569	7597	7626	7654	7682
17	7711	7739	7768	7796	7824	7853	7881	7909	7938	7966	7994	8023	8051	8079	8108	8136
18	8165	8192	8221	8249	8278	8306	8335	8363	8391	8420	8448	8476	8504	8533	8561	8590
19	8618	8646	8675	8703	8731	8760	8788	8816	8845	8873	8902	8930	8958	8987	9015	9043
20	9072	9100	9128	9157	9185	9213	9242	9270	9298	9327	9355	9383	9412	9440	9469	9497
21	9525	9554	9582	9610	9639	9667	9695	9724	9752	9780	9809	9837	9865	9894	9922	9950
22	9979	10007	10036	10064	10092	10120	10149	10177	10206	10234	10262	10291	10319	10347	10376	10404

Table 7
Approximate Metric and Imperial Equivalents

Useful approximate metric and imperial equivalents

    1 cm = 0.39 inches   1 in =   2.54 cm
    1 meter = 1.1 yards   1 ft = 30.48 cm

To convert centimeters to inches

  Divide the length in centimeters by 2.54.

  Example: The average newborn infant measures 50.8 cm:

$$= \frac{50.8}{2.54} = 20 \text{ inches}$$

To convert inches to centimeters

  Multiply the length in inches by 2.54.

  Example: The average newborn infant measures 20 inches:

$$= 20 \times 2.54 = 50.8 \text{ cm}$$

Table 8
Conversion of Inches to Centimeters

Inches	Centimeters	Inches	Centimeters	Inches	Centimeters
10	25.40	15	38.10	20	50.80
10½	26.67	15½	39.37	20½	52.07
11	27.94	16	40.61	21	53.34
11½	29.21	16½	41.91	21½	54.61
12	30.48	17	43.18	22	55.88
12½	31.75	17½	44.45	22½	57.15
13	33.02	18	45.72	23	58.42
13½	34.29	18½	46.99	23½	56.69
14	35.56	19	48.26	24	60.96
14½	36.83	19½	49.58		

Figure 1 Boys: Birth To 36 Months
Physical Growth NCHS Percentiles*

NAME_____ RECORD #_____

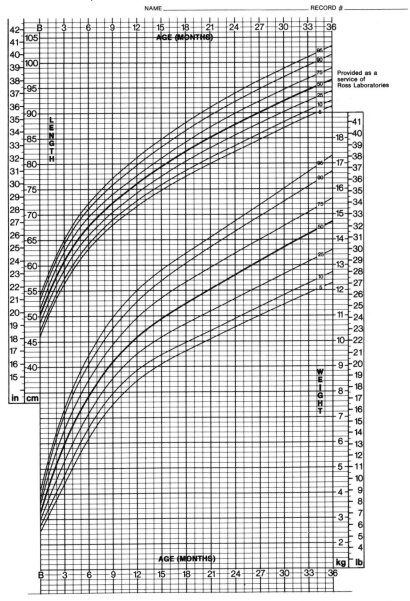

Provided as a
service of
Ross Laboratories

Source: Reprinted with permission from Ross Laboratories, Columbus, Ohio, © 1976.

*Adapted from National Center for Health Statistics: NCHS Growth Charts, 1976. Monthly Vital Statistics Report. Vol. 25, No. 3, Supp. (HRA) 76-1120. Health Resources Administration, Rockville, Maryland, June, 1976. Data from the Fels Research Institute, Yellow Springs, Ohio.

1047

Figure 2 Boys: Birth to 36 Months
Physical Growth NCHS Percentiles*

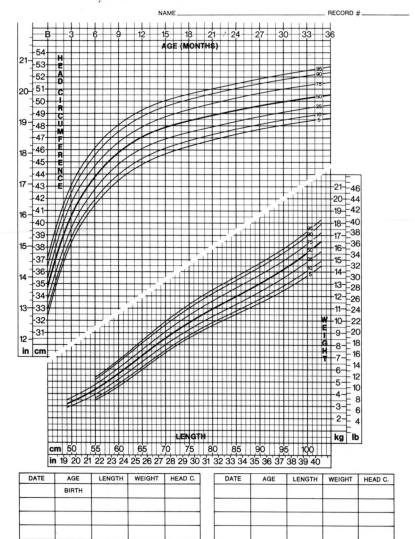

Source: Reprinted with permission from Ross Laboratories, Columbus, Ohio, © 1976.

---

*Adapted from National Center for Health Statistics: NCHS Growth Charts, 1976. Monthly Vital Statistics Report. Vol. 25, No. 3, Supp. (HRA) 76-1120. Health Resources Administration, Rockville, Maryland, June, 1976. Data from the Fels Research Institute, Yellow Springs, Ohio.

Figure 3   Girls: Birth To 36 Months
Physical Growth NCHS Percentiles*

NAME_____ RECORD #_____

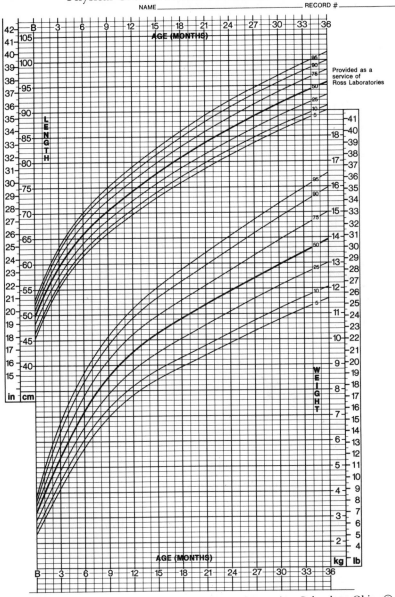

Provided as a
service of
Ross Laboratories

*Adapted from National Center for Health Statistics: NCHS Growth Charts, 1976. Monthly Vital Statistics Report. Vol. 25, No. 3, Supp. (HRA) 76-1120. Health Resources Administration, Rockville, Maryland, June, 1976. Data from the Fels Research Institute, Yellow Springs, Ohio.

Figure 4 Girls: Birth To 36 Months
Physical Growth NCHS Percentiles*

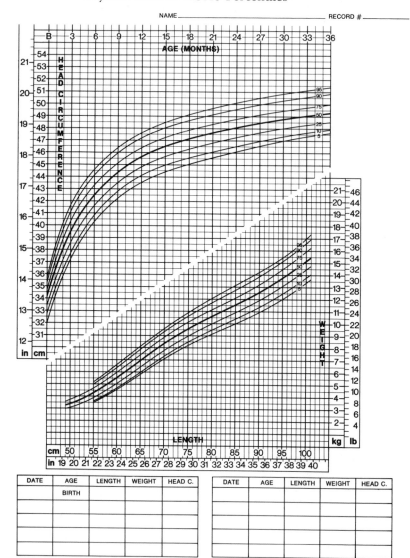

DATE	AGE	LENGTH	WEIGHT	HEAD C.
	BIRTH			

DATE	AGE	LENGTH	WEIGHT	HEAD C.

Source: Reprinted with permission from Ross Laboratories, Columbus, Ohio, © 1976.

*Adapted from National Center for Health Statistics: NCHS Growth Charts, 1976. Monthly Vital Statistics Report. Vol. 25, No. 3, Supp. (HRA) 76-1120. Health Resources Administration, Rockville, Maryland, June, 1976. Data from the Fels Research Institute, Yellow Springs, Ohio.

Figure 5 Boys: 2 To 18 Years
Physical Growth NCHS Percentiles*

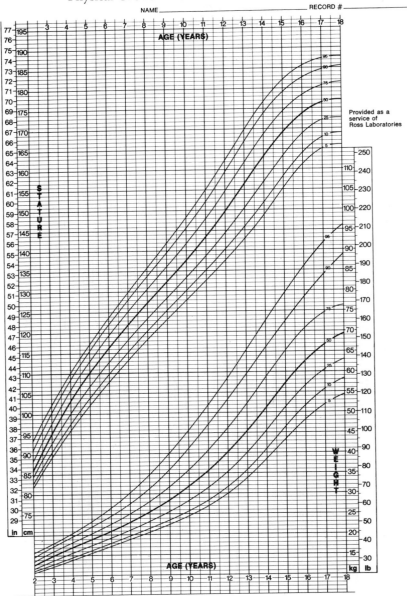

Source: Reprinted with permission from Ross Laboratories, Columbus, Ohio, © 1976.

*Adapted from National Center for Health Statistics: NCHS Growth Charts, 1976. Monthly Vital Statistics Report. Vol. 25, No. 3, Supp. (HRA) 76-1120. Health Resources Administration, Rockville, Maryland, June, 1976. Data from the Fels Research Institute, Yellow Springs, Ohio.

Figure 6 Boys: Prepubescent Physical Growth NCHS Percentiles*

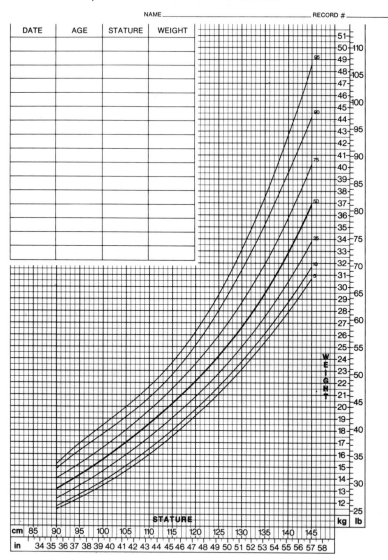

Source: Reprinted with permission from Ross Laboratories, Columbus, Ohio, © 1976.

*Adapted from National Center for Health Statistics: NCHS Growth Charts, 1976. Monthly Vital Statistics Report. Vol. 25, No. 3, Supp. (HRA) 76-1120. Health Resources Administration, Rockville, Maryland, June, 1976. Data from the Fels Research Institute, Yellow Springs, Ohio.

Figure 7 Girls: 2 To 18 Years
Physical Growth NCHS Percentiles*

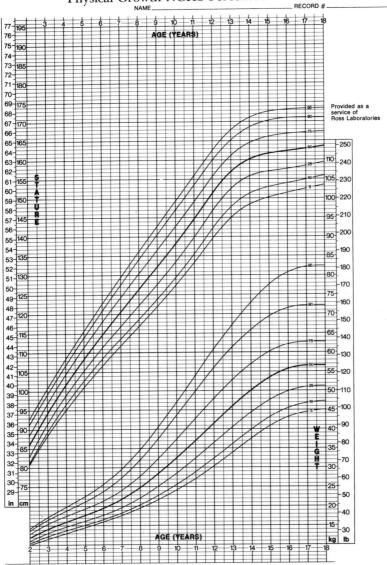

Source: Reprinted with permission from Ross Laboratories, Columbus, Ohio, ©
1976.

*Adapted from National Center for Health Statistics: NCHS Growth Charts, 1976.
Monthly Vital Statistics Report. Vol. 25, No. 3, Supp. (HRA) 76-1120. Health Resources Administration, Rockville, Maryland, June, 1976. Data from the Fels Research Institute, Yellow Springs, Ohio.

Figure 8 Girls: Prepubescent
Physical Growth NCHS Percentiles*

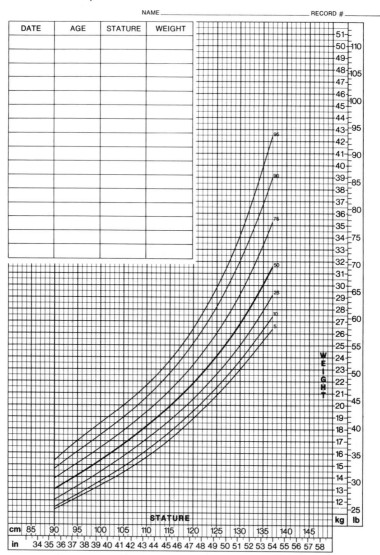

Source: Reprinted with permission from: Ross Laboratories, Columbus, Ohio, © 1976.

*Adapted from National Center for Health Statistics: NCHS Growth Charts, 1976. Monthly Vital Statistics Report. Vol. 25, No. 3, Supp. (HRA) 76-1120. Health Resources Administration, Rockville, Maryland, June, 1976. Data from the Fels Research Institute, Yellow Springs, Ohio.

Index